Quick Find Guide

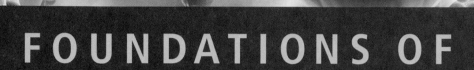

FOUNDATIONS OF
PERIODONTICS
FOR THE
DENTAL HYGIENIST

ENHANCED FIFTH EDITION

Jill S. Gehrig, RDH, MA
Dean Emeritus, Division of Allied Health
and Public Service Education
Asheville-Buncombe Technical Community College
Asheville, North Carolina

Daniel E. Shin, DDS, MSD
Director, Predoctoral Periodontics
Indiana University School of Dentistry
Indianapolis, Indiana

Donald E. Willmann, DDS, MS
Professor Emeritus, Department of Periodontics
University of Texas Health Science Center at San Antonio
San Antonio, Texas

JONES & BARTLETT
LEARNING

World Headquarters
Jones & Bartlett Learning
5 Wall Street
Burlington, MA 01803
978-443-5000
info@jblearning.com
www.jblearning.com

Jones & Bartlett Learning books and products are available through most bookstores and online booksellers. To contact Jones & Bartlett Learning directly, call 800-832-0034, fax 978-443-8000, or visit our website, www.jblearning.com.

20927-3

Production Credits

VP, Product Management: Amanda Martin
Product Manager: Sean Fabery
Product Specialist: Rachael Souza
Product Coordinator: Elena Sorrentino
Digital Project Specialist: Angela Dooley
Director of Marketing: Andrea DeFronzo
Marketing: Dani Burford
Production Services Manager: Colleen Lamy

VP, Manufacturing and Inventory Control: Therese Connell
Composition: S4Carlisle Publishing Services
Project Management: S4Carlisle Publishing Services
Cover Design: Kristin E. Parker
Senior Media Development Editor: Troy Liston
Rights Specialist: Rebecca Damon
Printing and Binding: LSC Communications

Library of Congress Cataloging-in-Publication Data
Library of Congress Cataloging-in-Publication Data unavailable at time of printing.

LCCN: 2020931321

6048

Printed in the United States of America
25 24 23 22 21   10 9 8 7 6 5 4

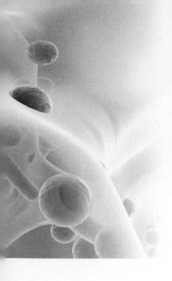

Liability Statement

This textbook endeavors to present an evidence-based discussion of periodontology based on information from recent research. Periodontology, however, is a rapidly changing science. The authors, editors, and publisher have made every effort to confirm the accuracy of the information presented and to describe generally accepted practices at the time of publication. However, as new information becomes available, changes in treatment may become necessary. The reader is encouraged to keep up with dental and medical research through the many peer-reviewed journals available to verify information found here and to determine the best treatment for each individual patient. The authors, contributors, editors, and publisher are not responsible for errors or omissions or for any consequences from application of the information in this book and make no warranty, express or implied, with respect to the contents of this publication.

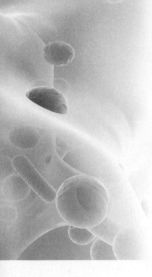

Contributors

Kimberly S. Bray, RDH, MS
Professor, Division of Dental
Hygiene
University of Missouri—Kansas
City School of Dentistry
Kansas City, Missouri

Delwyn Catley, PhD
Professor and Associate Director,
Center for Children's Healthy
Lifestyles and Nutrition
Children's Mercy Kansas City
University of Missouri—Kansas
City
Kansas City, Missouri

**Teresa Butler Duncan, RDH, BS,
MDH**
Assistant Professor
Department of Dental Hygiene
School of Dentistry
The University of Mississippi
Medical Center
Jackson, Mississippi

Pinar Emecen-Huja, DDS, PhD
Division of Periodontics
Department of Stomatology
College of Dental Medicine
Medical University of Carolina
Charleston, South Carolina

Richard Foster, DMD
Department Chair, Dental Science
Guilford Technical Community
College
Jamestown, North Carolina

Yusuke Hamada, DDS, MSD
Department of Periodontology and
Allied Dental Programs
Indiana University School of
Dentistry
Indianapolis, Indiana

Carol A. Jahn, BSDH, MS
Director of Professional Relations
and Education
Water Pik, Inc.
Fort Collins, Colorado

**Dr. Vanchit John, BDS, MDS,
DDS, MSD**
Chairman, Department of
Periodontology and Allied Dental
Programs
Indiana University School of
Dentistry
Indianapolis, Indiana

**Tawana K. Lee-Ware, DDS, MSD,
FABPD, FACI**
Department of Pediatric Dentistry
Indiana University School of
Dentistry
Indianapolis, Indiana

Sharon Logue, RDH, MPH
Dental Health Program
Virginia Department of Health
Richmond, Virginia

Robin B. Matloff, RDH, BSDH, JD
Professor Emeritus
Dental Hygiene Program
Mount Ida College
Newton, Massachusetts

Lisa L. Maxwell, LDH, MSM
Program Director, Dental Hygiene
Division
Department of Periodontology and
Allied Dental Programs
Indiana University School of
Dentistry
Indianapolis, Indiana

Craig S. Miller, DMD, MS
Chief, Division of Oral Diagnosis,
Oral Medicine and Maxillofacial
Radiology
University of Kentucky College of
Dentistry
Lexington, Kentucky

John Preece, DDS, MS
Professor (Retired)
Division of Oral and Maxillofacial
Radiology
Department of Dental Diagnostic
Science
University of Texas Health Science
Center at San Antonio
San Antonio, Texas

**Keerthana Satheesh, BDS,
DDS, MS**
Department of Periodontics
University of Missouri—Kansas
City School of Dentistry
Kansas City, Missouri

Robert Schifferle, PhD, DDS
Department of Periodontics and
Endodontics
Department of Oral Biology
University at Buffalo School of
Dental Medicine
Buffalo, New York

Carol Southard, RN, MSN
Tobacco Treatment Specialist
Pulmonary and Critical Care
Medicine
Northwestern Medicine
Chicago, Illinois

Rebecca Sroda, RDH, MA
Dean Emeritus, Health Sciences
South Florida State College
Avon Park, Florida

Dianne Glasscoe Watterson, RDH, MBA
Chief Executive Officer
Watterson Speaking/Consulting
LLC
Lexington, North Carolina

Karen Williams, RDH, MS, PhD
Department of Biomedical and
Health Informatics
University of Missouri—Kansas
City School of Medicine
Kansas City, Missouri

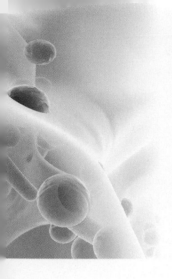

Preface for Course Instructors

The ancient Greek philosopher Heraclitus famously stated: *"There is nothing permanent except change."* This quotation serves as the basis for the evolution of each successive edition of our textbook. And, while some may view any semblance of change with a sense of apprehension, the authors of the fifth edition of *Foundations of Periodontics for the Dental Hygienist* see this as an opportunity to grow upon previous editions so as to improve the preparation of students for productive functioning in the rapidly evolving and highly demanding environment of clinical periodontology. ***One such exciting development in periodontology is the new classification of periodontal and peri-implant diseases and conditions developed jointly by the American Academy of Periodontology (AAP) and the European Federation of Periodontology (EFP) in 2017.***

The *Enhanced Fifth Edition* is written with three primary goals in mind. First and foremost, this textbook focuses on the dental hygienist's role in periodontics. Our second goal is to develop a book with an instructional design that facilitates the teaching and learning of the complex subject of periodontics—as it relates to dental hygiene practice—without omitting salient concepts or "watering down" the material. Third, we hope to help guide you, the teacher, in transmitting your expertise and knowledge in periodontology to your students. To accomplish all our goals, many of the complex theoretical concepts that are covered in this textbook are reinforced with clinical photographs/radiographs, illustrations, flow charts, and hypothetical case scenarios which, we hope, may provide your students with visualization aids that can assist in the learning process. Written primarily for dental hygiene students, *Foundations of Periodontics for the Dental Hygienist* also would be a valuable resource on current concepts in periodontics for the practicing dental hygienist or general dentist.

ONLINE INSTRUCTOR AND STUDENT RESOURCES

Qualified instructors can receive access to the following supplemental resources:

- A comprehensive Test Bank

- Slides in PowerPoint format

- Discussion Points for the classroom

- Class Activities that tie back to every chapter

- Lesson Plans to help plan your course

- Syllabus Conversion to assist in transitioning from the *Fourth* to *Fifth Edition*

ENHANCED FIFTH EDITION NEW CONTENT

- **New 2017 World Workshop on the Classification of Periodontal and Peri-Implant Diseases and Conditions**

- **Chapter 4: Classification of Periodontal and Peri-Implant Diseases and Conditions**

- **Chapter 6: Periodontal Health, Gingival Diseases and Conditions**

- **Chapter 7: Periodontitis**

- **Chapter 8: Other Conditions Affecting the Periodontium**

- **Chapter 9: Peri-Implant Health and Diseases**
  - In 2017, a joint collaborative effort by the American Academy of Periodontology and the European Federation of Periodontology was conducted to develop a revised periodontal diagnosis classification that aligns with emerging scientific evidence.
  - The revised classification system also introduces a new classification for peri-implant diseases and conditions that could be accepted worldwide.
  - The aforementioned chapters highlight many key aspects of the new classification system. Additionally, the chapters review the case definitions and diagnostic criteria for each category of periodontal and peri-implant disease and condition.

- **Chapter 11: Shared Decision-Making for Periodontal Care**
  - Shared decision-making is a collaborative process that recognizes a patient's right to make decisions about his or her care once fully informed about the options.
  - *Periodontal treatment is always based upon the best available scientific evidence, but many times there will be more than a single course of treatment that could benefit an individual patient.*
  - Shared decision-making is a process in which clinicians and patients work together to make treatment decisions that are best for the patient.

- **Chapter 23: Iatrosedation: Easing and Managing Pediatric Patient Fears**
  - Fear of dentistry is a worldwide health problem of considerable significance. In the United States it is estimated that 20 million people avoid the dental care because of fear.
  - The use of drugs is the traditional modality used to help the fearful patient. It must be recognized, however, that pharmacosedation does not reduce or eliminate fear.
  - Treatment of the fear syndrome requires a different technique, one with which the

fear is eliminated or significantly reduced by means of a relearning process.

- Iatrosedation is defined as: the act of making calm by the clinician's behavior. Behavior, in this sense, includes a broad spectrum of verbal and non-verbal communication techniques.

- **Chapter 31: Periodontal Disease in the Pediatric Population:** an important new chapter that presents content on periodontal disease in pediatric patients.
  - This chapter elaborates on the significance of pediatric oral health and explains why pediatric oral health is essential to child growth and development and to the general health and well-being of the child.
  - There is the need to ensure that messages of health promotion and disease prevention are brought home to both the pediatric individual and their caretakers.

Content Sequencing

The textbook is divided into nine major content areas:

Part 1: The Periodontium in Health

Part 2: Diseases Affecting the Periodontium

Part 3: Risk Factors for Periodontal Diseases

Part 4: Assessment and Planning for Patients With Periodontal Disease

Part 5: Implementation of Therapy for Patients With Periodontal Disease

Part 6: Health Maintenance in Treated Periodontal Patients

Part 7: Other Aspects of the Management of Patients With Periodontal Diseases

Part 8: Comprehensive Patient Cases

Part 9: Online Resources

TEXTBOOK FEATURES

The fifth edition of *Foundations of Periodontics for the Dental Hygienist* has many features designed to facilitate learning and teaching.

1. **Chapter Overview and Outline.** Each chapter begins with a concise overview of the chapter content. The outline makes it easier to locate material within the chapter. The outline provides the reader with an organizational framework with which to approach new material.

2. **Learning Objectives and Key Terms.** Learning objectives assist students in recognizing and studying important concepts in each chapter. Key terms are listed at the beginning of each chapter. One of the most challenging tasks for any student is learning a whole new dental vocabulary and gaining the confidence to use new terms with accuracy and ease. The "Key Terms" list assists students in this task by identifying important terminology and facilitating the study and review of terminology in each chapter. Terms are highlighted in bold type and clearly defined within the chapter.

3. **Instructional Design**
   - Each chapter is subdivided into sections to help the reader recognize major content areas.

- Chapters are written in an expanded outline format that makes it easy for students to identify, learn, and review key concepts.
- Material is presented in a manner that recognizes that students have different learning styles. Hundreds of illustrations and clinical photographs visually reinforce chapter content.
- Chapter content is supplemented in a visual format with boxes, tables, and flow charts.

4. **Focus on Patients.** "*Focus on Patients*" items allow the reader to apply chapter content in the context of clinical practice. The cases provide opportunities for students to integrate knowledge into their clinical work. Three types of scenarios help students apply content to the real-world setting:
   - Clinical Patient Care scenarios
   - Evidence in Action scenarios
   - Ethical Dilemma scenarios

5. **Patient Case Studies**
   - Chapter 37 presents five hypothetical patient scenarios. Patient assessment data pertinent to the periodontium challenges the student to interpret and use the information in periodontal care planning for the patient.
   - Chapter 38 (an online chapter) provides radiographs for six cases. These cases are intended to give students the opportunity to develop their critical thinking skills in analyzing and interpreting radiographs as it pertains to the hard tissues of the periodontium in health and disease.

6. **Glossary.** The glossary provides quick access to common periodontal terminology.

7. **Online Resources**
   - Chapter 38: Patient Cases: Radiographic Analysis
   - Instructor Resources
     - PowerPoint presentations for each chapter
     - Lesson plans
     - Test Bank
     - Image bank
     - Discussion topics and learning exercises
   - Student Resources
     - Animation: Anatomy of Periodontium in Disease

Foundations of Periodontics for the Dental Hygienist, Enhanced Fifth Edition strives to present the complex subject of periodontics in a reader-friendly manner. The authors greatly appreciate the comments and suggestions from educators and students about previous editions of this book. It is our sincere hope that this textbook will help students and practitioners alike to acquire knowledge that will serve as a foundation for the prevention and management of periodontal diseases.

Jill S. Gehrig, RDH, MA
Donald E. Willmann, DDS, MS
Daniel Shin, DDS, MSD

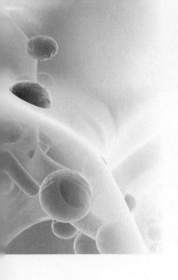

Acknowledgments

It is a great pleasure to acknowledge the following individuals whose assistance was indispensable to this *Enhanced Fifth Edition*:

- **Charles D. Whitehead** and **Holly R. Fischer,** MFA, the highly skilled medical illustrators, who created all the wonderful illustrations for the book.

- **Kevin Dietz,** a colleague and friend for his vision and guidance for all editions of this book.

- And with great thanks to our wonderful publishing team without whose expertise and support this book would not have been possible: **Jonathan Joyce, John Larkin,** and **Jennifer Clements.**

Jill S. Gehrig, RDH, MA
Donald E. Willmann, DDS, MS
Daniel Shin, DDS, MSD

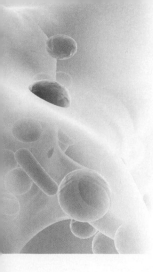

Contents

PART 3: RISK FACTORS FOR PERIODONTAL DISEASES

PART 4: ASSESSMENT AND PLANNING FOR PATIENTS WITH PERIODONTAL DISEASE

PART 5: IMPLEMENTATION OF THERAPY FOR PATIENTS WITH PERIODONTAL DISEASE

PART 6: HEALTH MAINTENANCE IN TREATED PERIODONTAL PATIENTS

PART 7: OTHER ASPECTS OF THE MANAGEMENT OF PATIENTS WITH PERIODONTAL DISEASES

PART 8: COMPREHENSIVE PATIENT CASES

PART 9: ONLINE RESOURCES

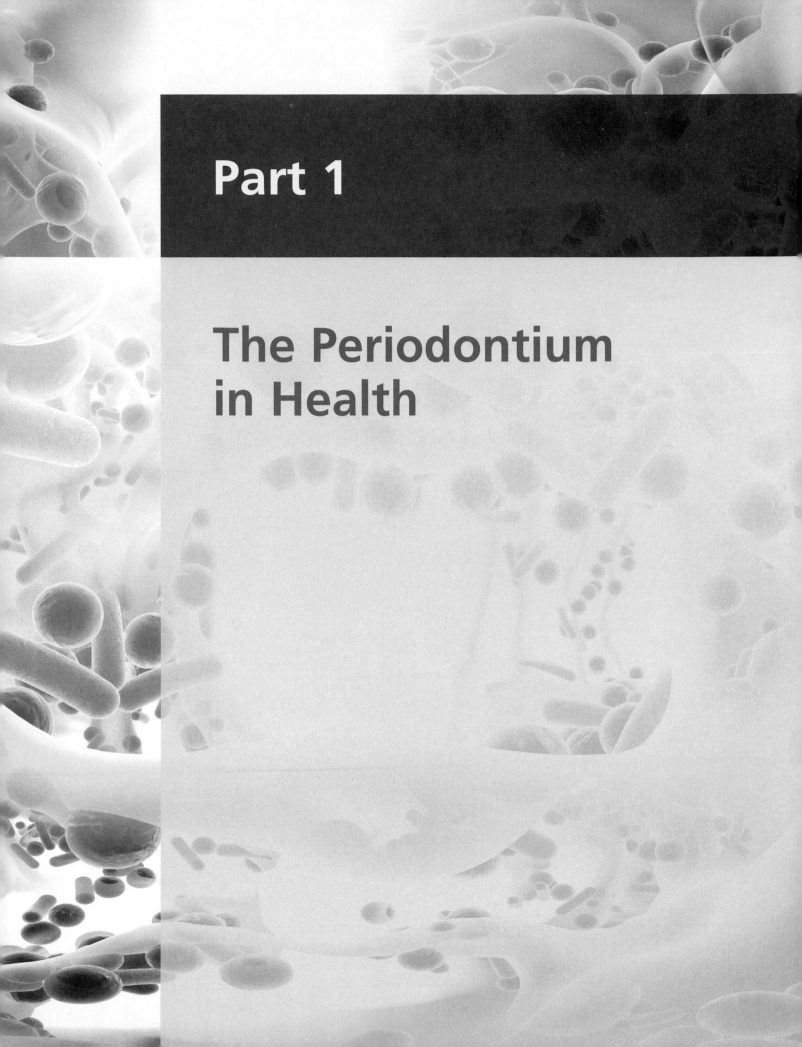

Part 1

The Periodontium in Health

1 Periodontium: The Tooth-Supporting Structures

Clinical Application.

Dental health care providers continuously interact with patients when making clinical decisions, performing clinical procedures, evaluating new techniques, and adapting to emerging treatment approaches. Nearly every action taken by a clinician requires a detailed knowledge of the anatomy of the tooth-supporting structures—the periodontium. Chapters 1 and 2 outline current knowledge about the anatomy of the periodontium. Chapter 1 deals with what is known about the fundamental structure of the complex system of tissues that support the teeth and can serve as a basis for organizing thoughts about additional anatomical information as it becomes available through additional research. Chapter 2 deals with the microscopic anatomy of these same structures.

Learning Objectives

- Identify the tissues of the periodontium on an unlabeled diagram depicting the periodontium in cross section.
- Describe the function that each tissue serves in the periodontium, including the gingiva, periodontal ligament, cementum, and alveolar bone.
- In a clinical setting or on a color photograph, identify the following anatomical areas of the gingiva: free gingiva, gingival sulcus, interdental gingiva, and attached gingiva.
- In a clinical setting or on a color photograph, identify the following boundaries of the gingiva: gingival margin, free gingival groove, and mucogingival junction.
- In a clinical setting, identify the free gingiva on an anterior tooth by inserting a periodontal probe to the base of the sulcus.
- In a clinical setting, compare and contrast the coral pink tissue of the attached gingiva with the darker, shiny tissue of the alveolar mucosa.
- In the clinical setting, use compressed air to detect the presence or absence of stippling of the attached gingiva.
- Identify the alveolar process (alveolar bone) on a human skull.
- Describe the position and contours of the alveolar crest of the bone in health.
- Describe the nerve and blood supply to the periodontium.
- Explain the role of the lymphatic system in the health of the periodontium.

Key Terms

Periodontium	Mucogingival junction	Gingival crevicular fluid	Periosteum
Gingiva	Free gingiva	Sharpey fibers	Innervation
Periodontal ligament	Attached gingiva	Alveolar process	Trigeminal nerve
Cementum	Stippling	Alveolar bone proper	Anastomose
Alveolar bone	Interdental gingiva	Alveolus	Lymphatic system
Gingival margin	Papillae	Cortical bone	Lymph nodes
Alveolar mucosa	Gingival col	Alveolar crest	
Free gingival groove	Gingival sulcus	Cancellous bone	

Section 1
Tissues of the Periodontium

The periodontium (peri = around and odontos = tooth) is the functional system of tissues that surrounds the teeth and attaches them to the jawbone (Figs. 1-1 and 1-2). The periodontium is also called the "supporting tissues of the teeth" and "the attachment apparatus." The tissues of the periodontium include the following:

1. Gingiva—the tissue that covers the cervical portions of the teeth and the alveolar processes of the jaws.
2. Periodontal ligament (PDL)—the fibers that surround the root of the tooth. These fibers attach to the bone of the socket on one side and to the cementum of the root on the other side.
3. Cementum—the thin layer of mineralized tissue that covers the root of the tooth.
4. Alveolar bone—the bone that surrounds the roots of the teeth. It forms the bony sockets that support and protect the roots of the teeth.

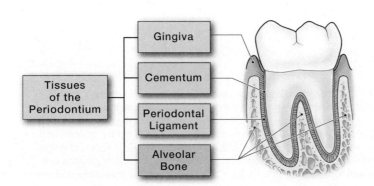

Figure 1-1. Tissues Comprising the Periodontium. A graphic representation of the periodontium in cross section.

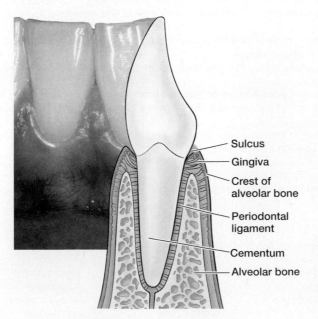

Figure 1-2. Healthy Periodontium. Clinical photograph and drawing depicting the structures of the periodontium.

TABLE 1-1	THE PERIODONTIUM
Structure	**Brief Description of Its Function**
Gingiva	• Provides a tissue seal around the cervical portion (neck) of the tooth • Covers the alveolar processes of the jaws • Holds the tissue against the tooth during mastication
Periodontal Ligament	• Suspends and maintains the tooth in its socket
Cementum	• Anchors the ends of the periodontal ligament fibers to the tooth so that the tooth stays in its socket • Protects the dentin of the root
Alveolar Bone	• Surrounds and supports the roots of the tooth

Each of the tissues of the periodontium plays a vital role in maintaining the health and function of the periodontium (Table 1-1). Knowledge of the periodontal tissues in health is a necessary foundation for understanding the concepts of (1) normal function of the periodontium, (2) disease prevention, and (3) the periodontal disease process.

Dental hygiene students usually are introduced to the tissues of the periodontium during the first semester or quarter of the dental hygiene curriculum. In the preclinical stages of the curriculum, mastering dental terminology and anatomy can sometimes be overwhelming and confusing. This chapter provides an opportunity to review this complex system of tissues known as the periodontium.

THE GINGIVA

1. Overview of the Gingiva
   A. **Description.** The gingiva is the part of the mucosa that surrounds the cervical portions of the teeth and covers the alveolar processes of the jaws (Fig. 1-3).
      1. The gingival margin is located coronal to the cementoenamel junction (CEJ) of each tooth and attaches to the tooth by means of a specialized type of epithelial tissue (junctional epithelium).
      2. It is composed of a thin outer layer of epithelium and an underlying layer of connective tissue.
      3. The gingiva is divided into four anatomical areas (Fig. 1-4):
         a. Free gingiva
         b. Gingival sulcus
         c. Interdental gingiva
         d. Attached gingiva
   B. **Function.** The gingiva protects the underlying tooth-supporting structures of the periodontium from the oral environment. The oral environment is exposed to a wide range of temperatures in food and drink, mechanical forces, and many oral bacteria. To accomplish these functions, the gingiva has several defense mechanisms, including the saliva and immune system.

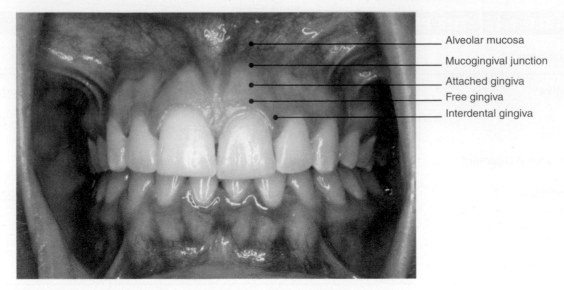

Alveolar mucosa
Mucogingival junction
Attached gingiva
Free gingiva
Interdental gingiva

Figure 1-3. The Gingival Tissues. Photograph of healthy gingival tissues showing the free, attached, and interdental gingiva.

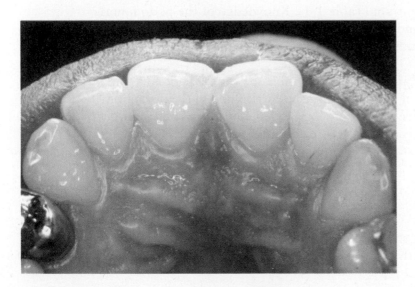

Figure 1-4. Gingival Tissue of the Palate. On the palate, the lingual gingiva is directly continuous with the keratinized masticatory mucosa.

C. **Boundaries of the Gingiva**
   1. The coronal boundary, or upper edge, of the gingiva is the **gingival margin** (Fig. 1-5).
   2. The apical boundary, or lower edge, of the gingiva is the alveolar mucosa. The **alveolar mucosa** can be distinguished easily from the gingiva by its dark red color and smooth, shiny surface.
D. **Demarcations of the Gingiva**
   1. The **free gingival groove** is a shallow linear depression that separates the free and attached gingiva (this line is rarely visible to the naked eye).
   2. The **mucogingival junction** is the clinically visible boundary where the pink attached gingiva meets the red, shiny alveolar mucosa. (Clinically visible means that this landmark is readily seen by the naked eye.)

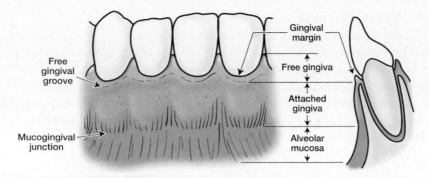

Figure 1-5. Boundaries of the Gingiva. Illustration showing the boundaries and anatomical areas of the gingiva.

2. **Free Gingiva.** The free gingiva is the unattached portion of the gingiva that surrounds the tooth in the region of the CEJ. The free gingiva is also known as the unattached gingiva or the marginal gingiva.
   A. **Location of the Free Gingiva**
      1. The free gingiva is located coronal to (above) the CEJ.
      2. It surrounds the tooth in a turtleneck or cuff-like manner.
      3. The free gingiva attaches to the tooth by means of a specialized epithelium—the junctional epithelium.
   B. **Characteristics of the Free Gingiva**
      1. The tissue of the free gingiva fits closely around the tooth but is not directly attached to it.
      2. This tissue, because it is unattached, may be gently retracted away from the tooth surface with a periodontal probe.
      3. The free gingiva also forms the soft tissue lateral wall of the gingival sulcus.
   C. **Contour of the Free Gingival Margin**
      1. The tissue of the free gingiva meets the tooth in a thin rounded edge called the gingival margin.
      2. The gingival margin follows the contours of the teeth, creating a scalloped (wavy) outline around them.
3. **Attached Gingiva.** The attached gingiva is continuous with the free gingiva and is the part of the gingiva that is tightly bound to the underlying cementum on the cervical-third of the root and to the periosteum (connective tissue cover) of the alveolar bone.
   A. **Location of the Attached Gingiva.** The attached gingiva lies between the free gingiva and the alveolar mucosa (Fig. 1-6).
   B. **Width of the Attached Gingiva**
      1. The attached gingiva is widest in the incisor and molar regions, ranging from 3.3 to 3.9 mm on the mandible and 3.5 to 4.5 mm on the maxilla (Fig. 1-7).
      2. The attached gingiva is narrowest in premolar regions (1.8 mm on mandible and 1.9 mm on maxilla).
      3. The width of the attached gingiva is not measured on the palate since clinically it is not possible to determine where the attached gingiva ends and the palatal mucosa begins (Fig. 1-4).
      4. It was once believed that a minimum 2-mm width of attached gingiva is necessary to maintain the health of the periodontium.[1] Currently, this concept is being reassessed and revisited.

C. Color of the Attached Gingiva
1. In health, the attached gingiva is pale or light coral pink.
2. The attached gingiva may be pigmented (Fig. 1-8). This pigmented tissue is known as physiologic pigmentation.
   a. Pigmentation occurs more frequently in dark-skinned individuals.[2]
   b. The pigmented areas of the attached gingiva may range from light brown to black.
   c. Pigmentation is due to an increased production of melanin (pigment) from melanocytes (melanin-producing cells found in the epidermal layer).

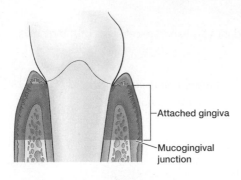

Figure 1-6. Location of the Attached Gingiva. The attached gingiva extends from the free gingival groove to the mucogingival junction.

Attached gingiva

Mucogingival junction

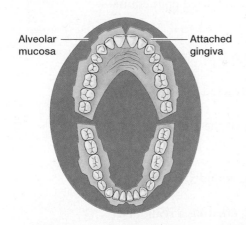

Alveolar mucosa

Attached gingiva

Figure 1-7. Mean Width of the Attached Gingiva. The attached gingiva is widest in the incisor and molar regions and narrowest in premolar regions.

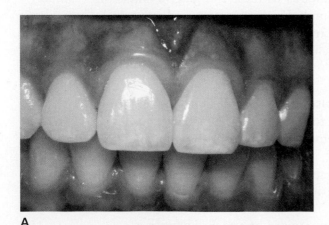
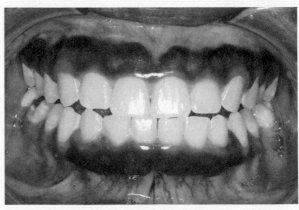

A   B

Figure 1-8. Color Variations of Normal Gingiva. The color of the normal gingiva varies among different persons. **A.** The color is a lighter, coral pink in individuals with fair complexions. **B.** In individuals with dark skin and hair, the gingiva may be pigmented. (Courtesy of Elizabeth Carr, University of Mississippi Medical Center, Jackson, MS.)

D. **Texture of the Attached Gingiva.** In health, the surface of the attached gingiva may have a dimpled appearance similar to the skin of an orange peel. This dimpled appearance is known as **stippling** (Fig. 1-9). Stippling acts to provide mechanical reinforcement to the gingiva. Stippling is seen only on the attached and interdental gingiva, not the marginal gingival. Healthy tissue, however, may or may not exhibit a stippled appearance as the presence of stippling varies greatly from individual to individual. Stippling is present in 40% of adults.

E. **Function of the Attached Gingiva**
1. The attached gingiva allows the gingival tissue to withstand the mechanical forces created during activities such as mastication, speaking, and toothbrushing.
2. The attached gingiva prevents the free gingiva from being pulled away (apically) from the tooth when tension is applied to the alveolar mucosa.

4. **Interdental Gingiva.** The **interdental gingiva** is the portion of the gingiva that fills the interdental embrasure between two adjacent teeth apical to the contact area (Fig. 1-10).

A. **Parts of Interdental Gingiva**
1. The interdental gingiva consists of two interdental **papillae**—one facial papilla and one lingual papilla (papilla = singular noun; papillae = plural noun).
   a. The lateral borders and tip of an interdental papilla are formed by the free gingiva from the adjacent teeth.
   b. The center portion of the interdental papilla is formed by the attached gingiva.
2. The **gingival col** is a valley-like depression in the portion of the interdental gingiva that lies directly apical to the contact area of two adjacent (touching) teeth and connects the facial and lingual papillae. *The col is not present if the adjacent teeth are not in contact* (i.e., there is a space between two adjacent teeth), there is no adjacent tooth (i.e., the lingual surface of the posterior-most tooth in the arch), or if the interdental gingiva has receded (Fig. 1-11).

B. **Function of Interdental Gingiva.** The interdental gingiva prevents food from becoming packed between the teeth during mastication.

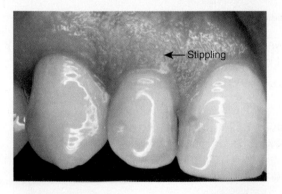

Figure 1-9. Gingival Stippling. In health, the surface of the attached gingiva may have a dimpled appearance known as gingival stippling.

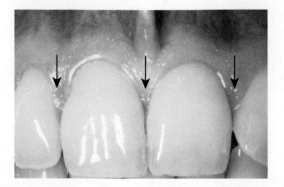

Figure 1-10. The Interdental Gingiva. The interdental tissue fills the area between two adjacent teeth.

5. **Gingival Sulcus.** The gingival sulcus is the *space* between the free gingiva and the tooth surface (Fig. 1-12).
   A. **Description.** The sulcus is a V-shaped, shallow space around the neck of a tooth.[3]
      1. The depth of a clinically healthy gingival sulcus is from 1 to 3 mm, as measured using a periodontal probe.
      2. Base of Sulcus. The base of the sulcus is formed by the junctional epithelium (a specialized type of epithelium that attaches to the tooth surface).
   B. **Gingival Crevicular Fluid.** The gingival crevicular fluid, also called the gingival sulcular fluid, is a fluid that seeps from the underlying connective tissue into the sulcular space.[4]
      1. Little or no fluid is found in the healthy gingival sulcus but the fluid flow increases in the presence of dental plaque biofilm and the resulting gingival inflammation.[5]
      2. Fluid flow increases in response to toothbrushing, mastication, or other stimulation of the gingiva. The flow is greatly increased when the gingiva is inflamed.
      3. If a filter strip is inserted into the sulcus, it absorbs the fluid in the sulcus. Using the filter strip, the amount of gingival crevicular fluid can be measured and used as an index of gingival inflammation.

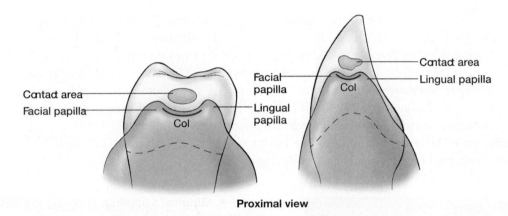

Proximal view

Figure 1-11. Interdental Col. Apical to the contact area between two teeth, the interdental gingiva has a concave (depressed) form. The concavity, the "col" is located between the facial and lingual papillae and extends beneath the contact area of two adjacent teeth.

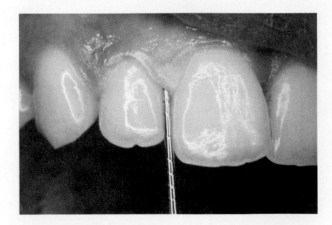

Figure 1-12. Gingival Sulcus. This photograph shows a periodontal probe inserted into the gingival sulcus, the space between the free gingiva and the tooth.

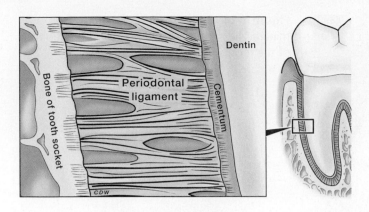

Figure 1-13. Periodontal Ligament.

- **On tooth side**, the ends of the periodontal ligament fibers are anchored in the cementum of the root.
- **On the bone side**, the ends of the periodontal ligament fibers are anchored in the alveolar bone of the tooth socket.

PERIODONTAL LIGAMENT

1. **Description**
   A. The periodontal ligament (PDL) is a layer of soft connective tissue that covers the root of the tooth and attaches it to the bone of the tooth socket (Fig. 1-13).
      1. The PDL is composed mainly of dense fibrous connective tissue.[3]
      2. The fibers of the PDL attach on one side to the root cementum and on the other side to the alveolar bone of the tooth socket.[6]
   B. The PDL not only connects the tooth to the alveolar process, but also supports the tooth in the socket and absorbs mechanical loads placed on the tooth, thus protecting the tooth in its socket.[7]
2. **Functions.** The PDL has five functions in the periodontium:
   A. Supportive function—suspends and maintains the tooth in its socket.
   B. Sensory function—provides sensory feeling to the tooth, such as pressure and pain sensations.
   C. Nutritive function—provides nutrients to the cementum and bone.
   D. Formative function—builds and maintains cementum and the alveolar bone of the tooth socket. The tissues of the PDL contain specialized cells such as fibroblasts, cementoblasts, and osteoblasts.
   E. Remodeling function—can remodel the alveolar bone in response to pressure, such as that applied during orthodontic treatment (braces).

ROOT CEMENTUM

1. **Description.** Cementum is a thin layer of hard, mineralized connective tissue that covers the surface of the tooth root (Fig. 1-14).
2. **Characteristics of Cementum**
   A. Cementum overlies and is attached to the dentin of the root. It is light yellow in color and softer than dentin or enamel. In terms of weight, it is composed of 50% to 55% organic substance—primarily, Type I collagen and noncollagenous matrix proteins—and 45% inorganic content (calcium and phosphate forms of hydroxyapatite and trace elements).
   B. Cementum is a bone-like tissue that is more resistant to resorption than bone.[8]
      1. Resistance to resorption (loss of substance) is an important characteristic of cementum that makes it possible for the teeth to be moved during orthodontic treatment.[9]

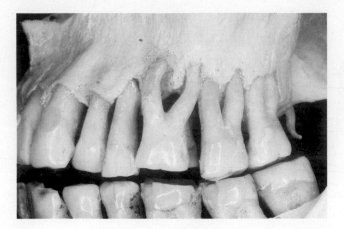

Figure 1-14. Cementum. Cementum is mineralized connective tissue that covers the root of the tooth; it is light yellow in color.

   2. The high resistance of cementum to resorption allows the pressure applied during orthodontics to cause resorption of the alveolar bone, for tooth movement, without resulting in root resorption.
   C. Cementum undergoes a continuous and slow physiologic process of resorption and repair throughout the lifetime of a tooth. This process allows for repair of existing cementum and deposition of new cementum. As a result, as an individual ages, the average thickness of cementum increases.
   D. There are two main types of cementum: cellular and acellular (Table 1-2).
   E. Cementum does not have its own blood or nutrient supply; it receives its nutrients from the PDL.
   F. Cementum is relatively permeable to extrinsic dyes, organic substances, inorganic ions, and bacteria. In periodontal disease, bacteria have been shown to invade the cementum.

3. **Functions of Cementum in the Periodontium.** Cementum performs several important roles in the periodontium, and, therefore, conservation of healthy cementum should be a goal of periodontal instrumentation.
   A. The primary function of cementum is to give attachment to the collagen fibers of the PDL. Cementum anchors the ends of the PDL fibers (via terminal endings known as **Sharpey fibers**) to the tooth. Without cementum, the tooth would fall out of its socket.
   B. The outer layer of cementum protects the underlying dentin and seals the ends of the open dentinal tubules.
   C. Cementum formation compensates for tooth wear at the occlusal or incisal surface due to attrition.
      1. Cementum is formed at the apical area of the root to compensate for occlusal attrition. This allows for the tooth to maintain its length. Consequently, the apical third of the root tends to be thicker (150 to 250 µ) than the coronal half of the root (16 to 60 µ).
      2. However, excessive deposition of cementum in the apical third of the root may result in an abnormality known as hypercementosis which can potentially obstruct the apical foramen. Radiographically, the characteristic hallmark of hypercementosis is a radiopaque thickening of the cementum that is enveloped by the radiolucent shadow of the PDL space and an intact lamina dura. In the absence of any pathology, hypercementosis does not pose a problem and does not require treatment.

TABLE 1-2	CHARACTERISTICS OF CEMENTUM	
	Acellular Cementum	**Cellular Cementum**
Time of Development	Forms before teeth are in occlusion	Forms after teeth have reached occlusion
Histologic Features	Is devoid of cells	Contains cementocytes
Location on Root	Covers cervical two thirds of root	Covers apical one third of root
Function	Plays important role in tooth support	Compensates for active eruption and normal tooth wear by continuous deposition of cementum

ALVEOLAR BONE

1. Description.
    A. The alveolar process or alveolar bone is the bone of the upper or lower jaw that surrounds and supports the roots of the teeth (Fig. 1-15).
    B. Bone is mineralized connective tissue and consists by weight of about 60% inorganic material, 25% organic material, and about 15% water.
    C. The existence of the alveolar bone is dependent on the presence of teeth; when teeth are extracted, in time, the alveolar bone resorbs. If teeth do not erupt, the alveolar bone does not develop.
2. **Function of the Alveolar Bone in the Periodontium.** The alveolar bone forms the bony sockets that provide support and protection for the roots of the teeth.
3. **Layers That Compose the Alveolar Process.** When viewed in cross section, the alveolar process is composed of three layers of hard tissue and covered by a thin layer of connective tissue (Figs. 1-16 and 1-17).
    A. The alveolar bone proper (or cribriform plate) is the thin layer of bone that lines the socket that surrounds the root of the tooth.
        1. The alveolus is the bony socket, a cavity in the alveolar bone that houses the root of a tooth (alveolus = singular; alveoli = plural) (Fig. 1-18).
        2. The alveolar bone proper has numerous holes (foramina) that allow blood vessels from the cancellous bone to connect with the vessels of the PDL space.
        3. The ends of the PDL fibers (Sharpey fibers) are embedded in the alveolar bone proper.

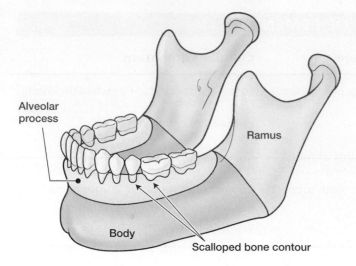

Figure 1-15. Alveolar Process. The alveolar process is the bone that surrounds and supports the roots of the teeth.

Alveolar process

Ramus

Body

Scalloped bone contour

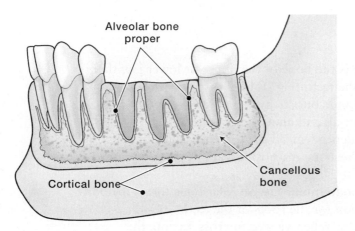

Figure 1-16. Layers of the Alveolar Process. A lateral section of the mandible reveals three bony layers: the alveolar bone proper, cancellous bone, and cortical bone.

Alveolar bone proper

Cortical bone

Cancellous bone

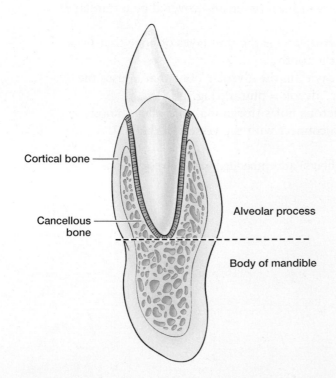

Figure 1-17. Cross Section of the Mandible. The *dotted line* indicates the boundary of the alveolar process with the body of the mandible.

Cortical bone

Cancellous bone

Alveolar process

Body of mandible

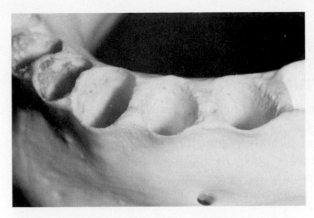

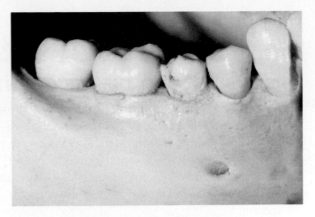

Figure 1-18. Alveoli of the Mandible. The alveoli are the sockets in the alveolar bone that house the roots of the teeth. (Courtesy of Dr. Don Rolfs, Wenatchee, WA.)

Figure 1-19. Bony Contours. The alveolar crest conforms to a scalloped line that follows the contours of the cementoenamel junctions. (Courtesy of Dr. Don Rolfs, Wenatchee, WA.)

B. The **cortical bone** (or cortical plate) is a layer of compact bone that forms the hard, outer wall of the mandible and maxilla on the facial and lingual aspects. This cortical bone surrounds the alveolar bone proper and gives support to the socket.
   1. The buccal cortical bone is thinner in the incisor, canine, and premolar regions; cortical bone is thicker in molar regions.
   2. Since the cortical plate is only on the facial and lingual sides of the jaw, it will not show up in a radiograph; only the cancellous bone and the alveolar bone proper can be seen on a radiograph.
   3. The **alveolar crest** is the coronal-most portion of the alveolar process.
      a. In health, the alveolar crest is located 1 to 2 mm apical to (below) the CEJs of the teeth (Fig. 1-19).
      b. When viewed from the facial or lingual aspect, the alveolar crest meets the teeth in a scalloped (wavy) line that follows the contours of the CEJs.
C. The **cancellous bone** (or **spongy bone**) is the lattice-like bone that fills the interior portion of the alveolar process (between the cortical bone and the alveolar bone proper). Cancellous bone is found mostly in the interproximal areas. Furthermore, a higher proportion of cancellous bone tends to exist in the maxilla than in the mandible while a higher proportion of cortical bone is found in the mandible. The cancellous bone is oriented around the tooth to form support for the alveolar bone proper.
D. The **periosteum** is a layer of connective soft tissue covering the outer surface of bone; it consists of an outer layer of collagenous tissue and an inner layer of fine elastic fibers.

Section 2
Nerve Supply, Blood Supply, and Lymphatic System

NERVE SUPPLY TO THE PERIODONTIUM

1. **Description.** The innervation of the periodontium—nerve supply to the periodontium—occurs via the branches of the trigeminal nerve—Cranial Nerve V (Fig. 1-20). Innervation to the maxilla (Fig. 1-21) is by the second branch of the trigeminal nerve (the maxillary nerve—Cranial Nerve V2) and the mandible by the third branch (the mandibular nerve—Cranial Nerve V3). The first branch (the ophthalmic nerve—Cranial Nerve V1) does not innervate regions of the oral cavity, so it will not be covered in this section.

   A. The second branch of the trigeminal nerve exists from the skull through the foramen rotundum and courses to the skin of the middle of the face to provide only sensory innervation to the maxilla. The third branch of the trigeminal nerve exits from the skull through the foramen ovale and courses to the lower face to provide both sensory and motor innervation.

   B. The trigeminal nerve is responsible for the sensory innervation of most of the skin of the front part of the face and head, the teeth, oral cavity, maxillary sinus, and nasal cavity.

   C. The motor function of the trigeminal nerve regulates movements of the mandible, such as jaw opening, jaw closing and excursive movements of the mandible—all key movements performed in the act of chewing and talking.

2. **Functions of the Nerve Supply to the Periodontium**

   A. Nerve receptors in the gingiva, alveolar bone, and PDL register pain, touch, and pressure.

   B. Nerves in the PDL provide information about movement and tooth position. These nerves provide the sensations of light touch or pressure against the teeth and play an important role in the regulation of chewing forces and movements. When biting down on something hard, it is the nerves of the PDL that are stimulated, allowing the individual to experience a sense of pressure with the teeth against the hard object.

3. **Innervation of the Periodontium**

   A. **Innervation of the Gingiva**

      1. Innervation of the gingiva of the maxillary arch is from the superior alveolar nerves (anterior, middle, and posterior branches), infraorbital nerve, and the greater palatine and nasopalatine nerves.

      2. Innervation of the gingiva of the mandibular arch is from the mental nerve, buccal nerve, and the sublingual branch of the lingual nerve (Fig. 1-22).

   B. **Innervation of the Teeth and Periodontal Ligament**

      1. Innervation of the teeth and PDL of the maxillary arch is from the superior alveolar nerves (anterior, middle, and posterior branches).

      2. Innervation of the teeth and PDL of the mandibular arch is from the inferior alveolar nerve.

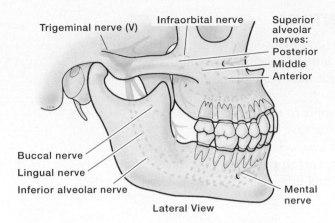

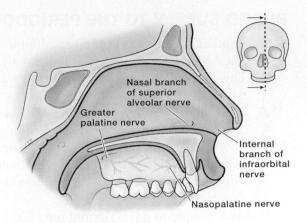

Figure 1-20. Nerve Supply to the Periodontium (Lateral View). The nerve supply to the periodontium is derived from the branches of the trigeminal nerve.

Figure 1-21. Nerve Innervation to the Palate (Midsagittal Section). The sensory nerves of the palate are branches of the maxillary nerve.

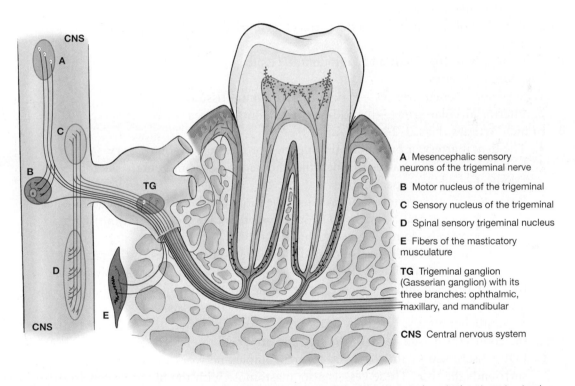

A Mesencephalic sensory neurons of the trigeminal nerve

B Motor nucleus of the trigeminal

C Sensory nucleus of the trigeminal

D Spinal sensory trigeminal nucleus

E Fibers of the masticatory musculature

TG Trigeminal ganglion (Gasserian ganglion) with its three branches: ophthalmic, maxillary, and mandibular

CNS Central nervous system

Figure 1-22. Innervation of Mandibular Teeth. Innervation of the gingiva and periodontium is via the mandibular nerve.

BLOOD SUPPLY TO THE PERIODONTIUM

1. **Description.** The vessels of the periodontium **anastomose** (join together) to create a complex *system of blood vessels* that supply blood to the periodontal tissues.
   A. This network of blood vessels acts as a unit, supplying blood to the soft and hard tissues of the maxilla and mandible.
   B. It is the proliferation of this rich blood supply to the gingiva that accounts for the dramatic color changes that are seen in gingivitis.
2. **Function.** The major function of the complex network of blood vessels of the periodontium is to transport oxygen and nutrients to the tissue cells of the periodontium and to remove carbon dioxide and other waste products from the cells for elimination.
3. **Vascular Supply to the Periodontium** (Fig. 1-23)
   A. Maxillary gingiva, PDL, and alveolar bone
      1. Anterior and posterior superior alveolar arteries
      2. Infraorbital artery
      3. Greater palatine artery
   B. Mandibular gingiva, PDL, and alveolar bone
      1. Inferior alveolar artery
      2. Branches of the inferior alveolar artery: the buccal, facial, mental, and sublingual arteries
4. **Vascular Supply to the Teeth and Periodontal Tissues**
   A. **The Major Arteries**
      1. Superior alveolar arteries—maxillary periodontal tissues
      2. Inferior alveolar artery—mandibular periodontal tissues
   B. **Branch Arteries** (Figs. 1-24 and 1-25)
      1. The dental artery: a branch of the superior or inferior alveolar artery
      2. Intraseptal artery: courses through the interdental bone and enters the tooth socket through rami perforantes.
      3. Rami perforantes: terminal branches of the intraseptal artery; they penetrate the tooth socket and enter the PDL space where they anastomose (join) with the blood vessels from the alveolar bone and PDL.
      4. Supraperiosteal blood vessels: located along the outer surfaces of the facial and lingual cortical plates. These vessels provide the main blood supply to the free and attached gingiva; these vessels anastomose with capillaries from the alveolar bone (intraseptal artery) and the PDL (PDL vessels).
      5. Subepithelial plexus: branches of the supraperiosteal blood vessels located in the connective tissue beneath the free and attached gingiva.
      6. PDL vessels: supply the PDL and form a complex network of vessels that surrounds the root. These vessels also anastomose with the blood vessels from the intraseptal artery and the supraperiosteal arterioles.
      7. Dentogingival plexus: a fine-meshed network of blood vessels located in the connective tissue beneath the gingival sulcus.

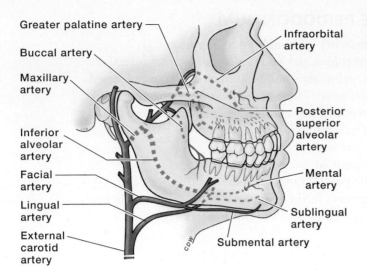

Greater palatine artery
Buccal artery
Maxillary artery
Inferior alveolar artery
Facial artery
Lingual artery
External carotid artery
Infraorbital artery
Posterior superior alveolar artery
Mental artery
Sublingual artery
Submental artery

Figure 1-23. Vascular Supply to the Periodontium. A complex network of blood vessels supplies blood to the periodontium.

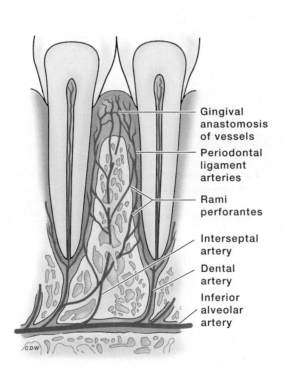

Gingival anastomosis of vessels
Periodontal ligament arteries
Rami perforantes
Interseptal artery
Dental artery
Inferior alveolar artery

Figure 1-24. Branch Arteries. The branch arteries supply blood to the teeth and periodontium.

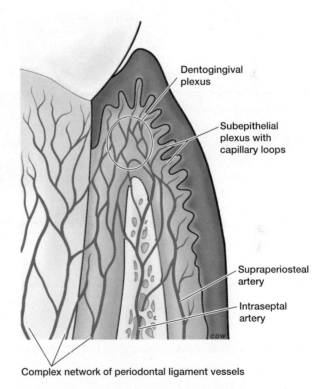

Dentogingival plexus
Subepithelial plexus with capillary loops
Supraperiosteal artery
Intraseptal artery
Complex network of periodontal ligament vessels

Figure 1-25. Network of Vessels. A fine network of vessels supplies blood to gingiva, gingival connective tissue, and periodontal ligament.

LYMPHATIC SYSTEM AND THE PERIODONTIUM

1. **Description.** The lymphatic system is a network of lymph nodes connected by lymphatic vessels that plays an important role in the body's defense against infection.
2. **Function.** Lymph nodes (pronounced: limf nodes) are small bean-shaped structures located on either side of the head, neck, armpits, and groin. These nodes filter out and trap bacteria, fungi, viruses, and other unwanted substances to safely eliminate them from the body.
3. **Lymph Drainage of the Periodontium.** The lymph from the periodontal tissues is drained to the lymph nodes of the head and neck (Fig. 1-26).
   A. Submandibular lymph nodes—drain most of the periodontal tissues
   B. Deep cervical lymph nodes—drain the palatal gingiva of the maxilla
   C. Submental lymph nodes—drain the gingiva in the region of the mandibular incisors
   D. Jugulodigastric lymph nodes—drain the gingiva in the third molar region

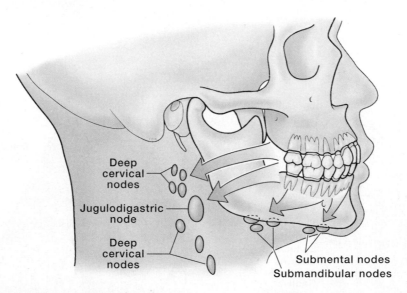

Figure 1-26. Lymphatic System of the Periodontium. The lymph from the periodontium is drained to the lymph nodes of the head and neck.

Chapter Summary Statement

The gingiva, periodontal ligament, cementum, and alveolar bone make up a system of tissues that surround the teeth and attach them to the alveolar bone. Each tissue of the periodontium plays a vital role in the functioning and retention of the teeth.

- The gingiva provides a tissue seal around the cervical portion of the teeth and covers the alveolar process.
- The periodontal ligament supports the tooth in its socket, provides nutrients and sensory feeling to the tooth, and maintains cementum and the alveolar bone of the tooth socket.
- The cementum anchors the periodontal ligament to the tooth and seals the ends of the open dentinal tubules. Cementum formation compensates for tooth wear due to occlusal attrition.
- The alveolar bone forms the bony sockets that provide support and protection for the roots of the teeth.

Section 3
Focus on Patients

Clinical Patient Care

CASE 1

A patient involved in an automobile accident receives a penetrating wound involving the oral cavity. The wound enters the alveolar mucosa near the apex of a lower premolar tooth and extends from the surface mucosa all the way through the tissues to the premolar tooth root. List the periodontal tissues most likely injured by this penetrating wound.

CASE 2

A patient who has lost a maxillary lateral incisor tooth is scheduled to have a dental implant placed. The dental implant placement will require the clinician to prepare a hole with a drill in the bone formerly occupied by the lateral incisor tooth. Name the types of bone that will most probably be penetrated by the drill.

CASE 3

A dentist injects a local anesthetic before working on a maxillary molar tooth. The injection results in complete loss of sensation in the molar tooth and in most of the gingiva surrounding the molar tooth. Name the nerves that most likely have been affected by the injection of the local anesthetic.

References

1. Lang NP, Loe H. The relationship between the width of keratinized gingiva and gingival health. *J Periodontol.* 1972;43(10): 623–627.
2. Ainamo J, Loe H. Anatomical characteristics of gingiva. A clinical and microscopic study of the free and attached gingiva. *J Periodontol.* 1966;37(1):5–13.
3. Cho MI, Garant PR. Development and general structure of the periodontium. *Periodontol 2000.* 2000;24:9–27.
4. Taylor JJ, Preshaw PM. Gingival crevicular fluid and saliva. *Periodontol 2000.* 2016;70(1):7–10.
5. Barros SP, Williams R, Offenbacher S, Morelli T. Gingival crevicular fluid as a source of biomarkers for periodontitis. *Periodontol 2000.* 2016;70(1):53–64.
6. Saygin NE, Giannobile WV, Somerman MJ. Molecular and cell biology of cementum. *Periodontol 2000.* 2000;24:73–98.
7. Huang L, Liu B, Cha JY, et al. Mechanoresponsive properties of the periodontal ligament. *J Dent Res.* 2016;95(4):467–475.
8. Diekwisch TG. The developmental biology of cementum. *Int J Dev Biol.* 2001;45(5–6):695–706.
9. Sodek J, McKee MD. Molecular and cellular biology of alveolar bone. *Periodontol 2000.* 2000;24:99–126.

 ## STUDENT ANCILLARY RESOURCES

A wide variety of resources to enhance your learning is available online:

- Audio Glossary
- Book Pages
- Animation: Anatomy of the Periodontium in Disease
- Chapter Review Questions and Answers

2 Microscopic Anatomy of the Periodontium

Clinical Application.
Dental health care providers continuously interact with patients when making clinical decisions, performing clinical procedures, evaluating new techniques, and adapting to emerging treatment approaches. Nearly every action taken by a clinician requires a detailed knowledge of the anatomy of the tooth-supporting structures—the periodontium. Chapter 1 dealt with what is known about the fundamental structure of the complex system of tissues that support the teeth. Chapter 2 deals with the microscopic anatomy of these same structures. The information presented in these two chapters can serve as a basis for organizing thoughts about additional anatomical information as it becomes available through additional research.

Learning Objectives

* Describe the histology of the tissues and the function that each serves in the human body.
* List and define the layers that comprise the stratified squamous epithelium of the skin.
* Define keratin and describe its function in the epithelium.
* Describe the composition and function of connective tissue.
* Describe the epithelial–connective tissue interface found in most tissues of the body, such as the interface between the epithelium and connective tissues of the skin.
* Define the term *cell junction* and describe its function in the epithelial tissues.
* Compare and contrast the terms *desmosome* and *hemidesmosome*.
* Identify the three anatomical areas of the gingival epithelium on an unlabeled drawing depicting the microscopic anatomy of the gingival epithelium.
* Describe the location and function of the following regions of the gingival epithelium: oral epithelium, sulcular epithelium, and junctional epithelium.
* State the level of keratinization present in each of the three anatomical areas of the gingival epithelium (keratinized, nonkeratinized, or parakeratinized).
* State which of the anatomical areas of the gingival epithelium have an uneven, wavy epithelial–connective tissue interface **in health** and which have a smooth junction in **health**.
* Identify the enamel, gingival connective tissue, junctional epithelium, internal basal lamina, external basal lamina, epithelial cells, desmosomes, and hemidesmosomes on an unlabeled drawing depicting the microscopic anatomy of the junctional epithelium and surrounding tissues.
* Define and describe the function of the supragingival fiber bundles and the periodontal ligament in the periodontium.
* Identify the fiber groups of the periodontal ligament on an unlabeled drawing.
* Define the terms *cementum* and *Sharpey fibers* and describe their function in the periodontium.
* State the three relationships that the cementum may have in relation to the enamel at the cementoenamel junction.
* Define the term *alveolar bone* and describe its function in the periodontium.

Key Terms

Histology	Keratinized epithelial cells	Cell junctions	Keratin	Periodontal ligament
Tissue	Nonkeratinized	Desmosome	Gingival crevicular fluid	(PDL)
Cells	epithelial cells	Hemidesmosome	Internal basal lamina	Fiber bundles of the PDL
Extracellular matrix	Connective tissue	Gingival epithelium	External basal lamina	Sharpey fibers
Epithelial tissue	Epithelial–connective	Oral epithelium (OE)	Collagen fibers	Cementum
Stratified squamous	tissue interface	Sulcular epithelium (SE)	Supragingival fiber	Cementum proteins
epithelium	Basement membrane	Junctional epithelium (JE)	bundles	OMG (overlap, meet, gap)
Basal lamina	Epithelial ridges	Keratinized	Dentogingival unit	Alveolar process
Keratinization	Connective tissue papillae	Parakeratinized	Periosteum	Bone remodeling

Section 1
Histology of the Body's Tissues

Histology is a branch of anatomy concerned with the study of the microscopic features of tissues. Knowledge of the microscopic characteristics of tissues is a prerequisite for understanding the microscopic anatomy of the periodontium. Section 1 reviews the microscopic anatomy of the epithelial and connective tissues of the body.

MICROSCOPIC ANATOMY OF A TISSUE

A **tissue** is a group of interconnected cells that perform a similar function within an organism. For example, muscle cells group together to form muscle tissue that functions to move parts of the body. The tissues and organs of the body are composed of several different types of cells and extracellular elements outside of the cells.

1. Cells
   A. Cells are the smallest structural unit of living matter capable of functioning independently.
   B. Cells group together to form a tissue.
   C. The four basic types of tissue are epithelial, connective, nerve, and muscle tissues.
2. **Extracellular Matrix.** Tissues are not made up solely of cells. A gel-like substance containing interwoven protein fibers surrounds most cells.
   A. The **extracellular matrix** is a mesh-like material that surrounds the cells (Fig. 2-1). It is like a structural and biomechanical scaffold for the cells. This material helps to hold cells together and provides a framework within which cells can migrate and interact with one another.
   B. The extracellular matrix consists of ground substance and fibers.
      1. The ground substance is a gel-like material that fills the space between the cells.
      2. The fibers consist of collagen, elastin, and reticular fibers. Collagens are the major proteins of the extracellular matrix.
   C. Amount of Extracellular Matrix
      1. In epithelial tissue, the extracellular matrix is sparse, consisting mainly of a thin mat called the basal lamina, which underlies the epithelium.
      2. In connective tissue, the extracellular matrix is more plentiful than the cells that it surrounds.

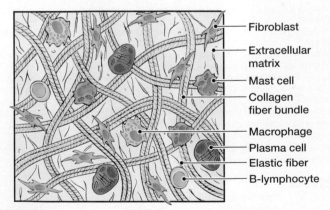

Figure 2-1. Extracellular Matrix. The extracellular matrix surrounds the cells of a tissue and is comprised of fibers and a gel-like substance.

MICROSCOPIC ANATOMY OF EPITHELIAL TISSUE

1. **Description.** The epithelial tissue is the tissue that makes up the outer surface of the body (skin or epidermis) and lines the body cavities such as the mouth, stomach, and intestines (mucosa). The skin and mucosa of the oral cavity are made up of stratified squamous epithelium—a type of epithelium that is comprised of flat cells arranged in several layers.

2. **Composition of Epithelial Tissue**
   A. **Plentiful Cells.** Most of the volume of epithelial tissue consists of many closely packed epithelial cells (Fig. 2-2). Epithelial cells are bound together into sheets.
   B. **Sparse Extracellular Matrix**
      1. The extracellular matrix is a minor component of the epithelial tissue existing mainly in the basal lamina.
      2. The basal lamina is a thin mat of extracellular matrix secreted by the epithelial cells. This basal lamina mat supports the epithelium (somewhat like the scaffolding of a building).

3. **Keratinization.** Keratinization—the process by which epithelial cells on the surface of the skin become stronger and waterproof.
   A. **Keratinized Epithelial Cells**
      1. Keratinized epithelial cells have no nuclei and form a tough, resistant layer on the surface of the skin.
      2. The most heavily keratinized epithelium of the body is found on the palms of the hands and soles of the feet.
   B. **Nonkeratinized Epithelial Cells**
      1. Nonkeratinized epithelial cells have nuclei and act as a cushion against mechanical stress and wear. Nonkeratinized epithelial cells are softer and more flexible.
      2. Nonkeratinized epithelium is found in areas such as the mucosal lining of the cheeks—permitting the mobility needed to speak, chew, and make facial expressions.

4. **Blood Supply.** Epithelial tissues are avascular—containing no blood vessels. The epithelial layer receives oxygen and nourishment from blood vessels located in the underlying connective tissue via a process known as diffusion (Fig. 2-2).

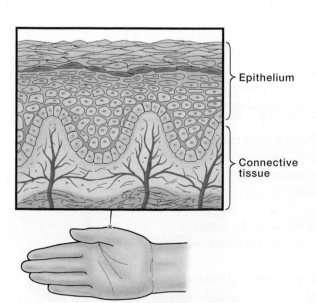

Epithelium

Connective tissue

Figure 2-2. Stratified Squamous Epithelium and Connective Tissue of the Skin. The epithelium of the skin consists of many closely packed epithelial cells and a thin basal lamina. The epithelium of the skin rests on a supporting bed of connective tissue. The epithelium does not contain blood vessels; nourishment is received from blood vessels in the underlying connective tissue.

MICROSCOPIC ANATOMY OF CONNECTIVE TISSUE

1. **Description.** Connective tissue fills the spaces between the tissues and organs in the body. It supports and binds other tissues. Connective tissue consists of cells separated by abundant extracellular substance.
2. **Composition of Connective Tissue**
   A. **Sparse Cells.** Connective tissue cells are sparsely distributed in the extracellular matrix.
      1. Fibroblasts ("fiber-builders")—cells that form the extracellular matrix (fibers and ground substance) and secrete it into the intercellular spaces
      2. Macrophages and neutrophils—phagocytes ("cell-eaters") that devour dying cells and microorganisms that invade the body
      3. Lymphocytes—cells that play a major role in the immune response
   B. **Plentiful Extracellular Matrix.** The extracellular matrix—a rich gel-like substance containing a network of strong fibers—is the major component of connective tissue. The network of the fiber matrix, rather than the cells, gives connective tissue the strength to withstand mechanical forces.
3. **Dental Connective Tissue.** All dental tissues of the tooth—cementum, dentin, alveolar bone, and the pulp—are specialized forms of connective tissue *except enamel*. Enamel is an epithelial tissue.

EPITHELIAL–CONNECTIVE TISSUE INTERFACE

1. **Description.** The epithelial–connective tissue interface is the boundary where the epithelial and connective tissues meet.
2. **The Basement Membrane and Basal Lamina**
   A. As discussed previously, the basal lamina is a thin layer secreted by the epithelial cells on which the epithelium sits. The term *basal lamina* often is confused with the term *basement membrane* and is sometimes used inconsistently in the literature.
   B. The basal lamina is not visible under the light microscope, but can be distinguished under the higher magnification of an electron microscope. The basal lamina assists the attachment of the epithelial cells to adjacent structures, such as the tooth surface.
   C. The term basement membrane specifies a thin layer of tissue visible with a light microscope beneath the epithelium. The basement membrane is formed by the combination of a basal lamina and a reticular lamina.
3. **Characteristics of the Epithelial–Connective Tissue Boundary**
   A. **Wavy Boundary.** In most places in the body, the epithelium meets the connective tissue in a wavy, uneven manner (Fig. 2-3).
      1. Epithelial ridges—deep extensions of epithelium that reach down into the connective tissue. The epithelial ridges are also known as rete pegs.
      2. Connective tissue papillae—finger-like extensions of connective tissue that project up and interlock with the epithelium.
   B. **Smooth Boundary**
      1. Some specialized epithelial tissues in the body meet the connective tissue in a smooth interface that has no epithelial ridges or connective tissue papillae.
      2. Some anatomical areas of the gingiva have an epithelial–connective tissue interface that is smooth.

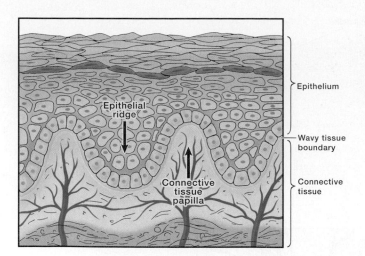

Figure 2-3. Wavy Epithelial–Connective Tissue Interface. In most cases, the epithelium meets the connective tissue at an uneven, wavy border. Epithelial ridges extend down into the connective tissue. Connective tissue papillae extend upward into the epithelium.

4. **Function of the Wavy Tissue Boundary**
   A. **Enhances Adhesion.** The wavy tissue interface enhances the adhesion of the epithelium to the connective tissue by increasing the surface area of the junction between the two tissues. This strong adhesion of the epithelium allows the skin to resist mechanical forces.
   B. **Provides Nourishment.** The wavy junction between the epithelium and connective tissue also increases the area from which the epithelium can receive nourishment from the underlying connective tissue. The epithelium does not have its own blood supply; blood vessels are carried close to the epithelium in the connective tissue papillae.

EPITHELIAL CELL JUNCTIONS

Neighboring epithelial cells attach to one another by specialized cell junctions that give the tissue strength to withstand mechanical forces and to form a protective barrier.

1. **Definition.** Cell junctions are cellular structures that mechanically attach a cell and its cytoskeleton to its neighboring cells or to the basal lamina.
2. **Purpose.** Cell junctions bind cells together so that they can function as a strong structural unit. Tissues, such as the epithelium of the skin that must withstand severe mechanical stresses, have the most abundant number of cell junctions.
3. **Types of Epithelial Cell Junctions**
   A. **Desmosome**—a specialized cell junction that connects two neighboring epithelial cells and their cytoskeletons together. You might think of desmosomes as being like the snaps used to close a denim jacket. Instead of fastening the front of a jacket together, desmosomes fasten epithelial cells together (Fig. 2-4A,B).
      1. A cell-to-cell connection
      2. An important form of cell junction found in the gingival epithelium
   B. **Hemidesmosome**—a specialized cell junction that connects the epithelial cells to the basal lamina (Fig. 2-4A,B). You might think of hemidesmosomes as specialized structures that represent half of a desmosome.
      1. A cell-to-basal lamina connection
      2. An important form of cell junction found in the gingival epithelium

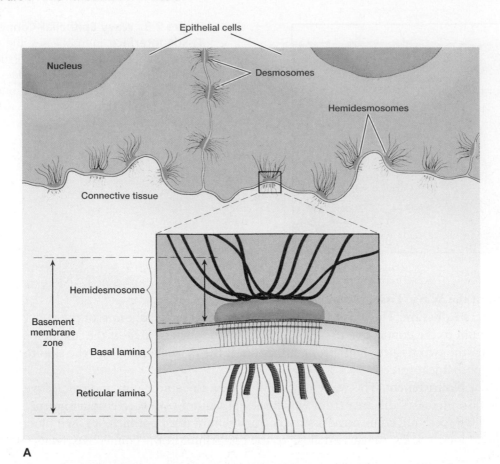

A

Figure 2-4A. The Epithelial–Connective Tissue Interface. The epithelial–connective tissue interface is the site of the basement membrane zone, a complex structure mostly synthesized by the epithelial cells. **Inset:** A representation of an electron micrograph showing the hemidesmosomal attachment to the basal lamina. (Adapted with permission from Rubin R, Strayer DS. *Rubin's Pathology: Clinicopathologic Foundations of Medicine*. 5th ed. Philadelphia, PA: Lippincott Williams & Wilkins; 2008.)

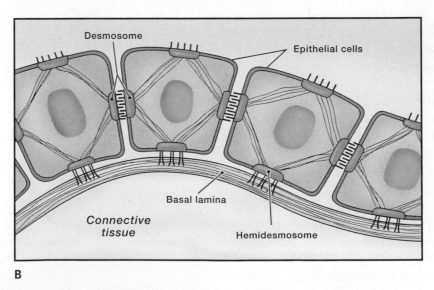

B

Figure 2-4B. Epithelial Cell Junctions. Epithelial cells attach to each other with specialized cell junctions called desmosomes. Hemidesmosomes attach the epithelial cells to the basal lamina.

Section 2
Histology of the Gingiva

Knowledge of the microscopic anatomy of the gingiva is a prerequisite for understanding the periodontium in health and in disease. At first glance, the microscopic anatomy of the periodontium may seem to be complicated.[1] The anatomy of the periodontium, however, is much like that of tissues elsewhere in the body. **The gingiva consists of an epithelial layer and an underlying connective tissue layer.** This section reviews the microscopic anatomy of the gingival epithelium, junctional epithelium, and gingival connective tissues.

MICROSCOPIC ANATOMY OF GINGIVAL EPITHELIUM

The gingival epithelium is a specialized stratified squamous epithelium that functions well in the wet environment of the oral cavity.[2] The microscopic anatomy of the gingival epithelium is like that of the epithelium of the skin. The gingival epithelium may be differentiated into three anatomical areas (Fig. 2-5):

1. Oral Epithelium (OE): epithelium that faces the oral cavity
2. Sulcular Epithelium (SE): epithelium that faces the tooth surface *without being in contact with the tooth surface*
3. Junctional Epithelium (JE): epithelium that attaches the gingiva to the tooth

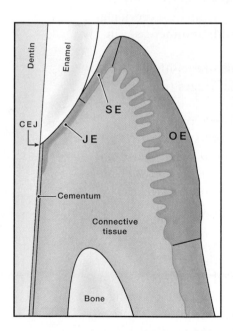

Figure 2-5. Three Areas of the Gingival Epithelium. The gingival epithelium has three distinct areas:

- **JE**—junctional epithelium at the base of the sulcus
- **SE**—sulcular epithelium that lines the sulcus
- **OE**—oral epithelium covering the free and attached gingiva

1. **Oral Epithelium (OE).** The oral epithelium covers the outer surface of the free gingiva and attached gingiva; it extends from the crest of the gingival margin to the mucogingival junction. The oral epithelium is the only part of the periodontium that is visible to the unaided eye.
   A. **Cellular Structure of the Oral Epithelium (OE)**
      1. The oral epithelium may be keratinized or parakeratinized (partially keratinized). Keratin is a tough, fibrous structural protein that occurs in the outer layer of the skin and the oral epithelium (Fig. 2-6).

2. The oral epithelium is stratified squamous epithelium that can be divided into cell layers (Fig. 2-6). The layers are listed below in order from the deepest layer to the most superficial layer.
   a. Basal cell layer (stratum basale): cube-shaped cells
   b. Prickle cell layer (stratum spinosum): spine-like cells with large intercellular spaces. The cells of both the basal and prickle cell layers attach to each other with desmosomes.
   c. Granular cell layer (stratum granulosum): flattened cells and increased intracellular keratin
   d. Keratinized cell layer (stratum corneum): flattened cells with extensive intracellular keratin.

   B. **Interface with Gingival Connective Tissue.** *In health, oral epithelium joins with the connective tissue in a **wavy interface** with epithelial ridges* (Figs. 2-7 and 2-8).

2. **Sulcular Epithelium.** Sulcular epithelium (SE) is the epithelial lining of the gingival sulcus. It is continuous with the oral epithelium and extends from the crest of the gingival margin to the coronal edge of the junctional epithelium.
   A. **Cellular Structure of the Sulcular Epithelium (SE)**
      1. The sulcular epithelium is a thin, nonkeratinized epithelium.[3]
      2. The sulcular epithelium has three cellular layers (Fig. 2-6):
         a. Basal cell layer
         b. Prickle cell layer
         c. Superficial cell layer: flattened cells without keratin
      3. The sulcular epithelium is permeable allowing fluid to flow from the gingival connective tissue into the sulcus. This fluid is known as the gingival crevicular fluid. The flow of gingival crevicular fluid is slight in health and increases in disease.
   B. **Interface with Gingival Connective Tissue.** In health, the sulcular epithelium joins the connective tissue at a **smooth interface** with no epithelial ridges (no wavy junction).

3. **Junctional Epithelium.** Junctional epithelium (JE) is the specialized epithelium that forms the base of the sulcus and joins the gingiva to the tooth surface. ***The gingiva surrounds the cervix of the tooth and attaches to the tooth by means of the junctional epithelium. The base of the sulcus is made up of the coronal-most cells of the junctional epithelium.*** In health, the JE attaches to the tooth at a level that is slightly coronal to the cementoenamel junction (CEJ).
   A. **Cellular Structure of the Junctional Epithelium (JE)**
      1. Keratinization of JE
         a. The junctional epithelium is a thin, nonkeratinized epithelium.
         b. Nonkeratinized epithelial cells of both the sulcular and junctional areas of the gingival epithelium make them a less effective protective covering. Thus, the sulcular and junctional areas provide the easiest point of entry for bacteria or bacterial products to invade the connective tissue of the gingiva.
      2. The junctional epithelium has only two cell layers (Figs. 2-6 and 2-7):
         a. Basal cell layer
         b. Prickle cell layer
      3. Length and Width of JE
         a. The junctional epithelium ranges from 0.71 to 1.35 mm in length.[4]
         b. The JE is about 15 to 30 cells thick at the coronal zone—the zone that attaches highest on the crown of the tooth.
         c. The JE tapers from 4 to 5 cells thick at the apical zone.

B. **JE Interface with Gingival Connective Tissue.** In health, the junctional epithelium has a *smooth tissue interface* with the connective tissue (no wavy junctions).

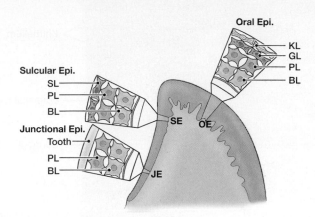

Figure 2-6. Cell Layers of the Gingival Epithelium. The cell layers of the oral, sulcular, and junctional epithelium. Illustration key: KL, keratinized cell layer; GL, granular cell layer; SL, superficial cell layer; PL, prickle cell layer; BL, basal cell layer.

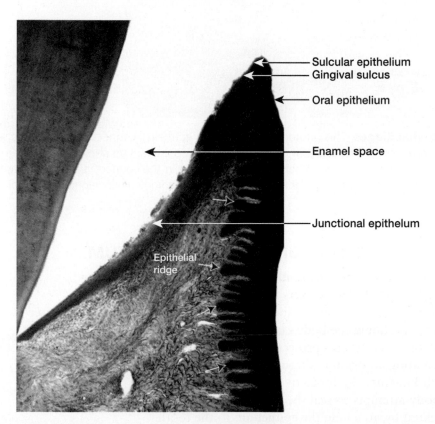

Figure 2-7. Human Gingiva. This photograph shows a decalcified longitudinal section of an incisor tooth as seen through an ordinary light microscope. All the calcium hydroxyapatite crystals have been extracted from the tooth and from its bony alveolus. Since enamel is composed almost completely of calcium hydroxyapatite crystals, only the space where enamel used to be—the enamel space—is represented in this photograph. The sulcular epithelium of the free gingiva borders a space known as the gingival sulcus. Observe the well-developed epithelial ridges (identified by label and arrows) of the oral epithelium. (Adapted with permission from Gartner LP, Hiatt JL. *Color Atlas and Text of Histology*. Philadelphia, PA: Lippincott Williams & Wilkins; 2013.)

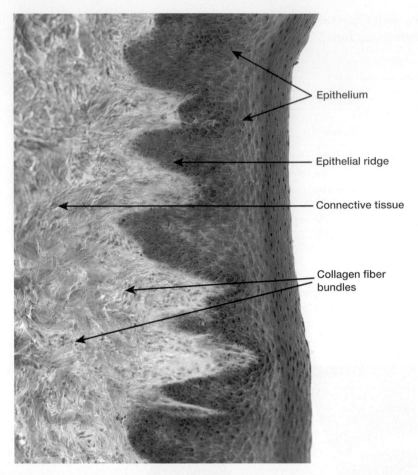

Epithelium

Epithelial ridge

Connective tissue

Collagen fiber bundles

Figure 2-8. Epithelial Ridges. This photograph shows the epithelial–connective junction as seen through an ordinary light microscope. The tall epithelial ridges of the epithelium (*in dark red*) project into the underlying connective tissue. Collagen fiber bundles are visible in the connective tissue. (Adapted with permission from Gartner LP, Hiatt JL. *Color Atlas and Text of Histology*. Philadelphia, PA: Lippincott Williams & Wilkins; 2013.)

WHY THE TEETH NEED A JUNCTIONAL EPITHELIUM

1. **The Teeth Create a Break in the Epithelial Protective Covering**
   A. **Protective Epithelial Sheet Covers the Body**
      1. A continuous sheet of epithelium protects the body by covering its outer surfaces and lining the body's cavities, including the oral cavity.
      2. The teeth penetrate this protective covering by erupting through the epithelium, thus creating an opening through which microorganisms can enter the body.
   B. **The Teeth Puncture the Protective Epithelial Sheet**
      1. The body attempts to seal the opening created when a tooth penetrates the epithelium by attaching the epithelium to the tooth.
      2. The word "junction" means "connection"; thus, the epithelium that is connected to the tooth is termed the "junctional epithelium."
2. **Functions of the Junctional Epithelium**
   A. **Epithelial Attachment.** The junctional epithelium provides an attachment between the gingiva and the tooth surface, thus providing a seal at the base of the gingival sulcus or periodontal pocket (Fig. 2-9).

B. Barrier. The junctional epithelium provides a protective barrier between the plaque biofilm and the connective tissue of the periodontium.

C. Host Defense. The epithelial cells play a role in defending the periodontium from bacterial infection by signaling the immune response.[5]

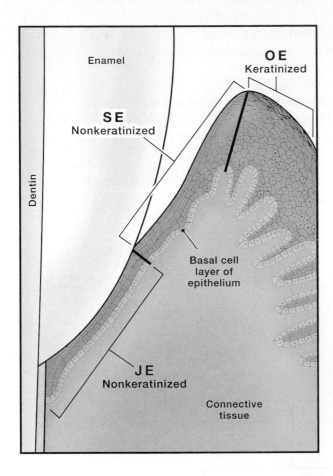

Figure 2-9. Microscopic Anatomy of the Three Areas of the Gingival Epithelium. Interface with Connective Tissue.

- **OE** (oral epithelium)—these epithelial cells form the outer layer of the free and attached gingiva.

- **SE** (sulcular epithelium)—these epithelial cells extend from the edge of the junctional epithelium coronally to the crest of the gingival margin.

- **JE** (junctional epithelium)—these epithelial cells join the gingiva to the tooth surface at the base of the sulcus.

ATTACHMENT OF THE CELLS OF THE JUNCTIONAL EPITHELIUM

1. **Microscopic Anatomy of Junctional Epithelium**
    A. **Components of the Junctional Epithelium (JE).** The junctional epithelium consists of:
        1. Plentiful Cells
            a. Layers of closely packed epithelial cells
            b. Desmosomes and hemidesmosomes—specialized cell junctions
        2. A Sparse Extracellular Matrix
            a. Internal basal lamina—a thin basal lamina between the junctional epithelium and the tooth surface.
            b. External basal lamina—a thin basal lamina between the junctional epithelium and the gingival connective tissue.
2. **Attachment of Junctional Epithelium to the Tooth Surface**
    A. **Attachment to the Tooth Surface**
        1. The JE cells next to the tooth surface form *hemidesmosomes* that enable these cells to attach to the *internal basal lamina* and the surface of the tooth.[6–9]

2. The internal basal lamina is a thin sheet of extracellular matrix adjacent to the tooth surface.
3. The epithelial cells physically attach to the tooth surface by four to eight hemidesmosomes per micron at the coronal zone and two hemidesmosomes per micron in the apical zone of the junctional epithelium.[10,11] The apical zone is the area of the junctional epithelium with the least adhesiveness.
4. The attachment of the hemidesmosomes and internal basal lamina to the tooth surface is not static; rather, the cells of the junctional epithelium can move along the tooth surface.

B. **Attachment to the Underlying Gingival Connective Tissue**
1. The epithelial cells of the JE attach to the underlying *gingival connective tissue* via *hemidesmosomes* and the *external basal lamina* (Fig. 2-10).[8,12,13]
2. In health, the junctional epithelium has a *smooth tissue interface* with the connective tissue (no wavy junctions).

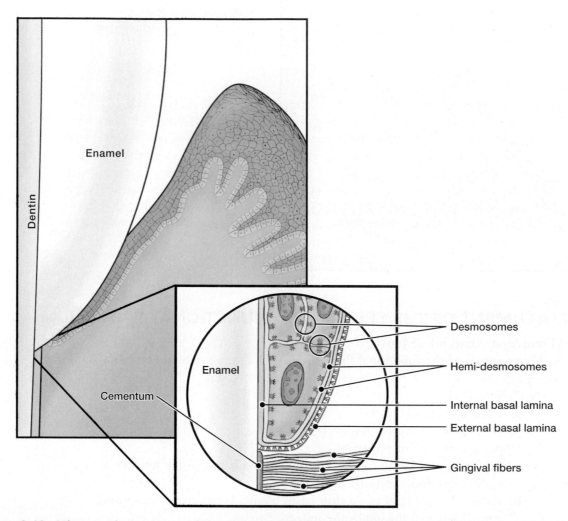

Figure 2-10. Microscopic Anatomy of the Junctional Epithelium (JE). Microscopic structures of the junctional epithelium include the epithelial cells, desmosomes, external and internal basal laminae, and hemidesmosomes.

MICROSCOPIC ANATOMY OF GINGIVAL CONNECTIVE TISSUE

1. **Function of Gingival Connective Tissue.** The gingival connective tissue of the free and attached gingiva provides solidity to the gingiva and attaches the gingiva to the cementum of the root and the alveolar bone.[14–16] The gingival connective tissue is also known as the lamina propria.

2. **Components of the Gingival Connective Tissue**
   A. **Cells**
      1. In contrast to the gingival epithelium (which has an abundance of cells and sparse extracellular matrix), the gingival connective tissue has an abundance of extracellular matrix and few cells (Fig. 2-11).
      2. Cells comprise about 5% of the gingival connective tissue.
      3. The different types of cells present in the gingival connective tissue are:
         a. Fibroblasts
         b. Mast cells
         c. Immune cells, such as macrophages, neutrophils, and lymphocytes.
      4. The fibers of the connective tissue are produced by the fibroblasts.
   B. **Extracellular Matrix**
      1. The major components of the connective tissue are collagen fibers, fibroblasts, vessels, and nerves that are embedded in the extracellular matrix. The matrix of the connective tissue is produced mainly by the fibroblasts.
      2. The matrix is the medium in which the connective tissue cells are embedded and it is essential for the maintenance of the normal function of the connective tissue. The transportation of water, nutrients, metabolites, oxygen, etc., to and from the individual connective tissue cells occurs within the matrix.
      3. Protein fibers account for about 55% to 65% of the gingival connective tissue. Most of these are collagen fibers that form a dense network of strong, rope-like cables that secure and hold the gingival connective tissues together.
      4. The collagen fibers enable the gingiva to form a rigid cuff around the tooth.
      5. Gel-like material between the cells makes up about 30% to 35% of the gingival connective tissue. This gel-like material helps to hold the tissue together.

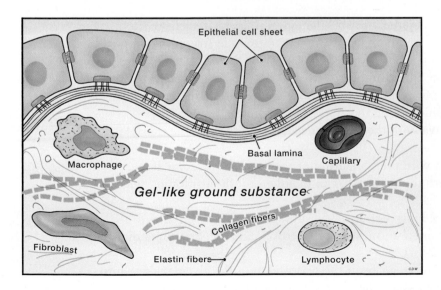

Figure 2-11. Microscopic Anatomy of Gingival Connective Tissue. The gingival connective tissue is comprised of a gel-like substance, protein fibers, and cells.

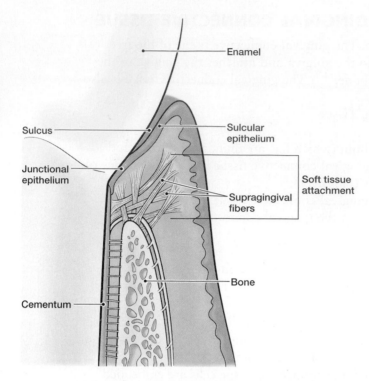

Enamel

Sulcus

Junctional epithelium

Cementum

Sulcular epithelium

Soft tissue attachment

Supragingival fibers

Bone

Figure 2-12. Supragingival Fibers of Gingival Connective Tissue. The gingival fibers are rope-like collagen fiber bundles in the gingival connective tissue. These fibers form a soft tissue attachment coronal to the alveolar bone.

3. **The Supragingival Fiber Bundles of the Gingival Connective Tissue.** The supragingival fiber bundles (gingival fibers) are a network of rope-like collagen fiber bundles in the gingival connective tissue (Fig. 2-12). These fibers are located coronal to (above) the crest of the alveolar bone.

A. **Characteristics of the Fiber Bundles**
   1. The fiber bundles are embedded in the gel-like extracellular matrix of the gingival connective tissue.
   2. The subgingival fiber bundles strengthen the attachment of the junctional epithelium to the tooth by bracing the gingival margin against the tooth surface.
   3. Together the junctional epithelium and the gingival fibers are referred to as the dentogingival unit. The dentogingival unit acts to provide structural support to the gingival tissue.

B. **Functions of the Gingival Fiber Bundles**
   1. Brace the free gingiva firmly against the tooth and reinforce the attachment of the junctional epithelium to the tooth.
   2. Provide the free gingiva with the rigidity needed to withstand the masticatory (chewing) forces.
   3. Unite the free gingiva with the cementum of the root and alveolar bone.
   4. Connect adjacent teeth to one another to maintain tooth positioning within the dental arch.

C. **Classification of Gingival Fiber Groups.** The supragingival fiber bundles are classified based on their orientation, sites of insertion, and the structures that they connect (Figs. 2-13 and 2-14).
   1. **Alveologingival fibers**—extend from the periosteum of the alveolar crest into the gingival connective tissue. These fiber bundles attach the gingiva to the bone. (The periosteum is a dense membrane composed of fibrous connective tissue that closely wraps the outer surface of the alveolar bone.)

2. **Circular fibers**—encircle the tooth in a ring-like manner coronal to the alveolar crest and are not attached to the cementum of the tooth.
3. **Dentogingival fibers**—embedded in the cementum near the CEJ and fan out into the gingival connective tissue. These fibers act to attach the gingiva to the teeth.
4. **Periosteogingival fibers**—extend laterally from the periosteum of the alveolar bone. These fibers attach the gingiva to the bone.
5. **Intergingival fibers**—extend in a mesiodistal direction along the entire dental arch and around the last molars in the arch. These fiber bundles link adjacent teeth into a dental arch unit.
6. **Intercircular fibers**—encircle several teeth. These fiber groups link adjacent teeth into a dental arch unit.
7. **Interpapillary fibers**—located in the papillae coronal to (above) the transseptal fiber bundles. These fiber groups connect the oral and vestibular interdental papillae of posterior teeth.
8. **Transgingival fibers**—extend from the cementum near the CEJ and run horizontally between adjacent teeth. These fiber bundles link adjacent teeth into a dental arch unit.
9. **Transseptal fibers**—pass from the cementum of one tooth, over the crest of alveolar bone, to the cementum of the adjacent tooth. These fiber bundles connect adjacent teeth to one another and secure alignment of teeth in the arch.

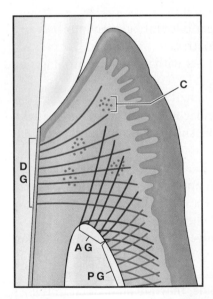

Figure 2-13. Supragingival Fiber Groups.

- C—circular
- AG—alveologingival
- DG—dentogingival
- PG—periosteogingival

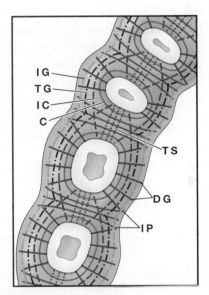

Figure 2-14. Supragingival Fiber Groups of the Mandibular Arch (Occlusal View, Looking Down on the Mandibular Arch).

- C—circular
- IG—intergingival
- IC—intercircular
- IP—interpapillary
- DG—dentogingival
- TG—transgingival
- TS—transseptal

4. The Periodontal Ligament Fibers of the Gingival Connective Tissue
   A. Definition. The periodontal ligament (PDL) is a thin sheet of fibrous connective tissue that surrounds the roots of the teeth and joins the root cementum with the socket wall. The thickness of the PDL space ranges from 0.05 to 0.25 mm depending on the age of the patient and the function of the tooth.[17,18]

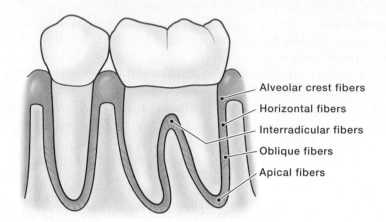

Alveolar crest fibers
Horizontal fibers
Interradicular fibers
Oblique fibers
Apical fibers

Figure 2-15. Principal Fiber Groups of the Periodontal Ligament. The fibers of the PDL are classified as the alveolar crest, horizontal, interradicular, oblique, and apical.

   B. Components of the Periodontal Ligament. The periodontal ligament consists of connective tissue fibers, cells, and extracellular matrix.
   1. Cells. The cells of the PDL are mainly fibroblasts with some cementoblasts and osteoblasts.
   2. Extracellular Matrix.
      a. The extracellular matrix of the PDL is similar to the extracellular matrix of other connective tissue. This rich gel-like substance contains specialized connective fibers.
      b. Fiber Bundles. The fiber bundles of the PDL are a specialized connective tissue that surrounds the root of the tooth and connects it to the alveolar bone. These fibers are the largest component of the PDL.
         1) The rope-like collagen fiber bundles of the PDL stretch across the space between the cementum and the alveolar bone of the tooth socket (Fig. 2-15).
         2) The collagen fiber bundles are anchored on one side in the cementum covering the tooth root; on the other side, they are embedded in the bone of the tooth socket.
      c. Blood Vessels and Nerve Supply. The PDL has a rich supply of nerves and blood vessels.
   C. Functions of the Periodontal Ligament
   1. Supportive function—the major function of the PDL is to anchor the tooth to its bony socket and to separate the tooth from the socket wall, so that the root does not traumatize the bone during mastication.
   2. Sensory function—the PDL is supplied with nerve fibers that transmit tactile pressure (such as a tap with dental instrument against tooth) and pain sensations.

3. Nutritive function—the PDL is supplied with blood vessels that provide nutrients to the cementum and bone.

4. Formative function—the PDL contains cementoblasts ("cementum builders") that produce cementum throughout the life of the tooth, while the osteoblasts ("bone builders") maintain the bone of the tooth socket.

5. Resorptive function—in response to severe pressure, cells of the PDL (osteoclasts) can induce rapid bone resorption and, sometimes, resorption of cementum.

D. **Principal Fiber Groups of the PDL.** The tooth is joined to the bone by bundles of collagen fibers that can be divided into the five groups based on their location and orientation (Fig. 2-15).

1. **Alveolar crest fiber group**—extend from the cervical cementum, running downward in a diagonal direction, to the alveolar crest. This fiber group resists horizontal movements of the tooth and prevents tooth extrusion.

2. **Horizontal fiber group**—located apical to the alveolar crest fibers. They extend from the cementum to the bone at right angles to the long axis of the root. This fiber group resists horizontal pressure against the crown of the tooth.

3. **Oblique fiber group**—located apical to the horizontal group. They extend from the cementum to the bone, running in a diagonal direction. This fiber group resists vertical pressures that threaten to drive the root into its socket.

4. **Apical fiber group**—extend from the apex of the tooth to the bone. This fiber group secures the tooth in its socket and resists forces that might lift the tooth out of the socket.

5. **Interradicular fiber group** (present only in the furcation region of multirooted teeth)—extend from the cementum in the furcation area of the tooth to the interradicular septum of the alveolar bone. These fiber groups help to stabilize the tooth in its socket.

E. **Sharpey Fibers of the Periodontal Ligament**

1. The ends of the PDL fibers that are embedded in the cementum and alveolar bone are known as **Sharpey fibers** (Figs. 2-16 and 2-17).

2. The attachment of the fiber bundles occurs when the cementum and bone are forming. As cementum forms, the tissue calcifies around the ends of the periodontal fibers (Sharpey fibers) surrounding them with cementum. The same process occurs during bone formation. As the bony wall of the tooth socket calcifies, it surrounds the ends of the periodontal fibers with bone. The ends of the fiber bundles become trapped in the bone that forms around them.

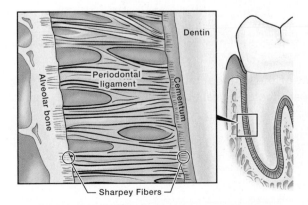

Figure 2-16. Sharpey Fibers. The ends of the periodontal ligament fibers that are embedded in the alveolar bone and the cementum are known as Sharpey fibers.

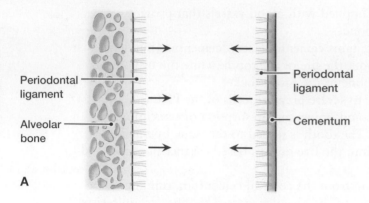

A. Fine collagen fibers arise from the root cementum. Similarly, collagen fibers arise from the alveolar bone proper.

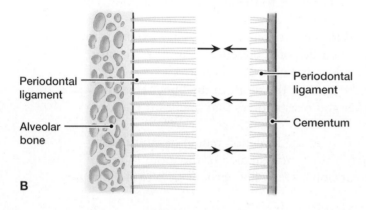

B. The fibers grow into the mid-portion of periodontal ligament space.

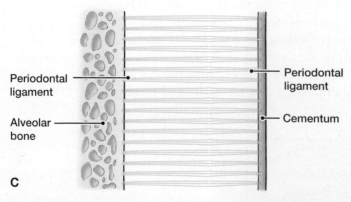

C. The fibers from the root cementum fuse with fibers from the alveolar bone proper.

Figure 2-17. Development of the Periodontal Ligament Fibers. Figures **A, B,** and **C** depict the stages in the development of the periodontal ligament between the alveolar bone and the cementum of the tooth root.

Section 3
Histology of Root Cementum and Alveolar Bone

Section 3 reviews the microscopic anatomy of the cementum and alveolar bone. Knowledge of the microscopic anatomy of these structures is a prerequisite to understanding the function of these structures in health and the alterations in disease.

MICROSCOPIC ANATOMY OF CEMENTUM

1. **Definition.** Cementum is a mineralized tissue that covers the roots of the teeth and serves to attach the tooth to alveolar bone via collagen fibers of the periodontal ligament (Fig. 2-18). Anatomically, cementum is part of the tooth, however, functionally it part of the periodontium.
   A. **Functions of Cementum**
      1. Its prime function is to attach the periodontal fibers to the root of the tooth.
      2. Cementum maintains the integrity of the root, helps to maintain the tooth in its functional position in the mouth, and is involved in tooth repair and regeneration.
         a. It seals and covers the open dentinal tubules and acts to protect the underlying dentin.
         b. Cementum is slowly formed throughout life.
            1. Constant cementum formation allows for continual reattachment of the periodontal ligament fibers.
            2. Cementum continues to grow in thickness throughout life to compensate for attrition of teeth at their occlusal or incisal surfaces.[19] Cementum is formed at the apical areas of the roots to compensate for loss of tooth tissues due to attrition and maintains the length of the root.
      3. Cementum is a key component of periodontal tissues, and its preservation is of paramount importance for the quality of healing at completion of periodontal treatment. Periodontal reattachment or new attachment as an end result of therapy strongly relies on the presence of cementum after root instrumentation.[20]
      4. Cementum may influence the activities of various types of periodontal cells. It is believed that molecules stored in the cementum matrix may induce periodontal ligament regeneration when needed.[20]

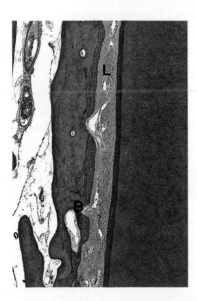

Figure 2-18. Cementum and Tooth Supporting Structures.

- A thin layer of cementum (appearing as a **blue band**) covers the dentin of the root.
- The periodontal ligament (**L**) holds the tooth in the bony socket of the alveolar bone (**B**).

(Used with permission from Mills SE. *Histology for Pathologists*. 3rd ed. Philadelphia, PA: Lippincott Williams & Wilkins; 2006, Figure 15–39, p. 423.)

B. **Components of Mature Cementum.** As in bone and dentin, the major organic component of cementum is collagen. Cementum contains collagen fibers embedded in an organic matrix.[21]

1. **Organic Portion**
   a. The organic matrix of cementum is composed of a framework of densely packed collagen fibers held together by the gel-like extracellular ground substance. These fibers are oriented more or less parallel to the long axis of the tooth.
   b. In addition to collagens, groups of proteins are present in cementum.
      1. Recent research suggests that these "cementum proteins" may have an important role in regulating the mineralization process associated with cementum formation.[22]
      2. There is still a great deal to learn about these cementum proteins. *From the current status of knowledge, it appears that cementum proteins may play an important role in future therapies to achieve regeneration of the periodontal structures.*[22]

2. **Mineralized Portion.** The mineralized portion of cementum is made up of hydroxyapatite crystals (calcium and phosphate).

3. **Vessels and Innervation.** Cementum contains no blood vessels or nerves. (Hypersensitivity of the root surface occurs when the cementum is removed exposing the dentin. It is the dentin that is sensitive to brushing, the touch of a dental instrument, or sudden temperature changes in the mouth (such as drinking hot coffee while eating ice cream.)

4. **Biologic Components.** From a biological perspective, the periodontium has been shown to contain biologically active mediators[21,23–26] and these molecules are elevated in alveolar bone and cementum.[26–29] It is believed that growth factor molecules are produced during cementum formation and then stored in the cementum matrix to induce periodontal ligament regeneration when needed.

C. **Conservation of Cementum During Periodontal Instrumentation.** Subgingival instrumentation during periodontal therapy results in the removal of root cementum, which can eventually lead to exposure of underlying dentin, pulp injury, and dentin hypersensitivity.[30]

1. **Historical Perspective.** Previously it was accepted that bacterial products penetrate the cementum of periodontally diseased root surfaces. This concept resulted in the intentional, aggressive removal of all or most cementum during periodontal instrumentation of root surfaces.[31,32] Overzealous instrumentation can result in removal of all cementum that may result in exposure of underlying dentin, tooth sensitivity, or even external root resorption. More specifically, in the past, the goal of periodontal therapy was to obtain a treated root surface with smooth and hard surface characteristics that was free of endotoxins.[31,33]

2. **Current Research**
   a. More recent studies show that bacterial products are not located within cementum[34,35] and removal of cementum is not necessary for a successful periodontal treatment.[36]
   b. The preservation of cementum on the root surface is further supported by Saygin et al. who report that cementum is necessary for new attachment and as a source of growth factors.[21,37]

c. Grzesik and Narayanan suggested that cementum plays an important regulatory role in periodontal regeneration.[38] From these studies, it can be concluded that nonaggressive removal of cementum is necessary for optimal periodontal health as well as for periodontal regeneration.

2. **Types of Cementum.** Functional, morphological, and histological differences appear to exist along the length of the root.[1,21,39] Cementum is classified as follows: intermediate, acellular, and cellular cementum.

A. **Intermediate Cementum.** Cementum located in the CEJ.

B. **Acellular (Primary) Cementum.** Acellular cementum is primarily responsible for attaching the tooth to the alveolar bone (Fig. 2-19).

1. Contains no living cells within its mineralized tissue (no cementocytes)
2. First cementum to be formed and covers approximately the cervical third or half of the root
3. No new acellular cementum is produced after the tooth reaches the occlusal plane
4. Thickness ranges from 30 to 230 microns
5. Sharpey fibers make up most of the structure of acellular cementum

C. **Cellular (Secondary) Cementum.** Cellular cementum is distinguished by the presence of living cells in its structure.

1. Contains cementocytes and fibroblasts within its mineralized tissue
2. Present in the apical and interradicular portions of the root
3. Formed after the tooth reaches the occlusal plane and is less calcified than acellular cementum
4. Deposited in intervals throughout the life of the tooth (thickness increases with age, where its increased thickness compensates for tooth attrition)
5. Thickness ranges from 150 to 200 microns
6. Sharpey fibers make up a smaller portion of cellular cementum

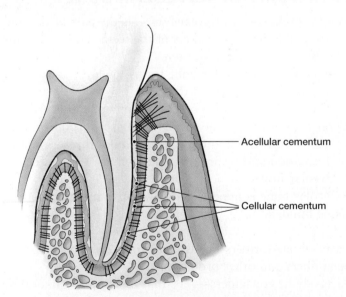

Figure 2-19. Types of Cementum. Acellular cementum covers approximately the cervical third or half of the root. New acellular cementum normally is not produced after the tooth has reached its occlusal plane. Cellular cementum covers the apical half of the root. It is continuously deposited throughout the life of the tooth after it has reached its occlusal plane and increases in thickness with age.

3. **Relationship of Cementum to Enamel at the CEJ.** The cementum covering the root may have any one of three relationships with the enamel of the tooth crown (Fig. 2-20).
   A. **Three Possible Arrangements of Enamel and Cementum**
      1. Overlap—the cementum overlaps the enamel for a short distance.
      2. Meet—the cementum meets the enamel.
      3. Gap—there is a small gap between the cementum and enamel (exposing the dentin in this area). The patient may experience discomfort (dentinal sensitivity) during instrumentation. The use of local anesthesia may be helpful during instrumentation, and desensitization of sensitive areas should be performed following instrumentation.
   B. These three relationships commonly are abbreviated as OMG (overlap, meet, gap).
   C. *In any one tooth, all three arrangements of the junction between the cementum and enamel may be present.*[19,21]

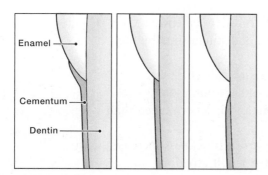

Figure 2-20. Three Patterns for the Arrangement of Cementum to Enamel at the Cementoenamel Junction. The cementum may (1) overlap the enamel, (2) meet the enamel, or (3) not meet, leaving a gap between the cementum and enamel.

Enamel

Cementum

Dentin

MICROSCOPIC ANATOMY OF ALVEOLAR BONE

1. **Definition.** The alveolar process—or alveolar bone—is the part of the maxilla and mandible that forms and supports the sockets of the teeth (Figs. 2-21 and 2-22).
2. **Function of Alveolar Bone in the Periodontium**
   A. **Protects Roots of Teeth.** The alveolar bone forms the bony sockets that provide support and protection for the roots of the teeth.
   B. **Changes in Response to Mechanical Forces and Inflammation.** Alveolar bone constantly undergoes periods of bone formation and resorption (loss) in response to mechanical forces on the tooth and inflammation of the periodontium. This process of bone formation and resorption is known as bone remodeling.
3. **Characteristics of Alveolar Bone**
   A. **Components.** Alveolar bone is mineralized connective tissue made by cells called osteoblasts ("bone builders").[21]
      1. Major Cell Types
         a. Osteoblasts—bone-formers—cells that produce the bone matrix consisting of collagen fibers and other protein fibers.
         b. Osteoclasts—bone consumers—cells that remove the mineral materials and organic matrix of alveolar bone.
      2. Extracellular Matrix
         a. Collagen fibers and gel-like substance forms the major component of the alveolar bone

b. The bone matrix is rigid because it undergoes mineralization by the deposition of minerals such as calcium and phosphate, which are subsequently transformed into hydroxyapatite.

B. Vessels and Innervation. The alveolar bone has blood vessels and nerve innervation.

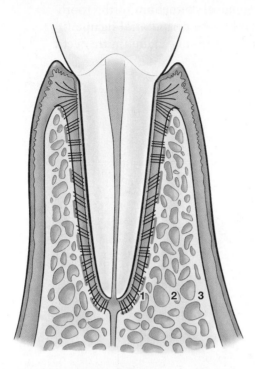

Figure 2-21. Anatomy of Alveolar Bone. (*1*), Alveolar bone proper; (*2*), trabecular bone; and (*3*), cortical (compact) bone.

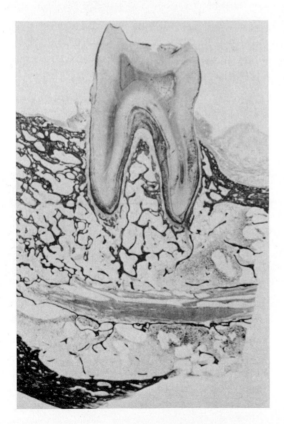

Figure 2-22. Histology of Alveolar Bone. A histologic section through a mandibular first molar and its alveolar process. (Used by permission from Melfi RC, Alley KE. *Permar's Oral Embryology and Microscopic Anatomy*. 10th ed. Philadelphia, PA: Lippincott Williams & Wilkins; 2000:215, Figure 9–20.)

Chapter Summary Statement

Knowledge of the microscopic anatomy of the periodontium is fundamental in understanding the (1) function of the periodontium in health and (2) changes that occur during the periodontal disease process. The junctional epithelium plays an important role in the health of the periodontium by attaching the gingival epithelium to the tooth via hemidesmosomes and an internal basal lamina. In health, the periodontal ligament, cementum, and alveolar bone act as a functional unit to support and maintain the teeth in the oral cavity.

Section 4
Focus on Patients

Clinical Patient Care

CASE 1

A clinician penetrates the oral mucosa with a needle before injecting a local anesthetic. The needle tip stops in the loose connective tissue underlying the surface structures. Name the layers of epithelium that have been penetrated by the needle.

CASE 2

A clinician finds it necessary to use a unique type of injection to achieve total anesthesia of a tooth being treated. The injection involves sliding a small-diameter needle into the PDL space to a point halfway down the tooth root. Name the PDL fibers most likely encountered by the needle tip during insertion.

CASE 3

Recession of the gingival margin exposes a portion of tooth root on a maxillary canine tooth. Microscopic examination of the cementum in the area of the crown margin on the canine will reveal what possible relationships between the level of cementum and the level of the tooth crown?

Evidence in Action: Clinical Relevance

Conservation of Cementum

Cementum is a key component of periodontal tissues, and its preservation is of paramount importance for the quality of healing at the completion of periodontal treatment. Conservation of cementum is ideal since loss of cementum is accompanied by exposure of the dentinal tubules and by a loss of attachment of PDL fibers to the root surface. Periodontal reattachment or new attachment as an end-result of therapy strongly relies on the presence of cementum after root instrumentation.

Research in the past 20 years has greatly advanced understanding of the cellular and molecular events involved in the developing periodontium. As understanding of the structure, function, and composition of cementum increases, so does the potential for new therapies for periodontal regeneration using molecules formed by these tissues.

Improper or aggressive periodontal instrumentation may reduce the thickness or eventually remove all the cementum over the root surface leading to a loss of growth factor reservoirs in the cementum. For this reason, it is strongly suggested that the root surface instrumentation should aim not only at thorough removal of calculus deposits but also at preserving root substance to improve healing following periodontal therapy.

References

1. Cho MI, Garant PR. Development and general structure of the periodontium. *Periodontol 2000.* 2000;24:9–27.
2. Bartold PM, Walsh LJ, Narayanan AS. Molecular and cell biology of the gingiva. *Periodontol 2000.* 2000;24:28–55.
3. Weinmann JP, Meyer J. Types of keratinization in the human gingiva. *J Invest Dermatol.* 1959;32(2, Part 1):87–94.
4. Listgarten MA. Electron microscopic study of the gingivo-dental junction of man. *Am J Anat.* 1966;119(1):147–77.
5. Dale BA. Periodontal epithelium: a newly recognized role in health and disease. *Periodontol 2000.* 2002;30:70–78.
6. Listgarten MA. The ultrastructure of human gingival epithelium. *Am J Anat.* 1964;114:49–69.
7. Schroeder HE. Ultrastructure of the junctional epithelium of the human gingiva. *Helv Odontol Acta.* 1969;13(2):65–83.
8. Schroeder HE, Listgarten MA. The gingival tissues: the architecture of periodontal protection. *Periodontol 2000.* 1997;13:91–120.
9. Thilander H, Bloom GD. Cell contacts in oral epithelia. *J Periodontal Res.* 1968;3(2):96–110.
10. Pollanen MT, Salonen JI, Uitto VJ. Structure and function of the tooth-epithelial interface in health and disease. *Periodontol 2000.* 2003;31:12–31.
11. Sabag N, Saglie R, Mery C. Ultrastructure of the normal human epithelial attachment to the cementum root surface. *J Periodontol.* 1981;52(2):94–95.
12. Schroeder HE, Listgarten MA. The junctional epithelium: from strength to defense. *J Dent Res.* 2003;82(3):158–161.
13. Schroeder HE, Theilade J. Electron microscopy of normal human gingival epithelium. *J Periodontal Res.* 1966;1(2):95–119.
14. Bartold PM. Connective tissues of the periodontium—preface. *Periodontol 2000.* 2000;24:7–8.
15. Bartold PM. Connective tissues of the periodontium. Research and clinical implications. *Aust Dent J.* 1991;36(4):255–268.
16. Wang Y, Wang Q, Arora PD, Rajshankar D, McCulloch CA. Cell adhesion proteins: roles in periodontal physiology and discovery by proteomics. *Periodontol 2000.* 2013;63(1):48–58.
17. Beertsen W, McCulloch CA, Sodek J. The periodontal ligament: a unique, multifunctional connective tissue. *Periodontol 2000.* 1997;13:20–40.
18. Ho SP, Marshall SJ, Ryder MI, Marshall GW. The tooth attachment mechanism defined by structure, chemical composition and mechanical properties of collagen fibers in the periodontium. *Biomaterials.* 2007;28(35):5238–5245.
19. Bosshardt DD, Selvig KA. Dental cementum: the dynamic tissue covering of the root. *Periodontol 2000.* 1997;13:41–75.
20. Bozbay E, Dominici F, Gokbuget AY, et al. Preservation of root cementum: a comparative evaluation of power-driven versus hand instruments. *Int J Dent Hyg.* 2018;16:202–209.
21. Saygin NE, Giannobile WV, Somerman MJ. Molecular and cell biology of cementum. *Periodontol 2000.* 2000;24:73–98.
22. Arzate H, Zeichner-David M, Mercado-Celis G. Cementum proteins: role in cementogenesis, biomineralization, periodontium formation and regeneration. *Periodontol 2000.* 2015;67(1):211–233.
23. Bartold PM, McCulloch CA, Narayanan AS, Pitaru S. Tissue engineering: a new paradigm for periodontal regeneration based on molecular and cell biology. *Periodontol 2000.* 2000;24:253–269.
24. Cochran DL, Wozney JM. Biological mediators for periodontal regeneration. *Periodontol 2000.* 1999;19:40–58.
25. MacNeil RL, Somerman MJ. Development and regeneration of the periodontium: parallels and contrasts. *Periodontol 2000.* 1999;19:8–20.

26. Nishimura K, Hayashi M, Matsuda K, Shigeyama Y, Yamasaki A, Yamaoka A. The chemoattractive potency of periodontal ligament, cementum and dentin for human gingival fibroblasts. *J Periodontal Res*. 1989;24(2):146–148.

27. Miki Y, Narayanan AS, Page RC. Mitogenic activity of cementum components to gingival fibroblasts. *J Dent Res*. 1987;66(8):1399–1403.

28. Nakae H, Narayanan AS, Raines E, Page RC. Isolation and partial characterization of mitogenic factors from cementum. *Biochemistry*. 1991;30(29):7047–7052.

29. Somerman MJ, Archer SY, Hassell TM, Shteyer A, Foster RA. Enhancement by extracts of mineralized tissues of protein production by human gingival fibroblasts in vitro. *Arch Oral Biol*. 1987;32(12):879–883.

30. Fischer C, Wennberg A, Fischer RG, Attstrom R. Clinical evaluation of pulp and dentine sensitivity after supragingival and subgingival scaling. *Endod Dent Traumatol*. 1991;7(6):259–265.

31. Jones WA, O'Leary TJ. The effectiveness of in vivo root planing in removing bacterial endotoxin from the roots of periodontally involved teeth. *J Periodontol*. 1978;49(7):337–342.

32. O'Leary TJ. The impact of research on scaling and root planing. *J Periodontol*. 1986;57(2):69–75.

33. Chace R. Subgingival curettage in periodontal therapy. *J Periodontol*. 1974;45(2):107–109.

34. Moore J, Wilson M, Kieser JB. The distribution of bacterial lipopolysaccharide (endotoxin) in relation to periodontally involved root surfaces. *J Clin Periodontol*. 1986;13(8):748–751.

35. Nakib NM, Bissada NF, Simmelink JW, Goldstine SN. Endotoxin penetration into root cementum of periodontally healthy and diseased human teeth. *J Periodontol*. 1982;53(6):368–378.

36. Nyman S, Westfelt E, Sarhed G, Karring T. Role of "diseased" root cementum in healing following treatment of periodontal disease. A clinical study. *J Clin Periodontol*. 1988;15(7):464–468.

37. Narayanan AS, Bartold PM. Biochemistry of periodontal connective tissues and their regeneration: a current perspective. *Connect Tissue Res*. 1996;34(3):191–201.

38. Grzesik WJ, Narayanan AS. Cementum and periodontal wound healing and regeneration. *Crit Rev Oral Biol Med*. 2002;13(6):474–484.

39. Zeichner-David M. Regeneration of periodontal tissues: cementogenesis revisited. *Periodontol 2000*. 2006;41:196–217.

 ## STUDENT ANCILLARY RESOURCES

A wide variety of resources to enhance your learning is available online:

- Audio Glossary
- Book Pages
- Chapter Review Questions and Answers

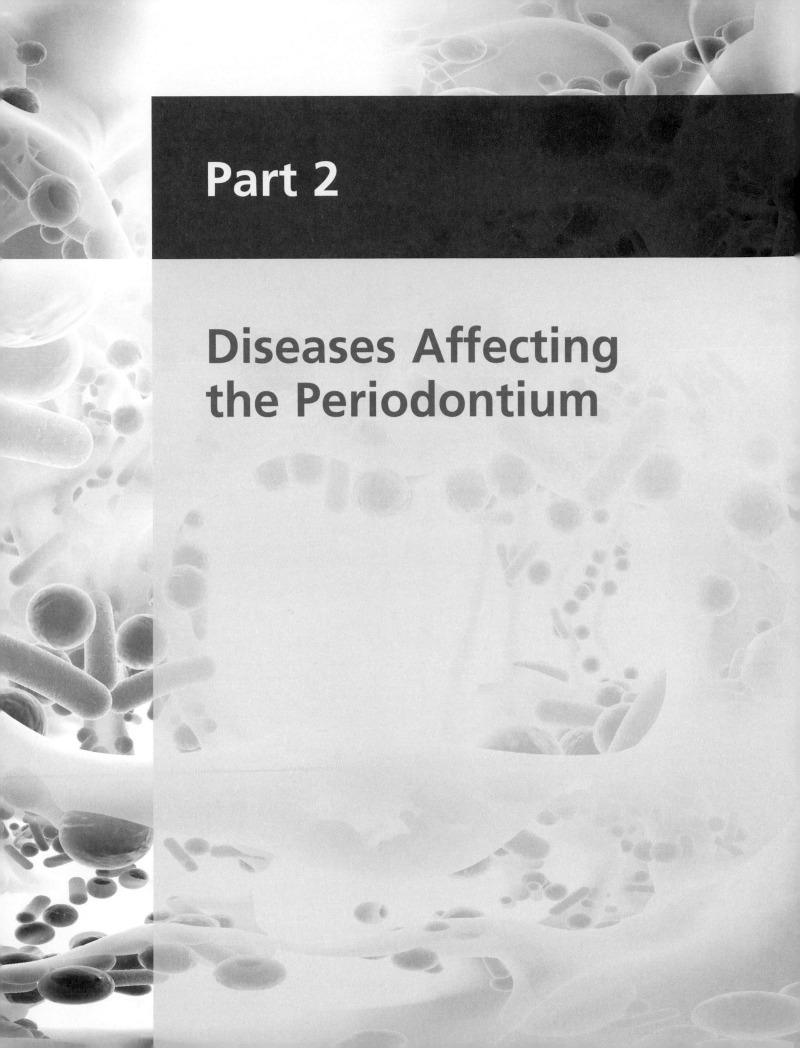

Part 2

Diseases Affecting the Periodontium

3 Overview of Diseases of the Periodontium

Clinical Application. Each of the various types of diseases that affect the periodontium will be discussed in detail in subsequent chapters of this book. To understand these upcoming detailed discussions, clinicians need to be aware of a few important ideas that relate to most of these disease conditions, and these topics are discussed in Chapter 3. This overview gives the student an understanding of the fundamental changes seen in the diseased periodontium and discusses concepts related to the epidemiology, occurrence, and progression of periodontal diseases.

Learning Objectives

- Define the term *disease progression*.
- Define the term *periodontal disease* and contrast it with the term *periodontitis*.
- Describe and contrast the (1) position of the junctional epithelium, (2) characteristics of the epithelial–connective tissue junction, and (3) position of the crest of the alveolar bone in health, gingivitis, and periodontitis.
- Explain why there is a band of intact transseptal fibers even in the presence of severe bone loss.
- Describe the progressive destruction of alveolar bone loss that occurs in periodontitis.
- Describe the pathway of inflammation that occurs in horizontal bone loss and contrast it with the pathway of inflammation that occurs in vertical bone loss.
- Contrast the characteristics of gingival and periodontal pockets.
- For patients in the clinical setting, identify visible clinical signs of health and periodontal disease for your clinic instructor.
- For a patient with periodontal disease, measure the probing depth of the sulci or pockets on the facial aspect of one sextant of the mouth. Using the information gathered visually and with the periodontal probe, explain whether this patient's disease is gingivitis or periodontitis.
- Given a drawing of a periodontal pocket, determine whether the pocket illustrated is a suprabony or infrabony pocket.
- Describe variables associated with periodontal disease that an epidemiologist might include in a research study.
- Define prevalence and incidence as measurements of disease within a population.
- Describe how clinical dental hygiene practice can be affected by epidemiological research.

Key Terms

Disease progression	Horizontal bone loss	Active disease site	Prevalence
Gingivitis	Vertical bone loss	Gingival pocket	National Health and
Reversible tissue damage	Osseous defect	Periodontal pocket	Nutrition Examination
Periodontitis	Infrabony defect	Suprabony pocket	Survey
Irreversible tissue damage	Osseous crater	Infrabony pocket	Centers for Disease Control
Apical migration of the	Furcation involvement	Intermittent disease	and Prevention
junctional epithelium	Attachment loss	progression theory	
Inflammation	Disease site	Epidemiology	
Alveolar bone loss	Inactive disease site	Incidence	

Section 1
The Periodontium in Health and Disease

THREE BASIC STATES OF THE PERIODONTIUM

Disease progression (pathogenesis) is the sequence of events that occur during the development of a disease or abnormal condition. The periodontium exists in three basic states: health, gingivitis, and periodontitis (Fig. 3-1). It is important to recognize the differences among health, gingivitis, and periodontitis (Figs. 3-2 to 3-4). This section provides an overview of these three basic states at the clinical and microscopic levels.

The term *periodontal disease* should not be confused with the term *periodontitis*. Gingivitis and periodontitis are the two basic categories of periodontal disease.[1–4]

- Gingivitis is a bacterial infection that is confined to the gingiva. The tissue damage that occurs in gingivitis results in reversible destruction to the tissues of the periodontium.
- Periodontitis is a bacterial infection of all parts of the periodontium including the gingiva, periodontal ligament, bone, and cementum. The tissue damage that occurs in periodontitis results in irreversible destruction to the tissues of the periodontium (Fig. 3-4).

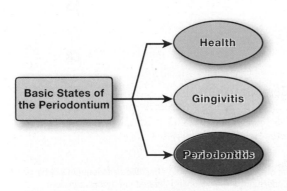

Figure 3-1. Three Basic States of the Periodontium. In the absence of disease, the periodontium is healthy. The two basic categories of periodontal disease are gingivitis and periodontitis.

TABLE 3-1	HISTOLOGIC CHANGES IN GINGIVITIS AND PERIODONTITIS			
State	**Junctional Epithelium**	**Connective Tissue Attachment**	**Periodontal Ligament Fibers**	**Alveolar Bone**
Health	JE coronal to CEJ Tight intercellular junctions	Intact; supragingival fiber bundles provide support to gingiva and JE	Intact; attach root to the bone of the tooth socket	Intact; supports and protects root of tooth
Gingivitis	JE at CEJ Widened intercellular junctions; epithelial extensions into connective tissue	Connective tissue damage	Intact	Intact
Periodontitis	JE apical to CEJ Widened intercellular junctions; epithelial extensions into connective tissue	Destruction of supragingival fiber bundles	Destruction of periodontal ligament fibers; exposure of cementum to pocket environment	Destruction of bone Eventual tooth loss

JE, Junctional epithelium; CEJ, cementoenamel junction.

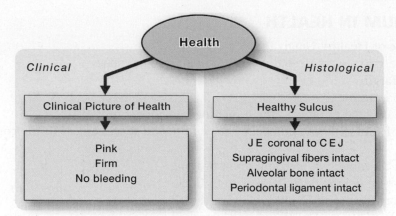

Figure 3-2. Characteristics of Healthy Periodontium. The clinical and histologic characteristics of the tissues of the periodontium in health.

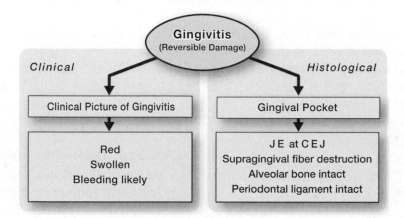

Figure 3-3. Characteristics of Gingivitis. The clinical and histologic characteristics of gingivitis. Some reversible tissue damage occurs in gingivitis.

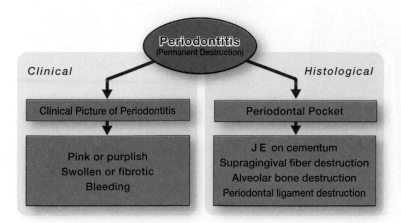

Figure 3-4. Characteristics of Periodontitis. The clinical and histologic characteristics of periodontitis. Permanent tissue damage occurs in periodontitis.

PERIODONTIUM IN HEALTH

1. **Clinical Picture of Healthy Gingiva**
   A. **Color:** Pink, may be pigmented, and is resilient in consistency.
   B. **Gingival Margin**
      1. Scalloped outline
      2. Located coronal to (above) the cementoenamel junction (CEJ).
   C. **Interdental Papillae:** Firm and occupy the embrasure spaces apical to the contact areas.
   D. **Absence of Bleeding:** No bleeding upon probing.
   E. **Sulcus:** Probing depths range from 1 to 3 mm.
2. **The Microscopic Picture of Healthy Gingiva** (Fig. 3-5)
   A. **Junctional Epithelium:** The JE is firmly attached by hemidesmosomes to the enamel slightly coronal to (above) the CEJ.
   B. **Epithelial–Connective Tissue Junction:** In health, the junctional epithelium has no epithelial ridges.
   C. **Gingival Fibers:** Intact supragingival fiber bundles support the junctional epithelium.
   D. **Alveolar Bone:** The crest of the alveolar bone is intact and located 2 to 3 mm apical to (below) the base of the junctional epithelium.
   E. **Periodontal Ligament Fibers:** Intact periodontal ligament fiber bundles stretch between the bony walls of the tooth socket and the cementum of the root.
   F. **Cementum:** Cementum is normal.

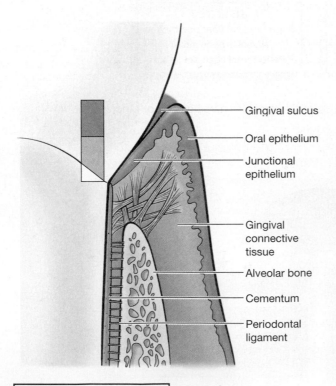

Gingival sulcus

Oral epithelium

Junctional epithelium

Gingival connective tissue

Alveolar bone

Cementum

Periodontal ligament

CEJ

Probing depth

Junctional epithelium

Figure 3-5. The Healthy Periodontium.
- **Plaque biofilm:** light accumulation
- **Junctional epithelium:** slightly coronal to the CEJ, no epithelial ridge formation
- **Supragingival fibers**: intact
- **Periodontal ligament fibers**: intact
- **Alveolar bone:** intact

Illustration Key: The white wedge indicates the location of the CEJ; the depth of the sulcus is shown by the blue vertical rectangle; the length of junctional epithelium is indicated by the pink vertical rectangle.

GINGIVITIS—REVERSIBLE TISSUE DAMAGE

1. **Characteristics of Gingivitis.** Gingivitis is *a type of periodontal disease* characterized by changes in the color, contour, and consistency of the gingival tissues (Fig. 3-6).
   A. **Onset of Gingivitis.** Gingivitis is observed clinically from 4 to 14 days after plaque biofilm accumulates in the gingival sulcus.[5]
      1. Acute gingivitis is a gingivitis that lasts for a short period of time. Acute gingivitis often is characterized by fluid in the gingival connective tissues that results in swollen gingiva.
      2. Chronic gingivitis is a gingivitis that lasts for months or years.
         a. When gingivitis is chronic, the body may attempt to repair the tissue damage by forming new collagen fibers in the gingival connective tissue.
         b. Excess collagen fibers lead to gingival tissues that are enlarged and fibrotic (leathery) in consistency.
         c. The excess collagen fibers conceal the redness caused by the increased blood flow, making the tissue appear less red.
   B. **Tissue Enlargement.** Gingival enlargement may be caused by swelling (acute gingivitis) or fibrosis (chronic gingivitis).
      1. Tissue enlargement causes the gingival margin to cover more of the crown of the tooth and results in deeper probing depths.
      2. This enlargement of the gingival tissue is said to produce a false or gingival pocket, known as a pseudopocket.
      3. A gingival pocket has a sulcus depth over 3 mm. This increased probing depth is caused solely by enlarged gingival tissue. Microscopically, the junctional epithelium remains in its normal position coronal to CEJ on the tooth in a gingival pocket.
   C. **Reversible Tissue Damage.** *The tissue damage in gingivitis is reversible tissue damage*—that is, with good patient self-care, the body can repair the damage.
   D. **Duration of Gingivitis.** In many cases, gingivitis may persist for years without ever progressing to the next stage, periodontitis. In some cases, a combination of risk factors may result in gingivitis progressing to periodontitis.
2. **Clinical Picture of Gingivitis**
   A. **Color:** In gingivitis, the gingival tissue usually is red or reddish-blue in color (Table 3-1).
      1. The blood flow increases in the gingival connective tissue and the gingival blood vessels become engorged with blood, causing the gingiva to appear red.
      2. If the gingivitis persists, the gingival blood vessels may become congested. This slow-moving blood flow causes the gingiva to have a bluish color.
   B. **Gingival Margin**
      1. The gingival margin is swollen and loses its knife-edge adaptation to the tooth.
      2. Gingival tissue may cover more of the crown of the tooth due to tissue swelling or fibrosis.
   C. **Interdental Papillae:** The interdental papillae often are bulbous and swollen.
   D. **Bleeding:** There is bleeding upon gentle probing.
   E. **Sulcus:** Probing depths may be greater than 3 mm due to swelling of the tissues. It is important to note that *there is NO apical migration of the junctional epithelium* in gingivitis.
3. **The Microscopic Picture of Gingivitis**
   A. **Junctional Epithelium:** The hemidesmosomes still attach to the enamel coronal to the CEJ (Fig. 3-6 and Table 3-2).
   B. **Epithelial–Connective Tissue Junction**
      1. The junctional epithelium extends epithelial ridges down into the connective tissue.

2. *Such extension of the epithelial ridges only can occur because destruction of the gingival fibers creates space for the growing epithelium.*

C. **Gingival Fibers:** Damage has occurred to the supragingival fiber bundles. This damage is reversible if the bacterial infection is brought under control.

D. **Alveolar Bone:** The bacterial infection has not progressed into the alveolar bone. There is no destruction of alveolar bone.

E. **Periodontal Ligament Fibers:** The bacterial infection has not progressed into the periodontal ligament fibers.

F. **Cementum:** The cementum covering the root of the tooth is normal.

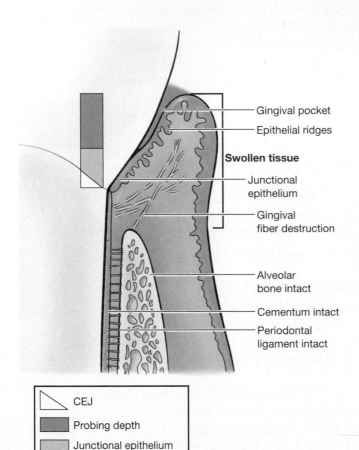

Gingival pocket
Epithelial ridges
Swollen tissue
Junctional epithelium
Gingival fiber destruction
Alveolar bone intact
Cementum intact
Periodontal ligament intact

CEJ
Probing depth
Junctional epithelium

Figure 3-6. Gingivitis.

• **Plaque biofilm:** increased numbers of bacteria
• **Junctional epithelium:** slightly coronal to the CEJ; the coronal portion of the JE detaches from the tooth; probing depth increases; epithelial ridges extend down into gingival connective tissue
• **Supragingival fibers:** some fiber destruction
• **Periodontal ligament fibers:** intact
• **Alveolar bone:** intact

Illustration Key: Note in this illustration that the JE, as indicated by the pink rectangle, is still coronal to the CEJ (white wedge). The blue rectangle has increased in depth due to the swelling of the gingival margin, so that the gingival tissue covers more of the crown of the tooth.

PERIODONTITIS—PERMANENT TISSUE DESTRUCTION

1. **Characteristics of Periodontitis.**
   A. **Extent of Tissue Destruction.**
      1. Periodontitis is *a type of periodontal disease* that is characterized by the (1) apical migration of the junctional epithelium, (2) loss of connective tissue attachment, and (3) loss of alveolar bone.[6]
      2. The tissue damage of periodontitis is permanent (irreversible tissue damage).
   B. **Process of Tissue Destruction.**
      1. The tissue destruction of periodontitis is not a continuous process. Rather, the disease process occurs in an intermittent manner with extended periods of disease inactivity followed by short bursts of destruction.[3]

2. Tissue destruction progresses at different rates throughout the mouth. Destruction does not occur in all parts of the mouth at the same time, but instead, destruction usually occurs in only a few specific sites (tooth surfaces) at a time.

2. **Clinical Picture of Periodontitis**
   A. **Color:** The gingival tissue shows visible alternations color, contour, and consistency.
      1. Edematous tissue (spongy tissue)—bluish- or purplish-red with a smooth, shiny appearance.
      2. Fibrotic tissue (firm, nodular tissue)—light pink with a leathery consistency. Beginning clinicians often mistakenly interpret this light pink color as a sign of tissue health.
   B. **Gingival Margin**
      1. The gingival margin may be swollen or fibrotic and does not have a close knife-edged adaptation to the neck of the tooth.
      2. The position of the gingival margin varies greatly in periodontitis. The margin may be apical to the CEJ (recession) resulting in a portion of the root being visible in the mouth.
   C. **Interdental Papillae:** The interdental papillae may not fill the interdental embrasure spaces.
   D. **Bleeding:** There often is bleeding upon probing, and suppuration (a discharge of pus) may be visible.
   E. **Pocket:** Probing depths are 4 mm or greater in depth because the junctional epithelium is attached to the root surface.
      1. Pus may be evident upon probing.
      2. Pain is usually absent; however, probing may cause some pain due to ulceration of the pocket epithelium.

3. **The Microscopic Picture of Periodontitis**
   A. **Junctional Epithelium**
      1. The junctional epithelium is located on the cementum, apical to—below—its normal location. Movement of the junctional epithelium apical to its normal location is termed the apical migration of the junctional epithelium.
      2. The coronal-most portion of the junctional epithelium detaches from the tooth surface. As the bacterial infection progresses, the apical portion of the junctional epithelium moves further in an apical direction along the root surface creating a periodontal pocket (Fig. 3-7 and Table 3-2).
      3. The extracellular matrix of the gingiva and the attached collagen fibers at the apical edge of the junctional epithelium are destroyed.
   B. **Epithelial–Connective Tissue Junction**
      1. The *junctional* epithelium proliferates and extends epithelial ridges into the connective tissue.
      2. The *sulcular* epithelium of the pocket wall thickens and extends epithelial ridges deep into the connective tissue. Small ulcerations of the pocket epithelium expose the underlying inflamed connective tissue.
   C. **Gingival Connective Tissue**
      1. Changes in the gingival connective tissue are severe. Collagen destruction in the area of inflammation is almost complete.
      2. There is widespread destruction of the supragingival fiber bundles, reducing them to fiber fragments. The destruction of the periodontal ligament fiber bundles makes it easier for the junctional epithelium to migrate apically along the root surface.

3. The transseptal fiber bundles, however, are regenerated continuously across the crest of bone. A band of intact transseptal fibers separates the site of inflammation from the remaining alveolar bone even in cases of extensive bone loss (Fig. 3-8).

4. Epithelium grows over the root surface in areas where the fiber bundles have been destroyed. *The loss of fiber attachment is permanent because the epithelium growing over the root surface prevents the reinsertion of the periodontal ligament fibers in the cementum.*

D. **Alveolar Bone:** There is permanent destruction of the alveolar bone that supports the teeth. Tooth mobility may be present.

E. **Periodontal Ligament Fibers:** There is permanent destruction of some or all of the periodontal ligament fiber bundles.

F. **Cementum:** Cementum within the periodontal pocket is exposed to dental plaque biofilm.

G. **Pulp:** Histologic studies of the dental pulp of patients with severe periodontitis show inflamed, edematous pulps, pulpal necrosis, vascular congestion, and dentin demineralization.[7,8]

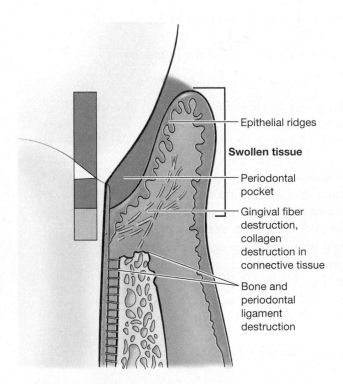

Epithelial ridges

Swollen tissue

Periodontal pocket

Gingival fiber destruction, collagen destruction in connective tissue

Bone and periodontal ligament destruction

CEJ

Probing depth

Junctional epithelium

Figure 3-7. Periodontitis.

- **Plaque biofilm:** vast numbers of bacteria
- **Junctional epithelium:** apical to the CEJ with attachment on cementum; a remnant of the JE persists at the base of the periodontal pocket: epithelial ridges extend down into gingival connective tissue
- **Supragingival fibers:** fiber destruction
- **Periodontal ligament fibers:** fiber destruction
- **Alveolar bone:** portions of alveolar bone destroyed

Illustration Key: Note the blue rectangle shows that the pocket in this illustration is increased by (1) the swollen gingival margin and (2) the location of the JE apical to (below) the CEJ. The level of the CEJ is indicated by the white wedge.

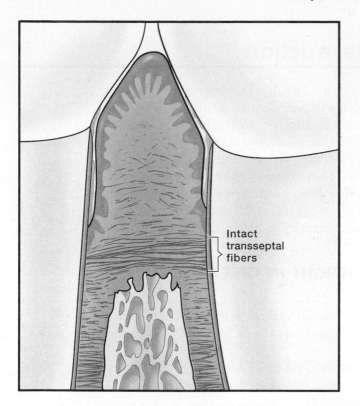

Figure 3-8. Band of Intact Transseptal Fibers. Even in the presence of severe horizontal bone loss, there is an intact band of transseptal fibers above the remaining alveolar bone.

TABLE 3-2	HISTOLOGIC CHANGES IN DISEASE
Disease State	**Histology**
Gingivitis	Epithelial ridges extend down into connective tissue Destruction of supragingival fiber bundles
Periodontitis	*Changes in Epithelial Tissues:* • Junctional epithelium located apical to the cementoenamel junction • Junctional epithelium grows along the root surface • Sulcular epithelium thickens and extends epithelial ridges down into the connective tissue *Changes in Connective Tissues and Alveolar Bone:* • Collagen destruction • Destruction of supragingival fiber bundles • Destruction of periodontal ligament fibers; transseptal fibers regenerate and remain intact • Junctional epithelium grows over the root surface in areas where the periodontal ligament fibers are destroyed • Root cementum is exposed to the plaque biofilm • Destruction of alveolar bone

Section 2
Pathogenesis of Bone Destruction

Inflammation is the body's response to injury or invasion by disease-producing organisms. The inflammatory process that occurs in periodontitis results in permanent destruction to the tissues of the periodontium, including the destruction of gingival connective tissue, periodontal ligament, and alveolar bone. **Alveolar bone loss** is the resorption of alveolar bone as a result of periodontitis. This section discusses the patterns of bone destruction that occur in periodontitis. *The pattern of bone destruction that occurs depends on the pathway of inflammation as it spreads from the gingiva into the alveolar bone.* It is important to understand the changes that occur in the alveolar bone because it is the reduction in bone height that eventually results in tooth loss.

CHANGES IN ALVEOLAR BONE HEIGHT IN DISEASE

1. **Reduction in Bone Height**
   A. **Bone Height in Health and Gingivitis.** In health and gingivitis, the crest of the alveolar bone is located approximately 2 mm apical to (below) the CEJs of the teeth (Fig. 3-9).
   B. **Bone Height in Periodontitis.** In periodontitis, the bone destruction may be severe (Fig. 3-10). As periodontal disease progresses (worsens), tooth loss may occur from lack of alveolar bone support (Fig. 3-11).

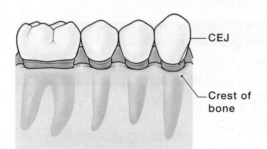

Figure 3-9. Level of Alveolar Crest in Health and Gingivitis. In health and gingivitis, the crest of the alveolar bone is located approximately 2 mm apical to the cementoenamel junction (CEJ).

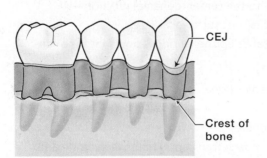

Figure 3-10. Level of Alveolar Crest in Disease. In periodontitis, the crest of the alveolar bone is located more than 2 mm apical to the cementoenamel junction.

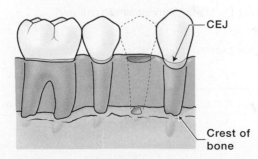

Figure 3-11. Level of Alveolar Crest as Disease Progresses. There is a progressive alveolar bone loss in periodontitis. Bone destruction may eventually lead to tooth mobility or loss due to insufficient bone support for the teeth.

PATTERNS OF BONE LOSS IN PERIODONTITIS

1. **Patterns of Bone Loss.** The two types of bone loss are (1) horizontal and (2) vertical bone loss.
   A. **Horizontal Bone Loss**
      1. Horizontal bone loss is the most common pattern of bone loss (Fig. 3-12).
      2. This type of bone loss results in a fairly even, overall reduction in the height of the alveolar bone.
      3. The alveolar bone is reduced in height, but the margin of the alveolar crest remains more or less perpendicular to the long axis of the tooth.
   B. **Vertical Bone Loss**
      1. Vertical bone loss is a less common pattern of bone loss (Fig. 3-13). Vertical bone loss is also known as angular bone loss.
      2. This type of bone loss results in an uneven reduction in the height of the alveolar bone.
      3. In vertical bone loss, the resorption progresses *more rapidly* in the bone next to the root surface. This uneven pattern of bone loss leaves a trench-like area of missing bone alongside the root.

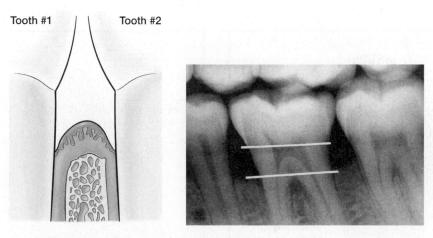

Figure 3-12. Horizontal Pattern of Bone Loss. Horizontal bone loss results in bone levels that are approximately at the same height on adjacent tooth roots. On a radiograph, if an imaginary line drawn between the CEJs of adjacent teeth is approximately parallel, then the bone loss is described as horizontal bone loss.

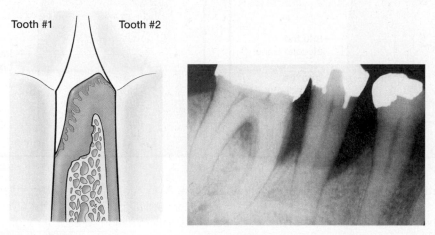

Figure 3-13. Vertical Pattern of Bone Loss. Vertical bone loss results in an uneven reduction in bone height on adjacent tooth roots, resulting in a trench-like area of missing bone alongside the root of one tooth. On a radiograph, if an imaginary line drawn between the CEJs of adjacent teeth is not parallel, then the bone loss is described as vertical bone loss.

2. Pathways of Inflammation into the Alveolar Bone
   A. Pathway of Inflammation in Horizontal Bone Loss
      1. In horizontal bone loss, inflammation spreads into the tissues in this order: (1) within the gingival connective tissue along the connective tissue sheaths surrounding the blood vessels, (2) into the alveolar bone, and (3) finally, into the periodontal ligament space (Fig. 3-14A).
      2. Inflammation usually spreads in this manner because it is the *path of least resistance*. The periodontal ligament fiber bundles act as an effective barrier to the spread of inflammation. Thus, the inflammation spreads into the alveolar bone and then into the periodontal ligament space.
   B. Pathway of Inflammation in Vertical Bone Loss
      1. In vertical bone loss, inflammation spreads into the tissues in this order (1) within the gingival connective tissue, (2) directly into the periodontal ligament space, and (3) finally, into the alveolar bone (Fig. 3-14B).
      2. Inflammation spreads in this manner whenever the crestal periodontal ligament fiber bundles are weakened and no longer present an effective barrier. Prior events such as occlusal trauma can be responsible for the weakened condition of the fiber bundles.

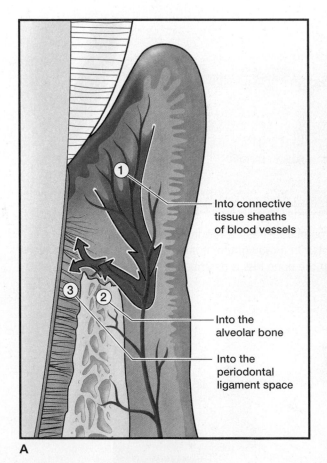

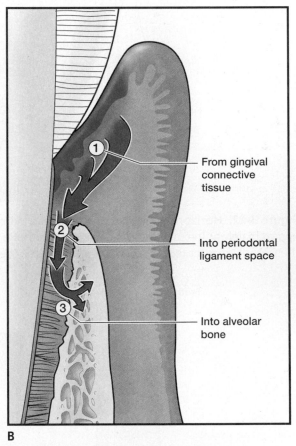

A   B

Figure 3-14. Pathway of Inflammation into Alveolar Bone. A. In horizontal bone loss, inflammation spreads through the tissues in this order: (*1*) Into the gingival connective tissue; (*2*) Into the alveolar bone; (*3*) Finally, into the periodontal ligament. **B.** In vertical bone loss, inflammation spreads through the tissues in this order: (*1*) Into the gingival connective tissue; (*2*) Into the periodontal ligament; (*3*) Finally, into the alveolar bone.

3. **Bone Defects in Periodontal Disease.** Periodontitis results in different types of defects in the alveolar bone. These bony defects are called **osseous defects**.
   A. **Infrabony Defects.**
      1. **Infrabony defects** result when bone resorption occurs in an uneven, oblique direction. In infrabony defects, the bone resorption primarily affects one tooth.
      2. Infrabony defects are classified on the basis of the number of osseous walls. Infrabony defects may have one, two, or three walls (Fig. 3-15).
   B. **Osseous Craters.** An **osseous crater** is a bowl-shaped defect in the interdental alveolar bone with bone loss nearly equal on the roots of two adjacent teeth (Fig. 3-16A,B).
      1. Whereas infrabony defects primarily affect one tooth, in craters the defect affects two adjacent root surfaces to a similar extent.
      2. The presence of an osseous crater causes dental plaque biofilm to collect and makes it difficult to clean the interdental area.

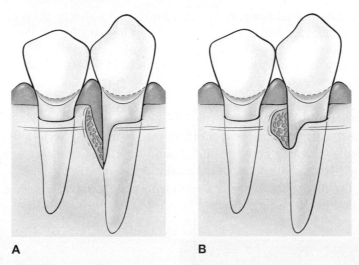

A   B

Figure 3-15. Osseous Defects. A. One-wall infrabony defect, looking from the canine tooth root distally toward the premolar, there is only "one" wall of bone remaining, and that is on the mesial surface of the premolar. The facial plate and lingual plate of bone are missing. **B.** Two-wall infrabony defect with facial plate of bone missing. The "two walls" of the bone surrounding this defect are the remaining lingual plate and bone on the mesial surface of the premolar tooth root.

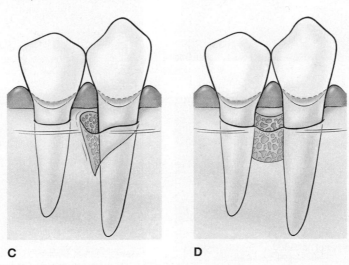

C   D

Figure 3-15. C. Three-wall infrabony defect. The "three walls" of remaining bone that surround this defect are the lingual plate, facial plate, and the bone on the mesial surface of the adjacent premolar root. **D.** Interproximal osseous crater with the lingual plate and facial plate of bone remaining. The bone between these plates is missing resulting in bone being lost on the mesial surface of the premolar and the distal surface of the adjacent canine. The term crater refers to the dip in the contour of the interproximal bone between the facial and lingual plates.

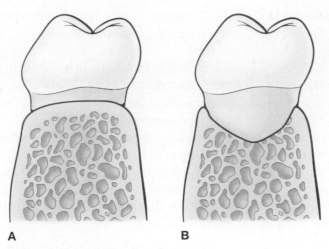

A   B

Figure 3-16. Contour of Interdental Bone. A. Normal contour of the alveolar bone on the proximal (mesial or distal) surface of a posterior tooth. Note that the bone contour from the facial to lingual is a relatively flat interproximal contour. **B.** Osseous crater on the proximal surface of a posterior tooth. Note that the contour of the bone from the facial to the lingual dips apically and forms what is described as a "crater" between the facial and lingual bone margins.

C. Bone Loss in Furcation Areas

1. **Furcation involvement** occurs on a multirooted tooth when periodontal infection invades the area between and around the roots, resulting in a loss of alveolar bone between the roots of the teeth.
2. Bone loss in the furcation area may be hidden by the gingival tissue or may be clinically visible in the mouth (Fig. 3-17).

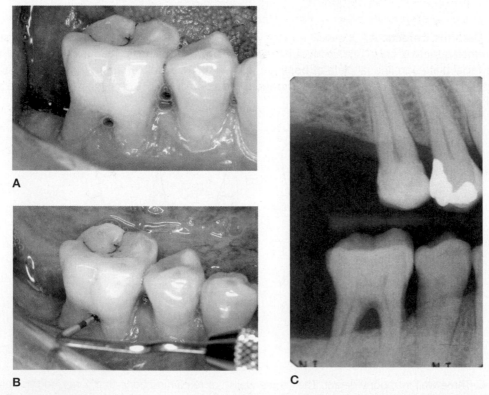

A

B   C

Figure 3-17. Furcation Involvement. A. Due to recession, the furcation involvement on this molar is clinically evident. **B.** A periodontal probe easily can be inserted between the two roots of this mandibular molar. **C.** A radiograph shows the extensive bone loss around this molar. (Images courtesy of Dr. Richard J. Foster, Guilford Technical Community College, Jamestown, NC.)

Section 3
Periodontal Pockets

CHARACTERISTICS OF PERIODONTAL POCKETS

1. **Attachment Loss in Periodontal Pockets**
   A. Attachment loss is the destruction of the fibers and bone that support the teeth.
   B. Tissue destruction does not spread only in an apical (vertical) direction but also in a lateral (side-to-side) direction.
   C. *A pocket on different root surfaces of the same tooth can have different depths.* The loss of attachment may vary from surface to surface of the tooth, with the base of the pocket exhibiting very irregular patterns of tissue destruction (Fig. 3-18).
2. **Disease Sites.** A disease site is an area of tissue destruction. A disease site may involve only a single surface of a tooth, for example, the distal surface of a tooth. The disease site may involve several surfaces of the tooth or all four surfaces (mesial, distal, facial, and lingual).
   A. Inactive disease site—a disease site that is stable, with the attachment level of the junctional epithelium remaining the same over time.
   B. Active disease site—a disease site that shows continued apical migration of the junctional epithelium over time.
   C. **Assessment of Disease Activity.** The disease activity of each site in the mouth should be assessed using a periodontal probe and recorded in the patient chart at regular intervals (scheduled check-up appointments).
   D. **Periodontal Pockets.** *A periodontal pocket is an area of tissue destruction left by the disease process.* The pocket is much like a demolished home that is left after a hurricane.
      1. The presence of a periodontal pocket does not indicate necessarily that there is active disease at that site. Likewise, a demolished house does not necessarily indicate that a hurricane still is pounding the shoreline. A demolished house may indicate that the hurricane is still active or that a hurricane passed through a day, a week, or a year ago.
      2. *The majority of pockets in most adult patients with periodontitis are inactive disease sites.*

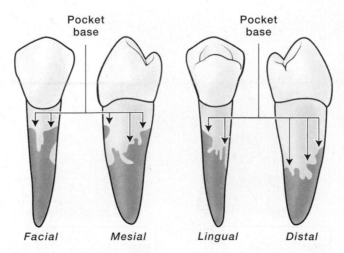

Figure 3-18. Irregular Pattern of Attachment Loss. The amount of attachment loss can vary greatly on different surfaces of the same tooth. The base of a pocket may exhibit very irregular patterns of destruction.

POCKET FORMATION

1. **Gingival Sulcus.** In health, the average histologic depth of the sulcus is 0.8 mm to 2.1 mm in depth.[9] The junctional epithelium is coronal to the CEJ and *attaches along its entire length to the tooth* (Fig. 3-19).
2. **Gingival Pockets.** A gingival pocket is a deepening of the gingival sulcus as a result of swelling or enlargement of the gingival tissue (Fig. 3-20A,B).
   A. **Why are gingival pockets often called "false" pockets?**
      1. Gingival pockets sometimes are referred to "pseudo-pockets," meaning "false pockets," because there is *no apical migration of the junctional epithelium.*
      2. *In gingivitis, however, the <u>coronal portion</u> of the junctional epithelium detaches from the tooth resulting in a slight increase in probing depth.*
   B. **What causes the increased probing depth of a gingival pocket?** The increased probing depth seen in a gingival pocket is due to (1) detachment of the coronal portion of the JE from the tooth and/or (2) increased tissue size due to swelling of the tissue.

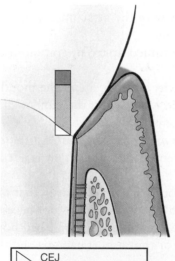

Figure 3-19. Gingival Sulcus. In health, the average clinical probing depth of gingival sulcus ranges from 1.3 mm to 2.7 mm (indicated by the blue rectangle). [Ainamo, 1966 #30]. *The junctional epithelium (JE) attaches along its entire length to the enamel of the tooth* (as represented by the pink rectangle). (From Ainamo J, Loe H. Anatomical characteristics of gingiva. A clinical and microscopic study of the free and attached gingiva. *J periodontol.* 1966;37(1):5–13.)

CEJ
Probing depth
Junctional epithelium

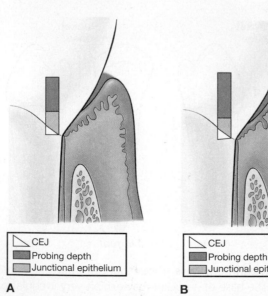

CEJ
Probing depth
Junctional epithelium

A

CEJ
Probing depth
Junctional epithelium

B

Figure 3-20. Gingival Pockets. A. There is no apical migration of the JE; however, the coronal portion of the JE detaches from the tooth resulting in increased probing depth. **B.** In some cases the gingival tissue swells, resulting in a pseudo-pocket.

3. **Periodontal Pockets**
   A. **A periodontal pocket is a pathologic deepening of the gingival sulcus.**
      1. Pocket formation occurs as the result of the (1) apical migration of the junctional epithelium, (2) destruction of the periodontal ligament fibers, and (3) destruction of alveolar bone.
      2. **Apical migration** is the movement of the cells of the junctional epithelium from their normal position—coronal to the CEJ—to a position apical to the CEJ. In health, the junctional epithelial cells attach to the enamel of the tooth crown. In periodontitis, the junctional epithelial cells attach to the cementum of the tooth root.
   B. **Two Types of Periodontal Pockets. The type of periodontal pocket is determined based on *the relationship of the junctional epithelium to the crest of the alveolar bone.***
      1. **Suprabony Pocket**
         a. **Suprabony pockets** occur when there is horizontal bone loss (Fig. 3-21).
         b. The junctional epithelium, forming the base of the pocket, is located *coronal* to (above) the crest of the alveolar bone.
      2. **Infrabony Pocket**
         a. **Infrabony pockets** occur when there is vertical bone loss (Fig. 3-22).
         b. The junctional epithelium, forming the base of the pocket, is located *apical* to (below) the crest of the alveolar bone. The base of the pocket is located within the cratered-out area of the bone alongside of the root surface.

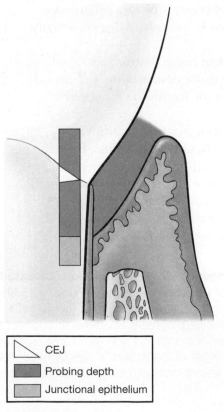

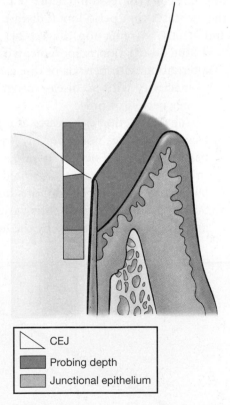

	CEJ
	Probing depth
	Junctional epithelium

	CEJ
	Probing depth
	Junctional epithelium

Figure 3-21. Suprabony Pocket. Characteristics of a suprabony pocket are (1) horizontal bone loss and (2) a pocket base located coronal to (above) the crest of the alveolar bone.

Figure 3-22. Infrabony Pocket. Characteristics of an infrabony pocket are (1) vertical bone loss and (2) a pocket base located below the crest of the alveolar bone within a trench-like area of the bone.

Section 4
Theories of Disease Progression

For years, clinical researchers have been trying to find an answer to the question, "How does untreated periodontal disease progress?" In this context, disease progression means that the disease gets worse. Data from ongoing studies suggest that the pattern of disease progression may vary from (1) one individual to another, (2) one site to another in a person's mouth, and (3) one type of periodontal disease to another.

1. **Historical Perspective on Disease Progression**
   A. **Continuous Progression Theory (Historical View of Disease Progression: Prior to 1980).** The continuous disease progression theory states that periodontal disease progresses throughout the entire mouth in a slow and constant rate over the adult life of the patient (Fig. 3-23).
      1. This past theory suggested that:
         a. All cases of untreated gingivitis lead to periodontitis.
         b. All cases of periodontitis progress at a slow and steady rate of tissue destruction.
      2. Research studies conducted in the early 1980s indicated that periodontal disease does not progress at a constant rate nor affect all areas of the mouth simultaneously. The continuous progression theory does not accurately reflect the complex nature of periodontal disease.

2. **Current Theory of Disease Progression**
   A. **Intermittent Progression Theory (Current View).** Intermittent disease progression theory states that periodontal disease is characterized by periods of disease activity and inactivity (remission) (Fig. 3-24).
      1. Tissue destruction is sporadic, with short periods of tissue destruction alternating with periods of disease inactivity (no tissue destruction). The period of inactivity with no disease progression may last for months or for a much longer period of time.
      2. Tissue destruction progresses at different rates throughout the mouth. Destruction does not occur in all parts of the mouth at the same time. Instead, tissue destruction occurs in only a few specific sites (tooth surfaces) at a time.
      3. In the majority of cases, untreated gingivitis does not progress to periodontitis.
      4. Different forms of periodontitis may progress at widely different rates.
      5. Susceptibility to periodontitis varies greatly from individual to individual and appears to be determined by the host response to periodontal pathogens.

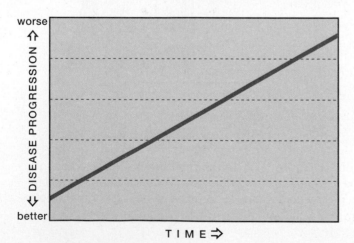

Figure 3-23. The Continuous Disease Model of Disease Progression (Prior to 1980). In the past, clinicians believed that periodontal disease progresses (worsens) throughout the entire mouth in a slow and constant rate over the life of the patient. It was believed that all cases of untreated gingivitis led to periodontitis.

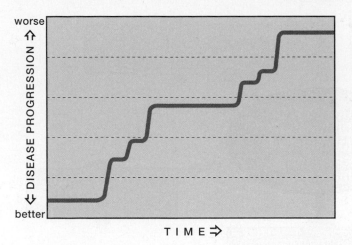

Figure 3-24. Intermittent Disease Progression Theory. Current research suggests that periodontal disease is characterized by periods of disease activity and inactivity. Furthermore, destruction does not occur in all parts of the mouth at the same time.

Section 5
Epidemiology of the Diseases of the Periodontium

Many generations of researchers have asked the question, "What causes periodontal disease?" while clinicians have asked, "What is the best care for my patients with periodontal disease?" This section discusses the study of disease in the population (epidemiology) and reviews historical and current perspectives on the causes and progression of periodontal disease.

1. **What is Epidemiology?**
   A. **Epidemiology** is the study of the health and disease within the total population (rather than an individual) and the behavioral, environmental, and genetic risk factors that influence health and disease. An epidemiologist assesses how much disease is prevalent in a given population, investigates possible causes and applies results to treatment recommendations. This translates into developing measures to prevent or control disease.
      1. Epidemiological research has three objectives: (1) to determine the amount and distribution of a disease in the total population and in subgroups, (2) to investigate the causes of a disease, and (3) to apply this knowledge to the control and prevention of disease.
      2. Through research of population groups, epidemiologists strive to identify the risk factors associated with disease such as race/ethnicity, heredity, gender, physical environment, systemic factors, socioeconomic status, and personal behavior.
      3. An understanding of the risk factors associated with a certain disease can lead to theories of the cause of that disease and then to treatment standards for patient care.
   B. **Epidemiology of Periodontal Disease**
      1. A large percentage of the adult population has periodontal disease. Epidemiologists study periodontal disease to determine its occurrence in the population and to identify risk factors for periodontal disease. Some of the questions epidemiologists ask when researching periodontal disease are illustrated in Figure 3-25.
      2. Epidemiological research also provides current information to the clinical dental hygienist about methods and behaviors that are successful in the treatment and prevention of periodontal disease. Current research also may define the level of risk a patient may have for periodontal disease.

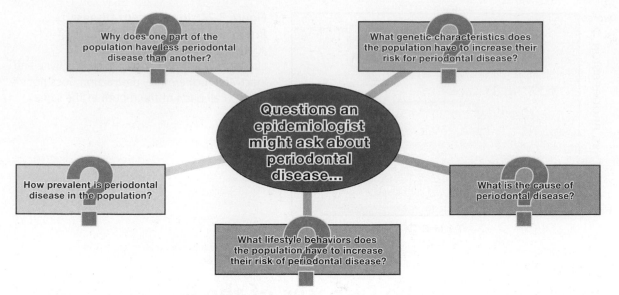

Figure 3-25. Researching Periodontal Disease. This diagram illustrates the types of questions asked by epidemiologists when studying periodontal disease.

3. Studies can be designed to look at the disparities or inequities of disease patterns. For instance, a study may explore why more periodontal disease is found in a specific segment of the population than in another group of people. Oral diseases occur disproportionately more among individuals with low socioeconomic status and poor general health.[10]

2. **Prevalence and Incidence of Disease**
   A. **Incidence and Prevalence**
      1. **Incidence** is the number of new disease cases in a population that occur over a given period of time. For example: A 2011 clinical study evaluated 250 white adult males with the Gingival Index (GI) to assess gingivitis. The results of this study indicated that 125 of the men had gingivitis. In 2012, a follow-up study evaluated the same population and the results were that 150 of the men exhibited clinical signs of gingivitis. Therefore, the incidence of new cases of gingivitis in this study population was 25 cases.
      2. **Prevalence** refers to the number of all cases (both old and new) of a disease that can be identified within a specified population at a given point in time. For example: Given the above example, the prevalence of gingivitis within the total 2011 study population was 50% (125/250). On the date of examination using the GI, the clinician does not know the length of time the men have had gingivitis, and cannot classify them as new cases of disease (or incidence).
   B. **Variables Associated with the Prevalence of Disease.** Research findings show that variables associated with the prevalence of periodontal disease include a person's gender, race, socioeconomic status, and age. The **National Health and Nutrition Examination Survey** (NHANES) is a program of studies to assess the health and nutritional status of adults and children in the United States. This survey protocol combines a survey with a physical examination. NHANES examines a nationally representative sample of about 5,000 persons each year.

1. Gender
   a. Males have a greater prevalence and severity of periodontal disease than females.[11] 2009–2010 NHANES reports periodontal disease in about 56% men versus 38% women.[12]
   b. There has been some speculation that females tend to practice better and more frequent self-care than males. These differences in self-care behaviors may lead to the greater prevalence of disease in males.
2. Race/ethnicity. Black and Hispanic males living in the United States have poorer periodontal health and a greater incidence of periodontal disease than White males. Results from the 2009-2010 NHANES indicate a disparity with the highest prevalence of periodontal disease in Mexican Americans when compared to other races.
3. Education and Socioeconomic Status
   a. There is a greater incidence of periodontal disease in individuals with less than a high school education and living below the federal poverty level.
   b. Underdeveloped countries have a higher incidence of periodontitis, possibly due to a lack of adequate information about disease prevention.
4. Age
   a. Research studies have shown that the severity of periodontal disease increases with age; however, the exact role that age plays in periodontal disease is difficult to assess.
      1) As a person grows older, the chances increase that he or she will be exposed to additional risk factors for periodontal disease. Systemic illness, medications, and stress may contribute to disease risk in this population. With less edentulism, the elderly population has a greater risk of developing periodontal disease. Results from the 2009-2010 NHANES indicate that 64% of adults over 65 years of age were found to have moderate to severe periodontitis.
      2) The higher incidence of periodontal disease in the elderly, therefore, may not be due to age, but rather other risk factors to which an individual has been exposed during his or her long life.
   b. Diminished dexterity is sometimes a problem in elderly individuals and can impact the individual's ability to perform self-care. Limited dexterity may also shorten the length of time that self-care is performed on a daily basis.
5. Behavior
   a. Tobacco use has been identified as a behavioral risk factor for the development of periodontal disease. Both smoking tobacco and the use of smokeless tobacco products negatively impact the periodontium.[13,14] The 2009-2010 NHANES found over 64% of current smokers examined had periodontal disease.
   b. With tobacco use as a risk factor, dental offices may consider stronger efforts towards including tobacco-cessation programs with patient education.
6. Access to Dental Care. Individuals who desire care or need care may not have access to dental care. Barriers to obtaining dental care include transportation, geographic distances to a dental office, financial expense of dental care, and time available to seek care.

C. **Measuring the Disease Prevalence**
1. The prevalence of periodontal disease in the US adult population is determined by performing clinical examinations on cross-sections of groups using indices. Indices measure the amount and severity of disease. Indices used to measure both gingivitis and periodontitis vary across epidemiological studies, as does the extent of disease present when a study begins. Refer to Table 3-3 for a list of indices commonly used to assess periodontal disease.
2. Prevalence is affected by new cases of disease (incidence), cures or deaths within a population, and the longer lives of subjects.
3. Historically, gingival indices have used criteria to measure variables of inflammation such as color changes, presence of edema, and bleeding upon probing. Clinical indices for measuring periodontitis include variable of probing depth, clinical attachment level (CAL), and interpretation of radiographic bone levels (BL). Many studies use sample groups numbering in the thousands. Several groups are then compared and statistically analyzed. Epidemiologists will have different approaches to research and will include different variables in studies. The selected population can be studied over time.

D. **Difficulties in Measurement of Periodontal Disease**
1. It is far easier to evaluate a population for prevalence and incidence of dental caries than for periodontal disease because caries lends itself for more objective measurement. The development and process of caries is well known and involves only tooth structure. The Centers for Disease Control and Prevention (CDC) has provided guidance and standardized methods for public health surveillance of dental caries for many years.
2. Periodontal disease, on the other hand, involves both hard and soft tissues and has multiple variables that must be considered. Determining the presence of gingivitis with or without the presence of periodontitis further complicates the assessment of disease. Assessment can include:
   a. Soft tissue color changes (redness)
   b. Tissue swelling (edema)
   c. Loss of periodontal ligament fibers that support the teeth
   d. Loss of alveolar bone/furcation involvement
   e. Bleeding upon probing/spontaneous bleeding
   f. Probing depths
3. The multiple variables used to define periodontal disease make the numbers for prevalence and incidence of periodontal disease less specific, more of a range, and more subject to change. NHANES most recently used the definition/classification of periodontal disease, as determined by the collaboration of CDC and the American Academy of Periodontology (AAP) to assess the population.
4. Historically national periodontal health surveys (NHANES) have used partial mouth examination protocols that may not accurately represent disease as periodontal disease is not evenly distributed in the entire mouth. For example, attachment loss can vary on tooth surfaces being examined. The 2009-2010 NHANES did use a full-mouth examination and is being described as the most comprehensive survey of periodontal health in the United States.[15]

TABLE 3-3	COMMONLY USED PERIODONTAL INDICES
Index	**Measurement**
Community and Periodontal Index of Treatment Needs (CPITN) (Federation Dentaire Internationale: Ainamo et al.)	Assesses probing depths and bleeding; developed to attain more uniform worldwide epidemiologic data; may be used for measuring group periodontal needs
Eastman Interdental Bleeding Index (EIBI) (Abrams, Caton, and Polson) (Caton and Polson)	Assesses presence of inflammation and bleeding in the interdental area upon toothpick insertion
Gingival Bleeding Index (GBI) (Carter and Barnes)	Assesses presence of gingival inflammation by bleeding from interproximal sulcus within 10 seconds of flossing
Gingival Index (GI) (Loe and Silness)	Assesses severity of gingivitis based on color, consistency, and bleeding on probing
Modified Gingival Index (MGI)	Similar to GI but assesses severity of gingivitis without probing; redefined scoring for inflammation
Periodontal Index (PI) (Russell)	Assesses the severity of gingival inflammation without probing
Periodontal Disease Index (PDI) (Ramfjord)	Assesses the severity of gingival inflammation, pocket depth, and the level of gingival attachment
Periodontal Screening and Recording (PSR) (American Academy of Periodontology and the American Dental Association)	Assesses periodontal health in a rapid manner including probing depths, bleeding, and presence of hard deposits

E. **What the Research Shows.** Research on periodontal disease indicates it is one of the most widespread diseases in adult Americans, with most individuals who have periodontal disease being unaware of its presence. The findings are based on data collected as part of CDC's 2009-2010 NHANES, designed to assess the health and nutritional status of adults and children in the United States. The 2009-2010 NHANES included for the first time a full-mouth periodontal examination to assess for mild, moderate, or severe periodontitis, making it the most comprehensive survey of periodontal health ever conducted in the United States. Researchers measured periodontitis because it is the most destructive form of periodontal disease. Gingivitis, the earliest stage of periodontal disease, was not assessed.

1. Prevalence or Periodontitis

a. A study titled Prevalence of Periodontitis in Adults in the United States: 2009 and 2010 estimates that 47.2%, or 64.7 million American adults, have mild, moderate, or severe periodontitis. In adults 65 and older, prevalence rates increase to 70.1%.[15] The findings also indicate disparities among certain segments of the US population. Periodontal disease is higher in men than women (56.4% vs. 38.4%) and is highest in Mexican Americans (66.7%) compared to other races. Other segments with high prevalence rates include current smokers (64.2%); those living below the federal poverty level (65.4%); and those with less than a high school education (66.9%).

    b. According to data from 2009-2010 NHANES, over 47% of the population had periodontitis:

        1) 8.7% had mild periodontitis

        2) 30.0% had moderate periodontitis

        3) 8.5% had severe periodontitis

    c. According to data from 2009-2010 NHANES, in adults over 65 years of age, 64% had moderate/severe periodontitis.

  2. Prevalence of Periodontitis

    a. The presence of periodontal disease is measured clinically in several ways. NHANES 2009-2010 used attachment loss and probing depths to assess periodontal disease. Loss of attachment is the term used to describe the destruction of periodontal ligament fibers and alveolar bone that support the teeth. Figure 5-3 shows that attachment loss of 4 mm or more affects approximately half of adults aged 50 to 59.[12]

    b. By age 60 to 69, less than half of all adults in the United States have retained 21 teeth or more.[12]

F. Public Health Surveillance of Periodontal Disease. The most recent NHANES data suggests that the amount of periodontal disease may have been underestimated in the general population.[15] Both AAP and CDC describe periodontal disease as a public health concern and are working toward improved disease surveillance. The CDC's Division of Oral Health and the Association of State and Territorial Dental Directors collaborate to monitor the burden of oral disease and track state data sources. As the World Health Organization and oral health professionals have reported, periodontal disease impairs the quality of life and general well-being for individuals and efforts are ongoing to create awareness of periodontal disease as a public health issue.[16]

Chapter Summary Statement

Periodontal pathogenesis is the sequence of events that occurs during the development of periodontal disease. The two types of periodontal disease are gingivitis and periodontitis.

- Gingivitis is a *reversible condition* that is characterized by changes in the color, contour, and consistency of the gingiva. There is no apical migration of the junctional epithelium or bone loss in gingivitis.
- Periodontitis results in some extent of *permanent tissue destruction* characterized by pocket formation, destruction of the periodontal ligament fibers, and resorption of alveolar bone. The pattern of alveolar bone loss and periodontal ligament destruction depends on the pathway that the inflammatory process takes as it spreads from the gingiva into the alveolar bone. It is the destruction of periodontal ligament fibers and resorption of alveolar bone that leads to tooth mobility and the possibility of tooth loss.

Epidemiological research of periodontal disease has three objectives: (1) to determine the amount and distribution of periodontal disease in a population, (2) to investigate the causes of periodontal disease, and (3) to apply this knowledge to the control of periodontal disease.

Advances in research have led to many changes in the understanding, prevention, and treatment of periodontal disease. In the future, ideas about causes and treatment will continue to be refined and changed as researchers delve further into the mysteries of periodontal disease.

Section 6
Focus on Patients

Clinical Patient Care

CASE 1

Your patient has 6- to 7-mm attachment loss on all surfaces of the maxillary first molar. Which of the tissues of the periodontium have experienced tissue destruction surrounding this tooth?

CASE 2

Your dental team provides appropriate therapy for a patient with periodontitis. When you began treatment, your initial findings were redness and edema (swelling) of the gingiva, bleeding on probing, periodontal pockets, and attachment loss. Successful control of the periodontal disease in the patient should not be expected to result in elimination of which of these initial clinical findings?

CASE 3

You find a newspaper article that estimates that in your home state 73% of state residents have some form of periodontal disease. You would like to use this statistic in a homework assignment. When you include this information in your homework assignment should you describe this statistic as incidence or prevalence of periodontitis?

CASE 4

Your dental team has a new patient who has gingivitis. The patient has poor daily self-care, generalized calculus deposits, poorly controlled diabetes mellitus, a history of smoking cigarettes, and inadequate dietary intake of calcium. In your patient counseling, how would you characterize the likelihood that the patient will develop periodontitis in the future and what might you tell the patient about this?

References

1. Armitage GC. Development of a classification system for periodontal diseases and conditions. *Ann Periodontol.* 1999;4(1):1–6.
2. Armitage GC. Periodontal diagnoses and classification of periodontal diseases. *Periodontol 2000.* 2004;34:9–21.
3. Armitage GC. Learned and unlearned concepts in periodontal diagnostics: a 50-year perspective. *Periodontol 2000.* 2013;62(1):20–36.
4. Armitage GC. Classifying periodontal diseases—a long-standing dilemma. *Periodontol 2000.* 2002;30:9–23.
5. The pathogenesis of periodontal diseases. *J Periodontol.* 1999;70(4):457–470.
6. Armitage GC, Cullinan MP. Comparison of the clinical features of chronic and aggressive periodontitis. *Periodontol 2000.* 2010;53:12–27.
7. Caraivan O, Manolea H, Corlan Puscu D, Fronie A, Bunget A, Mogoanta L. Microscopic aspects of pulpal changes in patients with chronic marginal periodontitis. *Rom J Morphol Embryol.* 2012;53(3 Suppl):725–729.
8. Fatemi K, Disfani R, Zare R, Moeintaghavi A, Ali SA, Boostani HR. Influence of moderate to severe chronic periodontitis on dental pulp. *J Indian Soc Periodontol.* 2012;16(4):558–561.
9. Ainamo J, Loe H. Anatomical characteristics of gingiva. A clinical and microscopic study of the free and attached gingiva. *J periodontol.* 1966;37(1):5–13.
10. U.S. Public Health Service; Office of the Surgeon General, National Institute of Dental and Craniofacial Research (U.S.). Oral Health in America: A Report of the Surgeon General. Rockville, MD: Department of Health and Human Services, U.S. Public Health Service; 2000.
11. Shiau HJ, Reynolds MA. Sex differences in destructive periodontal disease: a systematic review. *J Periodontol.* 2010;81(10):1379–1389.
12. Borrell LN, Talih M. Examining periodontal disease disparities among U.S. adults 20 years of age and older: NHANES III (1988-1994) and NHANES 1999-2004. *Public Health Rep.* 2012;127(5):497–506. doi: 10.1177/003335491212700505.
13. Kibayashi M, Tanaka M, Nishida N, et al. Longitudinal study of the association between smoking as a periodontitis risk and salivary biomarkers related to periodontitis. *J Periodontol.* 2007;78(5):859–867.
14. Laxman VK, Annaji S. Tobacco use and its effects on the periodontium and periodontal therapy. *J Contemp Dent Pract.* 2008;9(7):97–107.
15. Eke PI, Dye BA, Wei L, Thornton-Evans GO, Genco RJ; CDC Periodontal Disease Surveillance workgroup: James Beck GDRP. Prevalence of periodontitis in adults in the United States: 2009 and 2010. *J Dent Res.* 2012;91(10):914–920.
16. Dumitrescu AL. Editorial: Periodontal Disease—A Public Health Problem. *Front Public Health.* 2015;3:278.

 STUDENT ANCILLARY RESOURCES

A wide variety of resources to enhance your learning is available online:

- Audio Glossary
- Book Pages
- Animation: Anatomy of the Periodontium in Disease
- Chapter Review Questions and Answers

4 Classification of Periodontal and Peri-Implant Diseases and Conditions

Clinical Application. A periodontal disease classification system assists the clinician in diagnosing and treating periodontal and peri-implant diseases and conditions, communicating clinical findings accurately to other dental health care providers, and submitting information to dental insurance providers. In 2017, the American Academy of Periodontology (AAP) and the European Federation of Periodontology (EFP) developed a new classification scheme for periodontal and peri-implant diseases and conditions. This joint collaborative effort was undertaken to better align and update the classification system with our current understanding of periodontal and peri-implant diseases and conditions. Upcoming chapters will go into greater detail regarding the case definition and diagnostic criteria for each category. However, the purpose of this chapter is to provide the reader with a broad overview of the 2017 Classification of Periodontal and Peri-Implant Diseases and Conditions.

Learning Objectives

- Explain the importance of a classification system for periodontal disease.
- Name the three major categories of periodontal diseases and conditions.
- Explain why clinicians need to be familiar with terminology from the 1999 disease classification, such as chronic periodontitis and aggressive periodontitis.
- Be able to discuss some differences between the 2017 and the 1999 Classification Systems.
- Name the four subcategories of the Peri-Implant Diseases and Conditions category.

Key Terms

Classification system
American Academy of
  Periodontology

European Federation of
  Periodontology

2017 AAP/EFP Classification of
  Periodontal and Peri-Implant
  Diseases and Conditions

Section 1
Disease Classification Systems

A classification system is a grouping of similar entities on the basis of certain differing characteristics. An everyday example of a classification system is grouping motor vehicles into categories such as passenger cars, crossover vehicles, sport utility vehicles, and trucks. Classification systems provide a tool to study the etiology, pathogenesis, and treatment of periodontal diseases in an orderly manner.

Clinicians and researchers have struggled to develop a classification of the various forms of periodontal disease. Over the years, classification systems have changed in response to new scientific knowledge about the etiology and pathogenesis of periodontal diseases and conditions. In recent years, there have been several attempts to classify periodontal diseases. *A disease classification system, however, should not be regarded as a permanent structure. Rather, it is ever-changing and evolves with the development of new evidence-based knowledge. Thus, it is expected that systems of classification will change over time.* As more is learned about the nature of a disease, the disease classification system constantly is reassessed and redefined.

A periodontal classification system provides information necessary in (1) communicating clinical findings accurately to other dental health care providers, (2) formulating a diagnosis and devising an individualized treatment plan, (3) predicting treatment outcomes (prognosis), and (4) submitting information to dental insurance providers/carriers.

THE 2017 AAP/EFP CLASSIFICATION OF PERIODONTAL AND PERI-IMPLANT DISEASES AND CONDITIONS

The American Academy of Periodontology (AAP) and the European Federation of Periodontology (EFP) initiated the currently accepted classification system by organizing the *World Workshop on the Classification of Periodontal and Peri-Implant Diseases and Conditions* held in November 2017. This workshop brought together more than a hundred experts from across the world to review the scientific evidence and develop a new disease classification.

The previous classification of periodontal disease was developed nearly 20 years ago in 1999. Since then, periodontics has made notable advancements in the treatment and diagnosis of periodontal disease. Furthermore, peri-implantitis has emerged as a major new problem that was not accounted for in the 1999 classification system. The 2017 disease classification accounts for scientific advances in recent years and strives to standardize the definition of the diseases and conditions. The 2017 AAP/EFP Classification of Periodontal and Peri-Implant Diseases and Conditions is the most recent, internationally accepted classification system.[1]

Figure 4-1 presents a visual overview of the 2017 classification of periodontal and peri-implant diseases. Box 4-1 provides the link to the complete proceedings of the World Workshop.

Box 4-1 Link to the Complete Proceedings of World Workshop

The complete proceedings of the World Workshop on the Classification of Periodontal and Peri-Implant Diseases and Conditions is available free of charge online at https://onlinelibrary. wiley.com/toc/19433670/2018/89/S1.

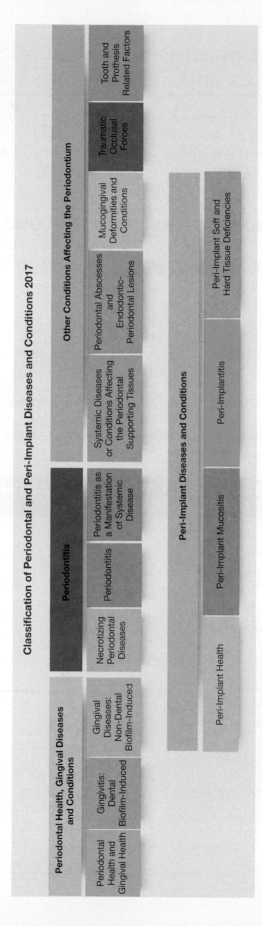

Figure 4-1. The 2017 AAP/EFP Classification of Periodontal and Peri-Implant Diseases and Conditions. A visual overview of the 2017 classification of periodontal and peri-implant diseases. (Used by permission of John Wiley & Sons from Kornman KS, Tonetti MS. Proceedings of the world workshop on the classification of periodontal and peri-implant conditions. *J Periodontol.* 2018;89(S1–S318):1–4.)

Section 2
The 2017 Classification of Periodontal and Peri-Implant Diseases and Conditions

Table 4-1 presents the 2017 Disease Classification for periodontal health, gingivitis, and gingival diseases and conditions. As shown in Figure 4-2, this broad category is subdivided into three subcategories: (1) periodontal and gingival health, (2) dental biofilm-induced gingivitis, and (3) nondental biofilm-induced gingival diseases. Each of these three major subcategories has several conditions listed under it (refer to Table 4-1).

HEALTH, GINGIVITIS, AND GINGIVAL DISEASES/CONDITIONS

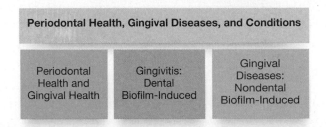

Figure 4-2. Classification of Periodontal Health, Gingivitis, and Gingival Diseases/Conditions. The 2017 Disease Classification of Periodontal Diseases and Conditions organization of periodontal and gingival health, dental biofilm-induced gingivitis, and nondental biofilm-induced gingival diseases.

TABLE 4-1	PERIODONTAL HEALTH, GINGIVITIS, AND GINGIVAL DISEASES/CONDITIONS

1. **Periodontal health and gingival health**
   a. Clinical gingival health on an intact periodontium
   b. Clinical gingival health on a reduced periodontium
      i. Stable periodontitis patient
      ii. Non-periodontitis patient
2. **Gingivitis—dental biofilm-induced**
   a. Associated with dental biofilm alone
   b. Mediated by systemic or local risk factors
   c. Drug-influenced gingival enlargement
3. **Gingival diseases—nondental biofilm-induced**
   a. Genetic/developmental disorders
   b. Specific infections
   c. Inflammatory and immune conditions
   d. Reactive processes
   e. Neoplasms
   f. Endocrine, nutritional, and metabolic diseases
   g. Traumatic lesions
   h. Gingival pigmentation

FORMS OF PERIODONTITIS

As shown in Figure 4-3, the major diagnostic category of periodontitis is subdivided into three forms. Table 4-2 presents the 2017 classification framework for periodontitis.

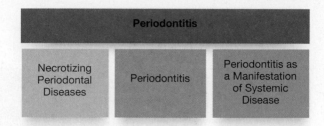

Figure 4-3. Three Major Forms of Periodontitis. The 2017 Disease Classification of Periodontal Diseases and Conditions subdivides the category of periodontitis into three major forms. Each of the three forms has two or more subcategories.

TABLE 4-2	FORMS OF PERIODONTITIS

1. **Necrotizing Periodontal Diseases**
   a. Necrotizing gingivitis
   b. Necrotizing periodontitis
   c. Necrotizing stomatitis

2. **Periodontitis as Manifestation of Systemic Diseases**

   Classification of these conditions should be based on the primary systemic disease according to the *International Statistical Classification of Diseases and Related Health Problems* (ICD) codes

3. **Periodontitis**
   a. *Stages*: Based on severity[a] and complexity of management[b]

   Stage I: Initial periodontitis

   Stage II: Moderate periodontitis

   Stage III: Severe periodontitis with potential for additional tooth loss

   Stage IV: Severe periodontitis with potential for loss of the dentition

   b. *Extent and distribution*[c]: localized, generalized; molar-incisor distribution

   c. *Grades*: Evidence or risk of rapid progression,[d] anticipated treatment response[e]

      i. Grade A: Slow rate of disease progression

      ii. Grade B: Moderate rate of disease progression

      iii. Grade C: Rapid rate of disease progression

[a]Severity: Interdental clinical attachment level (CAL) at site with greatest loss; Radiographic bone loss and tooth loss.
[b]Complexity of management: Probing depths, pattern of bone loss, furcation lesions, number of remaining teeth, tooth mobility, ridge defects, masticatory dysfunction.
[c]Add to Stage as descriptor: Localized <30% teeth, generalized ≥30% teeth.
[d]Risk of progression: direct evidence by periapical radiographs of CAL loss, or indirect (bone loss/age ratio).
[e]Anticipated treatment response: case phenotype, smoking, hyperglycemia (elevated levels of glucose in blood).

OTHER CONDITIONS AFFECTING THE PERIODONTIUM

As shown in Figure 4-4, this major diagnostic category is subdivided into five conditions. Table 4-3 presents the 2017 classification framework for other conditions affecting the periodontium.

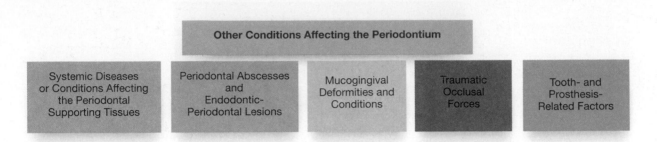

Figure 4-4. Other Conditions Affecting the Periodontium. The 2017 Disease Classification of Periodontal Diseases and Conditions includes a category for other conditions that may affect the health of the periodontium.

TABLE 4-3	OTHER CONDITIONS AFFECTING THE PERIODONTIUM

1. **Systemic diseases or conditions affecting the periodontal supporting tissues**
2. **Other periodontal conditions**
   a. Periodontal abscesses
   b. Endodontic-periodontal lesions
3. **Mucogingival deformities and conditions around teeth**
   a. Gingival phenotype
   b. Gingival/soft tissue recession
   c. Lack of gingiva
   d. Decreased vestibular depth
   e. Aberrant frenum/muscle position
   f. Gingival excess
   g. Abnormal color
   h. Condition of exposed root surface
4. **Traumatic occlusal forces**
   a. Primary occlusal trauma
   b. Secondary occlusal trauma
   c. Orthodontic forces
5. **Prostheses and tooth-related factors that modify or predispose to plaque-induced gingival diseases/periodontitis**
   a. Localized tooth-related factors
   b. Localized dental prostheses-related factors

PERI-IMPLANT DISEASES AND CONDITIONS

As shown in Figure 4-5, this major diagnostic category is subdivided into four subcategories. Table 4-4 presents the 2017 classification framework for peri-implant diseases and conditions.

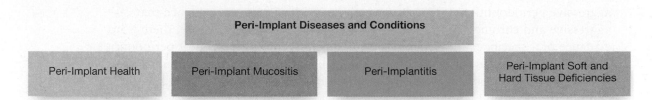

Figure 4-5. Peri-Implant Diseases and Conditions. The 2017 Disease Classification of Periodontal Diseases and Conditions subdivides the category of peri-implant diseases and conditions into four major subcategories.

TABLE 4-4	PERI-IMPLANT DISEASES AND CONDITIONS
1. **Peri-implant health**	
2. **Peri-implant mucositis**	
3. **Peri-implantitis**	
4. **Peri-implant soft and hard tissue deficiencies**	

COMPARISON OF THE 2017 AND 1999 CLASSIFICATION SYSTEMS

Much of the periodontal literature found in periodontal journals and textbooks is based on the earlier 1999 disease classification. For example, the classifications of chronic and aggressive periodontitis will appear in journal articles printed before June 2018. For this reason, readers need to be somewhat familiar with both the 1999 and 2017 classification systems. The 1999 disease classification is outlined in Table 4-5.[2]

TABLE 4-5	MAIN CATEGORIES: 1999 CLASSIFICATION OF PERIODONTAL DISEASES AND CONDITIONS
1. Gingival Diseases	
a. Plaque-Induced Gingival Diseases	
b. Non–Plaque-Induced Gingival Lesions	
2. Chronic Periodontitis	
3. Aggressive Periodontitis	
4. Periodontitis as a Manifestation of Systemic Diseases	
5. Necrotizing Periodontal Diseases	
6. Abscesses of the Periodontium	
7. Periodontitis Associated with Endodontic Lesions	
8. Developmental or Acquired Deformities and Conditions	

The 2017 classification system has several major features that distinguish it from the 1999 classification system. Several of these key differences will be briefly outlined below but, will be covered in greater detail in later chapters.

1. Forms of the disease that were previously recognized as "chronic" or "aggressive" are now grouped in the single disease entity known as "periodontitis." The 2017 classification system no longer has a chronic periodontitis category and a separate aggressive periodontitis category because there is little consistent evidence that aggressive and chronic periodontitis are different diseases. Furthermore, there is no evidence of a specific pathophysiology that is distinct for either form of periodontitis.
2. A classification system for periodontitis that is based on a multidimensional staging and grading system, similar to the system used for cancer classification. Using the combined staging and grading system, the provider can individualize patient-specific treatment modalities and treatment sequences which will enable him/her to optimize individual patient management and thus serve as the launch pad for personalized patient care.
3. A new classification for peri-implant diseases and conditions.

Chapter Summary Statement

This chapter presents an overview of the updated classification system of periodontal diseases and conditions and a new classification of peri-implant diseases and conditions. The 2017 classification represents the work of the worldwide community of scholars and clinicians in periodontology and implant dentistry.

Classification systems, like the one for periodontal diseases and conditions, group similar diseases and conditions into general categories. Classification systems provide a tool to study the etiology, pathogenesis, and treatment of periodontal diseases in an orderly manner. From the clinician's point of view, the classification system is a framework which provides a starting point for formulating a diagnosis and an individualized treatment plan. In addition, periodontal disease classifications assist the clinician in communicating with other dental health care providers and dental insurance providers.

Section 3
Focus on Patients

Clinical Patient Care

CASE 1

During the assessment of the periodontium, you note the following: apical migration of the junctional epithelium and attachment loss. The patient's medical history is normal; he takes no medications. According to the 2017 disease classification, would this patient be classified as having gingivitis, periodontitis, or periodontitis as a manifestation of systemic disease?

CASE 2

During the assessment of the periodontium, you note the following: bleeding, redness, and swelling of the tissue; abundant plaque biofilm, no apical migration of the junctional epithelium, and no attachment loss. The patient's medical history is normal; he takes no medications. According to the 2017 disease classification, would this patient be classified as having gingivitis, periodontitis, or periodontitis as a manifestation of systemic disease?

CASE 3

During the assessment of the periodontium, you note the following: bleeding, redness, and swelling of the tissue; abundant plaque biofilm, apical migration of the junctional epithelium, and attachment loss. The patient takes medication for diabetes. According to the 2017 disease classification, would this patient be classified as having gingivitis, periodontitis, or periodontitis as a manifestation of systemic disease?

References

1. Kornman KS, Tonetti MS. Proceedings of the world workshop on the classification of periodontal and peri-implant conditions. *J Periodontol.* 2018;89(S1–S318):1–4.
2. Armitage GC. Development of a classification system for periodontal diseases and conditions. *Ann Periodontol.* 1999;4(1): 1–6.

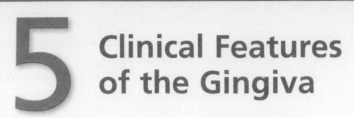

5 Clinical Features of the Gingiva

Clinical Application. A dental hygienist's ability to recognize the clinical features of both healthy and diseased gingiva plays a part in nearly every patient care visit. Knowledge of these clinical features continuously will be expanded throughout the hygienist's career. The outline of these features presented in this chapter provides a fundamental framework for recognition of clinical features and will allow a new clinician to enter a clinical setting with confidence.

Learning Objectives

- Describe characteristics of the gingiva in health.
- List clinical signs of gingival inflammation.
- Compare and contrast clinical features of healthy and inflamed gingival tissue.
- Explain the difference in color between acute and chronic inflammation.
- Differentiate between bulbous, blunted, and cratered papilla.
- Write a description of gingival inflammation that includes descriptors of duration, extent, and distribution of inflammation.

Key Terms

Stippling	Bulbous papilla	Extent of inflammation
Inflammation	Blunted papilla	Distribution of inflammation
Gingivitis	Cratered papilla	

Section 1
Clinical Features of Healthy Gingiva

It is important for clinicians to recognize the appearance of healthy gingiva and to recognize all of its variations in health. In addition, clinicians must be able to describe gingiva accurately when documenting the findings from a periodontal assessment. Careful choice of verbal descriptors documents the state of gingival health, or lack of it, and allows the clinician to focus on areas that may need additional treatment.

1. **Tissue Color and Contour in Health**
   A. **Tissue Color**
      1. Healthy gingival tissue has a uniform, pink color. The precise color depends on the number and size of blood vessels in the connective tissue and the thickness of the gingival epithelium. The shade of pink usually is lighter in persons with fair complexions and darker in individuals with dark complexions (Fig. 5-1).
      2. The coral pink of the gingiva is easily distinguished from the darker alveolar mucosa.
      3. Healthy tissue also can be pigmented. The pigmented areas of the attached gingiva may range from light brown to black.
   B. **Tissue Contour (Size and Shape)**
      1. In health, the gingival tissue lies snugly around the tooth and firmly against the alveolar bone (Fig. 5-2).
      2. The gingival margin is smoothly scalloped in an arched form as it flows across the tooth surface from papilla to papilla.
      3. The gingival margin meets the tooth with a tapered (knife edge), flat, or slightly rounded edge.
      4. Papillae come to a point and fill the space between teeth (Fig. 5-2).
      5. Teeth with a diastema—no contact between adjacent teeth—or large spaces between teeth will have flat papillae.

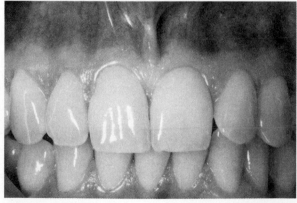 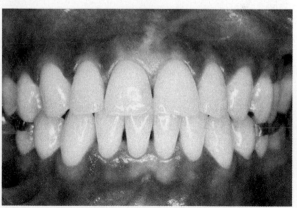

A   B

Figure 5-1. Tissue Color in Health. A. Periodontal health showing coral pink gingiva. Note the distinct difference in appearance between the keratinized gingiva and the nonkeratinized alveolar mucosa. **B.** Pigmentation of the gingiva showing how the gingiva can vary in color among patients.

2. Tissue Consistency and Texture in Health

A. Tissue Consistency

1. The attached gingiva is firmly connected to the underlying cementum and bone.
2. Healthy tissue is resilient (elastic). If gentle pressure is applied to the gingiva with the side of a probe, the tissue resists compression and springs back quickly. The attached gingiva will not pull away from the tooth when air is blown into the sulcus.

B. Surface Texture of the Tissue

1. In health, the surface of the attached gingiva is firm and may have a dimpled appearance similar to the skin of an orange peel (Fig. 5-3).
2. This dimpled appearance is known as stippling, appearing as minute elevations and depressions of the surface of the gingiva due to connective tissue projections within the epithelial tissue (connective tissue papillae). The presence of stippling is best viewed by drying the tissue with compressed air.
3. Healthy tissue may or may not exhibit a stippled appearance as the presence of stippling varies greatly from individual to individual.

3. Position of Gingival Margin in Health.

Ideally, the gingival margin is slightly coronal to the cementoenamel junction (CEJ) (Figs. 5-4 and 5-5). Patients with a previous history of bone loss, but healthy gingival tissue, may have a gingival margin that is apical to the CEJ (Fig. 5-6).

4. Absence of Bleeding in Health.

Healthy tissue does not bleed when disturbed by clinical procedures such as gentle probing of the sulcus.

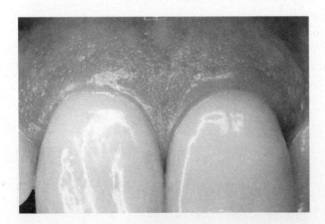

Figure 5-2. Contours of Healthy Gingiva. This tissue on the facial aspect of the maxillary anteriors exhibits all the characteristics of health, including a smoothly scalloped gingival margin, a tapered margin slightly coronal to the CEJ, and pointed papillae that completely fill the space between the teeth. (Courtesy of Dr. Don Rolfs, Wenatchee, WA.)

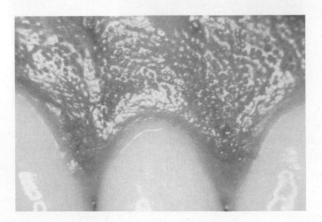

Figure 5-3. Stippling of Gingival Tissue. Healthy gingival tissue showing a stippled appearance. Stippling varies greatly from individual to individual. In some patients, healthy tissue may not exhibit a stippled appearance.

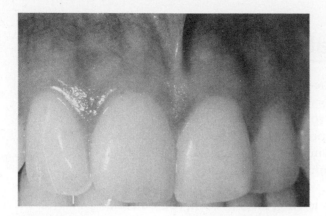

Figure 5-4. Position of the Margin in Health. In health, the gingival margin is slightly coronal to the cementoenamel junction. In anterior sextants, the margin is characterized by pronounced scalloping of the margin and pointed interdental papillae.

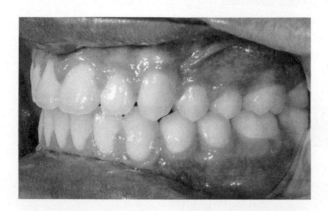

Figure 5-5. Gingiva in Posterior Sextants in Health. In posterior sextants, the tissue is characterized by a gently scalloped margin and papillae that fill the interdental embrasure spaces. (Used with permission from Langlais RP. *Color Atlas of Common Oral Diseases*. Philadelphia, PA: Wolters Kluwer; 2003.)

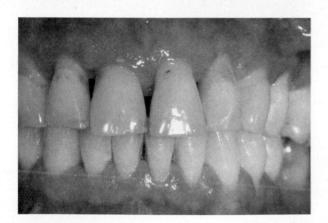

Figure 5-6. Health or Disease? This individual received periodontal treatment for periodontitis several years ago. The assessment at today's appointment reveals no inflammation and no additional attachment loss since beginning periodontal maintenance several years ago. Therefore, this tissue is considered healthy. The attachment loss is simply an indicator of previous disease activity. (Courtesy of Dr. Ralph Arnold.)

Section 2
Clinical Features of Gingival Inflammation

Gingival **inflammation** is the body's reaction to the bacterial infection of the gingival tissues by periodontal pathogens. The inflammatory response to this bacterial infection results in clinical changes in the gingival tissue involving the free and attached gingiva, as well as the papillae. Inflammation that is confined to gingival tissue with no effect on attachment level is called **gingivitis**, and is the mildest form of periodontal disease. Most patients are unaware they have a gingival infection because there usually is no discomfort.

A clinician with a trained eye can discern subtle differences in color, contour, and consistency even in gingival tissues that appear relatively healthy at first glance. The phrase "tissue talks" is a good phrase to remember when assessing the gingival tissue. Indications that the tissue is not healthy include such clinical observations as red, swollen tissue or papillae that do not fill the interdental space. Table 5-1 contrasts the characteristics of healthy versus inflamed gingival tissue.

TABLE 5-1	CHARACTERISTICS OF HEALTHY VERSUS INFLAMED GINGIVAL TISSUE	
	Healthy Tissue	**Gingivitis**
Color	Uniform pink color Pigmentation may be present	Acute: bright red Chronic: bluish red to purplish red

Contour	Marginal gingiva:
	   Meets the tooth in a tapered or slightly rounded edge
	Interdental papillae:
	   Pointed papilla fills the space between the teeth
		Marginal gingiva:
		   Meets the tooth in a rolled, thickened edge
		Interdental papillae:
		   Bulbous, blunted, cratered

Consistency	Firm Resilient under compression	Spongy, flaccid Indents easily when pressed lightly Compressed air deflects the tissue
Texture	Smooth and/or stippled	Tissue appears "shiny" Stretched appearance
Margin	Slightly coronal to the CEJ	Coronal to the CEJ (due to swellling)
Bleeding	No bleeding upon probing	Bleeding upon probing

1. **Characteristics of Gingivitis**
    A. **Tissue Color in Gingivitis.**
        1. Gingivitis is an inflammation of the gingiva often causing the tissue to become red and swollen, to bleed easily, and sometimes to become slightly tender.
        2. Inflammation results in increased blood flow to the gingiva causing the tissue to appear bright red. Figures 5-7 and 5-8 show examples of common clinical presentations of gingivitis.

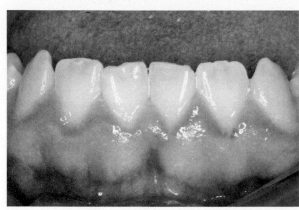
A

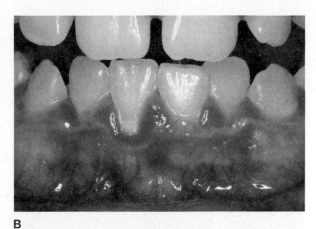
B

Figure 5-7. Color Changes in Gingivitis. A. Slight marginal redness is a clinical sign of early gingivitis. **B.** This gingival tissue shows more inflammation than seen in photograph **A.** The marginal and papillary gingival tissues are bright red in color. Note, also, the swelling of the marginal gingiva and papillae in this example. (Courtesy of Dr. Richard Foster, Guilford Technical Community College, Jamestown, NC.)

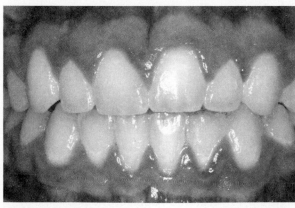
A

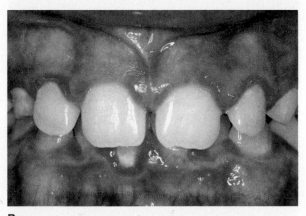
B

Figure 5-8. Color Changes in Gingivitis. A. This example shows subtle color changes in the marginal and papillary gingival tissues. **B.** In this example, the color changes are pronounced with fiery red marginal gingiva and papillae. (Courtesy of Dr. Richard Foster, Guilford Technical Community College, Jamestown, NC.)

B. Tissue Contour (Size and Shape) in Gingivitis

1. An increase of fluid within the tissue spaces—edema—causes enlargement of the gingival tissues. The normal scalloped appearance of the gingiva is lost if the gingival papillae are swollen.
2. Examples of types of changes in the appearance of the papillae are listed below.
   a. Bulbous papilla—a papilla that is enlarged and appears to bulge out of the interproximal space (Fig. 5-9).
   b. Blunted papilla—a papilla is flat and does not fill the interproximal space (Fig. 5-10).
   c. Cratered papilla—a papilla appears to have been "scooped out" leaving a concave depression in the midproximal area. Cratered papillae are associated with necrotizing gingivitis (Fig. 5-11).

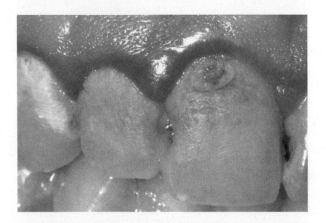

Figure 5-9. Bulbous Papillae. In gingivitis, the papillae may be enlarged and appear to bulge out of the interproximal space as seen in the papilla between the central and lateral incisors in this clinical photograph. (Courtesy of Dr. Ralph Arnold, San Antonio, TX.)

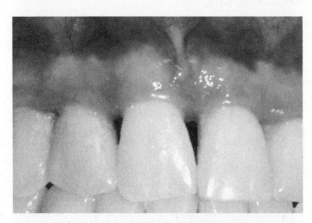

Figure 5-10. Blunted Papillae. In gingivitis, the papillae may be blunted and missing as seen in the papillae between the central and lateral incisors. (Courtesy of Dr. Don Rolfs, Wenatchee, WA.)

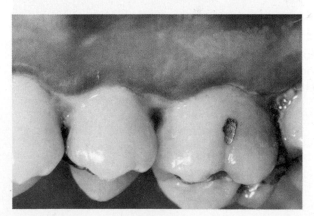

Figure 5-11. Cratered Papillae. The papillae may have a concave appearance in the midproximal area as seen in the papillae between second premolar and molar in this clinical photo. (Courtesy of Dr. Don Rolfs, Wenatchee, WA.)

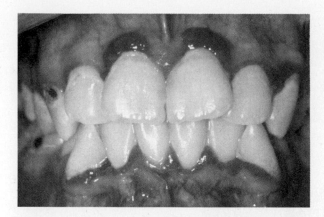

Figure 5-12. Soft, Spongy Tissue. Inflamed gingival tissue may be soft and spongy. The inflammatory fluids can cause the gingival tissues to feel somewhat like a moist sponge. (Courtesy of Dr. Ralph Arnold, San Antonio, TX.)

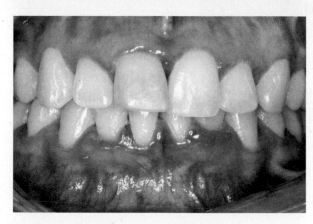

Figure 5-13. Smooth, Shiny Tissue. In gingivitis, fluid in the tissue can cause the tissue to appear smooth and shiny with a stretched appearance. (Courtesy of Dr. Richard Foster, Guilford Technical Community College, Jamestown, NC.)

2. **Tissue Consistency and Texture in Gingivitis**
   A. **Tissue Consistency in Gingivitis**
      1. Increased fluid in the inflamed tissue also causes the gingiva to be soft, spongy, and nonelastic (Fig. 5-12).
      2. When pressure is applied to the inflamed gingiva with the side of a probe, the tissue is easily compressed and can retain an imprint of the probe for several seconds.
      3. Inflamed gingival tissue loses its firm consistency becoming flaccid (soft, movable). When compressed air is directed into the sulcus, it readily deflects the gingival margin and papillae away from the neck of the tooth.
   B. **Surface Texture in Gingivitis**
      1. The increase in fluid due to the inflammatory response can cause the gingival tissues to appear smooth and very shiny (Fig. 5-13).
      2. The tissue almost has a "stretched" appearance that resembles plastic wrap that has been pulled tightly.
3. **Position of Margin in Gingivitis**
   A. In gingivitis, the position of the gingival margin may move more coronally (further above the CEJ).
   B. This change in the position of the gingival margin is due to tissue swelling and enlargement (Fig. 5-14).
4. **Presence of Bleeding in Gingivitis**
   A. Bleeding upon gentle probing is seen clinically before changes in color are clinically detectible (Fig. 5-15).
   B. In gingivitis, the sulcus lining becomes ulcerated and the blood vessels become engorged. The tissues bleed easily during probing or instrumentation.
   C. There is a direct relationship between inflammation and bleeding: the more severe the inflammation, the heavier the bleeding.

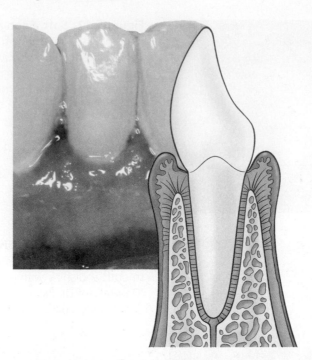

Figure 5-14. Tissue Margin in Gingivitis. The tissue swelling in gingivitis may cause the position of the gingival margin to move coronally—further above the CEJ—than in health. There is no destruction of periodontal ligament fibers or alveolar bone in gingivitis.

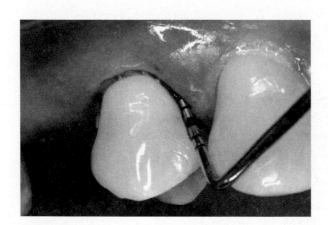

Figure 5-15. Bleeding on Probing. Bleeding is an important clinical indicator of inflammation. Inflammation results in ulceration of the sulcus/pocket wall causing the gingival tissues to bleed easily during gentle probing.

Section 3
Extent and Distribution of Inflammation

In documenting inflammation of the gingival tissues it is useful to note both the extent and distribution of the inflammation. Just documenting the presence of gingival inflammation is too vague, and does not identify severity of inflammation accurately enough to help establish a treatment plan.

1. **Gingival Inflammation**
    A. **Extent of Inflammation.** The extent of inflammation is the area of tissue that is affected by inflammation. The extent of inflammation is described as localized or generalized in the mouth.
       1. Localized inflammation is confined to the gingival tissue of a single tooth—such as the maxillary right first molar—or to a group of teeth—such as the mandibular anterior sextant.
       2. Generalized inflammation involves all or most of the tissue in the mouth.
    B. **Distribution of Inflammation.** The distribution of inflammation describes the area where the gingival tissue is inflamed.
       1. The inflammation may affect only the interdental papilla, the gingival margin and the papilla, or the gingival margin, papilla, and the attached gingiva.
       2. Table 5-2 summarizes how to describe the extent and distribution of inflammation of the gingival tissue. Figures 5-16 to 5-20 illustrate the use of this descriptive terminology.

TABLE 5-2	GINGIVAL INFLAMMATION
Extent	• Localized—inflammation confined to the tissue of a single tooth or a group of teeth • Generalized—inflammation of the gingival tissue of all or most of the mouth
Distribution	• Papillary—inflammation of the interdental papilla only • Marginal—inflammation of the gingival margin and papilla • Diffuse—inflammation of the gingival margin, papilla, and attached gingiva
Descriptions	Descriptive terms may be combined to create a verbal picture of the inflammation, such as: • "Localized marginal inflammation in the mandibular anterior sextant" • "Localized papillary inflammation on the maxillary right canine" • "Generalized marginal inflammation" • "Generalized diffuse inflammation"

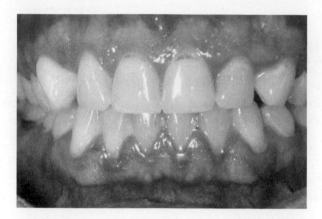

Figure 5-16. Localized Marginal Inflammation.
Note the redness and swelling of the marginal and papillary gingival tissues that are localized to the mandibular anterior sextant. (Courtesy of Dr. Ralph Arnold.)

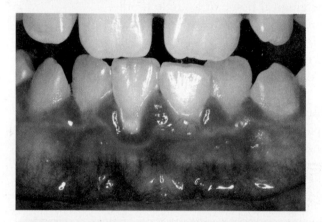

Figure 5-17. Localized Diffuse Inflammation.
Redness and edema of the gingival margin, papillae, and attached gingiva in the mandibular anterior sextant. (Courtesy of Dr. Richard Foster, Guilford Technical Community College, Jamestown, NC.)

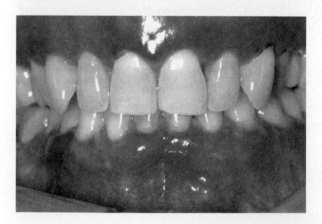

Figure 5-18. Generalized Diffuse Inflammation.
Diffuse inflammation of the gingival margin, papillae, and attached gingiva throughout the entire mouth. (Courtesy of Dr. Ralph Arnold.)

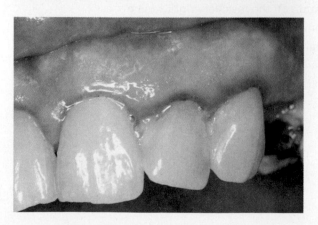

Figure 5-19. Localized Marginal Inflammation.
Note the reddened tissue color along the gingival margin, extending down into the papillae on these maxillary anterior teeth. (Courtesy of Dr. Richard Foster, Guilford Technical Community College, Jamestown, NC.)

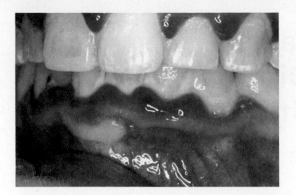

Figure 5-20. Localized Diffuse Inflammation.
Inflammation involving the gingival margin, papillae, and attached gingiva of the mandibular anterior sextant. (Courtesy of Dr. Richard Foster, Guilford Technical Community College, Jamestown, NC.)

Chapter Summary Statement

Clinicians must have a clear mental image of gingival health to recognize the signs of gingival inflammation when it occurs. Inflammation in the gingiva causes changes in the color, contour, and consistency of the gingiva that can be recognized even in the earliest stages by the trained clinician.

Section 4
Focus on Patients

Clinical Patient Care

CASE 1

A patient new to your dental team has been appointed with you for a dental prophylaxis. The patient has just relocated to your town. The patient tells you that he saw a dentist just before moving who told him that he has gingivitis. During your discussion with the patient, he asks if there is some way he can tell at home if he has gingivitis. How might you reply to this patient's question?

CASE 2

Reading through your patient's treatment notes from the previous visit, you notice the clinician documented "presence of gingival inflammation." Explain why this statement is not adequate in order to provide quality patient treatment. What would you add to the description to provide another clinician with a clear verbal description of the clinical features of the patient's gingival tissues?

 STUDENT ANCILLARY RESOURCES

A wide variety of resources to enhance your learning is available online:

- Audio Glossary
- Book Pages
- Chapter Review Questions and Answers

CHAPTER

6 Periodontal Health, Gingival Diseases and Conditions

Clinical Application.
Examination of the gingiva is part of every patient visit. In this context, a thorough clinical and radiographic assessment of the patient's gingival tissues provides the dental practitioner with invaluable diagnostic information that is critical to determining the health status of the gingiva. The dental hygienist is often the first member of the dental team to be able to detect the early signs of periodontal disease. In 2017, the American Academy of Periodontology (AAP) and the European Federation of Periodontology (EFP) developed a new worldwide classification scheme for periodontal and peri-implant diseases and conditions. Included in the new classification scheme is the category called "periodontal health, gingival diseases/conditions." Therefore, this chapter will first review the parameters that define periodontal health. Appreciating what constitutes as periodontal health serves as the basis for the dental provider to have a stronger understanding of the different categories of gingival diseases and conditions that are commonly encountered in clinical practice.

Learning Objectives

- Define periodontal health and be able to describe the clinical features that are consistent with signs of periodontal health.
- List the two major subdivisions of gingival disease as established by the American Academy of Periodontology and the European Federation of Periodontology.
- Compare and contrast the etiologic factors associated with dental biofilm-induced gingivitis and non–plaque-induced gingival diseases.
- List the conditions that are classified under the non–plaque-induced gingival diseases category.
- Describe the differences between an intact periodontium and a reduced periodontium.
- Differentiate papillary gingivitis, marginal gingivitis, and diffuse gingivitis.
- Describe the clinical signs of inflammation characteristic of moderate plaque-induced gingivitis.
- Describe how systemic factors can modify the host response to plaque biofilm and lead to gingival inflammation.

Key Terms

Periodontal health
Intact periodontium
Reduced periodontium
Periodontal health on an intact
   periodontium
Periodontal health on a
   reduced periodontium in a
   non-periodontitis patient
Periodontal health on a reduced
   periodontium in a successfully
   treated stable periodontitis patient

Plaque-induced gingivitis
Papillary gingivitis
Marginal gingivitis
Diffuse gingivitis
Acute gingivitis
Chronic gingivitis
Gingivitis on an intact periodontium
Gingival inflammation on a reduced
   periodontium in a successfully
   treated stable periodontitis
   patient

Pregnancy-associated pyogenic
   granuloma
Hyperglycemia
Drug-influenced gingival
   enlargements
Non–plaque-induced gingival
   diseases
Lichen planus

Section 1
Periodontal Health

The 2017 World Workshop defines **periodontal health** as simply "*a state free from inflammatory periodontal disease that allows an individual to function normally and avoid consequences (mental or physical) due to current or past disease.*"[1]

1. **Characteristics of Periodontal Health.** Clinically, periodontal health is characterized by the absence of bleeding on probing, erythema, edema, patient symptoms and attachment and bone loss.
2. **Categories of Periodontal Health**
   A. **Normal versus Reduced Periodontium.** The 2017 classification system recognizes that *periodontal health can occur either on an intact periodontium or on a reduced periodontium.*
      1. An intact periodontium—a periodontium with *no loss* of periodontal tissue (no loss of connective tissue or alveolar bone).
      2. A reduced periodontium—a periodontium with *pre-existing loss* of periodontal tissue but, is **not currently** undergoing loss of connective tissue/alveolar bone.
   B. **Three Categories of Periodontal Health.** The following describes the three categories of periodontal health as described by the 2017 World Workshop.
      1. Periodontal health on an intact periodontium—clinical signs characteristic of periodontal health coupled with an intact periodontium (Box 6-1, Fig. 6-1).
      2. Periodontal health on a reduced periodontium in a non-periodontitis patient—clinical signs of periodontal health on a periodontium with a pre-existing loss of connective tissue and/or loss of alveolar bone which is *attributed to non-periodontitis reasons* (Box 6-2, Fig. 6-2). For example, recession of the gingival margin that occurs from a history of traumatic toothbrushing or the deliberate removal of alveolar bone that occurs in surgical crown lengthening.
      3. Periodontal health on a reduced periodontium in a successfully treated stable periodontitis patient—clinical signs of periodontal health on a periodontium with a pre-existing loss of connective tissue and alveolar bone *which is attributed to periodontitis* but, has been successfully treated *and is currently stable* (Box 6-3, Fig. 6-3).

Box 6-1. Periodontal Health on an Intact Periodontium

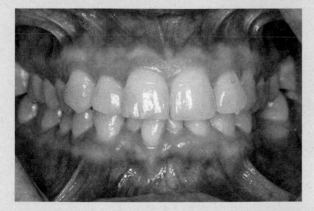
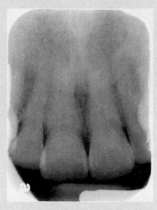

Figure 6-1. Periodontal Health on an Intact Periodontium. This patient exhibits no clinical signs of gingival inflammation and no previous loss of periodontal tissues. The dental radiograph does not reveal any changes in either the alveolar bone height or the architecture and morphology of the alveolar bone.

Box 6-2. Periodontal Health on a Reduced Periodontium in a Non-periodontitis Patient

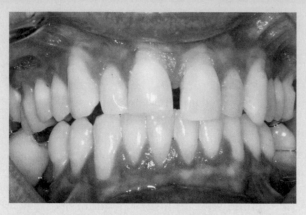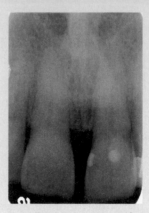

Figure 6-2. Periodontal Health on a Reduced Periodontium in a Non-periodontitis Patient. This is a 54-year-old male patient with a history of excessive frequent daily toothbrushing (he brushed five to six times a day with a hard-bristled toothbrush).

- Note the generalized recession of the gingival margin. However, there are no evident signs of clinical inflammation.
- The dental radiograph does not reveal any changes in either the alveolar bone height or the architecture and morphology of the alveolar bone.
- Treatment objectives for this case are to (1) address the patient's self-care habits and reinforce proper oral hygiene and (2) periodically monitor the patient's periodontal status to prevent further loss of tissue.

Box 6-3. Periodontal Health on a Reduced Periodontium in a Successfully Treated Periodontitis Patient

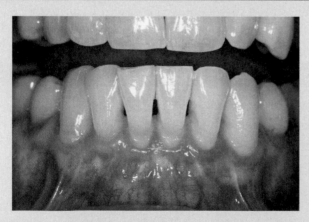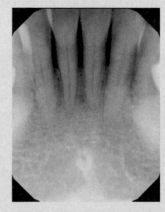

Figure 6-3. Periodontal Health on a Reduced Periodontium in a Successfully Treated Stable Periodontitis Patient. In 2016, this generalized periodontitis patient underwent nonsurgical and surgical periodontal therapy to control the disease. Eighteen months later, the above photo was taken to illustrate how healthy her gingiva looks following therapy and meticulous home care.

- The dental radiograph reveals loss of alveolar bone height.
- Future treatment objectives should be to (1) maintain the reduced periodontium in a healthy and stable state and (2) prevent the reactivation of periodontitis.

Section 2
Dental Plaque-Induced Gingival Conditions

As illustrated in Figure 6-4, gingival diseases and conditions are broadly classified as either (1) gingivitis that is dental biofilm-induced or (2) gingival diseases that *are not* dental biofilm-induced. This section discusses the first and most common of these, gingivitis that is dental biofilm-induced.[2]

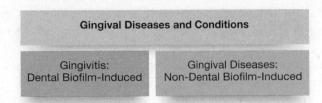

Figure 6-4. Gingival Diseases and Conditions. Gingival diseases and conditions are classified as either dental biofilm-induced or non–dental biofilm-induced.

CLASSIFICATION OF PLAQUE-INDUCED GINGIVITIS AND MODIFYING FACTORS

Plaque-induced gingivitis is an inflammatory response of the gingival tissues resulting from bacterial plaque biofilm accumulation located at and below the gingival margin. Löe and colleagues first described gingivitis in their landmark research in 1965.[3] The 2017 classification scheme for plaque-induced gingivitis is outlined in Table 6-1.[2] The severity of plaque-induced gingivitis can be influenced by various systemic and tooth-related factors.

TABLE 6-1	**CLASSIFICATION OF PLAQUE-INDUCED GINGIVITIS AND MODIFYING FACTORS**

A. **Associated with bacterial dental biofilm only**

B. **Potential modifying factors of plaque-induced gingivitis**
   1. Systemic conditions
      a) Sex and steroid hormones
         1) Puberty
         2) Menstrual cycle
         3) Pregnancy
         4) Oral contraceptives
      b) Hyperglycemia
      c) Leukemia
      d) Smoking
      e) Malnutrition
   2. Oral factors enhancing plaque biofilm accumulation
      a) Prominent subgingival restoration margins
      b) Hyposalivation (reduced saliva production)

C. **Drug-influenced gingival enlargements**

PLAQUE-INDUCED GINGIVITIS

1. **Characteristics of Plaque-Induced Gingivitis**
   A. **The Most Common Form of Periodontal Disease.** Plaque-induced gingivitis is by far the most common type of periodontal disease. It does not directly cause tooth loss; however, managing gingivitis is the primary strategy for preventing periodontitis.[4] Epidemiologic data show that plaque-induced gingivitis is prevalent at all ages in the population.[5,6]
      1. *The intensity of the clinical signs and symptoms of gingivitis may vary between individuals and within the dentition of an individual.*[7]
      2. Plaque-induced gingivitis differs between children and adults (for more detailed information regarding the periodontium of a child patient, refer to Chapter 31, Periodontal Disease in the Pediatric Population).
         a. Inflammation is not as intense in children versus young adults with the same quantity of plaque biofilm.[8–10]
         b. Adolescents may have elevated levels of certain bacteria: *Actinomyces, Capnocytophaga, Leptotrichia,* and *Selenomonas* species.[11]
         c. Children may have fewer pathogenic bacteria in their plaque biofilm, a thicker junctional epithelium, and a less developed immune response.[12,13]
         d. Gingival inflammation in adults is more pronounced even when similar amounts of plaque biofilms are present, perhaps attributed to age-related differences in cellular inflammatory response to plaque biofilm.[14,15]
      3. Local factors—such as dental restorations, appliances, root fractures, and tooth anatomy—act as sites for plaque biofilm retention and may contribute to progression of the disease.
   B. **Clinical Signs of Plaque-Induced Gingivitis**
      1. Common clinical signs of plaque-induced gingivitis include changes in gingival color, contour, and consistency. These common signs include redness (erythema), swelling (edema), bleeding, increased gingival crevicular fluid, and tenderness.[4,16]
      2. The earliest signs of gingivitis are seen in the papillary region. This is known as **papillary gingivitis**. Papillary gingivitis is gingival inflammation that involves the interdental papilla. If the papillary gingival inflammation extends into the adjacent gingival margin, the condition is known as **marginal gingivitis**. Marginal gingivitis involves the gingival margin and a portion of the contiguous attached gingiva. If the gingival inflammation affects all three parts of the gingiva—the interdental papilla, the marginal gingiva, and the attached gingiva—this is known as **diffuse gingivitis**.
      3. It should be noted that gingivitis is a *clinical* diagnosis. Thus, radiographs, alone, cannot be used to diagnose gingivitis.
   C. **Duration of Plaque-Induced Gingivitis**
      1. **Acute gingivitis**—gingivitis of a sudden onset and short duration, after which professional care and patient self-care returns the gingiva to a healthy state.
      2. **Chronic gingivitis**—long-lasting gingivitis; gingivitis may exist for years without ever progressing to periodontitis. Chronic gingivitis is typically painless and is more commonly encountered than acute gingivitis.
2. **Categories of Plaque-Induced Gingivitis**
   A. **Three Categories of Plaque-Induced Gingivitis.** The 2017 classification system recognizes that plaque-induced gingivitis can occur either on an intact periodontium or on a reduced periodontium. Table 6-2 summarizes the key clinical features for each category.

1. Gingivitis on an intact periodontium (Box 6-4, Fig. 6-5)—the presence of plaque-induced inflammation on an intact periodontium.
2. Gingivitis on a reduced periodontium in a non-periodontitis patient (Box 6-5, Fig. 6-6)—the presence of plaque-induced inflammation on a periodontium with pre-existing loss of connective tissue and/or loss of alveolar bone that can be attributed to non-periodontitis reasons.
3. Gingival inflammation on a reduced periodontium in a successfully treated stable periodontitis patient (Box 6-6, Fig. 6-7).

B. **Plaque-Induced Gingivitis on a Reduced Periodontium After Successful Treatment**
1. In someone successfully treated for periodontitis, if the extent of attachment loss present remains stable over months or years, then the presence of attachment loss is *not* an indication of active periodontitis.
2. Plaque-induced gingivitis on a reduced periodontium in a successfully treated periodontitis case is characterized by the return of bacteria-induced inflammation to the gingival margin on a reduced periodontium with *no evidence of progressive attachment loss*.[2] If a clinician is going to make the diagnosis of "gingivitis on a reduced but stable periodontium," it is necessary to demonstrate that attachment loss (loss of connective tissue and alveolar bone) is not ongoing.
3. The common clinical findings on a reduced periodontium are the same as plaque-induced gingivitis except for the presence of pre-existing attachment loss and therefore a higher risk of periodontitis. Due to this higher risk for recurrence of periodontitis, individualized professional care is of utmost importance for the patient with plaque-induced gingivitis on a reduced periodontium.[17]
4. Although a successfully treated periodontitis patient exhibits an absence of ongoing, progressive periodontitis, the patient cannot revert to being classified as a "gingivitis case on an intact periodontium."
   a. Periodontitis is an irreversible condition that results in a *permanent* loss of attachment and alveolar bone.
   b. A periodontitis patient remains a periodontitis patient for life—even following successful periodontal therapy—and requires lifelong supportive care to prevent recurrence of disease.[1]

TABLE 6-2	KEY FEATURES OF PERIODONTAL HEALTH AND DENTAL PLAQUE-INDUCED GINGIVITIS	
Intact Periodontium	**Health**	**Gingivitis**
Clinical attachment loss	No	No
Radiological bone loss	No	No
Reduced Periodontium, Non-periodontitis Patient	**Health**	**Gingivitis**
Clinical attachment loss	Yes	Yes
Radiological bone loss	Possible[a]	Possible[a]
Successfully Treated Stable Periodontitis Patient	**Health**	**Gingivitis**
Clinical attachment loss	Yes	Yes
Radiological bone loss	Yes	Yes

[a]Clinical attachment loss would be present on a reduced periodontium; however, bone loss may not be detectable on a radiograph.

Box 6-4. Plaque-Induced Gingivitis on an Intact Periodontium

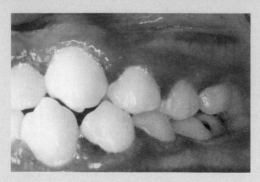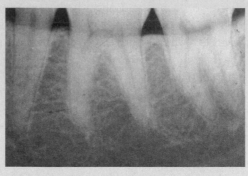

Figure 6-5. Plaque-Induced Gingivitis. Plaque-induced gingivitis on an intact periodontium in this patient has resulted in rolled gingival margins and enlarged papillae.

- Note how this plaque-induced gingivitis is affecting the interdental papilla and the marginal gingiva. This type of plaque-induced gingivitis would be classified as marginal gingivitis.
- The dental radiograph does not reveal any changes in either the alveolar bone height or the architecture and morphology of the alveolar bone.

Box 6-5. Plaque-Induced Gingivitis on a Reduced Periodontium in a Non-periodontitis Patient

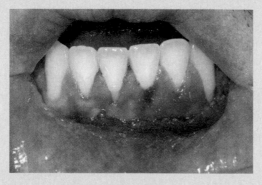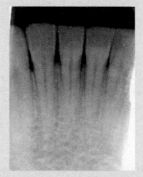

Figure 6-6. Plaque-Induced Gingivitis on a Reduced Periodontium in a Non-periodontitis Patient. On the clinical photograph, note all the visual signs of gingival inflammation, such as bleeding, swelling, and redness. This is a 17-year-old male patient who just completed orthodontic therapy to straighten teeth that were previously malaligned (crowded). The dental radiograph does not reveal any changes in either the alveolar bone height or the architecture and morphology of the alveolar bone.

- Orthodontists use different strategies to move teeth to an ideal alignment and position. However, one undesired consequence is that changes in the periodontal tissues may occur as a result of orthodontically induced movement of the teeth. This is apparent in cases where orthodontic therapy displaces the teeth in a buccal direction causing resorption of the overlying thin, delicate outer cortical plate. In the case above, post-orthodontic movement of the lower right central incisor and both canines have led to recession of the gingival margin (permanent loss of the marginal gingiva).
- Since the recession of the gingival margin is *not due to periodontitis*, the treatment objectives are to (1) remove the etiologic factors responsible for gingival inflammation, (2) reinforce oral hygiene, (3) avoid further loss of periodontal tissues (i.e., recession of the gingival margin), and (4) minimize the risk of the gingivitis converting into periodontitis.

Box 6-6. Plaque-Induced Gingivitis on a Reduced Periodontium in a Successfully Treated Periodontitis Case

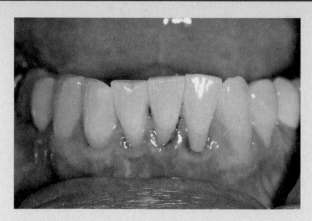
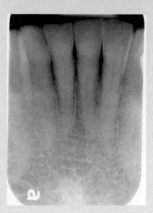

Figure 6-7. Plaque-Induced Gingivitis on a Reduced Periodontium in a Successfully Treated Stable Periodontitis Patient. This is a 68-year-old female patient who was successfully treated in the past for periodontitis. The dental radiograph reveals loss of alveolar bone height.

- By performing a comprehensive periodontal examination and comparing the present information with previous periodontal findings (such as past probing depths, CAL, bleeding upon probing scores, etc.), it is apparent that the periodontitis is not ongoing, but rather arrested (no additional loss of alveolar bone or connective tissue).
- However, note the visual signs of gingival inflammation—such as thickened marginal gingiva and slight gingival bleeding from the lower left incisors.
- In such a case, the treatment objectives are to (1) maintain the reduced periodontium in a healthy and stable state by removing the etiologic agents, (2) reinforce patient self-care and professional care to prevent the reactivation of periodontitis.

MODIFYING FACTORS OF PLAQUE-INDUCED GINGIVITIS

Several modifying factors may play a role in exacerbating the host inflammatory response to the plaque biofilm. These modifying factors can be subdivided into systemic factors that alter the host response to plaque biofilm or oral factors that contribute to increased plaque retention.

1. **Systemic Conditions as Modifying Factors**
    A. **Sex and Steroid Hormones.** The maintenance of a healthy balance within the periodontium involves a complex relationship with the endocrine system. Evidence suggests that tissue responses in the periodontium are influenced by the levels of sex hormones present at one time or another throughout a person's life cycle.[18,19] *The following conditions may modify plaque-induced gingivitis but are not considered diagnoses in and of themselves.*
        1. Puberty
            a. The dramatic rise in steroid hormone levels during puberty has a temporary effect on the inflammatory status of the gingiva.[18,19]
            b. Studies demonstrate an increase in gingival inflammation around the time of puberty in both genders.[20,21]

    c. Puberty-associated gingivitis has many of the clinical features of plaque-induced gingivitis; however, it is distinguished by clinical signs of *gingival inflammation in the presence of relatively small amounts of plaque biofilm.*[2] Thus, puberty-associated gingivitis is characterized by an exaggerated inflammatory response of the gingiva to a relatively small amount of plaque biofilm around the time of puberty. Figure 6-8 shows one example of puberty-associated gingivitis.

2. Menstrual Cycle

    a. Most clinical studies show there to be only modest observable inflammatory changes in the gingiva during ovulation.[20,21]

    b. Although there may be a few women who are extremely sensitive to hormonal changes in the gingiva during the menstrual cycle, in most women there will be no clinically evident inflammatory changes to the gingiva.[22–24]

3. Pregnancy

    a. During pregnancy, the levels of estrogen and progesterone continue to rise and reach their peak in the eighth month of gestation. High levels in both blood and saliva cause an exaggerated tissue response to plaque biofilm. Increased quantities of hormones also trigger gingival crevicular fluid flow, which may precipitate gingival inflammation.

    b. Gingival inflammation is significantly higher in the pregnant patient in response to even relatively small amounts of plaque biofilm and bleeding on probing or with toothbrushing is also increased.[3,25–28] Figure 6-9 shows a case of gingivitis associated with pregnancy.

    c. Gingivitis associated with pregnancy can spontaneously resolve postpartum.

    d. In some cases, a gingival papilla can react so strongly to plaque biofilm that a large, localized overgrowth of gingival tissue called a **pregnancy-associated pyogenic granuloma** (pregnancy tumor), may form on the interdental gingiva or on the gingival margin.[29]

        1) This condition is the result of an exaggerated tissue response to plaque biofilm or other irritants that usually occurs after the first trimester of pregnancy.

        2) The gingival mass is characterized by a mushroom-like tissue mass that most commonly occurs in the maxilla and interproximally (Fig. 6-10).

        3) A pregnancy-associated pyogenic granuloma is painless and noncancerous. However, if it grows to interfere with occlusion, painful ulceration of the pyogenic granuloma may occur.

        4) The tissue mass bleeds easily if disturbed and may appear to be covered with dark red pinpoint markings.

        5) The growth usually resolves after childbirth. Even though the growth spontaneously resolves after childbirth, the granuloma can be completely eliminated during the pregnancy stage by removing the plaque biofilm responsible for the enlargement.

4. Oral Contraceptives

    a. Early conceptive agents had high hormone concentrations that were associated with gingival inflammation.

    b. Current oral contraceptive concentrations are much lower than the original doses and current formulations of oral contraceptives do not induce clinical changes in the gingiva.[18,19,30]

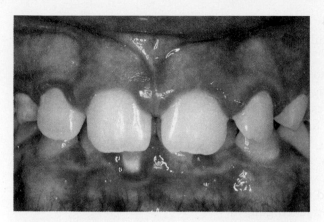

Figure 6-8. Gingivitis Associated with Puberty. Gingivitis associated with puberty is an exaggerated inflammatory response of the gingiva to a relatively small amount of plaque biofilm. The exaggerated response is modulated by hormones released during puberty. (Courtesy of Dr. Richard Foster, Guilford Technical Community College, Jamestown, NC.)

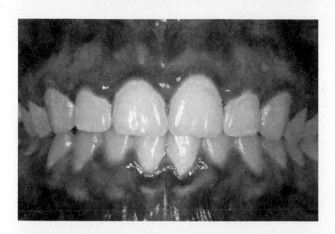

Figure 6-9. Gingivitis Associated with Pregnancy. Note the red gingiva and bulbous interdental papilla on this patient with gingivitis that is associated with pregnancy. (Courtesy of Dr. Richard Foster, Guilford Technical Community College, Jamestown, NC.)

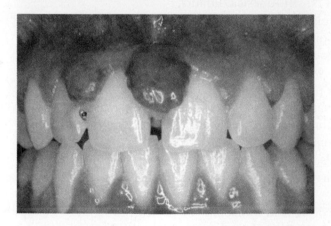

Figure 6-10. Pregnancy-Associated Pyogenic Granuloma. This mushroom-like mass of the gingiva bleeds easily if disturbed.

B. **Hyperglycemia.** Hyperglycemia is the presence of an abnormally high concentration of glucose in the circulating blood that occurs especially in individuals with diabetes mellitus.
   1. Gingivitis is often seen in children with poorly controlled diabetes mellitus.
   2. The level of glycemic control may be more important in determining the severity of the gingival inflammation than the amount of plaque biofilm present.[31,32] In other words, the inflammatory response of the gingiva to plaque biofilm is exacerbated by the high blood glucose levels.
C. **Leukemia.** Leukemia is cancer of the body's blood-forming tissues, including the bone marrow and the lymphatic system. Leukemia usually involves the white blood cells. In people with leukemia, the bone marrow produces abnormal white

blood cells, which do not function properly. Many types of leukemia exist. Some forms of leukemia are more common in children. Other forms of leukemia occur mostly in adults.

1. Gingivitis associated with leukemia is an exaggerated inflammatory response of the gingiva to plaque biofilm resulting in increased bleeding and tissue enlargement. Oral lesions may be the first clinical signs of leukemia; therefore, dental health care providers can be the first to suspect that a patient may have leukemia.
2. Gingival tissues appear swollen, spongy, shiny, and red to deep purple in appearance.[33,34] Figure 6-11 shows an example of gingivitis associated with leukemia. Typically, leukemia-associated gingivitis begins in the papillae and spreads to the marginal and then, the attached gingiva.
3. Tissues are very friable (tear easily) and tend to bleed with slight provocation.
4. Although plaque biofilm can exacerbate the gingival response to leukemia, the presence of biofilm is *NOT* a prerequisite for gingivitis in patients with leukemia.[33]

D. Smoking
1. Epidemiologic studies indicate that smoking is one of the major lifestyle risk factors for periodontal disease.[35]
2. Plaque biofilm accumulation and disease progression are exacerbated in smokers. Gingival fibrosis—the formation of an abnormal amount of fibrous tissue—is often observed in smokers.[36]
3. *Smokers have fewer clinical signs and symptoms of gingival inflammation than nonsmokers.*[36–39] Therefore, clinicians should be aware that smoking can mask gingivitis.

E. Malnutrition
1. Even with our adequate food supply in North America, infants, institutionalized individuals, and alcoholics are all at risk for vitamin deficiencies. However, the precise relationship between nutrition and periodontal disease is not fully understood.
2. The one nutritional deficiency that has well-documented effects on the periodontium involves the depletion of plasma ascorbic acid (vitamin C).
   a. Vitamin C—a substance found in many fruits and vegetables—is essential for the formation of collagen and fibrous tissue for normal intercellular matrices in teeth, bone, cartilage, connective tissue, and skin, and for the structural integrity of capillary walls.
   b. A lack of vitamin C can lead to scurvy, or less severe conditions, such as delayed healing of wounds.
3. Gingivitis associated with declining ascorbic acid levels may be difficult to detect clinically, and when it is detected, it usually has characteristics similar to plaque-induced gingivitis. Figure 6-12 shows an example of gingivitis in a patient with scurvy.

2. **Oral Factors That Enhance Plaque Biofilm Accumulation**
   A. **Prominent Subgingival Restoration Margins**
   1. A 26-year longitudinal study confirms that dental restorations margins placed apical to the gingival margin are detrimental to gingival health.
      a. The margins of prominent subgingival restorations promote gingivitis by increasing the local accumulation of bacterial plaque biofilms. Therefore, subgingival restoration margins need to be carefully designed in order to minimize biofilm retention.

B. **Hyposalivation**
   1. Hyposalivation—a decreased flow of saliva—may be caused by some health conditions/diseases such as Sjögren syndrome, anxiety, and poorly controlled diabetes. In addition, it is frequently observed as a side effect of medications, such as antihistamines, decongestants, antidepressant, and antihypertensive medications.
   2. Hyposalivation may cause progressive dental caries, taste disorders, halitosis, and inflammation of the oral mucosa, tongue, and gingiva.[40,41] Dryness of the mouth may make patient self-care more difficult and worsen gingival inflammation.

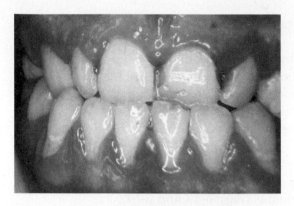

Figure 6-11. Gingivitis in an Adult with Leukemia. Note the red, swollen appearance of the gingiva in this patient with leukemia. (Courtesy of Dr. Ralph Arnold.)

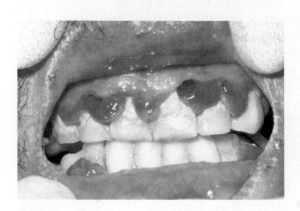

Figure 6-12. Ascorbic Acid-Deficiency Gingivitis. A photograph of a patient with scurvy. Scurvy is the clinical state arising from dietary deficiency of vitamin C (ascorbic acid). Note the bright red, swollen, and ulcerated gingival tissue. (Courtesy of Mediscan Company.)

DRUG-INFLUENCED GINGIVAL ENLARGEMENTS

1. **Drug-influenced gingival enlargements** are an increase in size of the gingiva associated with certain systemic medications, most commonly anticonvulsants, calcium channel blockers, and immunosuppressants.
   A. **Medications Associated with Gingival Enlargement**
      1. Anticonvulsants (e.g., Phenytoin, Celontin, Depakote). Anticonvulsants are used to manage epileptic seizures. In addition, some anticonvulsants are now used in the treatment of bipolar disorder.
      2. Immunosuppressants (e.g., cyclosporine). Immunosuppressant drugs suppress the natural immune responses. Immunosuppressants are given to transplant patients to prevent organ rejection or to patients with autoimmune diseases. The immunosuppressant stimulates fibroblast proliferation with excessive extracellular matrix accumulation in gingival tissues.[20]
      3. Calcium Channel Blocking Agents (e.g., amlodipine, nifedipine, verapamil). Calcium channel blocking agents relax the blood vessels and increase the supply of blood and oxygen to the heart while reducing its workload. Some

of the calcium channel blocking agents are used to relieve and control angina pectoris (chest pain). Some are also used to treat high blood pressure (hypertension). These drugs affect gingival connective tissues by stimulating an increase of fibroblasts and increasing the production of connective tissue matrix.

B. **Etiology**
   1. For drug-influenced gingival conditions, plaque biofilms in conjunction with the drug are necessary to produce gingival enlargements.
   2. However, not all individuals who take these medications will develop enlargements of the gingival tissues.

2. **Common Characteristics of Drug-Influenced Gingival Enlargements**
   A. **Onset of Tissue Enlargements**
      1. The onset of tissue enlargement usually occurs within 3 months of medication use. The severity of overgrowth is directly affected by level of patient self-care; scrupulous patient self-care can reduce the severity of the overgrowth but may not eliminate it.
      2. There is a higher prevalence of drug-influenced gingival enlargements in younger age groups.
   B. **Clinical Appearance**
      1. Gingival tissues in anterior sextants are most commonly affected, however, tissue enlargements can occur in posterior sextants (Figs. 6-13 and 6-14).
      2. The pattern of tissue enlargement is irregular, usually first observed in the papillae, beginning as a painless area of enlargement on the papilla and then proceeding to the marginal gingiva.
      3. Gingival enlargement is characterized by an increased flow of crevicular fluid from the sulcus and bleeding upon probing with no attachment loss.

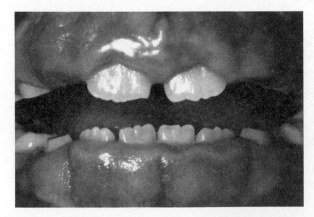

Figure 6-13. Phenytoin-Induced Gingival Enlargement. Massive-tissue overgrowth may be seen in phenytoin-induced gingival enlargement.

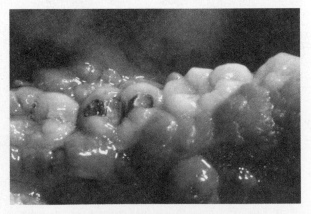

Figure 6-14. Cyclosporine-Induced Gingival Enlargement. Gingival changes seen in cyclosporine-induced gingival enlargement.

Section 3
Non–Plaque-Induced Gingival Diseases

A small percentage of gingival diseases—non–plaque-induced gingival diseases—are not caused by plaque biofilm and do not resolve after plaque biofilm removal. *It should be emphasized, however, that the presence of plaque biofilm could increase the severity of the gingival inflammation in non–plaque-induced lesions.*

Although non–plaque-induced gingival diseases are less common, these conditions are often painful and of major significance for patients. This section presents some examples of the small percentage of gingival disease in which plaque biofilm does not play a primary etiologic role. The 2017 classification scheme for non–plaque-induced gingival diseases and conditions is outlined in Table 6-3.

TABLE 6-3	CLASSIFICATION OF NON–PLAQUE-INDUCED GINGIVAL DISEASES AND CONDITIONS

1. **Genetic/developmental disorders**
   1.1 Hereditary gingival fibromatosis (HGF)
2. **Specific infections**
   2.1 Bacterial origin
   - Necrotizing periodontal diseases (*Treponema* spp., *Selenomonas* spp., *Fusobacterium* spp., *Prevotella intermedia*, and others)
   - *Neisseria gonorrhoeae* (gonorrhea)
   - *Treponema pallidum* (syphilis)
   - *Mycobacterium tuberculosis* (tuberculosis)
   - Streptococcal gingivitis (strains of streptococcus)

   2.2 Viral origin
   - Coxsackie virus (hand-foot-and-mouth disease)
   - Herpes simplex 1/2 (primary or recurrent)
   - Varicella-zoster virus (chicken pox or shingles affecting V nerve)
   - Molluscum contagiosum virus
   - Human papilloma virus (squamous cell papilloma, condyloma acuminatum, verruca vulgaris, and focal epithelial hyperplasia)

   2.3 Fungal
   - Candidosis
   - Other mycoses (e.g., histoplasmosis, aspergillosis)
3. **Inflammatory and immune conditions and lesions**
   3.1 Hypersensitivity reactions
   - Contact allergy
   - Plasma cell gingivitis
   - Erythema multiforme

   3.2 Autoimmune diseases of skin and mucous membranes
   - Pemphigus vulgaris
   - Pemphigoid
   - Lichen planus
   - Lupus erythematosus

   3.3 Granulomatous inflammatory conditions (orofacial granulomatosis)
   - Crohn's disease
   - Sarcoidosis

(continued)

TABLE 6-3	**CLASSIFICATION OF NON–PLAQUE-INDUCED GINGIVAL DISEASES AND CONDITIONS (*Continued*)**

4. **Reactive processes**
   4.1 Epulides
     • Fibrous epulis
     • Calcifying fibroblastic granuloma
     • Pyogenic granuloma (vascular epulis)
     • Peripheral giant cell granuloma (or central)

5. **Neoplasms**
   5.1 Premalignant
     • Leukoplakia
     • Erythroplakia
   5.2 Malignant
     • Squamous cell carcinoma
     • Leukemia
     • Lymphoma

6. **Endocrine, nutritional, and metabolic diseases**
   6.1 Vitamin deficiencies
     • Vitamin C deficiency (scurvy)

7. **Traumatic lesions**
   7.1 Physical/mechanical insults
     • Frictional keratosis
     • Toothbrushing-induced gingival ulceration
     • Factitious injury (self-harm)
   7.2 Chemical (toxic) insults
     • Etching
     • Chlorhexidine
     • Acetylsalicylic acid
     • Cocaine
     • Hydrogen peroxide
     • Dentifrice detergents
     • Paraformaldehyde or calcium hydroxide
   7.3 Thermal insults
     • Burns of mucosa

8. **Gingival pigmentation**
     • Gingival pigmentation/melanoplakia
     • Smoker's melanosis
     • Drug-induced pigmentation (antimalarials; minocycline)
     • Amalgam tattoo

DESCRIPTION OF SELECTED DISEASE DISORDERS

1. Genetic/Developmental Abnormalities

   A. **Hereditary Gingival Fibromatosis.** Hereditary gingival fibromatosis is a rare benign oral condition characterized by slow and progressive enlargement of both maxillary and mandibular attached gingiva. One example of a patient with hereditary gingival fibromatosis is pictured in Figure 6-15.[42] It may develop as an isolated disorder but can feature along with a syndrome. Compared to drug-related gingival overgrowth, hereditary gingival fibromatosis is a rare disease.

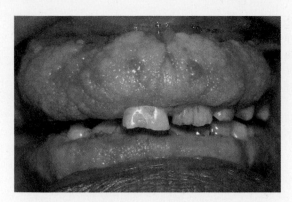

Figure 6-15. Hereditary Gingival Fibromatosis. A patient with gingival overgrowth of hereditary gingival fibromatosis.

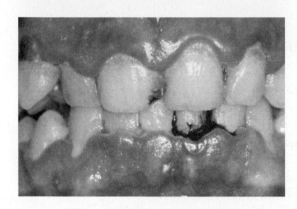

Figure 6-16. Necrotizing Gingivitis. This periodontal infection is characterized by a sudden onset, pain, and necrosis of interdental papillae (cratered, punched-out papillae).

2. **Infections of Bacterial Origin**
   A. **Necrotizing Periodontal Disease**
      1. Necrotizing gingivitis, necrotizing periodontitis, and necrotizing stomatitis are severe inflammatory periodontal diseases caused by bacterial infection in patients with specific underlying risk factors (poor oral self-care, smoking, stress, poor nutrition, compromised immune status). Necrotizing periodontal disease is the term encompassing necrotizing gingivitis, necrotizing periodontitis, and necrotizing stomatitis.
      2. Necrotizing gingivitis involves only gingival tissue and is characterized by no loss of periodontal attachment.[43]
      3. The clinical appearance of necrotizing periodontal disease is noticeably different than that of any other periodontal disease. Necrotizing periodontal disease is characterized by ulcerated and necrotic papillae and gingival margins, giving the appearance that the papillae and gingival margins have been "punched-out" or "cratered" (Fig. 6-16).
      4. Detailed content on necrotizing periodontal disease is found in Chapter 8, Other Periodontal Conditions.
   B. **Other Bacterial Infections.** Non–plaque-associated bacterial infections of the gingiva are uncommon. Gingival diseases in this category are characterized by a bacterial infection of the gingiva by a specific bacterium that is ***not commonly found*** in a typical bacterial plaque biofilm.
      1. Gingival diseases of specific bacterial origin occur on rare occasions when a bacterial infection overwhelms the host resistance. Examples include infections with *Neisseria gonorrhoeae*, *Treponema pallidum*, and streptococcal species.[44]
      2. The gingival lesions manifest as painful ulcerations, chancres or mucous patches, or atypical gingival inflammation (Fig. 6-17).

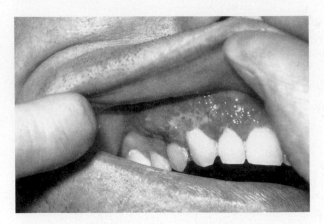

Figure 6-17. Atypical Mycobacterial Infection. This patient has an atypical bacterial infection of the gingiva. The fingers shown in this photograph are the patient's own. (Courtesy of Mediscan Company.)

DESCRIPTION OF SELECTED INFLAMMATORY AND IMMUNE CONDITIONS AND LESIONS

1. **Hypersensitivity Reactions: Intraoral Allergic Reactions.** Intraoral allergic reactions can be caused by ingredients in toothpastes, mouthwashes, or chewing gum.[45,46] These reactions are usually the result of a flavor additive or preservatives in the product. Flavor additives known to cause gingival reactions are cinnamon and carvone.
   A. **Occurrence of Intraoral Allergic Reactions**
      1. Allergic reactions occur most commonly in patients who have a history of allergic conditions such as hay fever, allergic skin rashes, or asthma.
      2. Allergic patients seem to be particularly sensitive to the flavoring agent. The flavoring agent in toothpastes and mouthwashes is usually the most allergenic component.
   B. **Clinical Manifestations.** The clinical manifestations of allergy are a diffuse fiery red gingivitis sometimes with ulcerations (Fig. 6-18).
   C. **Recognition and Treatment of Allergic Reaction**
      1. The dental clinician might suspect an intraoral allergic reaction in a patient with good self-care who previously has had healthy gingiva (especially if the patient has a history of allergies). The dental clinician should inquire if the patient is using a new toothpaste, mouthwash, or chewing gum.
      2. Advise the patient to change brands or flavors of gum, toothpaste, or mouthwash. Cessation of the allergen-containing product should result in a resolution of gingival inflammation.
      3. If necessary, the diagnosis of allergic response can be confirmed by a biopsy with a diagnosis of plasma cell gingivitis.
      4. When the manufacturer becomes aware of allergic reactions, the flavoring agent or additive causing the problem is usually altered. For this reason, the patient sometimes can switch back to the original product (after 6 to 12 months) and use it without problem.
2. **Erythema Multiforme**
   A. **Disease Characteristics**
      1. Erythema multiforme is an uncommon acute immune inflammatory disorder of the skin and/or oral mucosa.[47] The characteristic hallmarks of this condition are large, symmetrical red blotches, resembling a target, that appear on the skin in a circular pattern.

2. On mucous membranes, it begins as blisters and progresses to ulcers (Fig. 6-19). Oral involvement occurs in as many as 25% to 60% of cases and is sometimes the only involved site.
3. The exact cause is unknown, though may involve a hypersensitivity reaction.

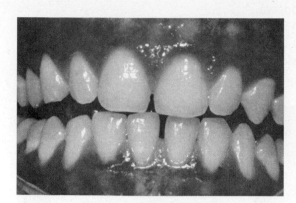

Figure 6-18. Allergic Reaction. Clinical signs of allergic reactions in the gingival tissues include redness extending from the gingival margin to the mucogingival junction.

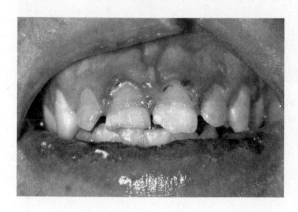

Figure 6-19. Erythema Multiforme. Erythema multiforme with ulcerations of the gingiva and crust formation of the lower lip. (Courtesy of Dr. Ralph Arnold, San Antonio, TX.)

3. **Oral Lichen Planus**
   A. **Disease Characteristics**
      1. Lichen planus (LIE-kun Play-nus) is a common inflammatory condition that can affect the skin, hair, nails, and mucous membranes.[48]
      2. On the skin, lichen planus usually appears as purplish, often itchy, flat-topped bumps, developing over several weeks. In the mouth and other areas covered by a mucous membrane, lichen planus forms lacy white patches, sometimes with painful sores. Figures 6-20 and 6-21 show two different presentations of lichen planus.
      3. The initial episode of oral lichen planus may last for weeks or months. Unfortunately, oral lichen planus is usually a chronic condition and can last for many years.
      4. *Symptoms usually can be managed, but people who have oral lichen planus need regular monitoring because they may be at risk of developing oral cancer in the affected areas. It is important to diagnose, treat, and follow patients through regular oral examinations.*[49,50]
      5. Good patient self-care can relieve the painful symptoms of the gingival lesions.[51]
   B. **Clinical Manifestations**
      1. Six types of clinical manifestations of oral lichen planus have been described: papular, reticular, plaque type, erythematous, ulcerative, and bulbous lesions.

    a. The reticular pattern is commonly found bilaterally on the buccal mucosa as lacy web-like, white threads that are slightly raised. These lines are sometimes referred to as Wickham's striae (Fig. 6-20).

    b. The ulcerative pattern can affect any mucosal surface, including the buccal mucosa, tongue, and gingiva. Ulcerative lichen planus is painful and associated with intense erythema of the gingiva.

2. Since the clinical appearance of lichen planus may mimic other types of non–plaque-induced gingival lesions, a biopsy and an oral pathology consultation will be required to determine the appropriate diagnosis.

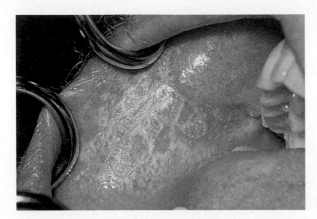

Figure 6-20. Lichen Planus of Buccal Mucosa. These delicate white lines arranged in a lacy web-like network are characteristic of the reticular pattern of lichen planus. (Used with permission from Langlais, RP, *Color Atlas of Common Oral Diseases*. Philadelphia, PA: Wolters Kluwer; 2016.)

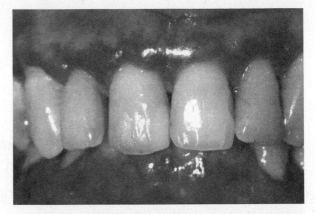

Figure 6-21. Oral Lichen Planus. Oral lichen planus of the maxillary gingiva. The gingival tissues are erythematous, ulcerated, and painful. (Courtesy of Dr. Ralph Arnold, San Antonio, TX.)

Chapter Summary Statement

This chapter reviews the criteria for periodontal health and gingival diseases/conditions as developed by the 2017 World Workshop on the Classification of Periodontal and Peri-Implant Diseases and Conditions. Periodontal health is defined as the absence of any clinical signs of inflammation. Periodontal health can occur on an intact periodontium, a reduced periodontium due to non-periodontitis reasons, or a reduced periodontium due to periodontitis.

    Plaque-induced gingivitis is the most common of the periodontal diseases. Clinically, plaque-induced gingivitis is characterized by gingiva that is red, swollen, bleeds easily, and is slightly tender. Gingival diseases are the mildest form of periodontal disease and patients with gingivitis can revert to a state of health. Like periodontal health, plaque-induced gingivitis can occur on an intact periodontium, reduced periodontium due to non-periodontitis reasons, or a reduced periodontium due to periodontitis. Plaque-induced gingivitis may also be modified by systemic factors, medications, or malnutrition.

    Non–plaque-induced gingival diseases are a group of uncommon gingival lesions that are *not caused by plaque biofilm*. Non–plaque-induced gingivitis can result from such diverse causes as bacterial, viral, or fungal infection, inflammatory conditions, allergic reactions, or trauma.

Section 4
Focus on Patients

Clinical Patient Care

CASE 1

You are scheduled to perform nonsurgical periodontal instrumentation on a patient with a diagnosis of localized severe plaque-induced gingivitis. At the time of the appointment, the patient informs you that she is pregnant. With this information in hand, what would be the most appropriate periodontal diagnosis?

CASE 2

A patient who has been cared for by your dental team suddenly exhibits poor self-care with quite a bit of plaque biofilm accumulation. This is unusual for this patient. Discussions reveal that the patient is having difficulty with brushing and flossing due to soreness of the mouth. Examination reveals numerous small mucosal ulcers. Further discussions reveal that the patient has been experiencing this soreness since she began using tartar control toothpaste. How might your dental team manage this patient's diminished effectiveness of self-care?

CASE 3

Your patient is a 12-year-old male, who despite good oral hygiene practices, presents with generalized marginal redness and bleeding upon probing. His demonstration of toothbrushing and flossing indicates high dexterity and an ability to remove plaque biofilm. In talking with his mother, she confirms that he practices daily oral hygiene. How would you explain the presence of gingival disease to this patient and what would you recommend to improve his gingival health?

CASE 4

Your patient reports a change in his medical history from last visit; he is now taking Depakote as a mood stabilizer. The drug reference manual states it is an anticonvulsant and may cause gingival enlargement. How will this new information alter your plan for dental hygiene care and patient education?

Ethical Dilemma

Lily E, a 17-year-old high school senior, who is a routine 6-month recall patient, is your first patient of the afternoon. She received her driver's license 3 months ago and has driven herself to today's appointment. You review her medical history, and she states there are *"no changes and that she has no chief complaint."*

As you are performing your intraoral examination, you notice that the tissue between the maxillary central incisors does not appear to be normal. You observe a mushroom-shaped gingival mass projecting from the gingival papilla. It appears red, and bleeds easily upon digital palpation. You ask Lily if it bothers her, but she denies any discomfort. She also states that she was not aware of any problem.

You are concerned that the lesion may be a pyogenic granuloma associated with pregnancy. You would like to discuss the possible implication of this lesion with Lily, but you are not sure how to proceed.

1. What is the best way for you to handle this ethical dilemma?
2. What is the best way to address/discuss Lily's treatment plan with her?
3. Under the ethical principle of confidentiality, can you discuss this with your employer dentist, without violating Lily's confidentiality?
4. Do you have the right to divulge your findings and concerns to her parents?
5. Can a 17-year-old consent to treatment, or must you receive parental consent?

References

1. Chapple ILC, Mealey BL, Van Dyke TE, et al. Periodontal health and gingival diseases and conditions on an intact and a reduced periodontium: Consensus report of workgroup 1 of the 2017 World Workshop on the Classification of Periodontal and Peri-Implant Diseases and Conditions. *J Periodontol.* 2018;89 Suppl 1:S74–S84.
2. Murakami S, Mealey BL, Mariotti A, Chapple ILC. Dental plaque-induced gingival conditions. *J Periodontol.* 2018;89 Suppl 1:S17–S27.
3. Loe H, Theilade E, Jensen SB. Experimental gingivitis in man. *J Periodontol.* 1965;36:177–187.
4. Tonetti MS, Chapple IL, Jepsen S, Sanz M. Primary and secondary prevention of periodontal and peri-implant diseases: Introduction to, and objectives of the 11th European Workshop on Periodontology consensus conference. *J Clin Periodontol.* 2015;42 Suppl 16:S1–S4.
5. Burt B, Research, Science and Therapy Committee of the American Academy of Periodontology. Position paper: epidemiology of periodontal diseases. *J Periodontol.* 2005;76(8):1406–1419.
6. Dye BA. Global periodontal disease epidemiology. *Periodontol 2000.* 2012;58(1):10–25.
7. Trombelli L, Scapoli C, Orlandini E, Tosi M, Bottega S, Tatakis DN. Modulation of clinical expression of plaque-induced gingivitis. III. Response of "high responders" and "low responders" to therapy. *J Clin Periodontol.* 2004;31(4):253–259.
8. American Academy of Periodontology—Research, Science and Therapy Committee. Periodontal diseases of children and adolescents. *Pediatric Dent.* 2008;30(7 Suppl):240–247.
9. Hamadneh N, Khan WA, Sathasivam S, Ong HC. Design optimization of pin fin geometry using particle swarm optimization algorithm. *PLoS One.* 2013;8(5):e66080.
10. Matsson L, Goldberg P. Gingival inflammatory reaction in children at different ages. *J Clin Periodontol.* 1985;12(2):98–103.
11. Yang NY, Zhang Q, Li JL, Yang SH, Shi Q. Progression of periodontal inflammation in adolescents is associated with increased number of Porphyromonas gingivalis, Prevotella intermedia, Tannerella forsythensis, and Fusobacterium nucleatum. *Int J Paediatr Dent* 2014;24(3):226–233.
12. Bimstein E, Matsson L. Growth and development considerations in the diagnosis of gingivitis and periodontitis in children. *Pediatric Dent.* 1999;21(3):186–1891.
13. Gafan GP, Lucas VS, Roberts GJ, Petrie A, Wilson M, Spratt DA. Prevalence of periodontal pathogens in dental plaque of children. *J Clin Microbiol.* 2004;42(9):4141–4116.
14. Fransson C, Berglundh T, Lindhe J. The effect of age on the development of gingivitis. Clinical, microbiological and histological findings. *J Clin Periodontol.* 1996;23(4):379–385.
15. Fransson C, Mooney J, Kinane DF, Berglundh T. Differences in the inflammatory response in young and old human subjects during the course of experimental gingivitis. *J Clin Periodontol.* 1999;26(7):453–460.
16. Suzuki JB. Diagnosis and classification of the periodontal diseases. *Dent Clin North Am.* 1988;32(2):195–216.
17. Heasman PA, McCracken GI, Steen N. Supportive periodontal care: the effect of periodic subgingival debridement compared with supragingival prophylaxis with respect to clinical outcomes. *J Clin Periodontol.* 2002;29 Suppl 3:163–172; discussion 95–96.
18. Mariotti A. Sex steroid hormones and cell dynamics in the periodontium. *Crit Rev Oral Biol Med.* 1994;5(1):27–53.
19. Mariotti A, Mawhinney M. Endocrinology of sex steroid hormones and cell dynamics in the periodontium. *Periodontol 2000.* 2013;61(1):69–88.

20. Hefti A, Engelberger T, Buttner M. Gingivitis in Basel schoolchildren. *SSO Schweiz Monatsschr Zahnheilkd.* 1981;91(12):1087–1092.

21. Sutcliffe P. A longitudinal study of gingivitis and puberty. *J Periodontal Res.* 1972;7(1):52–58.

22. Baser U, Cekici A, Tanrikulu-Kucuk S, Kantarci A, Ademoglu E, Yalcin F. Gingival inflammation and interleukin-1 beta and tumor necrosis factor-alpha levels in gingival crevicular fluid during the menstrual cycle. *J Periodontol.* 2009;80(12):1983–1990.

23. Becerik S, Ozcaka O, Nalbantsoy A, et al. Effects of menstrual cycle on periodontal health and gingival crevicular fluid markers. *J Periodontol.* 2010;81(5):673–681.

24. Shourie V, Dwarakanath CD, Prashanth GV, Alampalli RV, Padmanabhan S, Bali S. The effect of menstrual cycle on periodontal health—a clinical and microbiological study. *Oral Health Prev Dent.* 2012;10(2):185–192.

25. Arafat AH. Periodontal status during pregnancy. *J Periodontol.* 1974;45(8):641–643.

26. Figuero E, Carrillo-de-Albornoz A, Martin C, Tobias A, Herrera D. Effect of pregnancy on gingival inflammation in systemically healthy women: a systematic review. *J Clin Periodontol.* 2013;40(5):457–473.

27. Hugoson A. Gingivitis in pregnant women. A longitudinal clinical study. *Odontol Revy.* 1971;22(1):65–84.

28. Loe H, Silness J. Periodontal Disease in Pregnancy. I. Prevalence and Severity. *Acta Odontol Scand.* 1963;21:533–551.

29. Holmstrup P, Plemons J, Meyle J. Non-plaque-induced gingival diseases. *J Periodontol.* 2018;89 Suppl 1:S28–S45.

30. Preshaw PM. Oral contraceptives and the periodontium. *Periodontol 2000.* 2013;61(1):125–159.

31. Cianciola LJ, Park BH, Bruck E, Mosovich L, Genco RJ. Prevalence of periodontal disease in insulin-dependent diabetes mellitus (juvenile diabetes). *J Am Dent Assoc.* 1982;104(5):653–660.

32. Gusberti FA, Syed SA, Bacon G, Grossman N, Loesche WJ. Puberty gingivitis in insulin-dependent diabetic children. I. Cross-sectional observations. *J Periodontol.* 1983;54(12):714–720.

33. Dreizen S, McCredie KB, Keating MJ. Chemotherapy-associated oral hemorrhages in adults with acute leukemia. *Oral Surg Oral Med Oral Pathol.* 1984;57(5):494–498.

34. Lynch MA, Ship II. Initial oral manifestations of leukemia. *J Am Dent Assoc.* 1967;75(4):932–940.

35. Ryder MI. The influence of smoking on host responses in periodontal infections. *Periodontol 2000.* 2007;43:267–277.

36. Scott DA, Singer DL. Suppression of overt gingival inflammation in tobacco smokers—clinical and mechanistic considerations. *Int J Dent Hyg.* 2004;2(3):104–110.

37. Nociti FH, Jr., Casati MZ, Duarte PM. Current perspective of the impact of smoking on the progression and treatment of periodontitis. *Periodontol 2000.* 2015;67(1):187–210.

38. Peruzzo DC, Gimenes JH, Taiete T, et al. Impact of smoking on experimental gingivitis. A clinical, microbiological and immunological prospective study. *J Periodontal Res.* 2016;51(6):800–811.

39. Tatakis DN, Trombelli L. Modulation of clinical expression of plaque-induced gingivitis. I. Background review and rationale. *J Clin Periodontol.* 2004;31(4):229–238.

40. Mizutani S, Ekuni D, Tomofuji T, et al. Relationship between xerostomia and gingival condition in young adults. *J Periodontal Res.* 2015;50(1):74–79.

41. Wagaiyu EG, Ashley FP. Mouthbreathing, lip seal and upper lip coverage and their relationship with gingival inflammation in 11–14 year-old schoolchildren. *J Clin Periodontol.* 1991;18(9):698–702.

42. Dhadse PV, Yeltiwar RK, Pandilwar PK, Gosavi SR. Hereditary gingival fibromatosis. *J Indian Soc Periodontol.* 2012;16(4):606–609.

43. Riley C, London JP, Burmeister JA. Periodontal health in 200 HIV-positive patients. *J Oral Pathol Med.* 1992;21(3):124–127.

44. Rivera-Hidalgo F, Stanford TW. Oral mucosal lesions caused by infective microorganisms. I. Viruses and bacteria. *Periodontol 2000.* 1999;21:106–1024.

45. Calapai G, Miroddi M, Mannucci C, Minciullo P, Gangemi S. Oral adverse reactions due to cinnamon-flavoured chewing gums consumption. *Oral Dis.* 2014;20(7):637–643.

46. Skaare A, Kjaerheim V, Barkvoll P, Rolla G. Skin reactions and irritation potential of four commercial toothpastes. *Acta Odontol Scand.* 1997;55(2):133–136.

47. Shah SN, Chauhan GR, Manjunatha BS, Dagrus K. Drug induced erythema multiforme: two case series with review of literature. *J Clin Diagn Res.* 2014;8(9):ZH01–ZH04.

48. Camacho-Alonso F, Lopez-Jornet P, Bermejo-Fenoll A. Gingival involvement of oral lichen planus. *J Periodontol.* 2007;78(4):640–644.

49. Ingafou M, Leao JC, Porter SR, Scully C. Oral lichen planus: a retrospective study of 690 British patients. *Oral Dis.* 2006;12(5):463–468.

50. Mignogna MD, Fedele S, Lo Russo L, Mignogna C, de Rosa G, Porter SR. Field cancerization in oral lichen planus. *Eur J Surg Oncol.* 2007;33(3):383–389.

51. Stone SJ, McCracken GI, Heasman PA, Staines KS, Pennington M. Cost-effectiveness of personalized plaque control for managing the gingival manifestations of oral lichen planus: a randomized controlled study. *J Clin Periodontol.* 2013;40(9):859–867.

CHAPTER

7 Periodontitis

Clinical Application. In 2017, the American Academy of Periodontology (AAP) and the European Federation of Periodontology (EFP) developed a new worldwide classification scheme for periodontal and peri-implant diseases and conditions. Included in the new classification scheme is the category called "periodontitis." All dental health care providers are involved in recognizing this disease and in providing care designed to bring this disease under control. An understanding of the features and behavior of periodontitis is absolutely essential for every member of the dental team. This chapter only presents information on periodontitis. Chapter 8 discusses uncommon forms of periodontitis.

Learning Objectives

- In a clinical setting for a patient with periodontitis, describe to your clinical instructor the clinical signs of disease present in the patient's mouth.
- Define the term *clinical attachment loss* and explain its significance in the periodontal disease process.
- In the clinical setting, explain to your patient the warning signs of periodontal disease.
- Recognize and describe clinical and radiographic features of periodontitis.
- Describe the change or advancement—disease progression—typically seen in periodontitis.
- Explain how disease severity and complexity of management play a role in determining staging of periodontitis.
- List the primary criteria used to determine the grade of periodontitis.
- Define the meaning of the descriptors *recurrent* and *refractory* as they pertain to periodontitis.

Key Terms

Periodontitis	Site-specific	Pathophysiology
Clinical attachment loss	Compromised periodontal	Stage
Extent	maintenance	Grade
Localized	Recurrent form	Grade modifiers
Generalized	Refractory form	
Disease progression	Periodontitis case	

Section 1
Periodontitis

As discussed in Chapter 3, periodontitis is a bacterial infection of all parts of the periodontium including the gingiva, periodontal ligament, bone, and cementum. The tissue damage that occurs in periodontitis results in irreversible destruction to the tissues of the periodontium. As depicted in Figure 7-1, the AAP/EFP 2017 Classification of Periodontal and Peri-Implant Diseases and Conditions subdivides the category of periodontitis into three major forms.[1] This chapter discusses periodontitis. Content on necrotizing periodontal diseases is presented in Chapter 8, Other Conditions Affecting the Periodontium and periodontitis as a manifestation of systemic disease is discussed in Chapter 16, Systemic Risk Factors that Amplify Susceptibility to Periodontal Disease.

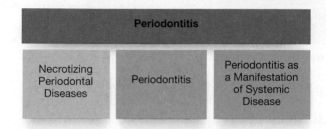

Figure 7-1. Three Major Forms of Periodontitis. The AAP/EFP 2017 Classification of Periodontal and Peri-Implant Diseases and Conditions subdivides the category of periodontitis into three major forms: necrotizing periodontal disease, periodontitis, and periodontitis as a manifestation of systemic disease.

DEFINITION OF PERIODONTITIS

Periodontitis is a complex microbial infection that triggers a host-mediated inflammatory response within the periodontium, resulting in progressive destruction of the periodontal ligament and supporting alveolar bone.[2] Periodontitis affects all parts of the periodontium—mainly the gingiva, periodontal ligament, bone, and cementum. It is the result of a complex interaction between the plaque biofilm that accumulates on tooth surfaces and the body's efforts to fight this infection.

Periodontitis is the number one cause of tooth loss in adults.[3] Moreover, according to the U.S. Centers for Disease Control and Prevention, approximately 47.2% of adults above the age of 30 years suffer from periodontitis and as a result, periodontitis is considered as a significant public health problem.[4]

- Periodontitis begins as plaque-induced gingivitis. Plaque-induced gingivitis is a reversible condition that can revert to a state of health. If left untreated, however, gingivitis may progress into periodontitis.
- *On the other hand, periodontitis is an irreversible condition that results in loss of attachment and alveolar bone. A periodontitis patient remains a periodontitis patient for life—even following successful periodontal therapy—and requires life-long supportive care to prevent recurrence of disease.*[2]
- Figure 7-2 depicts the disease characteristics of periodontitis.

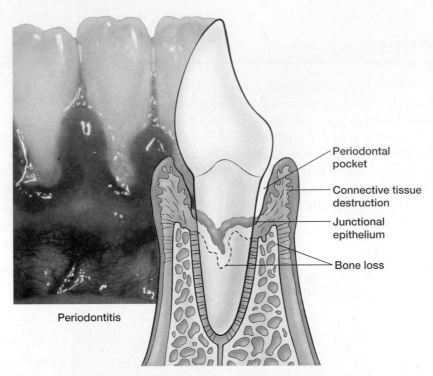

Periodontitis

Periodontal pocket

Connective tissue destruction

Junctional epithelium

Bone loss

Figure 7-2. Disease Characteristics of Periodontitis. Periodontitis is characterized by inflammation within the supporting tissues of the teeth, progressive destruction of the periodontal ligament, and loss of supporting alveolar bone.

CHARACTERISTICS OF PERIODONTITIS

1. **Alternative Terminology**
   - The 1999 disease classification subdivided periodontitis into two subgroups: chronic periodontitis and aggressive periodontitis.
   - Over the years, clinicians and researchers found it difficult to correctly differentiate between chronic and aggressive periodontitis.
   - There is little consistent evidence that aggressive and chronic periodontitis are different diseases, thus these two subdivisions were eliminated from the 2017 disease classification.[5,6]
   - *Since the 1999 disease classification was used for almost 20 years, however, much of the literature found in periodontal journals and textbooks uses the terminology "chronic periodontitis" and "aggressive periodontitis."*

2. **Signs and Symptoms of Periodontitis.** Clinical signs and symptoms of periodontitis include swelling, redness, gingival bleeding, periodontal pockets, bone loss, tooth mobility, suppuration (pus), moderate or heavy deposits of plaque biofilms and dental calculus. *However, the distinguishing features of periodontitis are the presence of alveolar bone loss and clinical attachment loss.*

   A. **Alterations in Color, Texture, and Size of the Marginal Gingiva**
      1. Reddish or Purplish Tissue. In periodontitis, the gingival tissue may appear bright red or purplish.
         a. In such cases, the clinical signs of periodontitis are very evident at the initial examination of the oral cavity. The gingiva appears swollen with the color ranging from pale red to magenta. Alterations in gingival contour and form are evident such as rolled gingival margins, blunted or flattened papillae.

  b. An example of periodontitis exhibiting this type of appearance is shown in Box 7-1, Figure 7-3A.

 2. Pale Pink Tissue. In periodontitis, the gingival tissue may appear pale pink and have an almost normal-looking appearance. An example of periodontitis exhibiting this type of appearance is shown in Box 7-1, Figure 7-3B.

  a. *The clinical appearance of the tissues is not a reliable indicator of the presence or severity of* **periodontitis.** Refer to Figures 7-4 to 7-6.

  b. In many patients, the changes in color, contour, and consistency may not be visible on inspection. At first glance, an inexperienced clinician may mistake the clinical appearance of periodontitis for one of health. Closer examination, however, will reveal firm, rigid (fibrotic) tissue, the presence of pocketing, and bleeding upon probing. Periodontitis exhibiting a fibrotic appearance is shown in Figure 7-6.

B. Bleeding, Crevicular Fluid, and Exudate

 1. Gingival bleeding is common, either spontaneous bleeding or bleeding in response to probing.

 2. Increased flow of gingival crevicular fluid or suppuration (pus) from periodontal pockets is common.

C. Plaque Biofilm and Calculus Deposits.

 1. Periodontitis is characterized by mature supra- and subgingival plaque biofilms and calculus deposits. Teeth with periodontitis usually have very complex and thick deposits of plaque biofilm on affected root surfaces.

 2. Although periodontitis is initiated and sustained by plaque biofilms, host factors determine the pathogenesis and rate of progression of the disease.

D. Loss of Attachment

 1. Clinical attachment loss is a measurement of the amount of destruction affecting tooth-supporting structures that have been destroyed around a tooth. Loss of attachment occurs in periodontitis and is characterized by (1) apical migration (relocation) of the junctional epithelium to the tooth root, (2) destruction of the fibers of the gingiva, (3) destruction of the periodontal ligament fibers, and (4) loss of alveolar bone support from around the tooth. The changes that occur in the alveolar bone in periodontal disease are significant because loss of bone height eventually can result in tooth loss.

 2. Clinical attachment loss of 1 to 2 mm at one or several sites can be found in nearly all members of the adult population.

 3. Clinical characteristics of attachment loss may include:

  a. Loss of alveolar bone support to the teeth

  b. Periodontal pockets or recession of the gingival margin

  c. Furcation involvement in multirooted teeth (Fig.7-7)

  d. Tooth mobility and/or drifting

 4. The loss of gingival/periodontal ligament fibers and alveolar bone is detected as clinical attachment loss by assessment of the dentition with a periodontal probe as measured from the cementoenamel junction (CEJ). Clinical attachment loss commonly is abbreviated as CAL. It has been well established that the extent of probe penetration is influenced by the inflammatory status of the periodontal tissue.[7-13] Refer to Figure 7-8.

E. **Localized or Generalized Inflammation.** In periodontitis, there is no consistent pattern to the number and types of teeth involved.

1. Localized inflammation may involve one site on a single tooth, several sites on a tooth, or several teeth. Generalized inflammation may involve the entire dentition.

2. In some cases, the site-specific nature of periodontitis may be apparent. For instance, a patient may present with areas of health in most sites interspersed with localized disease sites exhibiting clinical attachment loss.

F. **Contributing Factors**

1. Periodontitis may be modified by factors that increase the susceptibility of a patient to the disease. For instance, environmental factors, such as smoking, systemic factors, such as diabetes or HIV infection, and genetic factors can all contribute to increasing an individual's susceptibility to periodontitis.

2. Even local intraoral factors, such as tooth crowding or overhanging margins, may contribute to an increased susceptibility.

G. **Symptoms**

1. Periodontitis usually is painless. Therefore, an individual with periodontitis may be totally unaware of the disease, not seek treatment, and be unlikely to accept treatment recommendations.

2. Individuals may first become aware that something is wrong when they notice that their gums bleed when brushing; that spaces occur between the teeth; or that teeth have become loose.

3. Patients may complain of food impaction, sensitivity to hot or cold due to exposed roots, or dull pain radiating into the jaw.

3. **Onset of Periodontitis**

A. **Gingivitis as a Risk Factor for Periodontitis**

1. Findings from epidemiologic studies and clinical trials indicate that the presence of gingivitis may be regarded as a risk factor for periodontitis.[14,15]

2. Plaque-induced gingivitis precedes the onset of periodontitis. Plaque-induced gingivitis may remain stable for many years and, in most cases, never progress to become periodontitis. The level of host susceptibility and other contributing factors determines whether gingivitis progresses to periodontitis.

3. Gingivitis manifests only after days or weeks of plaque biofilm accumulation. In most cases, periodontitis requires longer periods (years) of plaque biofilm and calculus exposure to develop.[16]

B. **Age of Onset.** The onset of periodontitis may be at any age. It is most commonly detected in adults but, can occur in children and adolescents. The prevalence and severity of periodontitis increases with age.

4. **Patient Education: The Warning Signs of Periodontitis.**

A. **Pain Usually Not a Symptom of Periodontitis.** This absence of pain may explain why periodontitis is often advanced before the patient seeks treatment and why a patient may avoid treatment even after receiving a diagnosis of periodontitis.

1. The warning signs of periodontitis are red or swollen gingiva, bleeding during brushing, a bad taste in the mouth, persistent bad breath, sensitive teeth, loose teeth, and pus around teeth and gingiva.

2. Tools such as oral health self-evaluations distributed at health fairs or other events can be helpful in increasing the public's awareness of the signs and symptoms of periodontal disease.

Box 7-1. Periodontitis

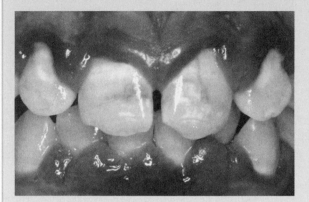

A

Figure 7-3A. Highly Visible Changes in the Gingiva. Periodontitis may exhibit many clinically visible signs, such as, changes in the contour and color of the gingiva.

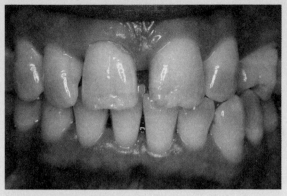

B

Figure 7-3B. Minimal Visible Changes in Gingiva. In this example of periodontitis, there are minimal visible tissue changes. Since periodontitis is a disease affecting the deeper tissues of the periodontium, the appearance of the surface tissue often is not a reliable indicator of disease severity.

Characteristics of Periodontitis

- Most commonly seen in adults, but can occur in children and adolescents
- Initiated and continued by plaque biofilms but host response plays an essential role in disease progression
- Signs and symptoms of inflammation include swelling, redness, gingival bleeding, periodontal pockets, bone loss, tooth mobility, suppuration (pus), moderate or heavy deposits of plaque biofilms and dental calculus
- Bone loss may be evident on radiographs
- Untreated periodontitis most commonly progresses slowly over time; however, in rare cases there is rapid disease progression
- Attachment loss may occur in one site of a single tooth, on several teeth, or the entire dentition
- It can be modified by other factors, such as smoking and poorly controlled diabetes

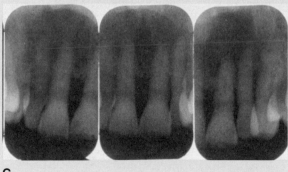

C

Figure 7-3C. Radiographic Evidence of Periodontitis. Dental radiographs of a patient with periodontitis reveal a horizontal pattern of alveolar bone loss.

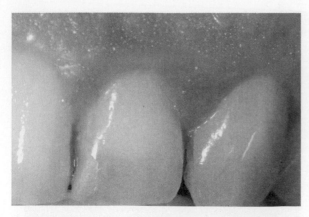 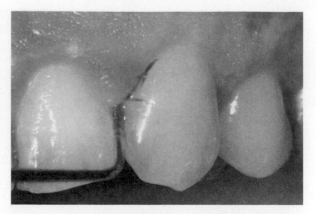

Figure 7-4. Health or Disease? The clinical appearance of the tissue in the photograph on the left suggests health. When assessed with a probe, however, a deep 7-mm pocket reveals bone loss on the mesiofacial of the canine. This example underscores the importance of a thorough periodontal assessment. (Courtesy of Dr. Don Rolfs, Wenatchee, WA.)

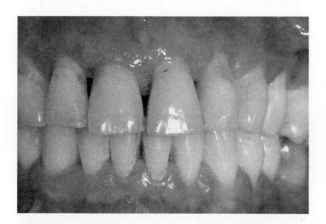

Figure 7-5. Health or Disease? This individual received periodontal treatment for periodontitis several years ago. The assessment at today's appointment reveals meticulous patient self-care and no additional attachment loss since beginning periodontal maintenance several years ago. Therefore, this tissue is considered healthy. The attachment loss is simply an indicator of previous disease. (Courtesy of Dr. Ralph Arnold, San Antonio, TX.)

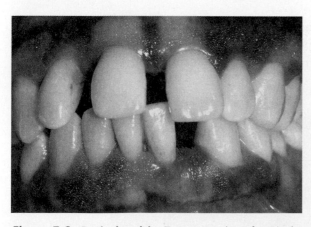 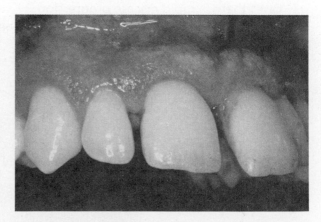

Figure 7-6. Periodontitis. Two examples of periodontitis showing firm, nodular (fibrotic) tissue changes.

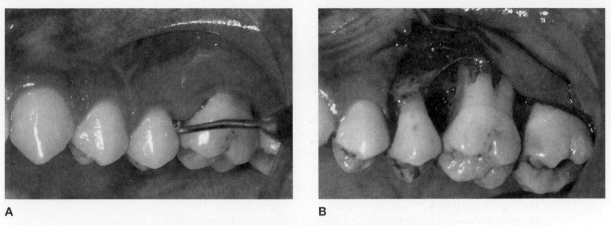

Figure 7-7. Attachment Loss. A. Assessment with a periodontal probe indicates severe loss of attachment on this molar tooth. **B.** The gingival tissue is lifted away from the molar during periodontal surgery to reveal severe loss of alveolar bone and furcation involvement. (Courtesy of Dr. Ralph Arnold, San Antonio, TX.)

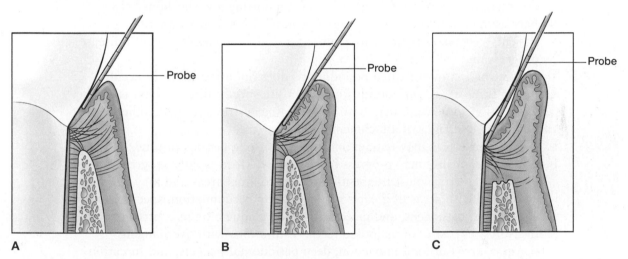

Figure 7-8. Diagrammatic Representation of Probe Tip Penetration Relative to the Periodontal Tissues. It has been established that the extent of probe penetration is influenced by the inflammatory status of the periodontal tissues.[7–13,17–23] **A.** In a healthy sulcus, the probe penetrates about one-third of the length of the junctional epithelium. **B.** With moderate inflammation within the tissues, the probe tip penetrates approximately half the length of the junctional epithelium. **C.** With severe inflammation within the tissues, the probe tip penetrates through the entire length of the junctional epithelium, and only stops when it encounters the most coronal intact collagen fibers in the gingival connective tissue.

EXTENT AND PROGRESSION OF PERIODONTITIS

1. **Extent of Destruction in Periodontitis**
   A. **Overview.** Extent is the distribution of the disease throughout the entire oral cavity. It can be thought of as the degree to which the disease has spread. It can be characterized based on the percentage of affected teeth which exhibit periodontal breakdown.
      1. Localized inflammation may involve one site on a single tooth, several sites on a tooth, or several teeth. A patient may simultaneously have areas of health adjacent to areas with periodontitis.
      2. Generalized inflammation may involve many teeth or the entire dentition.

B. **Localized or Generalized Extent**
 1. Localized periodontitis is periodontitis in which 30% or less of the teeth in the mouth have experienced attachment loss and bone loss.
 2. Generalized periodontitis is periodontitis in which more than 30% of the teeth in the mouth have experienced attachment loss and bone loss.

2. **Disease Progression**
 A. **Overview.** Disease progression refers to the change or advancement of periodontal destruction. For example, how does the amount of attachment loss and bone destruction seen today compare with what was observed several months ago? Is it the same, somewhat worse, or much worse?
 B. **Progression of Periodontitis.** In most cases, untreated periodontitis progresses at a slow to moderate pace.
  1. The current view is that the progression of untreated periodontitis in most individuals and at most disease sites is a continuous slow process, however, periods of remission and exacerbation occasionally may occur.
   a. In a limited number of individuals, periodontitis is characterized by rapid destruction of periodontal ligament and supporting alveolar bone.[5,24]
   b. Baer estimated that the loss of attachment in Grade C periodontitis patients progresses three or four times faster than in cases of typical disease progression.[25]
  2. Tissue destruction in untreated periodontitis does not affect all teeth evenly. Rather, in some cases, periodontitis may be a site-specific disease. That is, in the same dentition some teeth may have severe tissue destruction while other teeth are almost free of signs of attachment and bone loss.
   a. Some disease sites may remain unchanged for long periods of time.[16,24,26]
   b. Other disease sites may progress more rapidly. More rapidly progressing disease sites occur most frequently in interproximal areas and may be associated with areas of greater plaque biofilm accumulation, specific subgingival pathogens, and inaccessibility to plaque biofilm control measures (e.g., sites of malposed teeth, restorations with overhanging margins, areas of food impaction, deep periodontal pockets, and furcation areas).[26,27]
  3. *The desired outcome of periodontal therapy for periodontitis is to stop the progression of the disease to prevent further attachment loss.* Figures 7-9 to 7-11 show the clinical features before and after treatment for three different patients.
  4. The number of sites of attachment loss, bone loss, and/or deep pockets is a good predictor of future disease occurrence in an individual patient. The best predictor of disease progression is an individual's previous disease experience.

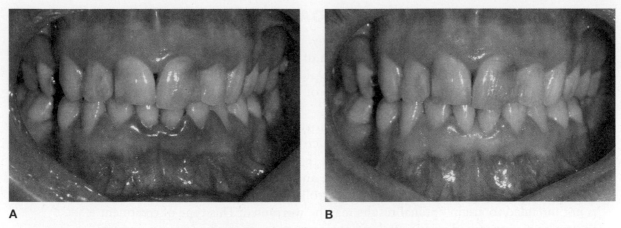

A   **B**

Figure 7-9.   Periodontitis: Before and After Periodontal Therapy. A. Note the tissue appearance before periodontal therapy. Clinical inflammation is particularly pronounced on the lower anterior sextant. **B.** The same individual after treatment. Note the decrease in inflammation in the mandibular anterior sextant.

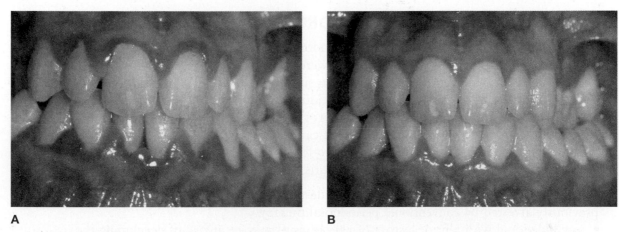

A   **B**

Figure 7-10.   Periodontitis: Before and After Periodontal Therapy. A. Prior to therapy, very inflamed tissue is evident. **B.** Much improved clinical picture at 3-month follow-up appointment. (Courtesy of Dr. Ralph Arnold, San Antonio, TX.)

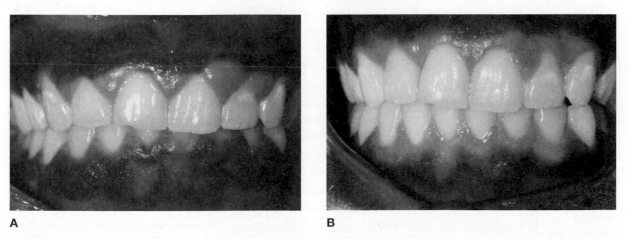

A   **B**

Figure 7-11.   Periodontitis: Before and After Periodontal Therapy. A. Very swollen gingival tissues pretreatment. **B.** The same individual after treatment. (Courtesy of Dr. Ralph Arnold, San Antonio, TX.)

THERAPEUTIC ENDPOINTS AND GOALS

1. **Therapeutic Endpoints of Periodontal Therapy.** The therapeutic endpoints of periodontal therapy should be (1) elimination of the microbial etiology and contributing factors that perpetuate periodontal inflammation, (2) preservation of the state of the teeth and periodontium in a state of health, function, and stability, and (3) prevention of disease reoccurrence.

2. **Treatment Goals.** Optimal treatment should focus on reinforcing daily self-care; periodontal instrumentation to remove the microbial etiology; elimination of local intraoral factors; periodontal surgery (if there is still persistent periodontal inflammation following nonsurgical therapy); and finally, adherence to a periodontal maintenance regimen after the disease is controlled. In certain cases, treatment that is not intended to attain optimal results may be warranted. This type of treatment is known as **compromised periodontal maintenance** and is typically done on patients who have serious health conditions, poor motivation/compliance, advanced age, or severe periodontal disease. In this case, the endpoint is compromised maintenance of a severely reduced periodontium.

RECURRENT AND REFRACTORY FORMS OF PERIODONTITIS

In previous classification systems, recurrent periodontitis and refractory periodontitis were thought to be distinct disease entities that were separate from periodontitis. However, current evidence has never been able to substantiate that, so recurrent periodontitis and refractory periodontitis are excluded from the 2017 classification system. Nevertheless, it is important for dental providers to understand that there are numerous and complex contributing factors that can stymie the successful management of the disease in the long-term. In such cases, two forms of periodontitis may arise: a *recurrent form* or a *refractory form* of periodontitis.

1. **Recurrent form** of periodontitis—a return of destructive periodontitis that had been previously arrested by conventional periodontal therapy.
   - Any individual with a prior history of periodontitis may be at risk of developing the recurrent form of the disease in the future.
   - Recurrence of periodontitis is a common event, especially in patients with poor self-care or who are noncompliant with routine professional care.
   - With recurrent disease, the patient and the dental practitioner must refocus their attention in arresting the disease and establishing patient adherence to the periodontal treatment, meticulous self-care, and frequent professional maintenance.

2. **Refractory form**—periodontitis in a patient who has been monitored over time and who exhibits continued attachment loss despite the following conditions: (a) the patient has received appropriate and continuous professional periodontal therapy, (b) the patient practices satisfactory self-care, and (c) the patient follows the recommended program of periodontal maintenance visits. Box 7-2, Figure 7-12 shows an example of a refractory form of periodontitis.
   - The etiology of the refractory form of periodontitis remains unknown but may be due to a complexity of unknown factors such as the emergence of opportunistic pathogens or compromised host response to the bacterial attack.
   - The designation "refractory" is applied to cases of periodontitis that do not respond favorably to conventional treatment.

- Since this form of periodontitis does not respond favorably to conventional therapy, periodontal therapy should be designed to slow down and control the progression of the disease.
- Treatment includes, but would not be limited to, patient education and behavior modification, periodontal instrumentation, use of systemic and/or local antibiotics, removal of periodontally hopeless teeth, correction of restorations that may be contributing to plaque retention, surgical therapy, and strict adherence to a periodontal maintenance regimen.
- It should be noted that despite the patient's and the dental clinician's best efforts, control of periodontitis may not be possible in some cases.

Box 7-2. Refractory Form of Periodontitis

Additional attachment loss in a patient despite all the following:

- Appropriate periodontal therapy
- A patient who practices satisfactory self-care
- An appropriate program of periodontal maintenance visits

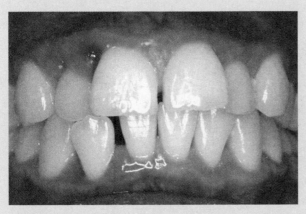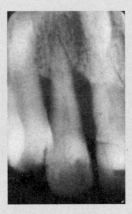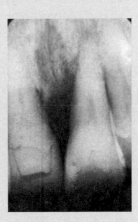

Figure 7-12. Refractory Form of Periodontitis. Periodontitis is considered refractory when the disease is not controlled by the conventional periodontal therapy normally recommended for patients with periodontitis. In a refractory case, the patient experiences additional attachment loss despite appropriate periodontal therapy and satisfactory self-care. The dental radiographs of a patient with refractory form of periodontitis reveal *continuing evidence of bone loss over time despite appropriate therapy.*

Section 2
Periodontitis Staging and Grading System

THE PERIODONTITIS CASE DEFINITION SYSTEM

1. Definition of a Patient as a Periodontitis Case
   A. **According to the 2017 classification system, a patient is a** periodontitis case **if:**
      1. *Interdental* clinical attachment loss is detectible at two or more nonadjacent teeth, **OR**
      2. Facial or lingual clinical attachment loss of 3 mm or more with pocketing greater than 3 mm is detectible at two or more teeth.
   B. Clinical Attachment in the Periodontitis Case Definition
      1. To be defined as a periodontal case, the observed CAL cannot be due to nonperiodontitis causes such as gingival recession of traumatic origin, dental caries extending to or apical to the CEJ, presence of CAL on the distal aspect of a second molar and associated with malposition or extraction of a third molar, an endodontic lesion draining through the marginal gingiva, and the occurrence of a vertical root fracture.
2. Identification of the Form of Periodontitis
   A. Pathophysiology
      1. As related to periodontal disease, pathophysiology is the study of the pathological manifestations of periodontitis. Pathophysiology does not deal directly with the treatment of disease, rather it explains the processes within the body that result in the signs and symptoms of periodontitis.
      2. Based on pathophysiology, three clearly different forms of periodontitis have been identified.[1]
         a. Necrotizing periodontitis
         b. Periodontitis as a direct manifestation of systemic diseases
         c. Periodontitis
   B. *Content on periodontitis is explained in this chapter. Chapter 8 presents content on necrotizing periodontitis and uncommon forms of periodontitis.*
3. The Periodontitis Staging and Grading System
   A. **Stage at Presentation.** An individual periodontitis case is defined as Stage I, II, III or IV.[6] The Stage at presentation of a periodontitis case is defined by (1) the disease severity and (2) complexity of management of the case. The staging system for periodontal cases is summarized in Table 7-1. When determining the stage of periodontitis, the clinician should keep in mind that there may be individual complexity factors or severity factors that may shift the stage to a higher level. For instance, if a patient has a Class II furcation, then that would shift the stage to either Stage III or Stage IV irrespective of other severity factors, such as CAL, radiographic bone loss, and tooth loss.
      1. **Stage I Periodontitis.** Stage I is characterized by the initial stages of attachment loss.
         a. Disease Severity
            1. Interdental CAL of 1 to 2 mm at the site of greatest loss
            2. Radiographic bone loss extending to the coronal one-third of the root
            3. No tooth loss due to periodontitis
         b. Complexity of Management
            1. Maximum probing depths of 4 mm or less
            2. Mostly horizontal bone loss
      2. **Stage II Periodontitis.** Stage II represents established periodontitis.

      a. Disease Severity
1. Interdental CAL of 3 to 4 mm at the site of greatest loss
2. Radiographic bone loss extending to the coronal one-third of the root
3. No tooth loss due to periodontitis

      b. Complexity of Management
1. Maximum probing depths of 5 mm or less
2. Mostly horizontal bone loss

3. Stage III Periodontitis. Stage III represents severe periodontitis with significant destruction to the attachment apparatus and potential tooth loss.

      a. Disease Severity
1. Interdental CAL 5 mm or greater at the site of greatest loss
2. Radiographic bone loss extending to the mid-third of the root and beyond
3. Tooth loss due to periodontitis of 4 or less teeth

      b. Complexity of Management—in addition to the Stage II complexity factors, one or more of the following complexity factors are characteristic of Stage III.
1. Maximum probing depths of 6 mm or greater
2. Vertical bone loss 3 mm or greater
3. Class II or III furcation involvement
4. Moderate alveolar ridge defect that complicates implant placement

4. Stage IV Periodontitis. Stage IV represents advanced periodontitis with extensive tooth loss and potential for loss of dentition.

      a. Disease Severity
1. Interdental CAL of 5 mm or greater at the site of greatest loss
2. Radiographic bone loss extending to the middle one-third of the root and beyond
3. Tooth loss due to periodontitis of 5 or more teeth

      b. Complexity of Management—in addition to the Stage III complexity factors, one or more of the following complexity factors are characteristic of Stage IV
1. Maximum probing depths of 6 mm or greater
2. Masticatory dysfunction
3. Secondary occlusal trauma, tooth mobility greater than Class II
4. Severe ridge defect of alveolar bone
5. Bite collapse, drifting, flaring of teeth
6. Less than 20 remaining teeth (10 opposing pairs)

B. Grade. Grade is an estimate of the future rate of progression of peridontitis (i.e., slow, moderate, or rapid).

- The grade of a patient's periodontitis is based on the availability of direct or indirect evidence of disease progression.
- Direct evidence is based on longitudinal observation available in the form of older diagnostic quality radiographs. Indirect evidence is based on the assessment of bone loss at the worst affected tooth in the dentition as a function of age.

- It should be noted that in many cases, longitudinal data is unavailable. So, the clinician must rely on indirect evidence of disease progression to assign a grade to an individual's periodontitis.
- As in staging, when determining the grade of an individual's periodontitis, the clinician should keep in mind that there may be individual risk factors that may shift the grade to a higher level. For instance, a patient who smokes less than 10 cigarettes/day but exhibits no evidence of CAL over the last 5 years would be classified as a Grade B.
- Grade modifiers are risk factors that may impact the rate of disease progression. Grade as an indication of disease progression is summarized in Table 7-2.
    1. **Grade A: Slow Rate of Disease Progression.**
        a. The primary criteria for a Grade A designation are:
            1. Direct evidence: *no* evidence of CAL or radiographic bone loss over a 5-year period
            2. Indirect evidence: Heavy biofilm deposits with low levels of tissue destruction
        b. The modifiers for Grade A are:
            1. Nonsmokers
            2. Normoglycemic patient
    2. **Grade B: Moderate Rate of Disease Progression.**
        a. The primary criteria for a Grade B designation are:
            1. Direct evidence: *less than 2 mm* of CAL or radiographic bone loss over a 5-year period
            2. Indirect evidence: Tissue destruction is in line with expectations given the amount of biofilm deposits
        b. The grade modifiers for Grade B are:
            1. Smoking *less than* 10 cigarettes a day and/or
            2. An HbA1c of less than 7% in patients with diabetes. (The HbA1c level is a measurement of the average blood glucose level over the past 2 to 3 months. A normal HbA1C level for nondiabetics is *below* 5.6%.)
    3. **Grade C: Rapid Rate of Disease Progression.**
        a. The primary criteria for a Grade C designation are:
            1. Evidence of 2mm *or more* of attachment loss over a 5-year period
            2. Tissue destruction exceeds expectations given the amount of biofilm deposits
        b. The grade modifiers for Grade C are:
            1. Smoking *10 or more* cigarettes a day and/or
            2. An HbA1c of 7% or greater in patients with diabetes.
   C. **Periodontal Diagnosis.** The periodontal diagnosis for an individual patient should include:
    1. Confirmation that patient is a periodontitis case based on detectable clinical attachment loss at two nonadjacent teeth
    2. Identification of the form of periodontitis as necrotizing periodontitis, periodontitis as a manifestation of systemic disease, or periodontitis
    3. Description of the presentation and aggressiveness of the disease by stage and grade

TABLE 7-1 | PERIODONTITIS STAGE

	Interdental CAL[a]	Radiographic Bone Loss	Tooth Loss	Probing Depth	Bone Loss	Other
Stage I	1 to 2 mm	Coronal third (>15% loss)	No tooth loss due to periodontitis	4 mm or less	Mostly horizontal bone loss	
Stage II	3 to 4 mm	Coronal third (15–33% loss)	No tooth loss due to periodontitis	5 mm or less	Mostly horizontal bone loss	
Stage III	5 mm or more	Extending to the mid-third of root or beyond	4 or less teeth lost due to periodontitis	6 mm or more	Vertical bone loss 3 mm or greater	
Stage IV	5 mm or more	Extending to the mid-third of root and beyond	5 or more teeth lost due to periodontitis	6 mm or more	Vertical bone loss 3 mm or greater	Need for complex rehabilitation

[a]Interdental clinical loss of attachment at the site of greatest loss.

TABLE 7-2	PERIODONTITIS GRADE	
	Disease Progression/ Characteristics	**Grade Modifiers**
Grade A	• No additional bone or attachment loss over past 5 years • Low levels of tissue destruction	• Nonsmoker • No history of diabetes
Grade B	• Evidence of *less than 2 mm* additional bone or attachment loss over a 5-year period • Tissue destruction in line with expectations	• Smoking *less than* 10 cigarettes a day and/or • An HbA1c of *less than* 7% in patients with diabetes
Grade C	• Evidence of *2 mm or more* of bone or attachment loss over a 5-year period • Tissue destruction exceeds expectations	• Smoking *10 or more* cigarettes a day and/or • An HbA1c of 7% or greater in patients with diabetes

EXAMPLES OF PERIODONTITS CASE STAGING AND GRADING

Boxes 7-3 to 7-10 (Figs. 7-13 to 7-20) provide examples of staging and grading for periodontitis cases.

Box 7-3. Case Example. Stage I Grade A Periodontitis

Clinical Findings

- 45 years of age
- Interdental CAL of 1 to 2 mm
- No tooth loss due to periodontitis
- No probing depths over 4 mm
- Horizontal bone loss
- No additional bone loss over last 5 years
- Nonsmoker
- No history of diabetes

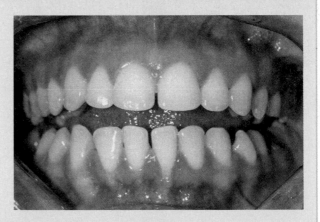

Figure 7-13. Clinical Findings. Clinical attachment readings indicate that this previously diagnosed periodontitis patient has not experienced any additional attachment loss over the past 5 years, indicating that a combination of good self-care and professional maintenance has stabilized the periodontium.

Box 7-4. Case Example. Stage III Grade C Periodontitis

Clinical Findings

- 28 years of age
- Interdental CAL of 3 to 4 mm
- No tooth loss due to periodontitis
- Probing depths of 5 mm or less
- Mostly horizontal bone loss extending past the middle one-third of the root
- Evidence of *2 mm or more* attachment loss over a 5-year period
- Tissue destruction exceeds expectations based on amount of biofilm present
- Smokes a pack of cigarettes a day (20 or more per day)
- Preserved masticatory function

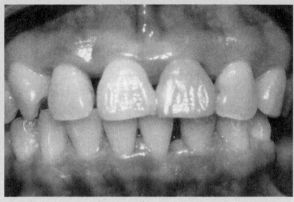

A

Figure 7-14A. Clinical Findings. This 28-year-old patient has experienced a rapid rate of loss of attachment over a 5-year period.

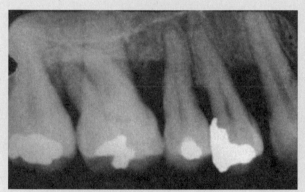

B

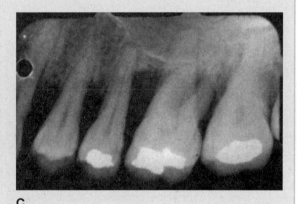

C

Figure 7-14B,C. Radiographic Characteristics. The patient's radiographs reveal severe horizontal bone loss around most teeth.

Box 7-5. Case Example. Stage III Grade C Periodontitis

Clinical Findings

- 20 years of age
- Interdental CAL of 3 to 4 mm
- No tooth loss due to periodontitis
- Probing depths of 4 mm or less
- Radiographic bone loss extends to the coronal third of root of the first molars
- Evidence of *2 mm or more* attachment loss over a 5-year period
- Tissue destruction exceeds expectations based on amount of biofilm present
- Possible grade modifiers: smoking or history of diabetes

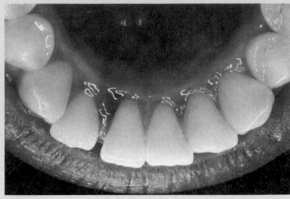

A

Figure 7-15A. Clinical Findings. The photo shows a patient with Stage III, Grade C periodontitis. Note that there are not any supragingival calculus deposits evident; thus, the tissue destruction exceeds expectations.

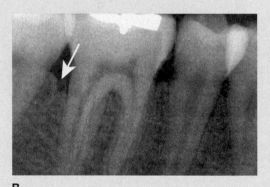

B

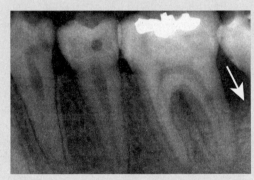

C

Figure 7-15B,C. Radiographic Characteristics of this Periodontitis Case. The patient's radiographs reveal a pattern of bone loss on the first molars that is similar on both sides of the mandibular arch. Note the angular defects (arrows) on the distal surfaces of the molars. Also note radiographic evidence of furcation involvement on both molars.

Box 7-6. Case Example. Stage III Grade C Periodontitis

Clinical Findings

- 5 years of age
- Interdental CAL of 3 to 4 mm
- No tooth loss due to periodontitis
- Probing depths of 4 mm or less
- Tissue destruction exceeds expectations based on amount of biofilm present

Due to the absence of longitudinal radiographic data on this 5-year-old patient, direct evidence of disease progression to assign a grade was not available. Instead, the following indirect evidence of progression was used to assign a grade to this patient's periodontitis: (1) amount of periodontal destruction exceeded given biofilm deposits, (2) early onset of disease, and (3) rapid progression that is not characteristic of the patient's age.

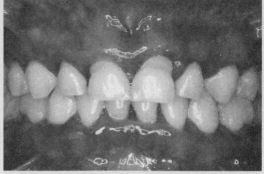

A

Figure 7-16A. Child with Grade C Periodontitis. Although very rare, children may exhibit periodontitis.

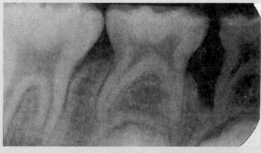

B

Figure 7-16B. Radiograph. Radiographic evidence of vertical bone loss in the patient shown in Figure 7-16A.

Box 7-7. Case Example. Stage IV Grade C Periodontitis

Clinical Findings

- 44 years of age
- Interdental CAL 5 mm or more
- 4 teeth lost due to periodontitis
- Probing depths 6 mm or more
- Radiographic bone loss extends to the mid-third of root
- Vertical bone loss
- Evidence of *2 mm or more* additional attachment loss over a 5-year period
- Smokes a pack of cigarettes a day
- Bite collapse with drifting of teeth and multiple teeth with Degree 2 mobility

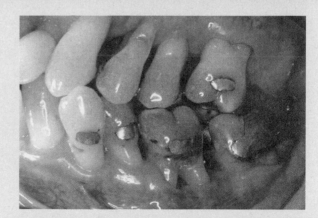

Figure 7-17. Grade C Disease Progression. An example of rapid disease progression despite good daily self-care by the patient.

Box 7-8. Case Example. Stage II Grade B Periodontitis

Clinical Findings

- 50 years of age
- Interdental CAL of 3 to 4 mm
- No tooth loss due to periodontitis
- Probing depths 5 mm or less
- Radiographic bone loss extends to the coronal third of root
- Mostly horizontal bone loss
- Evidence of *less than 2 mm* additional attachment loss over a 5-year period
- Nonsmoker
- No history of diabetes

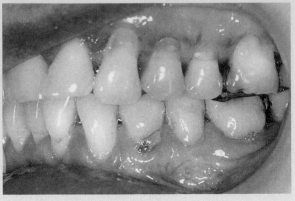

A

Figure 7-18A. Clinical Findings. The photo shows a patient with Stage II Grade B periodontitis. At her maintenance (recall) visit, she exhibits excellent self-care.

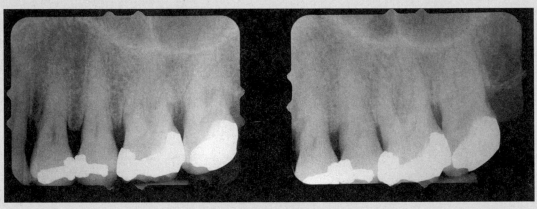

B

Figure 7-18B. Radiographic Characteristics of this Periodontitis Case. The patient's radiographs reveal bone loss that extends to the coronal thirds of the roots. However, over the past 5 years, she experienced less than 2 mm additional clinical attachment loss.

Box 7-9. Case Example. Stage III Grade B Periodontitis

Clinical Findings

- 47 years of age
- Interdental CAL 5 mm or more
- 4 teeth lost due to periodontitis
- Probing depths 6 mm or more
- Radiographic bone loss extends to the mid-third of root
- Some vertical bone loss
- Evidence of *less than 2 mm* of attachment loss over a 5-year period
- Nonsmoker
- History of diabetes with a long-term HbA1c levels less than 7%

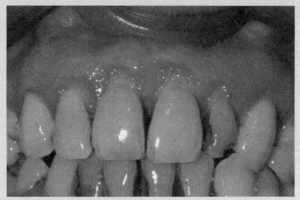

A

Figure 7-19A. Clinical Findings. The photo shows a patient with Stage III Grade B periodontitis. Clinical attachment readings for this patient have remained stable over the past 5 years at less than 2 mm CAL.

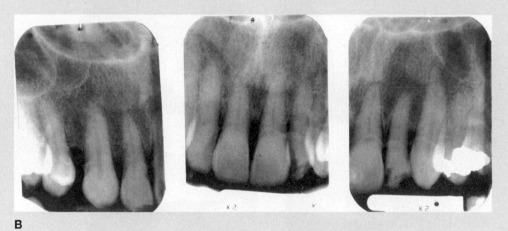

B

Figure 7-19B. Radiographic Characteristics of this Periodontitis Case. The patient's radiographs reveal bone loss that extends to the mid-thirds of the roots.

Box 7-10. Case Example. Stage IV Grade B Periodontitis

Clinical Findings

- 53 years of age
- Interdental CAL 5 mm or more
- More than 5 teeth lost due to periodontitis
- Probing depths 6 mm or more
- Radiographic bone loss extends to the mid-third of root
- Vertical bone loss
- Evidence of *less than 2 mm* additional attachment loss over a 5-year period
- Nondiabetic
- Smokes half a pack of cigarettes a day

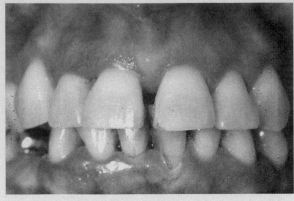

A

Figure 7-20A. Clinical Findings. The photo shows a patient with Stage IV Grade B periodontitis.

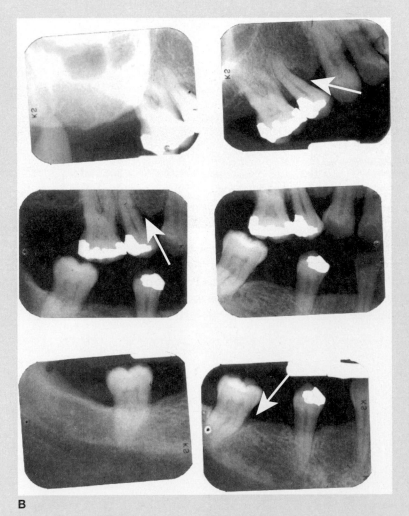

B

Figure 7-20B. Radiographic Characteristics of this Periodontitis Case. The patient's radiographs reveal vertical bone (indicated by *white arrows*).

Chapter Summary Statement

Periodontitis is a bacterial infection resulting in inflammation within the supporting tissues of the teeth, progressive destruction of the periodontal ligament, and loss of supporting alveolar bone.

- Periodontitis involves *irreversible* loss of attachment and alveolar bone.
- Periodontitis may involve one site of a tooth's attachment, several teeth, or the entire dentition. A patient can simultaneously have areas of health and areas with periodontitis.
- Untreated periodontitis usually is characterized by slow to moderate rates of disease progression and a favorable response to periodontal therapy. A limited number of periodontitis cases are characterized by rapid destruction of the attachment and rapid loss of supporting bone.
- The desired outcome of periodontal therapy for periodontitis is to stop the progression of the disease to prevent further attachment loss.

In 2017, the American Academy of Periodontology (AAP) and the European Federation of Periodontology (EFP) disease classification designated periodontitis cases using a staging and grading system.

Section 3
Focus on Patients

Clinical Patient Care

CASE 1

A new patient has a diagnosis of Periodontitis Stage II, Grade B. The patient tells you that it is hard for him to believe he has serious periodontal problems since he has never had any discomfort and has never even noticed any dental problems. How could you respond to the patient?

CASE 2

A patient who has recently moved to your city has an appointment with you regarding self-care instructions. The periodontal case diagnosis is Stage III, Grade B. In your discussion with the patient you learn that the patient is upset because she has been treated for periodontitis twice during the past decade in other dental offices. She is upset because now she needs periodontal treatment again, and she states she is confused about how this might be possible. How could you respond to this patient's concerns?

CASE 3

Mr. B. is a 60-year-old male who presents to your office for a periodontal evaluation. From your clinical and radiographic assessment, you note that there is generalized clinical attachment loss of 3 to 4 mm, probing depths of 5 mm or less, profuse bleeding upon probing, and radiographic bone loss in the coronal third. The patient's records indicate evidence of less than 2 mm of additional attachment loss over a 5-year period. What would be your periodontal diagnosis? How would you explain to the patient the significance of the *stage* and *grade* of his periodontitis?

CASE 4

While reading a journal article you find a reference to a periodontal disease called chronic periodontitis. Since this is not a disease category in the currently accepted disease classification system, how does this terminology relate to the current 2017 disease classification system?

Ethical Dilemma 1

Mrs. W. is a new patient in your general dentistry practice—having changed from another dental practice in your city. Mrs. W. states that she "decided to change to your dental office because her friend Cynthia is so happy with the care she receives here."

After completing a comprehensive periodontal assessment and obtaining Mrs. W's records from the previous dental practice, the dentist's diagnosis is periodontitis Stage II, Grade B. Members of the dental team clearly communicate this finding and offer recommendations for a treatment care plan. After asking some questions, Mrs. W. indicates that she is grateful that everything has been so clearly explained and that she can clearly see the problems and how the recommended care plan will help her.

After accepting the recommended care plan, Mrs. W. has several additional questions for you. She states that she has seen a dental hygienist and dentist in the other practice every 6 months for years, never missing an appointment. Mrs. W. states that the dental team in the other practice never told her that she has any dental problems and never suggested any treatment other than a 1-hour cleaning appointment once every 6 months. Mrs. W. states that she is upset that the other practice did not provide good care and wonders if she should sue them?

How can you respond to Mrs. W's concerns about the care she received in the other dental practice?

Ethical Dilemma 2

Your next patient, Josiah S., has recently relocated to your town, approximately 6 months ago, and is a new patient in your practice. He is a 45-year-old divorced male, who admits to smoking approximately 20 cigarettes per day, and drinks a nightly alcoholic cocktail. He works in sales, and due to his hectic travel schedule, tells you that he has had to cancel his last few dental hygiene appointments.

Your intraoral exam reveals that Josiah presents with moderate calculus and plaque biofilm. His gingival tissues appear red and swollen, have blunted papillae, and bleed readily upon probing. You take a full-mouth series of radiographs that show generalized horizontal bone loss throughout his mouth. You begin to probe his mouth, to determine his pocket readings, when he sits up in the dental chair, and demands that you stop. He states that he has always refused periodontal probing, as he just "can't stand the pain" and the last dental office abided by his wishes. He refuses to let you continue "poking around his gums" and asks that you just proceed to cleaning his teeth, so he can be on time for his 11:00 am business appointment.

1. What ethical principles are in conflict in this dilemma?
2. Do you have an ethical obligation to treat this patient?
3. What, if any alternatives, can you offer Josiah in terms of his treatment plan?

Ethical Dilemma 3

Your dental practice, which is within an urban city, has many long-standing patients. A number of the patients within the practice are on public assistance and struggle with money issues. Dr. Gordon is very generous and understanding about her patients' financial limitations, and often provides free dental services.

Your next patient of the morning is Jason S., a 14-year-old soccer player. His mother has made an emergency appointment, as he was hit in the mouth during a soccer practice today. His mother is concerned that Jason's front teeth may be lost as a result.

His mother reports that Jason had a thorough "cleaning" in another dental office 4 months ago. However, she brought Jason to your dental office today because it is closer to his school than the dental practice that they usually go to. Clinical examination reveals no trauma but some mobility, so you take radiographs. Clinically, Jason presents with no obvious signs or symptoms of disease, with lack of tissue inflammation and minimal amounts of plaque biofilm.

Jason's radiographs, however, show moderate vertical bone loss around the maxillary central incisors and mandibular central incisors. Bitewing radiographs also indicate moderate bone loss around the maxillary and mandibular first molars. Probe readings on his incisors and molars are in the 4 to 6 mm range. You are concerned that this amount of tissue destruction is unusual in a 14-year-old patient.

You present your findings to Dr. Gordon, who asks you to perform thorough periodontal instrumentation on Jason. You remind Dr. Gordon, that Jason had a dental hygiene appointment in another office 4 months ago and that his insurance only allows for periodontal instrumentation every 6 months. Dr. Gordon states that Jason is in dire need of this treatment and asks to you to instruct the office manager to delay submitting Jason's insurance claim until it is within the 6-month time frame.

1. Although you do not have all the information needed to classify Jason's periodontal condition, what do you suspect his case Stage and Grade might be? What are your biggest concerns about Jason's periodontium?
2. What ethical principles are in conflict in this dilemma?
3. What is the best way for you to handle this ethical dilemma?

References

1. Caton J, Armitage G, Berglundh T, et al. A new classification scheme for periodontal and peri-implant diseases and conditions—Introduction and key changes from the 1999 classification. *J Periodontol.* 2018;89 Suppl 1:S1–S8.

2. Chapple ILC, Mealey BL, Van Dyke TE, et al. Periodontal health and gingival diseases and conditions on an intact and a reduced periodontium: Consensus report of workgroup 1 of the 2017 World Workshop on the Classification of Periodontal and Peri-Implant Diseases and Conditions. *J Periodontol.* 2018;89 Suppl 1:S74–S84.

3. Pihlstrom BL, Michalowicz BS, Johnson NW. Periodontal diseases. *Lancet.* 2005;366(9499):1809–1820.

4. Eke PI, Dye BA, Wei L, Thornton-Evans GO, Genco RJ, Cdc Periodontal Disease Surveillance workgroup: James Beck GDRP. Prevalence of periodontitis in adults in the United States: 2009 and 2010. *J Dent Res.* 2012;91(10):914–920.

5. Fine DH, Patil AG, Loos BG. Classification and diagnosis of aggressive periodontitis. *J Periodontol.* 2018;89 Suppl 1:S103–S119.

6. Tonetti MS, Greenwell H, Kornman KS. Staging and grading of periodontitis: Framework and proposal of a new classification and case definition. *J Periodontol.* 2018;89 Suppl 1:S159–S172.

7. Anderson GB, Caffesse RG, Nasjleti CE, Smith BA. Correlation of periodontal probe penetration and degree of inflammation. *Am J Dent.* 1991;4(4):177–183.

8. Armitage GC. Periodontal diseases: diagnosis. *Ann Periodontol.* 1996;1(1):37–215.

9. Caton J, Greenstein G, Polson AM. Depth of periodontal probe penetration related to clinical and histologic signs of gingival inflammation. *J Periodontol.* 1981;52(10):626–629.

10. Fowler C, Garrett S, Crigger M, Egelberg J. Histologic probe position in treated and untreated human periodontal tissues. *J Clin Periodontol.* 1982;9(5):373–385.

11. Khan S, Cabanilla LL. Periodontal probing depth measurement: a review. *Compend Contin Educ Dent.* 2009;30(1):12–14, 16, 8–21; quiz 2, 36.

12. Lindhe J, Lang NP, Karring T. Clinical Periodontology and Implant Dentistry. 5th ed. Oxford; Ames, IA: Blackwell Munksgaard; 2008.

13. Tessier JF, Ellen RP, Birek P, Kulkarni GV, McCulloch CA. Relationship between periodontal probing velocity and gingival inflammation in human subjects. *J Clin Periodontol.* 1993;20(1):41–48.

14. Schatzle M, Loe H, Lang NP, Burgin W, Anerud A, Boysen H. The clinical course of chronic periodontitis. *J Clin Periodontol.* 2004;31(12):1122–1127.

15. Suda R, Cao C, Hasegawa K, Yang S, Sasa R, Suzuki M. 2-year observation of attachment loss in a rural Chinese population. *J Periodontol.* 2000;71(7):1067–1072.

16. Armitage GC. Learned and unlearned concepts in periodontal diagnostics: a 50-year perspective. *Periodontol 2000.* 2013;62(1):20–36.

17. Hancock EB, Wirthlin MR. The location of the periodontal probe tip in health and disease. *J Periodontol.* 1981;52(3):124–129.

18. Hefti AF. Periodontal probing. *Crit Rev Oral Biol Med.* 1997;8(3):336–356.

19. Listgarten MA, Mao R, Robinson PJ. Periodontal probing and the relationship of the probe tip to periodontal tissues. *J Periodontol.* 1976;47(9):511–513.

20. Magnusson I, Listgarten MA. Histological evaluation of probing depth following periodontal treatment. *J Clin Periodontol.* 1980;7(1):26–31.

21. Moriarty JD, Hutchens LH, Jr., Scheitler LE. Histological evaluation of periodontal probe penetration in untreated facial molar furcations. *J Clin Periodontol.* 1989;16(1):21–26.

22. Robinson PJ, Vitek RM. The relationship between gingival inflammation and resistance to probe penetration. *J Periodontal Res.* 1979;14(3):239–243.

23. Spray JR, Garnick JJ, Doles LR, Klawitter JJ. Microscopic demonstration of the position of periodontal probes. *J Periodontol.* 1978;49(3):148–152.

24. Armitage GC, Cullinan MP. Comparison of the clinical features of chronic and aggressive periodontitis. *Periodontol 2000.* 2010;53:12–27.

25. Baer PN. The case for periodontosis as a clinical entity. *J Periodontol.* 1971;42(8):516–520.

26. Lindhe J, Okamoto H, Yoneyama T, Haffajee A, Socransky SS. Longitudinal changes in periodontal disease in untreated subjects. *J Clin Periodontol.* 1989;16(10):662–670.

27. Kakuta E, Nomura Y, Morozumi T, et al. Assessing the progression of chronic periodontitis using subgingival pathogen levels: a 24-month prospective multicenter cohort study. *BMC Oral Health.* 2017;17(1):46.

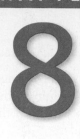

8 Other Conditions Affecting the Periodontium

Clinical Application.
This chapter highlights conditions and factors that can affect the periodontium other than the common varieties of periodontal diseases that were reviewed in Chapters 6 and 7. Familiarity with all forms of periodontal diseases is critical for all clinicians, since failure to recognize them may have a profound impact on the well-being of some patients. The importance of being able to recognize these conditions cannot be overstated since it is highly likely that a dental provider will encounter these conditions and factors in their clinical practice.

Learning Objectives

- Describe the clinical presentation of necrotizing periodontal diseases.
- Compare and contrast the tissue destruction that occurs in necrotizing gingivitis and necrotizing periodontitis.
- Compare and contrast the tissue destruction in periodontitis with that seen in necrotizing periodontitis.
- Explain the Miller and Cairo classification systems used to classify gingival recession.
- Name several local factors, such as tooth-related or prosthesis-related factors, that may contribute to the initiation and progression of periodontitis.

Key Terms

Necrotizing periodontal
  disease
Tissue necrosis
Necrotizing gingivitis
Necrotizing periodontitis

Necrotizing stomatitis
Pseudomembrane
Normal mucogingival
  condition
Periodontal biotypes

Mucogingival deformity
Recession of the gingival margin
Miller Classification System
Cairo Classification System

Please refer to these chapters for the following content:
Chapter 16: Systemic Risk Factors that Amplify Susceptibility to Periodontal Disease
Chapter 17: Local Factors Contributing to Periodontal Disease
Chapter 30: Acute Periodontal Conditions
Chapter 34: Impact of Periodontitis on Systemic Health

Section 1
Necrotizing Periodontal Diseases

Necrotizing periodontal diseases (NPD) include necrotizing gingivitis (NG), necrotizing periodontitis (NP), and necrotizing stomatitis. Studies suggest that necrotizing gingivitis, necrotizing periodontitis, and necrotizing stomatitis may represent different stages of the same disease because they have similar etiology and clinical characteristics.[1,2]

Necrotizing periodontal diseases present three typical clinical features: tissue necrosis, spontaneous bleeding (or pronounced bleeding after the slightest stimulation), and pain.[3,4] *They represent the most severe biofilm-related periodontal condition.*

1. **Necrotizing periodontal diseases** are a broad category of inflammatory destructive infections of the periodontal tissues that is characterized by **tissue necrosis** (localized tissue death). All forms of necrotizing periodontal diseases are painful infections characterized by tissue ulceration, swelling and sloughing of dead epithelial tissue from the gingiva, and fetid oral odor. The aforementioned signs and symptoms are unique to necrotizing periodontal diseases. Consequently, necrotizing periodontal diseases are considered to be a distinct family of disease which has unique clinical features that are separate from the typical clinical features of periodontitis.
   A. **Necrotizing gingivitis**—tissue necrosis that is limited to the gingival tissues (Box 8-1, Fig. 8-1).
   B. **Necrotizing periodontitis**—tissue necrosis of the gingival tissues combined with loss of attachment and alveolar bone loss (Box 8-2, Fig. 8-2).
      1. Necrotizing periodontitis is a painful infection characterized by necrosis of gingival tissues, periodontal ligament, and alveolar bone.
      2. Necrotizing periodontitis is an extremely rapid and destructive form of periodontitis that can produce loss of periodontal attachment within days.
   C. **Necrotizing stomatitis**—severe tissue necrosis that extends beyond the gingiva to other parts of the oral cavity, such as the tongue, cheek, and palate.
      1. Bone denudation may occur through the alveolar mucosa tissue.
      2. This is the most severe, yet rarest, form of necrotizing periodontal diseases.
2. **Alternative Terminology.** These conditions previously have been known as trench mouth, Vincent infection, acute necrotizing ulcerative gingivitis (ANUG), necrotizing ulcerative gingivostomatitis (NUG), and necrotizing ulcerative periodontitis (NUP). The terminology "ulcerative" was later eliminated because ulceration is secondary to the tissue necrosis that characterizes NPD.[5]
3. **Clinical Presentation of Necrotizing Periodontal Disease (NPD)**
   A. **Oral Signs and Symptoms.** The clinical appearance of necrotizing periodontal diseases is noticeably different than that of any other periodontal disease.[3,4,6] Figures 8-3 and 8-4 show examples of the clinical presentation of necrotizing periodontal diseases.
      1. NPD is a painful infection, primarily involving the interdental and marginal gingiva.
      2. NPD is characterized by ulcerated and necrotic papillae and gingival margins, giving the appearance that the papillae and gingival margins have been "punched-out" or "cratered." The ulcerated margin is bounded by a red halo.
      3. The necrotic areas of the gingiva are covered by a yellowish white or grayish tissue slough, which is termed a **pseudomembrane**.
         a. The pseudomembrane consists primarily of fibrin and necrotic tissue with leukocytes, erythrocytes, and masses of bacteria. (Fibrin is stringy protein formed during the process of blood clot formation.)

    b. The term, pseudomembrane, however, is misleading since the slough has no coherence and is not like a true membrane. It is easily wiped off with gauze, exposing an area of fiery red, shiny, hemorrhagic gingiva.

    c. The pseudomembrane may involve the gingiva of several teeth or it may cover the entire gingiva.

    d. The sloughing of dead gingival epithelial tissue exposes the underlying connective tissue.

4. Fiery red gingiva with spontaneous gingival bleeding or bleeding to gentle touch.

5. *The necrotizing lesions develop rapidly and are painful.* Intense oral pain that causes affected patients to seek dental treatment. This symptom is unusual since gingivitis and periodontitis normally are *not* painful.

6. The first lesions often are seen interproximally in the mandibular anterior sextant but, may occur in any interproximal papilla. Usually, the papillae swell rapidly and develop a rounded contour.

Box 8-1. Necrotizing Gingivitis (NG)

- Sudden onset
- Pain
- Necrosis of interdental papillae (cratered, punched-out papillae)
- Yellowish white or grayish tissue slough
- Fiery red gingiva with spontaneous bleeding

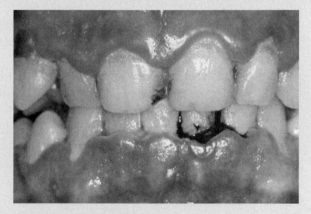

Figure 8-1. Necrotizing Gingivitis.

Box 8-2. Necrotizing Periodontitis (NP)

- The same signs and symptoms of NG
- The main difference is that NP leads to attachment loss and bone loss

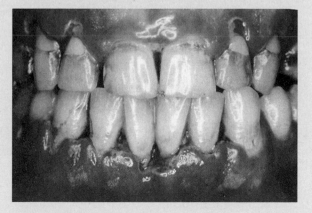

Figure 8-2. Necrotizing Periodontitis.

7. A pronounced fetid oral odor (bad breath) may be present, but can vary in intensity and in some cases, may not be very noticeable.
   a. The pain associated with necrotizing periodontal diseases usually causes the individual to stop brushing.
   b. Materia alba, plaque biofilm, necrotic tissue, blood, and stagnant saliva causes the distinctive fetid oral odor.
8. Necrotizing periodontal diseases may be associated with excessive salivation.
9. As tissue necrosis progresses, interproximal craters are formed.
   a. Within a few days, the involved interdental areas are often separated into one facial papilla and one lingual papilla with a necrotic depression between them.
   b. This central tissue destruction between the facial and lingual portions of a papilla results in a crater.
   c. Once interproximal craters are formed, the disease process usually involves the periodontal ligament and alveolar bone, resulting in loss of attachment.
   d. Deep craters in the interdental alveolar bone characterize necrotizing periodontitis.
   e. The deep periodontal pockets seen in other forms of periodontitis are not common in NP because the tissue necrosis destroys the marginal epithelium and connective tissue, resulting in gingival recession. Progression of the interproximal disease process often results in destruction of most of the interdental bone.
10. Due to the intense pain, it is often difficult for patients to eat or drink. As a result, the patient may become malnourished which may affect his/her overall well-being.

B. **Systemic Signs and Symptoms**
   1. Swelling of the lymph nodes, especially the submandibular and cervical lymph nodes, may occur in necrotizing periodontal diseases.
   2. Fever and malaise do not consistently accompany mild and moderate stages of necrotizing periodontal diseases. However, in more severe stages, there may be a high fever, increased pulse rate, loss of appetite, and general malaise.[7,8]

C. **Management.** Management of NPD is presented in Chapter 30, Acute Periodontal Conditions.

4. **Etiology of Necrotizing Periodontal Diseases**
   A. **Compromised Host Immune Response.** NPD are infectious conditions; however, a compromised host immune response is a critical component in the etiology of these diseases.[4] Both NG and NP appear to be related to diminished host response to bacterial infection.
   B. **Predisposing Factors for Necrotizing Periodontal Diseases**
      1. Poor self-care (plaque control)
      2. Emotional stress[9,10]
      3. Inadequate sleep, fatigue
      4. Alcohol use
      5. Caucasian background
      6. Cigarette smoking—most patients who experience necrotizing periodontal diseases are smokers.[8,11]
      7. Increased levels of personal stress
      8. Poor nutrition
         a. In North America, NPD is associated with poor eating habits of young adults, such as college students.
         b. In developing countries, NPD occurs in very young children and appears to be related to poor nutritional status, especially a low protein intake.

9. Pre-existing gingivitis or tissue trauma
10. Young age—this disease can occur at any age and is sometimes observed in young children. However, the reported mean age for necrotizing periodontal diseases in industrialized countries is between 22 and 24 years.[12]

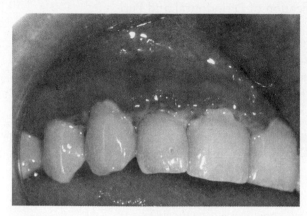
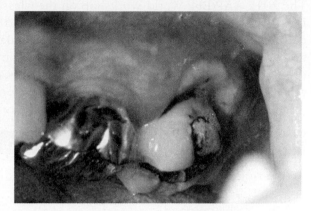

Figure 8-3. Necrotic Papillae and Gingival Margins. This patient with NPD exhibits the characteristic ulcerated, necrotic papillae and gingival margins. (Courtesy of Dr. Ralph Arnold.)

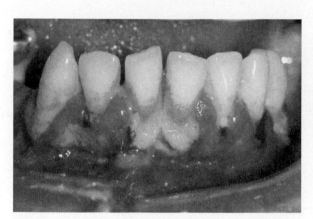
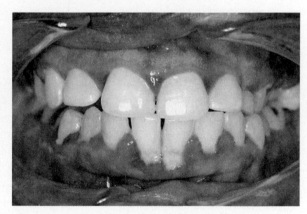

Figure 8-4. Necrotizing Periodontitis. Two examples of necrotizing periodontitis, characterized by the appearance of a pseudomembranous slough that covers the crest of the interdental papilla and extends to the marginal gingiva of the lower central incisors. (The photo on the left, courtesy of Dr. Ralph Arnold; Right-hand photo, courtesy of Dr. Richard Foster, Guilford Technical Community College, Jamestown, NC.)

Section 2
Mucogingival Deformities and Conditions Around Teeth

The 2017 AAP/EFP World Workshop on the Classification of Periodontal and Peri-Implant Diseases and Conditions modified the AAP 1999 classification of mucogingival deformities and conditions around teeth. The updated classification includes additional information such as periodontal biotype, recession severity, dimension of residual gingiva, presence of caries and noncarious cervical lesions, esthetic concerns of the patient, and presence of hypersensitivity. This new classification is summarized in Box 8-3.[13]

Box 8-3. Mucogingival Deformities and Conditions Around Teeth

1. Periodontal biotype
   a. Thin scalloped
   b. Thick scalloped
   c. Thick flat
2. Gingival/soft tissue recession
   a. Facial or lingual surfaces
   b. Interproximal (papillary)
   c. Severity of recession (Cairo RT1, 2, 3)
   d. Gingival thickness
   e. Gingival width
   f. Presence of carious and noncarious cervical lesions/cervical caries
   g. Patient esthetic concern
   h. Presence of hypersensitivity
3. Lack of keratinized gingiva
4. Decreased vestibular depth
5. Aberrant frenum/muscle position
6. Gingival excess
   a. Pseudopocket
   b. Inconsistent gingival margin
   c. Excessive gingival display
   d. Gingival enlargement
7. Abnormal color

---

1. **Normal Mucogingival Conditions**
   A. **Normal mucogingival condition** is defined as the absence of a diseased state. In other words, the absence of diseases/conditions such as gingivitis, periodontitis, and gingival recession.[13]
   B. **Periodontal Biotypes. Periodontal biotypes** describe individual differences in gingival anatomy and morphology. A recent systematic review classifies the "biotypes" in three categories.[14]
      1. *Thin scalloped* biotype is characterized by slender triangular-shaped tooth crowns, subtle cervical convexity (tissue scalloping), interproximal contact areas close to the incisal edge and a narrow zone of keratinized tissue, clear thin delicate gingiva, and a relatively thin alveolar bone.

2. *Thick flat* biotype is characterized by square⊠shaped tooth crowns, pronounced cervical convexity (tissue scalloping), large interproximal contact areas located more apically, a broad zone of keratinized tissue, thick, fibrotic gingiva, and a comparatively thick alveolar bone.

3. *Thick scalloped* biotype is characterized by thick fibrotic gingiva, slender teeth, narrow zone of keratinized tissue, and a pronounced gingival scalloping.

2. **Mucogingival Deformities.** Mucogingival deformities are a group of conditions that affect a large number of patients. A mucogingival deformity is defined as a significant alteration of the morphology, size and interrelationships between the gingiva and the alveolar mucosa that may involve the underlying bone.

A. **Recession of the Gingival Margin (also known as "gingival recession")**

   1. Recession of the gingival margin is the most common mucogingival deformity.

   2. Recession of the gingival margin is defined as the apical displacement of the gingival margin with respect to the cementoenamel junction (CEJ).[15]

   3. It is associated with attachment loss and with exposure of the root surface to the oral environment. Examples of recession of the gingiva are pictured in Figures 8-5 to 8-8.

B. **Risk Factors for Development of Recession of the Gingival Margin**

   1. A thin periodontal biotype

   2. An absence of attached gingiva[14,16,17]

      a. The presence of attached gingival tissue is considered important for the maintenance of gingival health.

      b. The current consensus is that about 2 mm of keratinized tissue and about 1 mm of attached gingiva are desirable around teeth to maintain periodontal health, even though a minimum amount of keratinized tissue is not needed to prevent attachment loss when optimal biofilm control is present.[17]

   3. Reduced thickness of the alveolar bone due to abnormal tooth position in the dental arch.

C. **The Miller Classification System for Recession of the Gingival Margin**

   1. For over 30 years, the Miller Classification System has been the most widely followed and most widely accepted gingival recession classification system.[18] The Miller classification system is based on the level of gingival margin with respect to the mucogingival junction and the underlying alveolar bone.

   2. The Miller classification system classifies gingival recession into four classes. Please refer to Chapter 20, Figure 20-3A–D for an illustration of the Miller classes.

      a. *Class I*: Marginal tissue recession, which does not extend to the mucogingival junction (MGJ). There is no periodontal loss (bone or soft tissue) in the interdental area, and 100% root coverage can be anticipated.

      b. *Class II*: Marginal tissue recession, which extends to or beyond the MGJ. There is no periodontal loss (bone or soft tissue) in the interdental area, and 100% root coverage can be anticipated.

      c. *Class III*: Marginal tissue recession, which extends to or beyond the MGJ. Bone or soft tissue loss in the interdental area is present or there is a malpositioning of the teeth, which prevents the attempting of 100% of root coverage. Partial root coverage can be anticipated.

      d. *Class IV*: Marginal tissue recession, which extends to or beyond the MGJ. The bone or soft tissue loss in the interdental area and/or malpositioning of teeth is so severe that root coverage cannot be anticipated.

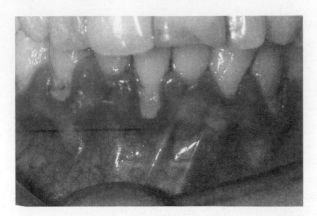

Figure 8-5. Recession of the Gingival Margin.
Recession on the mandibular central incisor extending to the mucogingival junction. (Courtesy of Dr. Ralph Arnold.)

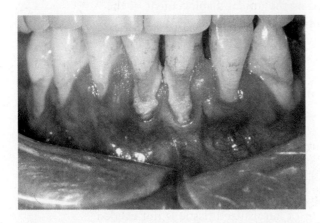

Figure 8-6. Recession of the Gingival Margin.
Recession on the mandibular central incisors extending to the mucogingival junction. (Courtesy of Dr. Ralph Arnold.)

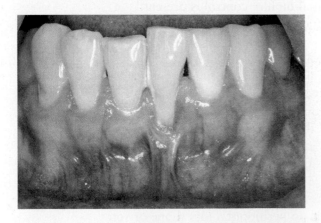

Figure 8-7. Frenum Attachment. Tension of the frenum may pull the gingiva away from the tooth and may be conducive to plaque biofilm accumulation and recession of the gingival margin. (Courtesy of Dr. Richard Foster, Guilford Technical Community College, Jamestown, NC.)

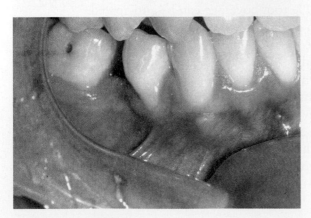

Figure 8-8. Frenum Attachment. Tension of a frenum may pull the gingiva away from the tooth and may be conducive to plaque biofilm accumulation and recession of the gingival margin. (Courtesy of Dr. Ralph Arnold.)

D. **The Cairo Classification System for Recession of the Gingival Margin**
1. In spite of its widespread use in dentistry, the Miller classification system has recently been subject to criticism for the following limitations:
   - From a clinical standpoint, it is sometimes difficult to identify the exact location of the apical extent of the recession defect with respect to the mucogingival junction. This makes it difficult to clinically differentiate a Miller class I from a Miller II.
   - The Miller classification does not clearly define the amount of interproximal soft/hard tissue loss needed to differentiate a Miller class III from a Miller IV.
   - The reliability of the Miller classification system is currently unavailable and has never been tested in a clinical setting.
2. Recently, a new classification system—The **Cairo Classification System**—for gingival recession has been proposed that is based on the CAL measurements at both buccal and interproximal sites.[19]
   a. Compared to the Miller classification system, the Cairo classification uses an objective identifiable criterion—namely, clinical attachment level—to classify the extent and severity of the soft tissue recession.
   b. Furthermore, because the Cairo classification uses an objective identifiable criterion that can be reliably measured, it is a more reliable gingival recession classification system that can be used in clinical practice.
3. The Cairo classification system classifies gingival recession into three types. These types are illustrated in Table 8-1, Figures 8-9 to 8-11.
   a. *Recession Type 1 (RT1):* Gingival recession with *no* loss of interproximal attachment. Interproximal CEJ is clinically not detectable at both mesial and distal aspects of the tooth. RT1 recession defects represent defects that are most likely associated with traumatic toothbrushing in healthy periodontal tissues.
   b. *Recession Type 2 (RT2):* Gingival recession associated with loss of interproximal attachment. The amount of interproximal attachment loss (measured from the interproximal CEJ to the depth of the interproximal sulcus/pocket) is less than or equal to the buccal attachment loss (measured from the buccal CEJ to the apical end of the buccal sulcus/pocket). RT2 represents a soft tissue defect that is most likely associated with periodontitis-induced horizontal bone loss.
   c. *Recession Type 3 (RT3):* Gingival recession associated with loss of interproximal attachment. The amount of interproximal attachment loss (measured from the *interproximal* CEJ to the apical end of the sulcus/pocket) is greater than the buccal attachment loss (measured from the buccal CEJ to the apical end of the buccal sulcus/pocket). Like RT2 recession defects, RT3 represents soft tissue recession defect that is most likely associated with periodontitis, albeit with much more severe interproximal attachment loss. In most cases, RT3 recession defects are associated with an interproximal infrabony defect.

TABLE 8-1	THE CAIRO CLASSIFICATION OF RECESSION OF THE GINGIVAL MARGIN

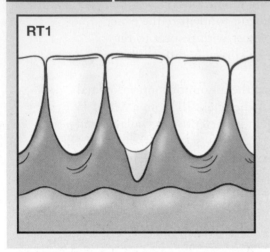

Figure 8-9. Recession Type 1 (RT1). Recession of the gingival margin on the facial aspect of the left central incisor:

- The level of clinical attachment loss on the facial aspect is 3 mm
- There is no detectable loss of interproximal attachment

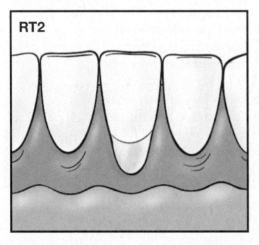

Figure 8-10. Recession Type 2 (RT2). Recession of the gingival margin on the facial aspect of the left central incisor:

- The level of clinical attachment loss on the facial aspect is 4 mm
- Interproximal attachment loss of 3 mm

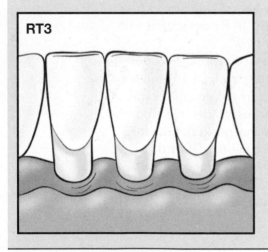

Figure 8-11. Recession Type 3 (RT3). Recession of the gingival margin on the facial aspect of the left central incisor:

- The level of clinical attachment loss on the facial aspect is 6 mm
- Interproximal attachment loss of 8 mm

Section 3
Tooth and Prosthesis-Related Predisposing Factors

Prosthetic factors (such as biologic width violation) and tooth-related factors (such as cervical enamel projections and enamel pearls, palatolingual grooves, or tooth malalignment) can have an adverse effect on the periodontium by enhancing plaque retention and contributing to the initiation and progression of periodontal disease (Figs. 8-12 and 8-13). Local factors such as orthodontic appliances (braces) or faulty dental restorations can lead to plaque biofilm retention and may impinge on the biologic width (Figs. 8-14 and 8-15). However, it is important to emphasize that a dental prosthetic factor and/or tooth-related factor alone does not initiate the disease process. Rather, they are local contributing factors that exacerbate the condition following onset of the disease. For more detailed information about how dental prosthetic factors and tooth-related factors contribute to plaque retention, the reader is referred to Chapter 17.

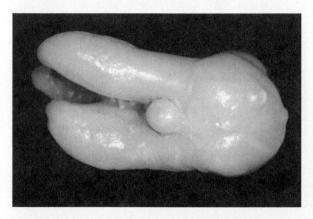 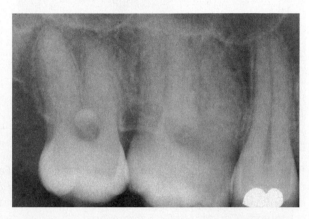

Figure 8-12. Enamel Pearl as Predisposing Factor. This maxillary second molar has an enamel pearl close to the entrance of a furcation. The enamel pearl is a plaque retentive anatomical factor that predisposes a tooth to attachment loss. Although not clear on the radiograph, this tooth exhibited alveolar bone loss on the facial aspect. (Courtesy of Dr. Ralph Arnold.)

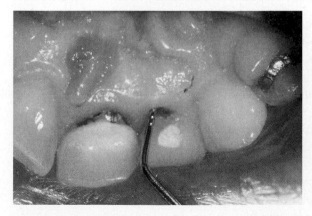 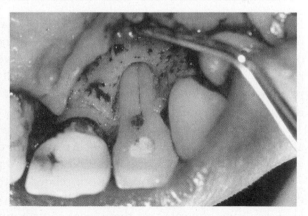

Figure 8-13. Palatolingual Groove. This patient has a deep periodontal pocket on the lingual of the maxillary lateral incisor. Periodontal surgery reveals a palatolingual groove as the predisposing factor for bone loss at this site. (Courtesy of Dr. Ralph Arnold.)

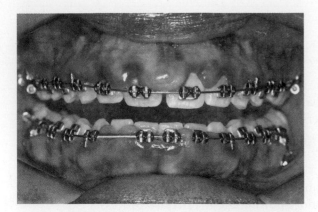

Figure 8-14. Orthodontic Appliances as a Predisposing Factor. Infrequent self-care and plaque biofilm accumulation results in severe soft tissue inflammation in this individual with orthodontic appliances. (Courtesy of Dr. Richard Foster, Guilford Technical Community College, Jamestown, NC.)

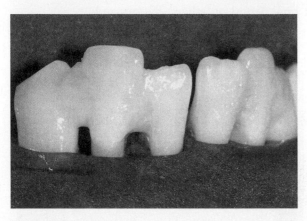

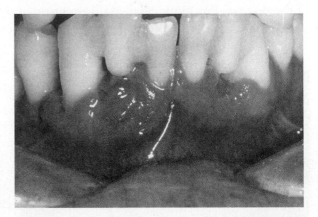

Figure 8-15. Dental Appliances as a Predisposing Factor. The photo to the left shows anterior teeth with a rubber dam in place. The splinting of these mandibular anterior teeth may lead to plaque biofilm accumulation if the patient is unable to perform adequate plaque control or if the splint is improperly placed and/or poorly contoured. (Courtesy of Dr. Ralph Arnold.)

Chapter Summary Statement

Necrotizing periodontal diseases present three characteristic clinical features: tissue necrosis, bleeding, and pain. They represent the most severe biofilm-related periodontal condition. NPDs are infectious conditions; however, a compromised host immune response is a critical component in the etiology of these diseases. Although necrotizing periodontal diseases are relatively uncommon, recognition of NPD is important because they require immediate management.

Mucogingival deformities and recession of the gingival margin are conditions that affect a large number of patients. There is an increased risk of development of recession in individuals with thin periodontal biotypes and poor self-care.

Dental prosthetic factors or tooth-related factors can thwart the combined and concerted efforts of patients and providers in successfully controlling the disease process. Understanding the role that these local contributing factors play in the disease process and reinforcing patient self-care, motivation, and compliance can be helpful in limiting the potential negative effects associated with these plaque retentive prosthetic-related factors and tooth-related factors.

Section 4
Focus on Patients

Clinical Patient Care

A new patient comes to the dental office on an emergency basis. The patient complains of severe pain in his gums and reports that he was unable to eat over the weekend due to the pain. A clinical examination reveals necrotic papillae and gingival margins, cratered papillae, a yellowish tissue slough, spontaneous bleeding, and no loss attachment or bone loss. Which type of periodontal disease does this patient exhibit?

References

1. Novak MJ. Necrotizing ulcerative periodontitis. *Ann Periodontol.* 1999;4(1):74–78.
2. Rowland RW. Necrotizing ulcerative gingivitis. *Ann Periodontol.* 1999;4(1):65–73; discussion 78.
3. Herrera D, Alonso B, de Arriba L, Santa Cruz I, Serrano C, Sanz M. Acute periodontal lesions. *Periodontol 2000.* 2014;65(1):149–177.
4. Herrera D, Retamal-Valdes B, Alonso B, Feres M. Acute periodontal lesions (periodontal abscesses and necrotizing periodontal diseases) and endo-periodontal lesions. *J Periodontol.* 2018;89 Suppl 1:S85–S102.
5. Feller L, Lemmer J. Necrotizing gingivitis as it relates to HIV infection: a review of the literature. *Periodontal Prac Today.* 2005;2:31–37.
6. Malek R, Gharibi A, Khlil N, Kissa J. Necrotizing ulcerative gingivitis. *Contemp Clin Dent.* 2017;8(3):496–500.
7. Shields WD. Acute necrotizing ulcerative gingivitis. A study of some of the contributing factors and their validity in an Army population. *J Periodontol.* 1977;48(6):346–349.
8. Stevens AW, Jr., Cogen RB, Cohen-Cole S, Freeman A. Demographic and clinical data associated with acute necrotizing ulcerative gingivitis in a dental school population (ANUG-demographic and clinical data). *J Clin Periodontol.* 1984;11(8):487–493.
9. da Silva AM, Newman HN, Oakley DA. Psychosocial factors in inflammatory periodontal diseases. A review. *J Clin Periodontol.* 1995;22(7):516–526.
10. Hildebrand HC, Epstein J, Larjava H. The influence of psychological stress on periodontal disease. *J West Soc Periodontol Periodontal Abstr.* 2000;48(3):69–77.
11. Gaggl AJ, Rainer H, Grund E, Chiari FM. Local oxygen therapy for treating acute necrotizing periodontal disease in smokers. *J Periodontol.* 2006;77(1):31–38.
12. Horning GM, Cohen ME. Necrotizing ulcerative gingivitis, periodontitis, and stomatitis: clinical staging and predisposing factors. *J Periodontol.* 1995;66(11):990–998.
13. Cortellini P, Bissada NF. Mucogingival conditions in the natural dentition: Narrative review, case definitions, and diagnostic considerations. *J Periodontol.* 2018;89 Suppl 1:S204–S213.
14. Zweers J, Thomas RZ, Slot DE, Weisgold AS, Van der Weijden FG. Characteristics of periodontal biotype, its dimensions, associations and prevalence: a systematic review. *J Clin Periodontol.* 2014;41(10):958–971.
15. Pini Prato G. Mucogingival deformities. *Ann Periodontol.* 1999;4(1):98–101.
16. Kassab MM, Cohen RE. The etiology and prevalence of gingival recession. *J Am Dent Assoc.* 2003;134(2):220–225.
17. Kim DM, Neiva R. Periodontal soft tissue non-root coverage procedures: a systematic review from the AAP Regeneration Workshop. *J Periodontol.* 2015;86(2 Suppl):S56–S72.
18. Miller PD, Jr. A classification of marginal tissue recession. *Int J Periodontics Restorative Dent.* 1985;5(2):8–13.
19. Cairo F, Nieri M, Cincinelli S, Mervelt J, Pagliaro U. The interproximal clinical attachment level to classify gingival recessions and predict root coverage outcomes: an explorative and reliability study. *J Clin Periodontol.* 2011;38(7):661–666.

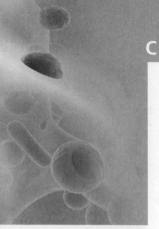

CHAPTER

9 Peri-Implant Health and Diseases

Clinical Application. According to the American Academy of Implant Dentistry, over 3 million Americans have dental implants. To add to this, the popularity of dental implants appears boundless as estimates project this number to grow by 500,000 per year. Yet, while dental implants have high success rates, they are not without risks. At any time during its lifespan, biological and/or mechanical complications could arise and jeopardize the survival of the dental implant. Consequently, as the number of patients with dental implants increases worldwide, dental health care providers, especially dental hygienists, will inevitably encounter patients with dental implants and must be able to distinguish peri-implant health versus peri-implant disease. This chapter focuses on several key aspects that encompass this broad topic: (1) the anatomical components of the dental implant; (2) the differences between the periodontium surrounding a natural tooth and the peri-implant tissues surrounding an implant; (3) the classification of peri-implant diseases and conditions developed by the 2017 AAP/EFP World Workshop on the Classification of Periodontal and Peri-Implant Diseases and Conditions; and (4) guidelines for the clinical monitoring and maintenance of peri-implant tissues.

Learning Objectives

- Describe the components of a conventional dental implant and restoration.
- Compare and contrast the periodontium of a natural tooth with the peri-implant tissues that surround a dental implant.
- Define and distinguish the key differences between peri-implant health, peri-implant mucositis, and peri-implantitis.
- Define the terms osseointegration and biomechanical forces as they apply to dental implants.
- Describe an appropriate maintenance interval for a patient with dental implants.
- In the clinical setting, select appropriate self-care aids for a patient with dental implants.

Key Terms

Dental implant
Implant body
Implant abutment
Biocompatible

Peri-implant tissues
Biological seal
Osseointegration
Peri-implant health

Peri-implant mucositis
Peri-implantitis
Biomechanical forces

Section 1
Anatomy of the Dental Implant and Surrounding Peri-Implant Tissues

Before reviewing the newly developed AAP/EFP classification on peri-implant diseases and conditions, it is important to review the essential components that make up the dental implant and the basic anatomy of the surrounding peri-implant hard and soft tissues. A **dental implant** is a nonbiologic (artificial) device surgically inserted into the jawbone to replace a missing tooth or provide support for a prosthetic denture. Over the past 30 years, research has validated the success of implant placement as a feasible option to replace missing teeth in partially or fully edentulous patients.[1] The dental hygienist plays an important role in patient education and professional maintenance of the dental implant. Understanding the basic concepts of implantology and the anatomy of the peri-implant tissues is a prerequisite for distinguishing peri-implant health from peri-implant diseases and is critical to understanding the significance of performing effective maintenance on patients with dental implants.

1. **The Dental Implant System.** Dental implant systems are used to replace individual teeth or support a fixed bridge or removable denture (Figs. 9-1 and 9-2).

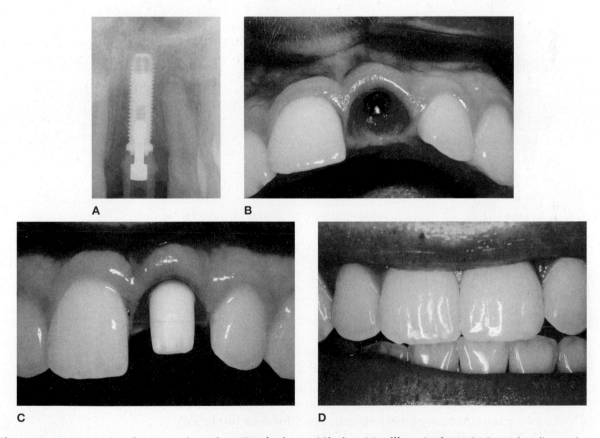

Figure 9-1. Example of a Dental Implant Replacing a Missing Maxillary Incisor. A. Dental radiograph showing the implant body surrounded by healthy bone. **B.** Clinical photograph showing the abutment post penetrating the gingiva. **C.** Clinical photograph of the abutment in place on the dental implant body. Note the healthy color and contour of the peri-implant soft tissue—its appearance is indistinguishable from the healthy periodontal tissue surrounding the neighboring natural teeth. **D.** Clinical photograph of the final prosthetic crown supported by the dental implant. Note that the prosthetic crown provides an esthetic appearance nearly identical to the adjacent natural incisor tooth. (Courtesy of Rodger A. Lawton, DMD, FACP, Northwest Center for Prosthodontics, Olympia, WA.)

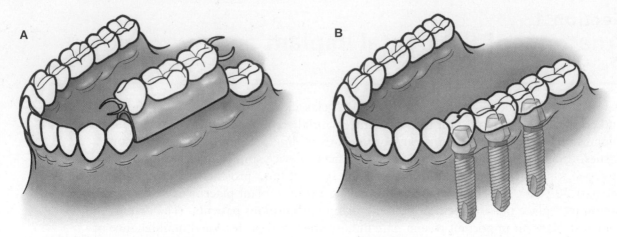

Figure 9-2. Replacement of Missing Teeth. A. Extracted teeth replaced by a traditional removable partial denture. **B.** Missing teeth replaced by three individual dental implants.

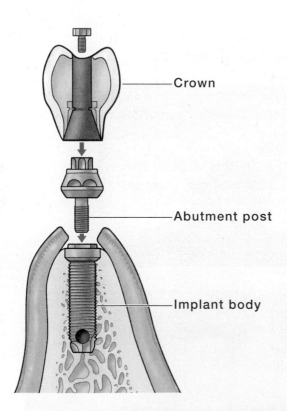

Figure 9-3. The Dental Implant System. The components of a dental implant system are the implant body, the abutment post, and the crown (or other prosthesis). The implant body is placed into living alveolar bone. The abutment post extends into or through living gingival tissue into the mouth. A crown or other prosthesis is connected to the abutment either by a screw or by dental cement.

A. **Components of an Implant System.** The components of a dental implant system are (1) the implant body (also known as the implant fixture), (2) the abutment, and (3) a prosthetic crown or prosthesis (Fig. 9-3). Clinical photographs of implant bodies and abutment posts are shown in Figures 9-4 and 9-5. Figure 9-6 shows a patient case with healing abutments for four implants.

1. **The Implant Body**

   a. An **implant body** is the portion of the implant system that is surgically placed into the living alveolar bone. Figure 9-7 depicts the steps in the surgical placement of a dental implant body. Refer to Chapter 29, Periodontal Surgical Concepts for the Dental Hygienist, for a more in-depth discussion on implant surgery.

b. The implant body acts as the "root" of the implant restoration. The implant body usually is threaded like a screw. These threads provide a greater surface area for contact with the alveolar bone.

1) The metal commonly used for dental implants is titanium or titanium alloy. Titanium is an ideal material for dental implants because it is a bone-friendly metal that is biocompatible and because it is a poor conductor of heat and electricity.

2) Titanium has several disadvantages, however. First, it is softer than other dental restorative metals, and thus scratches easily. Second, there is the biologic possibility that some individuals may exhibit unfavorable immunologic reactions to titanium particles released from titanium implants due to corrosion that takes place in the surrounding host tissues.[2] These disadvantages have cast suspicion on the biological compatibility and the mechanical superiority of titanium.

3) Lately, implant manufacturers are looking into using other types of nonmetallic materials—such as ceramics—as an alternative to titanium. One such ceramic material is zirconia (Fig. 9-4). The biocompatibility and physical and mechanical characteristics of zirconia are similar, if not superior, to titanium. Moreover, the white color of zirconia implants has the potential for better esthetic outcomes in patients with a thin gingiva compared to the grayish color of titanium. As implant manufacturers move to using zirconia as an implant substrate (material), it is important for the dental hygienist to be aware of the many changes that are coming down the pipeline in the implant market.

2. **The Abutment**

a. The **implant abutment** is a titanium post that attaches to the implant body and protrudes partially or completely through the gingival tissue into the mouth.

b. The abutment supports the restorative prosthesis (crown or denture).

c. The titanium abutment is extremely **biocompatible** (not rejected by the body) and allows tissue healing around the abutment.

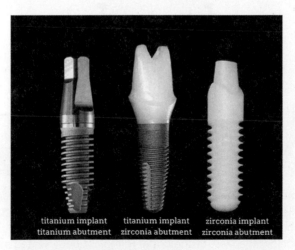

titanium implant   titanium implant   zirconia implant
titanium abutment   zirconia abutment   zirconia abutment

Figure 9-4. Differences in Esthetic Appearance of Titanium Versus Zirconia. Esthetic differences between titanium and zirconia are quite apparent from this figure. Titanium has a grayish dark color which could potentially show through a thin gingiva, and even detract from the most beautifully made implant crown. Zirconia, however, is more esthetically pleasing because of its whitish color which does not shine through the gingiva and is therefore not visibly apparent through the thin gingiva. Combining a zirconia abutment with a zirconia implant adds more to improving the esthetics of the implant restoration since it eliminates the problem of trying to match the shade of adjacent teeth while masking the color of an underlying titanium abutment.

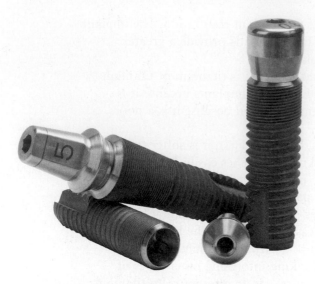

Figure 9-5. Implants and Components. Examples of screw-shaped titanium implant bodies and abutment posts.

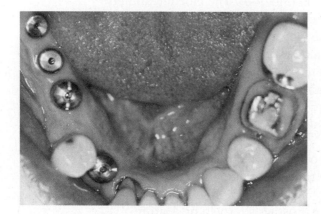

Figure 9-6. Abutments. This photograph shows the healing abutments for four implants.

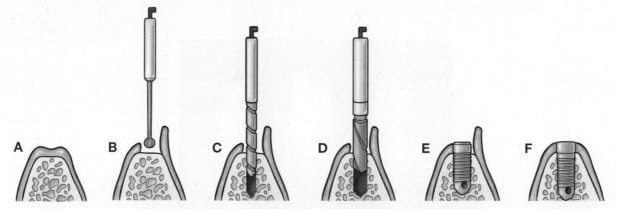

Figure 9-7. Surgical Placement of a Dental Implant. A. Edentulous alveolar ridge. **B.** Initial osteotomy site established. **C** and **D.** Drills of increasing diameters used to prepare the osteotomy site to the size of the planned implant. **E.** Implant body seated in the osteotomy. The top of the implant body may be placed slightly above, level with, or slightly below the crest of the bone. **F.** Implant body seated in bone with cover screw attached. At the end of placement surgery, the implant can be covered with gingiva or left exposed to the oral cavity, as shown here. A healing time of several weeks to months is allowed so that osseointegration can occur.

2. **The Peri-Implant Tissues.** The peri-implant tissues are the hard and soft tissues that surround the dental implant (Fig. 9-8). The peri-implant tissues are similar in many ways to the periodontium of a natural tooth, but there are some important differences (Table 9-1).
   A. **Implant-to-Epithelial Tissue Interface**
      1. The epithelium adapts to the abutment post, or to the implant itself, creating a **biological seal**. The union of the epithelial cells to the abutment or implant surface is very similar to that of the epithelial cells to the natural tooth surface.
      2. The biological seal functions as a barrier between the implant and the oral cavity.
      3. As with a natural tooth, a sulcus lined by sulcular epithelium and junctional epithelium surrounds the abutment or in some cases, the top of the implant body.
   B. **Implant-to-Connective Tissue Interface**
      1. *The implant-to-connective tissue interface is significantly different from that of the connective tissue surrounding a natural tooth.*
      2. The implant surface lacks cementum, so the gingival fibers and the periodontal ligament cannot insert into the titanium surface as they do into the cementum of a natural tooth.
         a. On a natural tooth:
            1) The supragingival fibers brace the gingival margin against the tooth and strengthen the attachment of the junctional epithelium to the tooth. The supragingival fibers insert into the cementum.
            2) The periodontal ligament suspends and maintains the tooth in its socket.
            3) The periodontal ligament fibers also serve as a physical barrier to bacterial invasion.
         b. On an implant:
            1) The connective tissue fiber bundles support the healthy gingiva against the abutment. The connective tissue fiber bundles in the gingiva around an implant have been shown to be either (1) oriented parallel to the implant surface or (2) encircling the implant abutment.[3] The fibers do not attach to the dental implant.
            2) There are no periodontal ligament fibers to provide protection for the dental implant. *Therefore, periodontal pathogens can create inflammation and destroy bone much more rapidly along a dental implant than along a natural tooth with its protective barrier of periodontal ligament fibers.*[4]
            3) Since there are no gingival or periodontal ligament fibers inserting into the titanium surfaces, a periodontal probe will pass more easily through the tissues to the alveolar bone surrounding the implant.
      3. Keratinized gingival tissue may or may not be present around the dental implant.
   C. **Implant-to-Bone Interface**
      1. **Osseointegration** is the direct contact of the living bone with the surface of the implant body (with no intervening periodontal ligament). In other words, an osseointegrated implant is functionally ankylosed to surrounding bone without the periodontal ligament (PDL). Osseointegration is the major determinant for implant success.

2. Clinically, osseointegration is regarded as successful if there is:
   a. An absence of clinical mobility of the implant
   b. No discomfort or pain when the implant is in function
   c. No increased bone loss or radiolucency surrounding the dental implant on a radiograph
   d. Less than 0.2 mm of bone loss annually after the first year in function.[5]

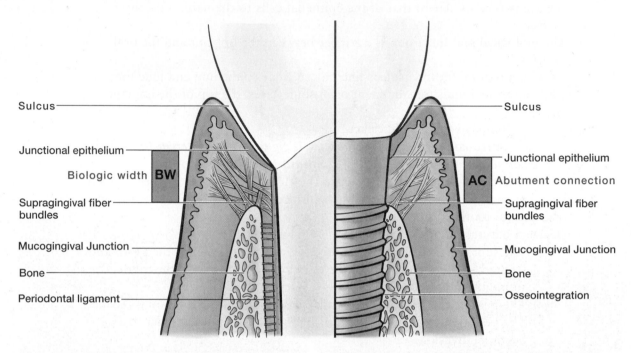

Figure 9-8. Comparison of Periodontium Interface With a Natural Tooth Versus a Dental Implant. The implant lacks the periodontal ligament connection to the alveolar bone and the gingival fibers do not insert into the titanium.

TABLE 9-1	TISSUES SURROUNDING A DENTAL IMPLANT
Tissues	**Peri-Implant Tissues**
Junctional epithelium	Attaches to the implant surface or abutment surface (biologic seal)
Connective tissue fibers	Run parallel to or encircle the implant and abutment surface
Periodontal ligament	No periodontal ligament
Cementum	No cementum
Alveolar bone	In direct contact with the implant surface (osseointegration)

Section 2
Peri-Implant Health, Diseases, and Conditions

The 2017 AAP/EFP World Workshop on the Classification of Periodontal and Peri-Implant Diseases and Conditions developed a new category of peri-implant diseases and conditions. Four key case definitions and diagnostic criteria were introduced: (1) peri-implant health; (2) peri-implant mucositis; (3) peri-implantitis; and (4) peri-implant soft and hard tissue deficiencies.[6]

1. **Peri-Implant Health**
   A. **Peri-implant health** is characterized by an *absence* of erythema, bleeding on probing, swelling, and suppuration. Clinically, there are no visual differences between healthy peri-implant tissues and healthy periodontal tissues. Figure 9-9 shows an example of peri-implant health.
   B. Probing depths may be deeper at a healthy *implant* site compared to a healthy *tooth* site, but this may be due to the orientation of the connective tissue fibers which offer less tissue resistance to probe penetration.

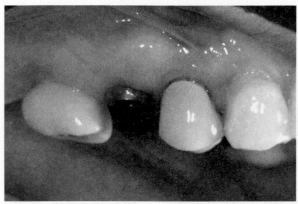

A

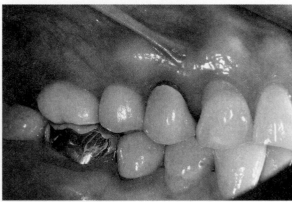

B

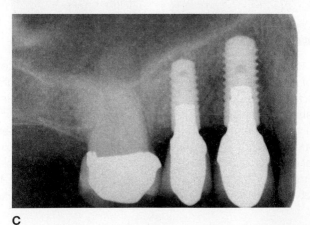

C

Figure 9-9. Healthy Peri-Implant Tissues. A. Clinical photograph 3 months after the implant body was surgically placed. Note the healthy color, contour, and tone of the peri-implant tissue. **B.** One-year clinical photograph. Note there are no visual differences between the healthy appearance of the peri-implant tissues and the healthy periodontal tissues surrounding the adjacent natural teeth. **C.** One-year radiographic follow-up. Note the absence of bone loss around both implants. (The implant in the maxillary first premolar position was placed 5 years prior.)

2. **Peri-implant mucositis** (also called peri-implant gingivitis) is a plaque biofilm-induced inflammation of the soft tissues—with no loss of supporting bone—that is localized in the mucosal tissues surrounding a dental implant.[7] Figure 9-10 shows an example of peri-implant mucositis on the maxillary left lateral incisor tooth.
   A. Peri-implant mucositis is reversible if the etiologic factors are removed.[8] On the other hand, if the etiologic factors are not removed, peri-implant mucositis *may* progress to peri-implantitis.
   B. Peri-implant mucositis has been reported to occur in about 80% of subjects and 50% of implant sites, while peri-implantitis has been reported to occur in 28% to 56% of subjects and 12% to 43% of sites.[9] The reported prevalence, however, varies widely and change as implant designs evolve.
   C. According to the 2017 AAP/EFP World Workshop, a diagnosis of peri-implant mucositis requires:
      1. Visual inspection demonstrating the presence of peri-implant signs of inflammation (red as opposed to pink, swollen tissue as opposed to no swelling, soft as opposed to firm tissue consistency)
      2. Presence of bleeding and/or suppuration upon probing (**Note**: in the absence of inflammatory changes, a local dot of bleeding resulting from traumatic probing should *not* be considered as a clinical sign of peri-implant disease.)
      3. Increased probing depths compared to previous measurements
      4. Absence of bone loss

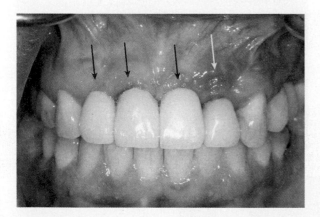
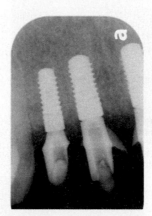
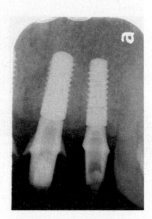

Figure 9-10. Peri-Implant Health and Peri-Implant Mucositis. Note the absence of any clinical signs of peri-implant inflammation of the implants in the maxillary right lateral, maxillary right central, and maxillary left central incisor positions (*black arrows*). However, note the clinical sign of peri-implant inflammation associated with the maxillary left lateral incisor implant (*yellow arrow*). The accompanying 12-month post-cementation periapical radiographs reveal no bone loss around the maxillary implants. Thus, based on the clinical and radiographic presentation, a diagnosis of peri-implant health was made for the maxillary right-sided implants and the maxillary left central incisor implant while a diagnosis of peri-implant mucositis was made for the maxillary left lateral incisor implant. If the etiologic factors are completely removed, the peri-implant mucositis observed around the maxillary left lateral incisor implant can revert to peri-implant health.

3. **Peri-implantitis** is essentially chronic periodontitis affecting the soft and hard tissues surrounding a functioning osseointegrated dental implant, characterized by a plaque biofilm-induced inflammation in the peri-implant mucosal tissues and *progressive* loss of supporting alveolar bone.[10]

   A. The onset of peri-implantitis may occur early during follow-up and may progress in a nonlinear and accelerating pattern.

   B. Peri-implantitis lesion can be diagnosed by the detection of radiographic bone loss around the implant (Figs. 9-11 and 9-12).

   1. The implant does not become mobile until the final stages of peri-implantitis. In fact, in most cases, the patient is unaware that they have peri-implantitis until the implant becomes mobile.

   2. An implant that exhibits mobility is an indication that it has lost osseointegration. If this is observed, the implant should be removed.[11,12]

   C. Differences in the prevalence of peri-implantitis have been reported by a number of research studies. The prevalence reported in these studies ranges from a prevalence of 6.61% to 47%.[13,14]

   D. According to the 2017 AAP/EFP World Workshop, a diagnosis of peri-implantitis requires:

   1. Visual inspection demonstrating the presence of peri-implant signs of inflammation (red as opposed to pink, swollen tissue as opposed to no swelling, soft as opposed to firm tissue consistency)

   2. Presence of bleeding and/or suppuration upon probing (**Note**: in the absence of inflammatory changes, a local dot of bleeding resulting from traumatic probing should not be considered as a clinical sign of peri-implant disease.)

   3. Increased probing depths compared to previous measurements

   4. Progressive bone loss seen by examining the bone levels between two radiographs taken at different time periods (i.e., comparison of radiograph taken at baseline vs. radiograph taken 12 months after cementation of the implant prosthesis)

   5. In the absence of initial radiographs and probing depths (lack of baseline recordings), radiographic evidence of bone level ≥ 3 mm and/or probing depths ≥ 6 mm in conjunction with profuse bleeding represents peri-implantitis.

4. **Hard and Soft Tissue Deficiencies**

   A. Following tooth loss, bone resorption naturally takes place. This will result in hard tissue deficiencies. To correct the deficiency, hard tissue augmentation must be performed either before implant surgery or simultaneously with implant surgery.

   B. Another common type of deficiency seen with implants is soft tissue recession. This may be due to malpositioning of implants, lack of buccal bone, thin soft tissue, lack of keratinized tissue, status of attachment of the adjacent teeth, and surgical trauma. Figure 9-13 shows an example of a clinical deficiency in which recession of the gingival margin results in the implant collar being clinically visible.

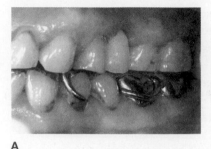

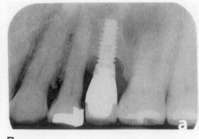

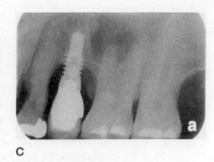

A

B

C

Figure 9-11. Peri-Implantitis (implant in the maxillary left second premolar position). A. Note the clinical signs of peri-implant soft tissue inflammation. Clinical evaluation reveals bleeding upon probing and peri-implant probing depths ranging from 7 to 10 mm. The clinical photograph was taken 18-months post-crown cementation and corresponds to radiograph depicted in **C. B.** Previous periapical radiograph taken at the 12-month post-crown cementation appointment. Note that at 12-months, the radiograph reveals loss of supporting bone. Nonsurgical therapeutic intervention was attempted at this stage, but proved to be ineffective. **C.** 18-month post-crown cementation. By comparing this radiograph against the 12-month radiograph (**B**), one can appreciate the progressive nature of bone loss that has occurred between the two different time periods. If surgical therapeutic intervention is not performed, the implant will inevitably be lost. (Case Courtesy of Dr. Taakaki Kishimoto, Indianapolis, IN.)

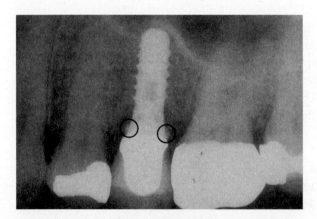

Figure 9-12. Peri-Implantitis. This radiograph shows a titanium implant supporting a single crown. Note the residual cement near the crown margin. This has become a contributing factor for peri-implantitis since bone loss is evident on the radiograph.

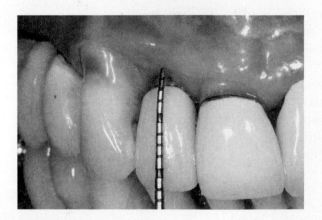

Figure 9-13. Soft Tissue Deficiency. This patient presented with the chief complaint: "*I can see the top of my implant!*" Clinical evaluation reveals an apical shift of the peri-implant gingival tissue, and 2 mm of the implant collar exposed. To resolve the patient's chief complaint, soft tissue augmentation may be performed to cover the exposed implant surface.

Section 3
Recognition of Peri-Implant Diseases

The two forms of peri-implant diseases—peri-implant mucositis and peri-implantitis—share a common primary etiology—bacterial infection. Biomechanical factors, the patient's medical history control, and smoking status are additional factors that can lead to peri-implant diseases.

1. **Etiology and Risk Factors**
   A. **Etiology: Bacterial Infection**
      1. Peri-implant mucositis—like gingivitis—occurs primarily as a result of a plaque-biofilm infection. It develops from healthy peri-implant mucosa following accumulation of bacterial biofilm around an osseointegrated implant.
      2. Peri-implantitis—like periodontitis—occurs primarily as a result of an overwhelming bacterial infection and the subsequent host immune response.[15] Peri-implant mucositis is considered to be a precursor of peri-implantitis. However, it should be kept in mind that peri-implant mucositis does *not* always convert into peri-implantitis. Similar to our current understanding of the conversion of gingivitis to periodontitis, the conditions leading to the conversion from peri-implant mucositis to peri-implantitis are still not understood.
      3. It appears that periodontal disease in both the peri-implant tissues and periodontium in natural teeth progresses in a similar fashion. *The rate of tissue destruction, however, tends to be more rapid in peri-implant tissues than in periodontal tissues.*
      4. No *single* microorganism has ever been implicated to be the causative agent of peri-implantitis. Rather, human cross-sectional studies have indicated that peri-implantitis is a polymicrobial infection (an infection that is related to several types of microorganisms) that is associated with several bacterial species associated with periodontitis.[16-20] A recent study identified a cluster of seven bacterial species that could be associated with peri-implantitis: *Tannerella forsythia, Porphyromonas gingivalis, Treponema socranskii, Staphylococcus aureus, Staphylococcus anaerobius, Streptococcus intermedius,* and *Streptococcus mitis.* The total bacterial load of these seven species was four times higher in implants with peri-implantitis compared to healthy implants. Thus, it was concluded that the bacterial burden may be an important factor in peri-implantitis.[21]
   B. **Risk Factors.** The risk factors identified for each patient are essential in forecasting the prognosis of the implants and these factors should be included in the determination of the appropriate maintenance interval. As in the treatment of periodontal disease, each patient must be assessed for the presence of risk factors that may lead to peri-implant disease or its progression. Risk factors that should be considered include previous history of periodontal disease, ineffective self-care, residual cement, smoking, and biomechanical overload.[15]
      1. **History of Previous Periodontal Disease.** Several systematic reviews indicated that peri-implantitis is a more frequent finding in patients with a history of periodontitis compared to patients without a history of periodontitis.[22-25]
      2. **Poor Plaque Biofilm Control/Lack of Regular Maintenance Therapy.** Like natural teeth, there is evidence that poor plaque control and lack of regular maintenance therapy are risk factors for peri-implant diseases.
      3. **Smoking.** Four systematic reviews concluded that there is an increased risk for peri-implantitis in smokers.[23,26-28]
      4. **Residual Cement.** Implant-supported crowns commonly are held in place with cement. Residual cement—may be left behind because of implant positioning

that may hamper access to the subgingival space.[29] Residual cement may induce inflammation due to its rough surface topography providing an environment for bacterial attachment.[30]

5. **Biomechanical Overload**

   a. Collectively, the forces placed on an implant have been called biomechanical forces to underscore the importance of both "biological" and "mechanical" aspects of controlling those forces to achieve long-term success with implants.

   b. Biomechanical forces on implants are influenced by a variety of factors that must be assessed by the clinician. Factors that influence the biomechanical forces include how much occlusal force is placed on the implant(s), the position of the implant, the number of implants supporting a prosthesis, and the distribution of the occlusal forces among the implants and remaining teeth.

   c. Since dental implants do not have a periodontal ligament, forces placed on an implant are transmitted directly to the alveolar bone.[31,32] It is critical to minimize forces placed on an implant to avoid damage to the surrounding alveolar bone.

      1) Around a natural tooth the periodontal ligament helps absorb some of the forces placed on the tooth. These forces placed on natural teeth can arise from chewing food, supporting a dental appliance, or perhaps from habits such as bruxing.

      2) Dental implants lack the protective features of the periodontal ligament that is found on natural teeth. Instead, as mentioned above, an osseointegrated dental implant is in direct contact with the alveolar bone that completely supports it. If the osseointegrated implant is subjected to excessive occlusal overload, these forces will be transmitted to the surrounding alveolar bone and irreversibly traumatize the bone support. If the occlusal overload is not controlled at its early stages, then loss of osseointegration may occur.

   d. Both bacterial plaque-related causes and excess biomechanical forces can contribute to the development of peri-implant disease. Both should be assessed and controlled at each implant maintenance appointments.

2. **Detection of a Failing Implant**

   A. **Clinical Signs of a Failing Implant**

      1. **Soft Tissue Indicators.** Clinical signs of a failing implant include the presence of a peri-implant pocket, bleeding after gentle probing, and or suppuration from the pocket. The surrounding gingival tissue may or may not be swollen. Pain is usually not present.

      2. **Implant Mobility**

         Absence of mobility is a very important clinical criterion for dental implants. *The presence of mobility presently is the best indicator for diagnosis of implant failure.*[4]

         a. Implants should not be mobile if osseointegrated and healthy.[33,34]

            1) Implant mobility may indicate a lack of osseointegration.

            2) In some instances, mobility of an implant restoration may indicate the presence of a loose abutment or the rupture of the cement seal on cemented restorations rather than loss of osseointegration. Mobility also can result from a loosening of the internal screw that attaches the abutment to the implant or the restoration and therefore is not the result of peri-implant disease (Fig. 9-14).

            3) Severe mobility accompanied with discomfort also might indicate fracture of the implant itself.

4) Long-term mobility or misfit between the prosthetic components (e.g., screws between the crown and implant) may lead to persistent inflammation, bone loss, and the eventual complete failure of the implant.

b. The technique for assessing mobility of a dental implant is similar to that used to assess a natural tooth. Two instruments with *plastic handles* are used to grasp the *implant restoration* and apply force back and forth in the facial and lingual direction. Remember that the implant *restoration* can be mobile while the implant itself is healthy and not mobile.

c. Radiographic evaluation is recommended when any mobility is noted. Loose internal screws or components will often be seen as a gap between the implant components on a radiograph.

B. **Radiographic Signs of a Failing Implant**

1. Radiographic signs of peri-implantitis include vertical destruction of the crestal bone around the implant—which assumes the shape of a saucer—while the bottom portion of the implant remains osseointegrated.[35]

2. Another radiographic indicator of peri-implantitis is wedge-shaped defects along the implant.[35]

3. A peri-implant radiolucency usually indicates bone loss adjacent to the implant and is a key indicator of a failing implant (Fig. 9-15).

3. **Treatment Modalities for Failing Implants**

A. There are various methods available for the treatment of peri-implantitis including nonsurgical periodontal instrumentation, the use of antiseptics, local and/or systemic antibiotics, and access flap surgery.[35]

1. All these treatment modalities have been used with varying degrees of success, but at this time, there is no standard protocol for the treatment of peri-implantitis.[35]

2. Surgical treatment in which the lost bone is reestablished through bone grafting shows promising results.[35]

B. Nonsurgical periodontal instrumentation of peri-implantitis lesions with adjunctive local delivery of microencapsulated minocycline or chlorhexidine may be beneficial to patients with peri-implantitis.[17,36–39]

C. The available evidence suggests that subgingival glycine powder air polishing for biofilm removal may reduce clinical signs of peri-implant mucosal inflammation to a greater extent than periodontal instrumentation with plastic curettes combined with adjunctive irrigation with chlorhexidine.[40]

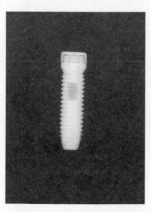

Figure 9-14. Loose Internal Screw. Radiograph of an abutment post with a loose internal screw. (Courtesy of Natalie A. Frost, DDS, MS, Omaha, NE.)

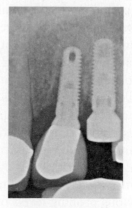

Figure 9-15. Peri-Implant Radiolucency. A peri-implant radiolucency with advanced bone loss adjacent to the implant. (Courtesy of Natalie A. Frost, DDS, MS, Omaha, NE.)

Section 4
Clinical Monitoring of Peri-Implant Health and Diseases

Routine monitoring of dental implants—as a part of a comprehensive periodontal examination and maintenance—is essential to the early detection and the effective management of peri-implant diseases.

1. **Probing**
   A. Initial probing of the implant should be done once the final restoration has been installed.[15,41]
      1. In the past, routine periodontal probing of dental implants was not recommended by some authors. More recent literature, however, suggests routine probing should be part of implant maintenance.[15,41] Yet, while probing depths alone (without having previous measurements to compare against) provide very little valuable information regarding the health of the peri-implant tissues, *changes* in probing depths (reflected by comparing probing depths to previous measurements) can be used to detect changes in tissue/attachment health and can alert the clinician for the need of therapeutic intervention. Probing around osseointegrated implants does not appear to have detrimental effects on the soft tissue seal and, hence, does not seem to jeopardize the longevity of oral implants.[42]
      2. Some implant surgeons recommend that probing should be avoided until postoperative healing is complete, approximately 3 months after abutment connection.
      3. A probing technique with light force (0.25 N, tip diameter of 0.45 mm) should be used since the biological seal is weakly adherent to the titanium surface.[42] Heavy probing force will be invasive since the probe easily can penetrate through the biological seal and introduce bacteria into the peri-implant environment.[43–45] The depth of penetration of the probe tip also is dependent on the health (or inflammatory stage of the peri-implant tissues) and the thickness of the tissue around the abutment.
      4. Commercially available plastic probes have long been used when investigating the depth of the peri-implant sulcus.[4] Recent literature recommends the use of conventional metal periodontal probes if probing pressures are kept light.[46] Light lateral forces on the probe will protect against damaging titanium surfaces. However, plastic probes are more flexible and sometimes advantageous in probing excessive contours and angles found in implant restorations.
      5. Unlike natural teeth, it is *not* possible to define a range of probing depths compatible with peri-implant health. However, peri-implant probing is still an essential component of the complete oral examination as it is the primary means of detecting clinical signs of inflammation.
   B. Clinical attachment levels can be used to monitor peri-implant health.
      1. To interpret probe readings, the clinician must have baseline data recording previous probing levels of attachment, and a fixed reference point for repeatable probing comparisons.
         a. Initial probing of the implant should be done once the final restoration has been installed. Probing depth should be recorded and defined as the depth of probe penetration from the base of the implant sulcus to the crest of the mucosa. Similar to assessing natural teeth, the level of the crestal soft tissue

attachment can be measured using a fixed reference point on the margin of the implant crown and should be noted as the clinical attachment level.

    b. *Changes in probing attachment levels over time may be more important than the initial findings as implants may have deeper soft tissue probing depths.* Due to variation in the depth of surgical placement, the tissue thickness at the site, as well as different lengths of the abutments and the connective tissue interface with the abutment, probing depths may be deeper than the 1- to 3-mm depths that are considered normal with natural teeth.

2. The depth of penetration of the probe tip also is dependent on the health (or inflammatory stage of the peri-implant tissues) and the thickness of the tissue around the abutment.

2. Bleeding and Suppuration

  A. Bleeding on probing is a good indicator of current tissue inflammation and should be recorded.

    1. Lack of bleeding on gentle probing is useful in predicting tissue health around implants.

    2. Elimination of the bleeding on probing in peri-implant mucositis is important and should be accomplished with improved biofilm removal by the clinician and the patient.

    3. Increasing probing depth and bleeding are indicators for the need to perform an additional radiographic examination.[9,47]

  B. Any suppuration should also be recorded at specific sites. Suppuration may be detected by probing, or by gently compressing the tissue over the implant with a gloved finger and observing for pus being expressed from the opening of the sulcus or pocket.

3. Radiographs

  A. Maintenance of bone levels around dental implants is an important criterion for determining treatment success. Radiographic evaluation of bone height and topography is necessary for the longitudinal monitoring of peri-implant stability.[44,45,47]

    1. Vertical bone loss of less than 0.2 mm annually following the implant's first year of function is a criterion utilized to determine treatment success.

    2. Baseline radiographs should include the day of surgical implant placement, the day of final prosthesis insertion, and periodically during implant maintenance.[15] Bone remodeling during the first year after the final prosthesis insertion is expected, and then there should be less than 0.2 mm of bone loss annually thereafter.

    3. The shape and amount of bone remodeling following the final prosthesis insertion is different for different implant systems and configurations.

    4. If prior radiographs are not available, use 2.0 mm of bone loss from the expected bone level for the implant at that time point as the "decision point" for the diagnosis of peri-implantitis.[46]

    5. Radiographs made on the day of the final prosthesis insertion (or re-cementation) should be reviewed for the presence of remaining excess cement. Cements that are visible radiographically should be used for implant restorations, especially if the margins and probable location of excess cements are subgingival.

    6. Radiographs also allow for the evaluation of the fit of the prosthesis and the integrity and adaptation of the different implant components.

  B. Dental implants should be evaluated radiographically at least once a year and should be checked more often in patients in whom periodontal breakdown around an implant was noted at a previous visit.

Section 5
Clinical Guidelines for Maintenance of Patients With Dental Implants

One of the most important factors in the long-term success of dental implants is the maintenance of the health of the peri-implant tissues. Successful maintenance requires the active participation of the patient and the dental team.

1. **Considerations for Implant Maintenance**
   A. **Goals of Maintenance Therapy for Dental Implants**
      1. Maintenance of Alveolar Bone Support
         a. Alveolar bone support is evaluated by use of good-quality radiographs taken with a long-cone paralleling technique at specific time intervals.
         b. The bone height and density around the implants is compared with previous radiographs of the site.
      2. Control of inflammation
         a. Patient and professional biofilm control is important for proper gingival health.
         b. Patient self-care must be reevaluated and, if necessary, reinforced each time the patient is seen for maintenance. The better the patient self-care, the better the possibilities of maintaining stable results.
      3. Maintenance of a Healthy and Functional Implant
         a. Implant components should be checked for prosthesis integrity (such as mobility, loose screws, cement washout, material wear); implant, screw, or abutment fracture; unseating of attachments and proper adaptation of all components.
         b. *Any mobility of an implant or its restorative components requires immediate consultation with a dentist or specialist.*
      4. **Maintenance of a Healthy and Functional Periodontium Surrounding Neighboring Teeth**
         a. It is theorized that the natural teeth in a partially edentulous mouth act as a reservoir of periodontal pathogens that colonize the implants.
         b. This finding makes meticulous self-care of dental implants *and* natural teeth even more critical for the partially edentulous patient than for the fully edentulous patient.
   B. **Patient Provided Information.** Before beginning an examination, it is very important to obtain information from the patient related to implant-supported restorations or prostheses. The patient can often identify problems for clinicians that are otherwise difficult to find. Implant patients should be encouraged to share their perceptions of any changes in the fit, tightness, or feel of the implant restoration including the occlusion. Helpful questions to ask the patient include:
      1. Questions About Daily Self-Care of Implant-Supported Restorations/Prosthesis
         a. *Are you able to clean around the neck portions of your implant(s) easily?*
         b. *Do you still have enough cleaning aids to perform daily oral self-care?*
      2. Questions Concerning Patient Satisfaction. General questions regarding the patient's satisfaction with the implant-supported restorations/prosthesis are part of a quality management concept for maintenance.
         a. *Are you satisfied with the way your implant(s) function(s)?*
         b. *Are you satisfied with the appearance of your implant(s)?*

3. Questions Regarding Patient-Perceived Changes Since Last Appointment
   a. *Do you feel like any part of the implant(s) is/are loose?*
   b. *Do the gums around your implant(s) bleed?*
   c. *Do you notice a bad taste coming from your implant(s)?*
   d. *Have you noticed any changes in your implant(s)?*

C. **The Dental Implant Maintenance Visit**
   1. Modern dental implants may be difficult to recognize intraorally since their restorations often have the same appearance as the crowns and fixed bridges used to restore natural teeth (Fig. 9-16). *For this reason, dental implants should be clearly noted in the chart so that all dental team members are alerted to the exact location of the dental implant in the patient's mouth.* Also, the patient's radiographs should be updated annually and reviewed before the start of periodontal instrumentation.
   2. The following may be included in a maintenance visit however, each maintenance visit should be individualized based on previous examinations, history, and judgment of the clinician: evaluation of peri-implant tissue health, examination of prosthesis/abutment components, evaluation of implant stability, occlusal examination, assessment of patient's self-care, radiographic examination, and treatment (e.g., periodontal instrumentation).

2. **Guidelines for Professional Recall and Maintenance**
   A. **Maintenance Frequency**
      1. Patients with implant-borne restorations—fixed or removable—should be advised to obtain a professional dental examination at least every 6 months as a lifelong regimen.[48] Maintenance intervals should be determined on an individual basis, because there is a lack of data detailing precise intervals.
         a. A 3-month maintenance interval is usually appropriate for the first year following restoration of the implant. The clinician, however, must determine the best interval for each specific case.
         b. After the initial 12-month period, a 3- to 6-month maintenance interval may be used.[49] Periodontal maintenance appointments should be scheduled as frequently as necessary to keep the periodontium and peri-implant tissues healthy.
            1) Patients categorized at higher risk based on age, ability to perform oral self-care, biological or mechanical complications of implant-borne restorations should be advised to obtain a professional examination more often than every 6 months.[48]
            2) The risk factors identified for each patient are essential in the estimation of the prognosis for the implants and these factors should be included in the determination of the appropriate maintenance interval. The following are indications for more frequent maintenance intervals.
               a) Reduced Bone Support Around Implants. Reduced bone support indicates that close monitoring of bone support is needed or the dental implant might be lost.
               b) Inflammation. A patient who has signs of inflammation around implants, even in the presence of good biofilm control, needs more frequent maintenance visits.
               c) Host Response. Systemic conditions or diseases, such as diabetes, may affect the host-bacterial interaction. A shorter maintenance interval is needed for these patients.

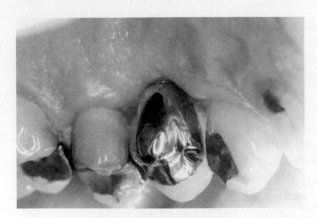

Figure 9-16. Fixed Prosthetic Crown. The first premolar in this photo is a prosthetic crown supported by a dental implant. During an intraoral examination, it would be difficult to distinguish between a crown that is supported by a natural tooth and a crown supported by a dental implant.

B. **Guidelines for Professional Maintenance.** A panel comprised of experts appointed by the American College of Prosthodontists (ACP), American Dental Association (ADA), Academy of General Dentistry (AGD), and the American Dental Hygienists Association (ADHA) met to establish new clinical practice guidelines for recall and maintenance of patients with implant-borne dental restorations.[48] These guidelines for professional maintenance are summarized in Table 9-2.

1. Previous research indicated that scratching of the implant surface was a significant cause of implant failure. This belief led to a recommendation that only plastic and graphite instruments be used on titanium surfaces. Exclusive use of polymer instruments is no longer recommended for several reasons:

   a. Investigation of failing implants shows that *residue left on the implant body is one significant reason for implant failure.* Residues may include cement, calculus deposits, or debris left from forceful use of polymer (plastic, graphite, resin) instruments.

   b. Modern implant material, itself, is very rough and porous. The implant companies make rough, porous implant material for better osseointegration of the implant to the bone. Rough surfaces are very common on portions or all of the implant body. These surfaces are usually intended to be adjacent to bone and not exposed to the oral environment. If an intentionally rough surface becomes exposed to the oral cavity—due to pocket formation or recession of the gingival margin—it needs to be instrumented as part of implant maintenance.

2. Removal of subgingival cement or calculus deposits requires a slender instrument working-end made of a metal compatible with the implant—in other words, a titanium instrument. *The new guidelines from the American College of Prosthodontics state that implants should be instrumented with like metals—titanium on titanium—so as to not leave any residue behind.*[48]

   a. Standard dental restorative materials, for example, gold and porcelain, can be cleaned with conventional periodontal instruments. Care must be taken, however, not to use these instruments apical to the margin of the prosthetic crown where titanium might be contacted.

   b. Titanium instruments are recommended for removal of subgingival calculus deposits and residual dental cement.

      1) The working-ends of titanium instruments are slender and have cutting edges that can be sharpened. The working-ends of polymer instruments are bulky and not well suited for subgingival instrumentation.

      2) The quality of titanium instruments varies from manufacturer to manufacturer. Gordon J. Christensen's *Dental Hygiene Clinicians Report*,

March/April 2018, rates the features and performance of titanium instruments (https://www.cliniciansreport.org).

   c. Residual dental cement is a frequent finding when restorations have been cemented to abutments. Cement deposits are typically located subgingivally. Some of the advanced cement formulations used today strongly adhere to the surface of the implant which makes removal very difficult. If removal efforts are not successful, surgical access is highly recommended.

C. **Special Considerations for Polishing**
   1. *Implants, abutments, and components do not require routine polishing.*
      a. When indicated, polishing of the implant restoration can be accomplished with rubber cups and nonabrasive polishing paste or by supragingival air polishing.[50,51]
      b. Polishing has been shown to improve titanium surfaces *that have previously been roughened or scratched. However, if no surface alterations are noted, the titanium surfaces should not be polished.*
      c. A systematic review by Louropoulou indicates that *for rough implant surfaces*, air abrasives are the instruments of choice, if surface integrity needs to be maintained. Air polishing with glycine powder may be considered a better method to remove plaque biofilm from dental implants because glycine is less aggressive than sodium bicarbonate powder.[50,51]
   2. Air polishing **with glycine powder** for the removal of biofilm from titanium surfaces is a relatively new technology with clinical research supporting its safety and efficacy for use in the treatment of peri-implant disease. Glycine-based powders are biocompatible and gentle on the soft tissues of the oral cavity and subgingival epithelium.[52–54]

TABLE 9-2	GUIDELINES FOR RECALL AND MAINTENANCE OF DENTAL IMPLANTS
Patient recall	Patients with implant-borne restorations—fixed or removable—should be advised to obtain a professional dental examination at least every 6 months as a lifelong regimen.
Professional maintenance	Meticulous patient self-care is an important factor for long-term implant health; instruction in self-care techniques for natural teeth, implant-borne restorations or implant abutments should be part of every maintenance visit. • Professionals should recommend appropriate oral topical agents and self-care aids suitable for the patient's at-home maintenance needs. • Chlorhexidine gluconate is the oral topical agent of choice when an antimicrobial agent is indicated. Dental professionals should use periodontal instruments compatible with the type and material of the implants, abutments, and restorations and powered instruments such as glycine powder air polishing.

3. **Patient Self-Care of Dental Implants**
   A. **Considerations**
      1. Meticulous self-care is of the utmost importance in preventing peri-implant disease. *An individualized self-care routine should be developed for each patient.*
      2. Some patients undergoing implant therapy may have had a long history of dental neglect and/or poor plaque biofilm control.
      3. The dental hygienist can assist the patient in maintaining dental implants by providing self-care education appropriate for implants and home care devices that are effective and simple to use.
   B. **Care of Fixed Prosthetic Restorations**
      1. A fixed prosthetic crown is an artificial tooth that fits over the abutment. These are made from a variety of routinely encountered restorative materials.
      2. Self-Care Challenges
         a. The single tooth prosthesis (crown) can present a challenge for biofilm control in that the patient may quickly begin to regard it to be just the same as a natural tooth.
            1) In fact, these restorations often have different designs and unusual contours that require focused self-care attention. The better the patient understands the design and contours etc. that must be cleaned, the better the oral hygiene effectiveness will be.
            2) Self-care practices must be modified to include aids that can effectively clean the altered morphology of the peri-implant region.
         b. The crown covering the implant abutment is larger in circumference than the abutment and will have contours added to it to make it look and function like a natural tooth.
            1) The "bulky" contours of the crown may contact the tissue and then "dip in" to meet the abutment at or below the gingival margin.
            2) Dental floss or tufted dental floss should be adapted along the margin of the crown and then pulled gently back and forth to direct it into the sulcus and around the abutment (Fig. 9-17).
         c. In some cases, the restoration may be similar to a fixed bridge (e.g., a pontic supported by two dental implants). Tufted dental floss, specially designed interdental brushes, and water flossers are effective cleaning devices for deplaquing the large embrasure spaces and into the sulci of these fixed bridge-type restorations.

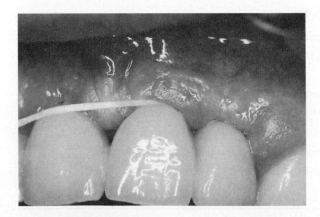

Figure 9-17. Implant Self-Care. Dental floss is used to clean a single implant with a prosthetic crown. The "bulky" contours of the crown may contact the tissue and then "dip in" to meet the abutment at or below the gingival margin.

    d. Restoration of multiple tooth replacement situations can involve complex, denture-like prostheses which are attached to multiple implants and which are not removable by the patient.

        1) These prostheses can be removed by either the dentist or specialist at which time cleaning access is optimal.

        2) Daily care by the patient requires an individualized plan and a combination of devices to overcome the limited access often encountered.

3. Techniques and Devices

    a. Standard multitufted, soft nylon bristle, manual toothbrushes can be used effectively by patients having sufficient dexterity and understanding of the task.

    b. Powered toothbrushes are safe for titanium surfaces and these devices are particularly helpful for implant patients in general.

    c. Interdental brushes can be effective in biofilm removal and may effectively clean the peri-implant sulcus.[55]

        1) *Note that interdental brushes used to clean implants and components should have a soft protective coating on the twisted wire that secures the bristles.*

        2) The use of a standard interdental brush (that does not have a plastic or nylon coating on the twisted wire) should be avoided since the exposed wire could scratch titanium.

    d. Dental floss can be used with dental implants. Patients must be instructed to gently use floss subgingivally. Flosses with expanded spongy or fluffy sections along with a stiffer, floss threader section (tufted floss) are particularly helpful.

    e. Oral irrigators may be safely used to remove plaque biofilm from dental implants.

        1) In a study, Magnuson et al.[56] compared the efficacy of a manual toothbrush paired with either traditional dental floss or a water flosser. The study results demonstrate that the water flossing group had statistically significantly greater reduction in bleeding than the dental floss group. The authors conclude that water flossing may be a useful adjunct to implant maintenance.

        2) Patients should be instructed to use the lowest setting and direct the flow through the interdental contacts or perpendicular to the implants rather than directly into the implant sulcus.

    f. Daily use of an antimicrobial mouth rinse is beneficial for many patients.[48] The entire mouth can be rinsed twice daily after brushing. Or, if that is not acceptable to the patient, the mouth rinse can be applied topically to each implant area twice daily with a cotton-tipped applicator or with gauze.

C. Care of a Removable Prosthesis

    1. An implant-supported removable prosthesis is similar to a traditional full denture except that in the case of implants, it is attached to the abutments by devices such as O-rings, magnets, or clips (Fig. 9-18).

        a. This type of prosthesis can also be designed as an implant- and tissue-supported prosthesis or as an overdenture.

        b. The patient can remove the prosthesis to clean it, the attachment devices, the abutments, and the remainder of the mouth.

2. **Techniques and Tools**
   a. Selection of cleaning devices for the abutments that support a removable prosthesis should be based on the knowledge that implant components are made from titanium, which is a relatively soft metal.
   b. Cleaning devices must be selected for ease of use by each individual patient, and the recommendation of fewer, rather than more, devices is best. The cleaning aids that are recommended should be demonstrated for the patient and then evaluated by the hygienist to verify their effective use by the patient.
   c. In some cases, a metal bar connects the abutments and is used to attach the prosthetic denture in the mouth. Tufted dental floss or an unfolded 2 × 2 gauze square can be useful in cleaning underneath the metal bar and around the abutments (Fig. 9-19).

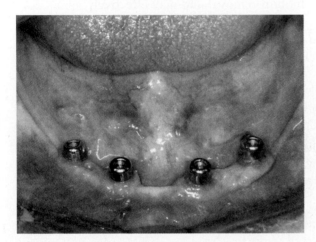
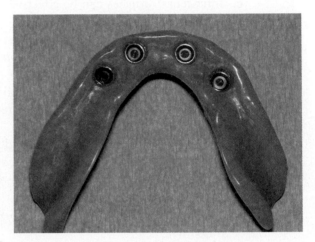

Figure 9-18. Implant Supported Removable Prosthesis. Abutment posts on the mandibular arch. An implant supported removable prosthesis is attached to the abutment posts by O-rings, magnets, or clips. (Courtesy of Rodger A. Lawton, DMD, FACP, Olympia, WA.)

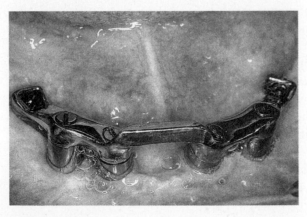
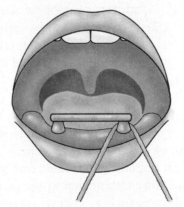

Figure 9-19. Abutments Joined by Metal Bar. Tufted dental floss is useful in cleaning the implant abutments and underneath the connecting metal bar.

Chapter Summary Statement

As dental implant therapy becomes more common, dental hygienists will care for increasing numbers of patients with implants, and as such, a significantly higher incidence of peri-implant diseases is inevitable. The primary goals of treatment for peri-implant diseases are to stop disease progression and maintain the implant in function with healthy peri-implant tissues. To be able to accomplish this, the dental hygienist must be able to distinguish between peri-implant health and peri-implant diseases.

Frequent professional maintenance is the most important step in the early detection and management of peri-implant diseases. An important role of the dental hygienist is to educate patients about the importance of meticulous self-care and frequent maintenance visits.

Implant restorations necessitate customized self-care instructions and devices. Implant maintenance appointments should include monitoring of plaque biofilm levels, examination of soft tissues, assessment of the restorative integrity, reinforcement of patient self-care measures, periodontal instrumentation of implant abutments and prostheses, and radiographic examination.

Section 6
Focus on Patients

Clinical Patient Care

CASE 1

A patient returns to you for his regular 3-month periodic recall. He is completely edentulous and wears an implant-supported maxillary denture and an implant-supported mandibular denture. Figures 9-20 and 9-21 are the clinical photograph and the radiograph of the implants.

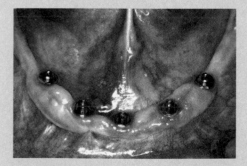
Figure 9-20. Clinical Photograph: Case I.

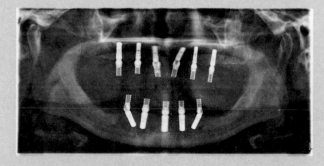
Figure 9-21. Radiograph: Case I.

Based on the patient's presentation, what would be the peri-implant diagnosis? What steps would you take to perform a thorough and complete peri-implant evaluation? What type of home care recommendations would you give to the patient? (*Assume that the clinical and radiographic presentation of the peri-implant tissues in the mandibular arch is representative of the maxillary implants.*)

CASE 2

While you are performing nonsurgical therapy on a periodontitis patient, the patient tells you that he is thinking about having all of his teeth removed, since they are not healthy anyway, and just having some implants placed. He tells you that this would be easier, since he would not have to worry about the implants like he does his teeth. How should you respond?

CASE 3

You are scheduled to record the information needed to make a periodontal diagnosis for a patient new to your dental team. Radiographs have not yet been ordered for the patient. As you begin your probing, the patient informs you that she has two dental implants. Visual examination of the patient's dentition does not immediately reveal which teeth are replaced by the implants. How should you proceed?

CASE 4

At a maintenance visit for one of your team's patients you note obvious mobility of a crown supported by an implant. How should you (the dental hygienist) proceed?

References

1. Cochran DL, Nummikoski PV, Schoolfield JD, Jones AA, Oates TW. A prospective multicenter 5-year radiographic evaluation of crestal bone levels over time in 596 dental implants placed in 192 patients. *J Periodontol*. 2009;80(5):725–733.
2. Pettersson M, Kelk P, Belibasakis GN, Bylund D, Molin Thoren M, Johansson A. Titanium ions form particles that activate and execute interleukin-1beta release from lipopolysaccharide-primed macrophages. *J Periodontal Res*. 2017;52(1):21–32.
3. Lang NP, Karring T, Lindhe J; European Federation of Periodontology; European Association of Osseointegration; Swiss Society of Periodontology. Proceedings of the 3rd European Workshop on Periodontology: implant dentistry: Charter House at Ittingen, Thurgau, Switzerland, January 30-February 3, 1999. Berlin; Chicago, IL: Quintessence; 1999:615.
4. Silverstein L, Garg A, Callan D, Shatz P. The key to success: maintaining the long-term health of implants. *Dent Today*. 1998;17(2):104, 106, 108–111.
5. Albrektsson T, Zarb G, Worthington P, Eriksson AR. The long-term efficacy of currently used dental implants: a review and proposed criteria of success. *Int J Oral Maxillofac Implants*. 1986;1(1):11–25.
6. Berglundh T, Armitage G, Araujo MG, et al. Peri-implant diseases and conditions: Consensus report of workgroup 4 of the 2017 World Workshop on the Classification of Periodontal and Peri-Implant Diseases and Conditions. *J Periodontol*. 2018;89(Suppl 1):S313–S318.
7. Heitz-Mayfield LJA, Salvi GE. Peri-implant mucositis. *J Periodontol*. 2018;89(Suppl 1):S257–S266.
8. Salvi GE, Aglietta M, Eick S, Sculean A, Lang NP, Ramseier CA. Reversibility of experimental peri-implant mucositis compared with experimental gingivitis in humans. *Clin Oral Implants Res*. 2012;23(2):182–190.
9. Lang NP, Berglundh T; Working Group 4 of Seventh European Workshop on Periodontology. Peri-implant diseases: where are we now?—Consensus of the Seventh European Workshop on Periodontology. *J Clin Periodontol*. 2011;38(Suppl 11):178–181.
10. Schwarz F, Derks J, Monje A, Wang HL. Peri-implantitis. *J Periodontol*. 2018;89(Suppl 1):S267–S290.
11. Mahesh L, Kurtzman GM, Shukla S. Microbiology of peri-implant infections. *J Hosp Infect*. 2009;72(2):104–110.
12. Pye AD, Lockhart DE, Dawson MP, Murray CA, Smith AJ. A review of dental implants and infection. *J Hosp Infect*. 2009;72(2):104–110.
13. Atieh MA, Alsabeeha NH, Faggion CM, Jr., Duncan WJ. The frequency of peri-implant diseases: a systematic review and meta-analysis. *J Periodontol*. 2013;84(11):1586–1598.
14. Derks J, Tomasi C. Peri-implant health and disease. A systematic review of current epidemiology. *J Clin Periodontol*. 2015;42(Suppl 16):S158–S171.
15. Peri-implant mucositis and peri-implantitis: a current understanding of their diagnoses and clinical implications. *J Periodontol*. 2013;84(4):436–443.
16. Heitz-Mayfield LJ, Lang NP. Comparative biology of chronic and aggressive periodontitis vs. peri-implantitis. *Periodontol 2000*. 2010;53:167–181.
17. Mombelli A, Lang NP. Antimicrobial treatment of peri-implant infections. *Clin Oral Implants Res*. 1992;3(4):162–168.
18. Quirynen M, De Soete M, van Steenberghe D. Infectious risks for oral implants: a review of the literature. *Clin Oral Implants Res*. 2002;13(1):1–19.
19. Renvert S, Roos-Jansaker AM, Lindahl C, Renvert H, Rutger Persson G. Infection at titanium implants with or without a clinical diagnosis of inflammation. *Clin Oral Implants Res*. 2007;18(4):509–516.

20. Shibli JA, Martins MC, Lotufo RF, Marcantonio E, Jr. Microbiologic and radiographic analysis of ligature-induced peri-implantitis with different dental implant surfaces. *Int J Oral Maxillofac Implants.* 2003;18(3):383–390.

21. Persson GR, Renvert S. Cluster of bacteria associated with peri-implantitis. *Clin Implant Dent Relat Res.* 2014;16(6):783–793.

22. Karoussis IK, Kotsovilis S, Fourmousis I. A comprehensive and critical review of dental implant prognosis in periodontally compromised partially edentulous patients. *Clin Oral Implants Res.* 2007;18(6):669–679.

23. Klokkevold PR, Han TJ. How do smoking, diabetes, and periodontitis affect outcomes of implant treatment? *Int J Oral Maxillofac Implants.* 2007;22(7):173–202.

24. Schou S, Holmstrup P, Worthington HV, Esposito M. Outcome of implant therapy in patients with previous tooth loss due to periodontitis. *Clin Oral Implants Res.* 2006;17(Suppl 2):104–123.

25. Van der Weijden GA, van Bemmel KM, Renvert S. Implant therapy in partially edentulous, periodontally compromised patients: a review. *J Clin Periodontol.* 2005;32(5):506–511.

26. Heitz-Mayfield LJ, Huynh-Ba G. History of treated periodontitis and smoking as risks for implant therapy. *Int J Oral Maxillofac Implants.* 2009;24:39–68.

27. Hinode D, Tanabe S, Yokoyama M, Fujisawa K, Yamauchi E, Miyamoto Y. Influence of smoking on osseointegrated implant failure: a meta-analysis. *Clin Oral Implants Res.* 2006;17(4):473–478.

28. Strietzel FP, Reichart PA, Kale A, Kulkarni M, Wegner B, Kuchler I. Smoking interferes with the prognosis of dental implant treatment: a systematic review and meta-analysis. *J Clin Periodontol.* 2007;34(6):523–544.

29. Linkevicius T, Puisys A, Vindasiute E, Linkeviciene L, Apse P. Does residual cement around implant-supported restorations cause peri-implant disease? A retrospective case analysis. *Clin Oral Implants Res.* 2012;24(11):1179–1184.

30. Wilson TG, Jr. The positive relationship between excess cement and peri-implant disease: a prospective clinical endoscopic study. *J Periodontol.* 2009;80(9):1388–1392.

31. Hudieb MI, Wakabayashi N, Kasugai S. Magnitude and direction of mechanical stress at the osseointegrated interface of the microthread implant. *J Periodontol.* 2011;82(7):1061–1070.

32. Rungsiyakull C, Rungsiyakull P, Li Q, Li W, Swain M. Effects of occlusal inclination and loading on mandibular bone remodeling: a finite element study. *Int J Oral Maxillofac Implants.* 2011;26(3):527–537.

33. Ericsson I, Lindhe J. Probing depth at implants and teeth. An experimental study in the dog. *J Clin Periodontol.* 1993;20(9):623–627.

34. Lang NP, Wetzel AC, Stich H, Caffesse RG. Histologic probe penetration in healthy and inflamed peri-implant tissues. *Clin Oral Implants Res.* 1994;5(4):191–201.

35. Mahesh L, Kurtzman GM, Bali P, Shukla S. Treatment of peri-implantitis. *Inside Dentistry.* 2013;9(3):84–90.

36. Porras R, Anderson GB, Caffesse R, Narendran S, Trejo PM. Clinical response to 2 different therapeutic regimens to treat peri-implant mucositis. *J Periodontol.* 2002;73(10):1118–1125.

37. Renvert S, Lessem J, Lindahl C, Svensson M. Treatment of incipient peri-implant infections using topical minocycline microspheres versus topical chlorhexidine gel as an adjunct to mechanical debridement. *J Int Acad Periodontol.* 2004;6(4 Suppl):154–159.

38. Renvert S, Polyzois I, Persson GR. Treatment modalities for peri-implant mucositis and peri-implantitis. *Am J Dent.* 2013;26(6):313–318.

39. Schar D, Ramseier CA, Eick S, Arweiler NB, Sculean A, Salvi GE. Anti-infective therapy of peri-implantitis with adjunctive local drug delivery or photodynamic therapy: six-month outcomes of a prospective randomized clinical trial. *Clin Oral Implants Res.* 2013;24(1):104–110.

40. Flemmig TF, Arushanov D, Daubert D, Rothen M, Mueller G, Leroux BG. Randomized controlled trial assessing efficacy and safety of glycine powder air polishing in moderate-to-deep periodontal pockets. *J Periodontol.* 2012;83(4):444–452.

41. Heitz-Mayfield LJ, Needleman I, Salvi GE, Pjetursson BE. Consensus statements and clinical recommendations for prevention and management of biologic and technical implant complications. *Int J Oral Maxillofac Implants.* 2014;29:346–350.

42. Etter TH, Hakanson I, Lang NP, Trejo PM, Caffesse RG. Healing after standardized clinical probing of the peri-implant soft tissue seal: a histomorphometric study in dogs. *Clin Oral Implants Res.* 2002;13(6):571–580.

43. Bader H. Implant maintenance: a chairside test for real-time monitoring. *Dent Econ.* 1995;85(6):66–67.

44. Cochran D. Implant therapy I. *Ann Periodontol.* 1996;1(1):707–791.

45. Papaioannou W, Quirynen M, Nys M, van Steenberghe D. The effect of periodontal parameters on the subgingival microbiota around implants. *Clin Oral Implants Res.* 1995;6(4):197–204.

46. Sanz M, Chapple IL; Working Group 4 of the VIII European Workshop on Periodontology. Clinical research on peri-implant diseases: consensus report of Working Group 4. *J Clin Periodontol.* 2012;39(Suppl 12):202–206.

47. Lindhe J, Meyle J, Group D of European Workshop on Periodontology. Peri-implant diseases: Consensus Report of the Sixth European Workshop on Periodontology. *J Clin Periodontol.* 2008;35(8 Suppl):282–285.

48. Bidra AS, Daubert DM, Garcia LT, et al. Clinical Practice Guidelines for Recall and Maintenance of Patients with Tooth-Borne and Implant-Borne Dental Restorations. *J Prosthodont.* 2016;25(Suppl 1):S32–S40.

49. Eskow RN, Smith VS. Preventive peri-implant protocol. *Compend Contin Educ Dent.* 1999;20(2):137–142, 44, 46 passim; quiz 54.

50. Cochis A, Fini M, Carrassi A, Migliario M, Visai L, Rimondini L. Effect of air polishing with glycine powder on titanium abutment surfaces. *Clin Oral Implants Res.* 2013;24(8):904–909.

51. Louropoulou A, Slot DE, Van der Weijden FA. Titanium surface alterations following the use of different mechanical instruments: a systematic review. *Clin Oral Implants Res.* 2012;23(6):643–658.

52. Petersilka GJ, Steinmann D, Haberlein I, Heinecke A, Flemmig TF. Subgingival plaque removal in buccal and lingual sites using a novel low abrasive air-polishing powder. *J Clin Periodontol.* 2003;30(4):328–333.

53. Sahrmann P, Ronay V, Schmidlin PR, Attin T, Paque F. Three-dimensional defect evaluation of air polishing on extracted human roots. *J Periodontol.* 2014;85(8):1107–1114.

54. Sculean A, Bastendorf KD, Becker C, et al. A paradigm shift in mechanical biofilm management? Subgingival air polishing: a new way to improve mechanical biofilm management in the dental practice. *Quintessence Int.* 2013;44(7):475–477.

55. Mengel R, Buns CE, Mengel C, Flores-de-Jacoby L. An in vitro study of the treatment of implant surfaces with different instruments. *Int J Oral Maxillofac Implants.* 1998;13(1):91–96.

56. Magnuson B, Harsono M, Stark PC, Lyle D, Kugel G, Perry R. Comparison of the effect of two interdental cleaning devices around implants on the reduction of bleeding: a 30-day randomized clinical trial. *Compend Contin Educ Dent.* 2013;34Spec No 8:2–7.

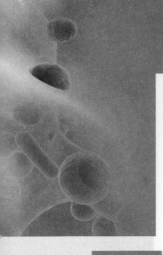

10 Clinical Decision-Making for Periodontal Care

Clinical Application. Members of the dental team are equipped with a broad array of skills that can be called upon when caring for patients with periodontal disease. All members of the dental team should be comfortable in providing many of the periodontal therapies when indicated. However, it is vital for the clinician to understand how to make decisions related to patient care to be an effective member of the health care team. This chapter outlines guidelines for decision-making by dental health care providers including those related to arriving at a periodontal diagnosis, sequencing periodontal treatment, obtaining consent for treatment, and the ongoing need for decision-making.

Learning Objectives

- List the three fundamental diagnostic questions used when assigning a periodontal diagnosis.
- List the two fundamental diagnostic questions used when assigning a peri-implant diagnosis.
- Explain how to arrive at appropriate answers to each of the fundamental diagnostic questions.
- Explain the difference between the terms "signs" of a disease versus "symptoms" of a disease.
- List several overt and hidden signs of periodontal inflammation.
- Define the term silent disease.
- Describe what is meant by the term clinical attachment loss.
- Describe the elements of a well-written diagnosis for periodontitis.
- List the phases of treatment.
- Explain why a patient's diagnosis and treatment plan may require modifications at a later point in time.

Key Terms

Clinical decision-making
Signs of periodontal disease
Symptoms of periodontal disease
Silent disease
Overt signs
Hidden signs

Natural level of the gingival attachment
Clinical attachment loss
Master treatment plan
Assessment and preliminary therapy phase

Nonsurgical periodontal therapy phase
Surgical therapy phase
Restorative therapy phase
Periodontal maintenance phase

Section 1
Guidelines for Arriving at a Periodontal Diagnosis

Clinical decision-making is the process whereby all members of the dental team use the information gathered during the comprehensive periodontal assessment to arrive at an appropriate diagnosis and identify treatment strategies that meet the individual needs of the patient.

The first step in planning periodontal treatment is assigning a correct periodontal diagnosis (or correct diagnoses, if the patient has more than one known periodontal condition in his/her mouth). Determination of a periodontal diagnosis can be simplified by asking and answering three fundamental clinical questions in a systematic manner (Fig. 10-1). These three fundamental questions can be used to guide the dental team through the diagnostic process. Many decisions, including assigning a periodontal diagnosis and planning nonsurgical/surgical therapy, revolve around the answers to these fundamental questions.

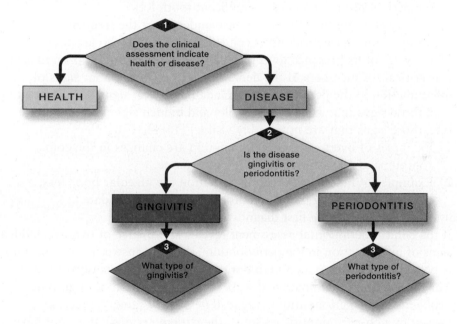

Figure 10-1. Decision Tree for Determining a Periodontal Diagnosis. A decision tree illustrating the three fundamental questions for determining an initial periodontal diagnosis.

1. **Answering Fundamental Diagnostic Questions When Assigning a Periodontal Diagnosis**
   A. **The First Fundamental Diagnostic Question is:** *"Does the clinical assessment indicate periodontal health or inflammatory disease in the periodontium?"*
      1. The answer to the first question should be based on the clinical signs of inflammation that are noted and recorded during the clinical assessment, and by its very nature is not usually difficult for members of the dental team to answer.
         a. Signs of Periodontal Disease. The dental team should be familiar with the difference between the *signs* of a disease and the *symptoms* of a disease. Signs of periodontal disease are the features of a disease that can be observed or are measurable by clinicians.
            1) Examples of periodontal disease signs might include gingival erythema (redness), gingival edema (swelling), bleeding on gentle probing, loss of attachment, tooth mobility, or loss of alveolar bone support.

2) While some of these signs are easily detectable by the clinician (i.e., gingival erythema or gingival redness); other signs require careful assessment to identify (i.e., loss of attachment, furcation involvement).

b. Symptoms of Periodontal Disease. Symptoms of periodontal disease are features of a disease that are noticed by the patient.

1) For example, symptoms of Stage IV periodontitis might include loose teeth, difficulty in mastication (chewing), profuse gingival bleeding, or a bad taste in the mouth.

2) It should be noted that in many patients the early symptoms of periodontitis are so subtle that they go undetected or unnoticed by the patient until the disease has progressed to such an advanced state that it causes serious complications that affect the survivability of the tooth. As such, some clinicians refer to periodontitis as a silent disease because of the lack of, or "silence," of early symptoms that are not obvious to the patient until the disease has progressed to cause considerable damage to the periodontium and causes significant tooth loss.

3) Calling periodontitis a silent disease underscores the frequent observation that periodontitis can exist in patients who are totally unaware of its presence until the symptoms become more pronounced.

c. It is critical for members of the dental team to recognize that signs of inflammation in the periodontium include both overt signs of inflammation (i.e., those signs that are readily visible) and hidden signs of inflammation (i.e., those signs that are not readily visible) (Table 10-1).

1) Examples of overt signs of inflammation are changes in the color, contour, and consistency of the gingival tissue.

2) Examples of hidden signs of inflammation are alveolar bone loss, bleeding on probing, and sometimes purulence or exudate.

2. Health as an answer to the first diagnostic question

a. If the clinical periodontal assessment reveals an absence of overt or hidden signs of inflammation in the periodontium, then the answer to Question no. 1 is periodontal health (i.e., a periodontium free of inflammation).

b. This means that inflammatory disease is not present and, though other problems in the periodontium *may well be present* (gingival recession caused by non-periodontitis reasons), the patient certainly does not have either gingivitis or periodontitis.

3. Inflammatory disease as an answer to the first diagnostic question

a. If the clinical periodontal assessment reveals either overt or hidden signs of inflammation in the periodontium, then the answer to Question no. 1 is, of course, inflammatory disease.

b. This means that some type of inflammatory disease is present (i.e., some type of gingivitis or periodontitis) and that further diagnostic decisions related to this inflammatory disease will need to be made by the team.

4. Additional diagnostic measures

a. Note that even in the absence of any inflammatory disease in the periodontium some patients will require further examination to help in the diagnostic decision-making process.

b. For example, a patient with no inflammation in the periodontium at all but with severe gingival recession accompanied by cervical abrasion of the teeth may need to be evaluated for possible history of traumatic tooth brushing.

TABLE 10-1	SIGNS OF INFLAMMATION IN THE PERIODONTIUM
Overt (Readily Visible) Signs	**Hidden Signs**
• Color changes in the gingiva • Contour changes in the gingiva • Changes in consistency in the gingiva	• Bone loss • Purulence (exudate) • Bleeding on probing

B. The Second Fundamental Diagnostic Question is: *"If the clinical assessment indicates inflammatory disease, is the disease gingivitis or is it periodontitis?"*
   1. Using Attachment Loss to Answer Fundamental Diagnostic Question no. 2
      a. The answer to this second fundamental question is based on the clinical evidence of attachment loss as determined from the findings recorded during the clinical assessment.
         1) The natural level of the gingival attachment to the tooth is slightly coronal to (or in a sense above) the level of the cementoenamel junction (CEJ).
         2) Clinical attachment loss or attachment loss refers to migration of the junctional epithelium to a position apical to (or in a sense below) the level of the CEJ.
      b. Gingivitis. If the clinical assessment reveals no attachment loss in the presence of inflammation, then the answer to Question no. 2 is gingivitis. The reader is referred to Chapter 6 to review the various categories and subcategories of gingivitis.
      c. Periodontitis. If the clinical assessment reveals attachment loss in the presence of inflammation, then the answer to Question no. 2 is periodontitis. The reader is referred to Chapter 7 to review the various stages and grades of periodontitis.
   2. It is important for the dental team to use dental radiographs as well as the clinical findings during the clinical assessment process.
      a. In most patients with periodontitis, alveolar bone loss will be evident on the radiographs.
      b. However, even before there is radiographic evidence of alveolar bone loss, clinical attachment loss should be apparent and detectable by an alert clinician.
      c. The members of the dental team must make every effort to detect periodontitis before there is obvious radiographic evidence of alveolar bone loss.
C. The Third Fundamental Diagnostic Question is: *"If the patient has gingivitis, what type of gingivitis?"* or *"If the patient has periodontitis, what type of periodontitis?"*
   1. The classification of various types of gingival diseases/conditions and the various types of peridontal diseases are covered in previous chapters of this textbook (Chapters 6 to 9).
   2. The dentist will use these disease classifications to assign a specific periodontal diagnosis based on the clinical features outlined in those chapters.
D. Classification of Peri-Implant Diseases and Conditions
   1. One of the key features to the 2017 classification system is the introduction of the categories of peri-implant health, peri-implant mucositis, and peri-implantitis that can be accepted worldwide.
   2. Determination of a proper peri-implant classification can be simplified by asking and answering two fundamental clinical questions in a systematic manner (Fig. 10-2).

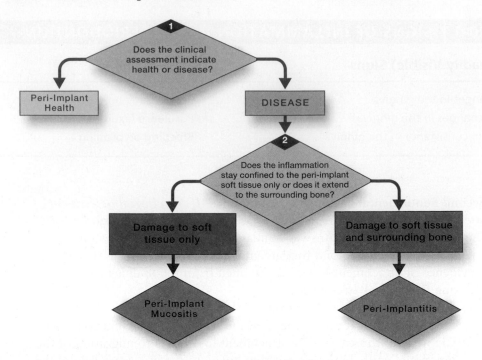

Figure 10-2. Decision Tree for Determining a Peri-Implant Diagnosis. A decision tree illustrating fundamental questions for determining an initial peri-implant diagnosis.

2. **Recognizing the Need for Flexibility When Assigning a Periodontal Diagnosis**
   A. **Flexibility.** The members of the dental team must be aware of the need for some flexibility when assigning a periodontal diagnosis, since more than one periodontal condition may be found in a patient.
      1. *Flexibility* in this case refers to a realization that the important fundamental decision as to the presence of either gingivitis or periodontitis in a patient may not describe the overall periodontal condition of that patient.
      2. Other periodontal conditions may indeed be present, and this finding must be noted when documenting a periodontal diagnosis in addition to any fundamental decision about the presence of gingivitis or periodontitis.
   B. **Other Findings.** Examples of some of these other periodontal conditions might be recession of the gingival margin, occlusal trauma, or aberrant frenum position.
3. **Thorough Documentation of the Periodontal Diagnosis.** Documenting the periodontal diagnosis is a critical skill for the dental team, and adhering to a standard format for such documentation is helpful. The following are some guidelines for documenting periodontal diagnoses.
   A. **Diagnostic Term.** As part of the diagnosis, the clinician should include the correct diagnostic term as outlined in the classification scheme, such as gingivitis or periodontitis (as discussed in Chapters 6–9).
   B. **Disease Stage.** When assigning a periodontitis diagnosis, the clinician should classify the disease using a multidimensional *staging* system. Staging of periodontitis defines the severity (according to the level of interdental clinical attachment loss, radiographic bone loss, and tooth loss), complexity of management, and extent and distribution of the disease. For more information about the staging of periodontitis, the reader is referred to Chapter 7 of this textbook.

1. Table 10-2 shows how the terms Stage I (initial periodontitis), Stage II (moderate periodontitis), Stage III (severe periodontitis with potential for tooth loss), and Stage IV (advanced periodontitis with extensive tooth loss and potential for loss of dentition) should be used as a part of the documentation of a periodontitis diagnosis.

2. Note that the term *clinical attachment loss* (CAL) is used to underscore that these measurements are clinical measurements and may not coincide exactly with precise histologic measurements.

C. **Disease Grading.** In addition to using the multidimensional staging system, the clinician should classify the disease using a multidimensional *grading* system. Grading should be used as an indicator of the anticipated rate of periodontitis progression. For more information about grading, the reader is referred to Chapter 7 of this textbook.

1. Table 10-2 shows how the terms Grade A (slow rate of periodontitis progression), Grade B (moderate rate of periodontitis progression), and Grade C (rapid rate of periodontitis progression) should be used as part of documentation of a periodontitis diagnosis.

2. The primary criteria for grading periodontitis are either direct or indirect evidence of progression. Whenever available, direct evidence should be used, and is based on longitudinal data (i.e., comparing radiographic bone loss or CAL that has occurred at two different time periods); in its absence, indirect estimation is made using bone loss as a function of age at the most affected tooth or case presentation (radiographic bone loss expressed as percentage of root length divided by the age of the subject, RBL/age).

3. Note that both staging and grading only applies to the the classification of periodontitis and should not be used to classify other periodontal diseases/conditions or peri-implant diseases/conditions detailed in the new classification system.

D. **Disease Extent.** When assigning a stage to the periodontitis, a descriptive modifier such as localized pattern, generalized pattern, or molar/incisor pattern of the disease, should be added to describe the number and the distribution of teeth affected with detectable periodontal breakdown.

1. Table 10-2 also shows how the terms localized, generalized, and molar/incisor pattern should be used as part of documentation of the extent of periodontitis.

2. Examples of appropriate periodontal diagnoses might be *generalized Stage I, Grade A periodontitis* or *localized Stage IV, Grade C periodontitis*. Table 10-3 provides some examples of well-written periodontal diagnoses.

4. **Using the ADA Case Type System for Periodontal Patients**

A. **Case Types**

1. Although the case type system is somewhat limited in value, it may be useful to assign a periodontal case type to periodontal patients when reporting to insurance carriers or to third-party payers.

2. Assigning a periodontal case type is included in the initial decision making process in most dental offices and is included here as additional information related to assigning a periodontal diagnosis.

   a. Case Type I.   Patients with gingivitis only
   b. Case Type II. Patients with slight (mild) periodontitis
   c. Case Type III. Patients with moderate periodontitis
   d. Case Type IV. Patients with severe periodontitis

B. **Limited Value of Case System.** The value of the case type system is very limited because the case type alone does not specify the precise periodontal disease classification.

1. The case type system fails to specify the precise disease extent. For example, a Case Type III patient could either be a patient who has localized periodontitis, localized to one sextant of the mouth, or a patient with generalized periodontitis throughout the entire mouth.
2. Furthermore, a patient with Case Type III does not provide any information regarding the staging of the condition. In other words, the case type system does not define any specific factors that may influence the complexity of controlling current disease, such as a deep vertical defect.
3. The case type system does not give the clinician much flexibility in assigning periodontal diagnosis. For instance, a Case Type III implies that the patient has moderate periodontitis but, may not reflect other types of periodontal conditions affecting the periodontium.
4. It is important for all members of the dental team to use the formal periodontal diagnosis (e.g., generalized Stage I, Grade C periodontitis) when describing the periodontal status of a patient and to use the case type only as a supplemental description if called for.

TABLE 10-2	USE OF MODIFIERS IN DOCUMENTING DISEASE STAGE, GRADE, AND EXTENT	
	Descriptive Modifier	**Definition**
Disease Stage	Stage I	Initial periodontitis
	Stage II	Moderate periodontitis
	Stage III	Severe periodontitis with potential for tooth loss
	Stage IV	Advanced periodontitis with extensive tooth loss and potential for loss of dentition
Disease Grading	Grade A	Slow rate of anticipated disease progression
	Grade B	Moderate rate of anticipated disease progression
	Grade C	Rapid rate of anticipated disease progression
Disease Extent	Localized	30% or less of the teeth in the mouth are involved
	Generalized	More than 30% of the teeth in the mouth are involved
	Molar/incisor pattern	Only molars and incisors exhibit periodontal breakdown

TABLE 10-3	EXAMPLES OF A WELL WRITTEN PERIODONTAL DIAGNOSIS		
Extent	**Stage**	**Grade**	**Name of Disease**
Localized	Stage I	Grade A	Periodontitis
Localized	Stage III	Grade C	Periodontitis
Generalized	Stage II	Grade B	Periodontitis
Generalized	Stage IV	Grade A	Periodontitis
Molar/incisor pattern	Stage I	Grade C	Periodontitis

Section 2
Guidelines for Periodontal Treatment Sequencing

1. **The Periodontal Master Treatment Plan.** The master treatment plan is a sequential outline of the measures to be carried out by the dentist, the dental hygienist, or the patient to eliminate disease and restore a healthy periodontal environment. It can be thought of as a blueprint of all treatment strategies recommended to attain and maintain the long-term periodontal health of the patient and should involve all members of the health care team and the patient.
   - The master treatment plan can be used to coordinate and to sequence all treatment and educational measures employed.
   - Although some of the treatment included in the master treatment plan may not involve the dental hygienist directly, it is important that the hygienist understand how all phases of treatment contribute to the goal of restoring a healthy periodontium.

2. **Understanding the Phases of Periodontal Treatment.** The master treatment plan can be sequenced into phases. An overview of the sequence of phases of treatment is presented in Figure 10-3 as well as in the discussion below. Refer to Table 10-4 for examples of components of each of the phases in the management of periodontal patients. It should be noted that individual treatment phases may overlap one another, especially in the management of patients who need both restorative and periodontal therapy.
   A. **Assessment and Preliminary Therapy Phase**
      1. The assessment and preliminary therapy phase includes: (1) assessment data collection; and (2) urgent care for any acute conditions such as emergency dental care. Details of the clinical periodontal assessment are discussed in Chapter 20, and periodontal emergencies are discussed in Chapter 30.
      2. This phase of care also has been referred to as emergency therapy by some authors.
   B. **Nonsurgical Periodontal Therapy Phase**
      1. The nonsurgical periodontal therapy phase of treatment includes all the *nonsurgical* measures used to control gingivitis and periodontitis.
         a. This phase includes intensive nonsurgical periodontal instrumentation and comprehensive patient educational measures.
         b. This phase can also include measures to minimize the impact of local contributing factors.
      2. The nonsurgical periodontal therapy phase has also been called *initial periodontal therapy, Phase I therapy, bacterial control*, and *anti-infective therapy*.
   C. **Surgical Therapy Phase**
      1. The surgical therapy phase of treatment includes any needed periodontal surgery to control or eliminate periodontal disease that cannot be managed by nonsurgical therapy alone. The surgical phase also includes the placement of dental implants to replace missing teeth and reestablish form and function of the oral dentition.
      2. The surgical therapy phase of care has also been called *Phase II* therapy. Periodontal surgical procedures are discussed in Chapter 29.
      3. If the periodontal health can be reestablished solely by nonsurgical periodontal therapy, then this phase of treatment is not indicated for the patient.

D. **Restorative Therapy Phase**
   1. The restorative therapy phase of treatment may include placement of dental restorations and replacement of missing teeth by fixed or removable prostheses.
   2. The restorative therapy phase of care has also been called *Phase III* therapy.
E. **Periodontal Maintenance Phase**
   1. The periodontal maintenance phase of treatment includes all measures used by the dental team and the patient to keep periodontitis from recurring once the inflammatory disease is brought under control.
   2. The objective of the periodontal maintenance phase is to maintain the teeth functioning throughout the life of the patient and may be needed for the rest of the patient's life.
   3. The periodontal maintenance phase of care has also been called *Phase IV* therapy. Periodontal maintenance is discussed in detail in Chapter 33.

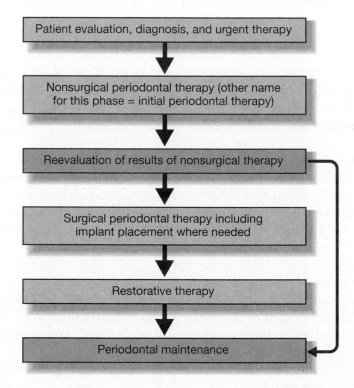

Figure 10-3. Sequencing of Treatment Phases. This flow chart provides an overview of the sequence of the normal phases of treatment for a patient. After periodontal instrumentation has been completed, reevaluation of results is typically done 4 to 6 weeks after initial therapy. The reevaluation allows the clinician to revisit the periodontium and reassess its response to initial therapy. If periodontitis has been successfully arrested, then a stable state has been achieved, and the patient can be enrolled in a periodontal maintenance program. If, however, periodontitis remains active in spite of initial therapy, then the patient should be referred to a specialist to initiate surgical periodontal therapy. Note: for healthy patients or gingivitis patients with a reduced periodontium, the reevaluation is done at each recall visit.

TABLE 10-4	EXAMPLES OF MEASURES AND PROCEDURES PERFORMED AT EACH PHASE OF THERAPY
Phase	**Measures and Procedures**
Assessment phase and preliminary therapy	Health history Comprehensive oral examination Assessment data collection Radiographs as indicated Diagnosis of oral conditions Treatment of urgent conditions Planning of nonsurgical therapy Referral for care of medical conditions Extraction of hopeless teeth
Nonsurgical periodontal therapy	Self-care education Nutritional counseling Nicotine cessation counseling Periodontal instrumentation Antimicrobial therapy Correction of local risk factors Fluoride therapy Caries control and temporary restorations Occlusal therapy Minor orthodontic treatment Reevaluation of Phase I therapy
Surgical therapy	Periodontal surgery Endodontic surgery Dental implant placement
Restorative therapy	Dental restorations, fixed and removable prostheses Reevaluation of overall response to treatment
Periodontal maintenance	Ongoing care at specified intervals

Section 3
The Need for Ongoing Decision-Making

Since most patients are monitored for many years or even decades by the members of the dental team, clinical decision-making and treatment planning is best described as an ongoing, evolving process over time. The aim of periodontal therapy is to preserve the periodontium during the patient's lifetime.

- In addition, the periodontium consists of dynamic and continuously changing tissues (even in the absence of disease) that is subject to physiologic tissue remodeling or pathologic periodontal destruction throughout the lifetime of the tooth. Therefore, an individual's plan for periodontal care frequently requires adjustment over time because of these changes.
- *The dental team must be aware that a perfectly sensible periodontal diagnosis and plan for therapy at one point in time may require modification at a later date, and this fact must be communicated to the patient.*

Chapter Summary Statement

This chapter outlines guidelines that can be helpful to the members of the dental team during the management of patients with periodontal diseases. These guidelines include those related to arriving at a periodontal diagnosis, periodontal treatment sequencing, and the need for ongoing decision-making.

Section 4
Focus on Patients

Clinical Patient Care

CASE 1

Periodontal assessment of a new patient reveals generalized bleeding on probing but very little gingival erythema (redness) and very little gingival edema (swelling). How would you answer the first fundamental diagnostic question for this patient?

CASE 2

Periodontal assessment of a new patient reveals definite signs of inflammation in the periodontium. Explain how to answer the second diagnostic question for this patient.

CASE 3

Periodontal assessment of a new patient reveals localized signs of gingival inflammation but no attachment loss. The findings also include a site of gingival recession and toothbrush abrasion on the facial surface of a canine tooth. At this site of recession, there is no sign of inflammation of the gingiva. How should this site of gingival recession due to traumatic brushing affect the basic diagnostic questions?

CASE 4

Following thorough clinical assessment of the periodontal condition of a patient, you are convinced that the patient has periodontitis. Explain how you would determine the severity of the periodontitis.

Suggested Readings

American Academy of Periodontology. Guideline for periodontal therapy. *Pediatr Dent.* 2016;38(6):397–401.
Azouni KG, Tarakji B. The trimeric model: a new model of periodontal treatment planning. *J Clin Diagn Res.* 2014;8(7):ZE17–ZE20.
Bailey DL, Barrow SY, Cvetkovic B, et al. Periodontal diagnosis in private dental practice: a case-based survey. *Aust Dent J.* 2016;61(2):244–251.
Krebs KA, Clem DS, 3rd; American Academy of Periodontology. A report from the American Academy of Periodontology. Guidelines for the management of patients with periodontal diseases. *Compend Contin Educ Dent.* 2006;27(12):654–658.
Lindhe J, Lang NP, Berglundh T, et al. *Clinical Periodontology and Implant Dentistry.* Chichester, West Sussex; Ames, Iowa: John Wiley and Sons, Inc.; 2015.
Newman MG, Takei HH, Klokkevold PR, Carranza FA. *Carranza's Clinical Periodontology.* St. Louis, MO: Saunders Elsevier; 2015.
Sweeting LA, Davis K, Cobb CM. Periodontal Treatment Protocol (PTP) for the general dental practice. *J Dent Hyg.* 2008;82(Suppl 3):16–26.

 STUDENT ANCILLARY RESOURCES

A wide variety of resources to enhance your learning is available online:

- Audio Glossary
- Book Pages
- Chapter Review Questions and Answers

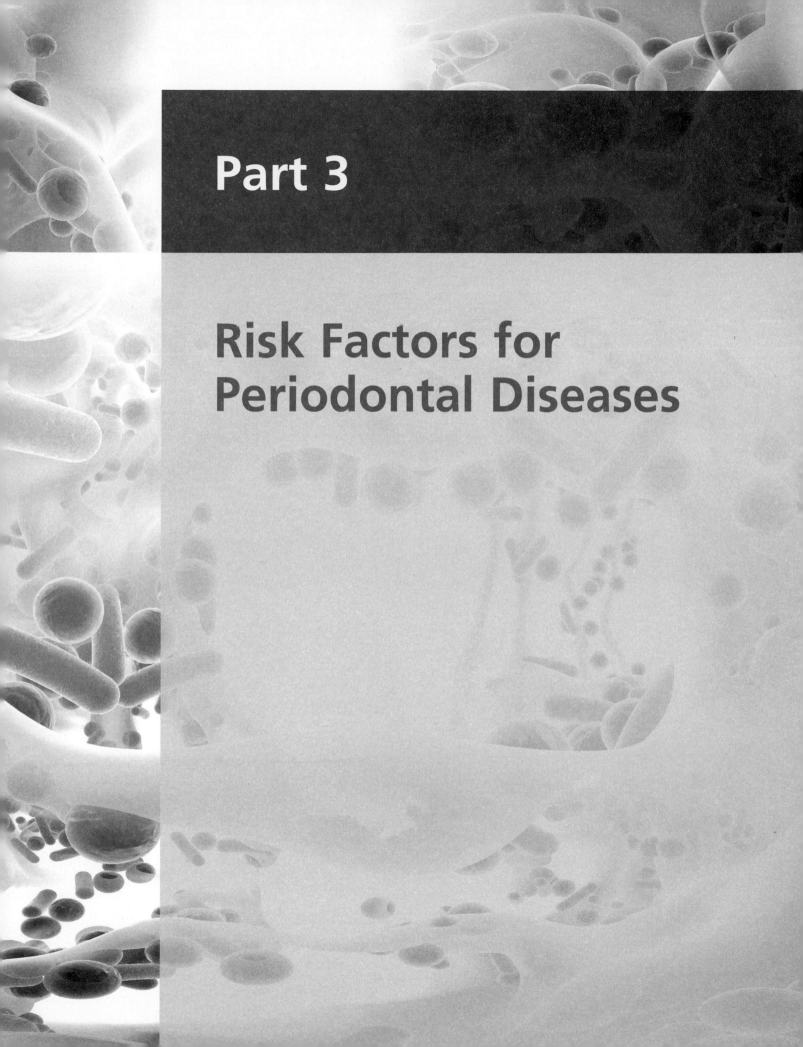

Part 3

Risk Factors for Periodontal Diseases

11 Shared Decision-Making for Periodontal Care

Clinical Application.
Periodontal treatment is always based upon the best available scientific evidence, but many times there will be more than a single course of treatment that could benefit an individual patient. To successfully participate in clinical decisions, patients need information about their oral conditions and treatment options. Dental health care providers must be able to work collaboratively and communicate effectively with their patients. Well-informed patients tend to have more realistic expectations of periodontal treatment outcomes and their role in maintaining periodontal health. This chapter discusses shared decision-making, decision aids, and informed consent.

Learning Objectives

- Define shared decision-making.
- Explain key steps for engaging in shared decision-making.
- Describe how patient decision aids facilitate shared decision-making.
- Describe the importance of informed consent to successful periodontal care.
- List guidelines for obtaining informed consent.
- Describe two formats for documenting informed consent.

Key Terms

Shared decision-making
Evidence-based
   health care
Systematic review

Cochrane Database of
   Systemic Reviews
SHARE approach
Patient decision aids

Informed consent
Reasonable patient
   standard
Informed refusal

Section 1
Shared Decision-Making

In the past, medical and dental health care providers took responsibility not only for being well informed about the benefits and harms of treatment options, but also for judging their value in the best interests of their patients. More recently, a shared decision-making approach is being advocated in which the patient is recognized as a mutual expert for judging the value of treatments. Shared decisions—as opposed to clinicians making decisions on behalf of patients—is gaining increasing importance in health care policy.[1-5] Shared decision-making has been called the "crux of patient-centered care" and is identified as a key part of change for improved quality in health care.[6]

1. **What is shared decision-making?** Shared decision-making is a collaborative process that recognizes a patient's right to make decisions about his or her care once fully informed about the options. *Periodontal treatment is always based upon the best available scientific evidence, but many times there will be more than a single course of treatment that could benefit an individual patient.* Shared decision-making is a process in which clinicians and patients work together to make treatment decisions that are best for the patient. The optimal decision considers evidence-based information about periodontal care options, the clinician's knowledge and experience, and the patient's informed preferences. As depicted in Figure 11-1, shared decision-making involves agreement between the clinician and patient on the patient's care plan.

   A. **When is shared decision-making appropriate?** Shared decision-making is appropriate for any dental health decision where there is more than one reasonable option.

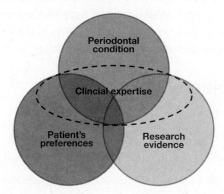

Figure 11-1. Shared Decision-Making Model for Evidence-Based Decisions. In shared decision-making, the patient's knowledge and preferences are considered, alongside the clinician's expertise, and the decisions they reach—in agreement with each other—are founded on valid evidence on effective treatment options.

   B. **What is evidence-based information?**
   1. Evidence-based health care is a systematic approach to clinical problem solving which allows the integration of the best available research evidence with clinical expertise and patient values.[7]
   2. A systematic review summarizes the results of available carefully designed health care studies (controlled trials) and provides a high level of evidence on the effectiveness of health care interventions.

   3. The Cochrane Database of Systemic Reviews
      a. Many dental clinicians do not have the expertise needed to do their own systematic reviews. Fortunately, there is a trustworthy resource—the Cochrane Database of Systemic Reviews—for busy practitioners who want to integrate high-quality science into patient care.
      b. The Cochrane organization, previously known as the Cochrane Collaboration, is an independent, nonprofit, nongovernmental organization consisting of a group of volunteers in more than 130 countries. The group was formed to organize medical research information in a systematic way to facilitate the choices that health professionals, patients, policy makers, and others face in health care interventions according to the principles of evidence-based care.

2. Characteristics of Shared Decision-Making. A key characteristic of shared decision-making on the dental health care provider's part is the conscientious offering of care options for the patient's consideration.[8] In addition to the patient, shared decision-making also may involve a team of health professionals, involve significant others (partners, family members) and differ across cultural, social, and age groups. As illustrated in Figure 11-2, a dental health care provider should be able to inform patients and engage them in shared decision-making by being able to do the following[9,10]:

  A. Develop a partnership with a patient.
  B. Establish the patient's preferences for his or her role in decision-making (degree of involvement of self and others, such as family members).
  C. Elicit and respond to the patient's ideas, concerns, and expectations of periodontal therapy.
  D. Identify choices and evaluate the research evidence in relation to the individual patient.
  E. Help the patient reflect on and assess the impact of alternative decisions with regard to his or her values.
  F. Develop a periodontal care plan in partnership with the patient.
  G. Document the agreed-upon periodontal care plan, and complete arrangements for follow-up.

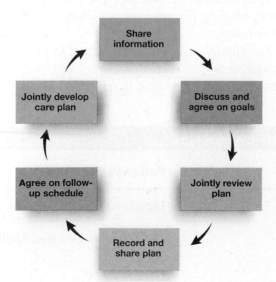

Figure 11-2. Shared Care Planning. A depiction of the steps in shared care planning.

3. **A Mutual Decision: Why Patients' Preferences Matter**
   A. **An Ethical Imperative**
      1. The most important reason for practicing shared decision-making is that it is the right thing to do. Communication of unbiased and understandable information on options, uncertainties, risks, and benefits of each option is an ethical necessity. Failure to do so should be taken as evidence of poor quality care.
      2. No treatment is 100% reliable and there are very few clinical situations where there is just one course of action that should be followed in all cases.
         a. In many situations, there is no single "right" care decision because choices about periodontal care come with pros and cons. There usually is a choice between undergoing a procedure or not, or—more commonly—a choice between different options.
         b. In circumstances where there are several options leading to different outcomes, the "right" decision depends on a patient's own unique set of needs, expectations, and outcome goals.[11] The decision might be whether to:
            • Undergo a diagnostic procedure such as a full series of radiographs
            • Undergo a periodontal surgical procedure
            • Increase frequency of recall/maintenance appointments
            • Take a medication
            • Undertake a lifestyle change such as quitting smoking
   B. **Two Sources of Expertise.** At the heart of shared decision-making is the recognition that clinicians and patients bring different but equally important forms of expertise to the decision-making process (Table 11-1). Shared decision-making is appropriate for any dental health decision where there is more than one reasonable option.
      1. The clinician is an expert in dental care such as knowledge of the diagnosis, likely course of the disease, treatment options, and the range of possible outcomes.
      2. The patient is an expert on his or her own life, circumstances, and what matters most to him or her. The patient knows about the impact of the condition on his/her daily life, personal attitude toward risk, values, and preferences. For example, referring to Table 11-1, the dental health care provider may suggest counseling for smoking cessation. The patient's perspective might be as follows:
         • Patient's experience of condition: aware of coughing in morning, but not concerned about cough
         • Patient's social circumstances: immediate family members all smoke

TABLE 11-1	SHARING EXPERTISE
Clinician's Expertise	**Patient's Expertise**
Diagnosis of condition	Experience of condition
Disease etiology	Circumstances (finances, family values)
Prognosis	Attitude to risk
Treatment options	Values
Outcome probabilities	Preferences

- Patient's attitude to risk: feels that smoking does not present a health risk since her grandfather smoked heavily and lived to be 90 years of age
- Patient's values: enjoys smoking especially in social situations and believes smoking helps to control her weight
- Patient's preferences: is not interested in quitting

C. Improved Treatment Outcomes

1. Research studies show that patients frequently do not understand recommended treatment options, or risks and benefits. An international Cochrane Review reported consistent evidence that as patients are better informed, they make better informed decisions and feel more confident about their choices.[12]

2. On the other hand, the evidence suggests that clinicians do not fully grasp the treatment outcomes that patients prefer (Fig. 11-3). Several studies document substantial gaps between the outcomes patients prefer and the outcomes clinicians *think* patients prefer.[13–16]

3. Figure 11-4 depicts the problems created by lack of information by patients and misconceptions of clinicians that result in poor decision quality. Shared decision-making helps the patient understand what the provider is trying to do (the goals of treatment).

4. When patients participate in decision-making and understand what they need to do, they are more likely to follow through. Shared decisions can result in a course of action for which the patient understands the need to take responsibility (e.g., meticulous daily self-care for biofilm control). In this case, patients are more likely to make behavioral changes if they have made the decision for themselves.

5. Shared decision-making facilitates a trusting relationship between the clinician and patient and increases patient and provider satisfaction.

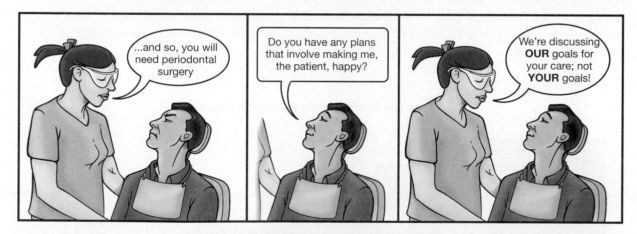

Figure 11-3. Treatment Outcomes. The evidence suggests that the outcomes that clinicians prefer may differ from those of their patients.

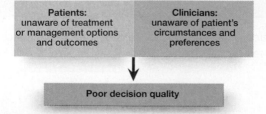

Figure 11-4. The Clinical Decision Problem. Less than ideal care results when patients do not understand the proposed treatment and clinicians are unaware of the patient's circumstances and preferences.

Section 2
A Model for Shared Decision-Making in Periodontal Care

The concept of engaging patients in decision-making to improve the quality of health care is firmly grounded in the Institute of Medicine report: Crossing the Quality Chasm.[17] The Institute of Medicine defines patient-centered care as "care that is respectful of and responsive to individual patient preferences, needs, and values" and that ensures "patient values guide all clinical decisions."

Several studies suggest that many health care professionals believe that patients are not interested in taking an active role in care planning.[18–21] Evidence suggests, however, that many patients would prefer to be given more information and would like to be involved in decision-making about their health care.[19,20]

THE SHARE APPROACH: ESSENTIAL STEPS OF SHARED DECISION-MAKING

The U.S. Department of Health and Human Services, Agency for Healthcare Research and Quality (AHRQ) developed a model to support the training of health care professionals on how to engage patients in their health care decision-making. AHRQ's SHARE Approach is a five-step process for shared decision-making that includes exploring the benefits and risks of each care/treatment option through meaningful discussion about what matters most to the patient.[22] The mnemonic "SHARE" is a learning device to assist in remembering the five steps (Fig. 11-5).

The five steps are intended to serve as prompts to help health care providers ensure that they are engaging patients in a meaningful discussion of treatment options. The dialog is an individualized process with each individual patient and some steps may overlap with one another. The SHARE Approach usually begins with inviting the patient to play an active role in the decision-making process.

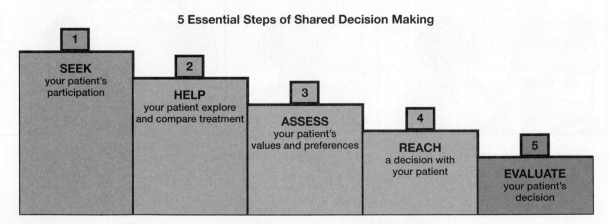

Figure 11-5. The SHARE Approach. The five essential steps of the SHARED decision-making model—Seek, Help, Assess, Reach, Evaluate—developed by the U.S. Department of Health and Human Services, Agency for Healthcare Research and Quality.[22]

STEP 1: SEEK YOUR PATIENT'S PARTICIPATION

Many patients are not aware that they can participate in health care decisions or that there may be different care options. Some patients may not want—or be ready—to participate in care decisions.[20,21] Clinicians should respect a patient's preference not to participate in the decision-making process or to delegate the decision to a family member or caregiver.

- Summarize the periodontal condition. Describe the problem clearly.
- Ask the patient to participate. Help the patient understand that he or she is being invited to ask questions and discuss options. Inviting patients to participate lets them know that they have options and that their goals and concerns are a key part of the decision-making process.
- If appropriate, include family members and caregivers in discussions. Ask if the patient would like to have family members or caregivers participate in the discussion.
- Remind the patient that his or her participation is important. For example, say, "*What is your next question?*" or "*I would like your input.*" Box 11-1 provides several examples of "conversation starters" to facilitate patient participation.

Box 11-1. Conversation Starters for Step 1

"Now that you understand the problem with the tissues that support your teeth, it is time for us to think about what to do next."

"I want to go over all the options so we can decide together what is best for you."

"There is good information about how these treatment outcomes differ that I'd like to discuss with you before we decide on an approach that is best for you."

If the patient wants the clinician to make the decision for them, the following might be useful to try: *"I am happy to share my views and help you make a good decision. Before I do, would you like more details about your options?"*

STEP 2: HELP YOUR PATIENT EXPLORE AND COMPARE TREATMENT OPTIONS

Letting the patient know that there are several options for home care or treatment is helpful in building a trusting patient–clinician relationship. Clinicians should guide patients through the benefits and risks of each option. Box 11-2 provides several examples of "conversation starters" to facilitate patient participation.

- Describe each option in plain language. Avoid using technical or dental jargon (e.g., say, "both sides" instead of "bilateral").
- Clearly communicate the benefits and risks of all options.
- Offer evidence-based decision aid tools whenever possible. (Decision Aids are discussed in Section 3 of this chapter.)
- After presenting information about options, make sure that the patient understands the information. Ask the patient to summarize the options in his or her own words.

> ## Box 11-2. Conversation Starters for Step 2
>
> *"Let me list the options for removing plaque biofilm from between your teeth before we get into more detail about them."*
>
> *"Here are some choices we can consider. Treatments have different consequences ... some will matter more to you than other people..."*
>
> *"These options will have different implications for the health status of your mouth. Let me tell you what the research says about the benefits and risks of these two treatment options."*
>
> *"The options that I just described are not always effective for everyone."*
>
> *"We've talked about your treatment options. To make sure I've explained things well, would you tell me how they're different?"*

STEP 3: ASSESS YOUR PATIENT'S VALUES AND PREFERENCES

Several studies document substantial gaps between the outcomes patients prefer and the outcomes health care providers *think* patients prefer.[21,23] Additionally, several researchers have shown that treatment decisions change after patients become well informed. An international Cochrane Review reports consistent evidence that as patients become better informed, they make different decisions and feel more confident in their decisions.[2,24,25] Box 11-3 provides several examples of "conversation starters" to facilitate patient participation.

- Assist patients in evaluating options based on their goals and concerns. To understand patients' preferences, ask them what is important to them and what they are concerned about.
- Encourage the patient to talk about what matters most to him or her. For example, how important it is to relieve the symptoms he or she is experiencing. What matters most might be recovery time, cost, or having a certain level of functioning.
- Listen to the patient. Encourage the patient to continue talking. For example, "Go on," or "Tell me more about that."
- Show empathy and interest in the effect that a problem is having on the patient's life. For example, say, "That sounds really upsetting."
- Agree on what is important to your patient.

> ## Box 11-3. Conversation Starters for Step 3
>
> *"As you think about your options, what matters most to you?"*
>
> *"Is there anything that may get in the way of doing this?"*
>
> *"Tell me more about your fear that you will lose your teeth no matter what you do."*
>
> *"It sounds like you are upset that your previous dental hygienist did not tell you about the loss of bone support around your molar teeth."*

STEP 4: REACH A DECISION WITH YOUR PATIENT

Deciding may take time, especially if the treatment is irreversible, such as periodontal surgery. Box 11-4 provides several examples of "conversation starters" to facilitate patient participation.

- Help the patient move to a decision. Ask if he or she is ready to decide or if he or she has additional questions.

- Confirm the decision with the patient.
- Assist patients to follow through on the decision. Lay out the next steps and the timing of these actions for patients, check for understanding, and discuss any possible challenges with carrying out the decision.
- Assist patients in managing barriers to implementing their decisions.

Box 11-4. Conversation Starters for Step 4

"Are you ready to decide?" "Do you have more questions?" "Are there more things that we should discuss to help you make your decision?"

"Now that we've discussed your treatment options, which treatment do you think is right for you?"

"So, we have talked about two options for removing the plaque biofilm and calculus: a series of four shorter appointments treating one fourth of your mouth at a time or a series of two longer appointments treating one half of your mouth at a time. Would one of these options work better for you in taking time away from your office?"

"Now that I've shown you two options for removing plaque biofilm from between your teeth—an interdental brush or a water flossing device—which one do you think will work best for you at home?"

"We discussed two options—surgery or frequent professional care with the hygienist. There is good evidence about how these treatment options differ that I'd like to discuss with you before we decide on an option that is best for you."

STEP 5: EVALUATE YOUR PATIENT'S DECISION

Once a decision has been made, it is important to follow-up with the patient on how he or she is doing. Since periodontal disease is a chronic condition, treatment decisions should be revisited at frequent intervals. Box 11-5 provides several examples of "conversation starters" to facilitate patient participation.

- Make plans to review the decision in the future. Remind the patient that decisions may be revisited and some may be changed if they are not working well. For example, a patient may decide against having periodontal surgery—at first—but may reconsider that decision at the next maintenance appointment.
- Monitor the extent to which the treatment decision is implemented. For example, the patient may decide to use an interdental brush for biofilm control, however, discover that he finds the brush too time-consuming to use.
- Revisit the decision with your patient to determine if other decisions need to be made.

Box 11-5. Conversation Starters for Step 5

"Can we talk at your next appointment in 3 months to see how you are doing?"

"Let's review how things are going for you in 3 months."

"If you feel things are not improving, please call immediately so we can plan a different approach."

"If you find that you do not like using this interdental brush, we have other options."

Section 3
Decision Aids for Periodontal Patients

Often there will be more than a single option for periodontal treatment that could benefit an individual patient. Patients need clear, comprehensive information about periodontal conditions and treatment or maintenance options to play an effective role in the decision-making process. Clear and consistent research shows that most patients want to be informed and involved in decisions about their care.[26]

Patient decision aids are the best known and proven tools to support shared decision-making.[12] *Patient decision aids* are information resources—such as, written materials, videos, or web-based tools—designed to facilitate shared decision-making and patient participation in health care decisions. Patient decision aids provide an evidence-based guide for patients: they present the decision to be taken, the options available, and the associated outcomes (including benefits, harms, and uncertainties).[27] Findings show that when patients use decision aids they (1) improve their knowledge of options, (2) feel more informed and clearer about what matters most to them, (3) have more accurate expectations of possible benefits and harms, and (4) participate more in decision-making.[12] *Patient decision aids are different from more traditional patient information materials because they do not tell the patient what to do. Instead they set out the facts and help the patient to deliberate about the options.* Box 11-6 provides an example of a conversation starter for introducing a patient decision aid. Box 11-7 summarizes the information that patient decision aids usually contain. Figures 11-6A,B and 11-7A,B provide two examples of patient decision aids.

Box 11-6. Conversation Starters When Introducing a Decision Aid

"This decision aid is designed to help you understand your options in more detail."

Box 11-7. Typical Information for Patient Decision Aids

- A description of the condition and symptoms (e.g., gingivitis)
- The likely prognosis (disease progression) with and without treatment
- The treatment and self-management options and outcome probabilities
- What's known from the evidence and not known (uncertainties)
- The most frequent complications of the treatment options

Patient Decision Aid: A Diagnosis of Gingivitis

This two-page decision aid is intended to help you and your dental health care professional decide how to best manage your periodontal disease. You can use it on your own—or with the assistance of your dental health care provider—to help you decide what is right for you now. The main options are presented in the table below.

Frequently asked Questions	No Treatment	Self-Care Instruction	Professional Treatment	Nicotine Cessation
What does the treatment involve?	No treatment means that you decide not to have any treatment at this time	Instruction in techniques and devices to remove plaque biofilm at home	Professional removal of plaque biofilms and tartar from your teeth	Counseling to assist you in giving up nicotine products or electronic cigarettes ("vaping")
What are the potential benefits of this option?	No benefit	An important component in limiting or controlling gum disease; "self-help"	A necessary component to contain or control disease (limiting gum disease and loss of supporting bone); decrease likelihood of worsening gum disease	Improved success of periodontal treatment; improved oral health and systemic well-being
What happens if I decide not to have this treatment?	Continuing inflammation (such as swelling, redness, bleeding) of gum tissues; potential worsening of disease	Continuing inflammation (such as swelling, redness, bleeding) of gum tissues; potential worsening of disease	Continuing inflammation (such as swelling, redness, bleeding) of gum tissues; potential worsening of disease	Continued use associated with worsening of gum disease and general health risks

A

Figure 11-6A. Patient Decision Aid for Diagnosis of Gingivitis. Page one of a sample patient decision aid for a diagnosis of gingivitis.

Frequently asked Questions	No Treatment	Self-Care Instruction	Professional Treatment	Nicotine Cessation
What are the possible risks/side effects of this treatment?	Continuing inflammation (such as swelling, redness, bleeding) of gum tissues; potential worsening of disease	No known risks for self-care instruction by a professional	Gums may bleed during procedure; slight discomfort in some patients (easily controlled by topical anesthesia applied directly to the gum tissue with a cotton swab)	No known risks to stopping nicotine use; If medications are used, side effects are possible; consult with your physician to learn more about options for nicotine cessation
How will this treatment impact my ability to work?	None	Short office visit for instruction; instruction can be combined with other care	1-hour appointment	Short office visit for counseling: counseling session can be combined with other treatment
Are there other treatment options?		No reasonable alternative for most patients	No reasonable alternative for most patients	No reasonable alternative for most patients

B

Figure 11-6B. Patient Decision Aid for Diagnosis of Gingivitis. Page two of a sample patient decision aid for a diagnosis of gingivitis.

Patient Decision Aid: A Diagnosis of Stage I, Grade A Periodontitis

This 2-page decision aid is intended to help you and your dental health care professional decide how to best manage your periodontal disease. You can use it on your own—or with the assistance of your dental health care provider—to help you decide what is right for you now. The main options are presented in the table below.

Frequently asked Questions	No Treatment	Self-Care Instruction	Professional Treatment	Local Anesthesia	Nicotine Cessation	Frequent Maintenance Care
What does the treatment involve?	No treatment means that you decide not to have any treatment at this time	Instruction in techniques and devices to remove plaque biofilm at home	Professional removal of plaque biofilms and tartar from your teeth	Local anesthesia ("numbing shot")	Counseling to assist you in giving up nicotine products or electronic cigarettes ("vaping")	Follow-up care at frequent intervals to assist you in maintaining the health of your gums and supporting bone
What are the potential benefits of this option?	No benefit	An important component in limiting or controlling disease; "self-help"	A necessary component to contain or control disease (limiting gum disease and loss of supporting bone)	Pain control and increased comfort during treatment	Improved success of periodontal treatment; improved oral health and systemic well-being	Continuing care to limit and control disease (limiting gum disease and loss of supporting bone)
What happens if I decide not to have this treatment?	Worsening disease to be expected; potential tooth loss	Worsening disease to be expected; potential tooth loss	Worsening disease to be expected; potential tooth loss	Pain during treatment	Continued use associated with worsening of periodontal disease and general health risks	Worsening disease to be expected; potential tooth loss

A

Figure 11-7A. Patient Decision Aid for Diagnosis of Stage I, Grade A Periodontitis. Page one of a sample patient decision aid.

Frequently asked Questions	No Treatment	Self-Care Instruction	Professional Treatment	Local Anesthesia	Nicotine Cessation	Frequent Maintenance Care
What are the possible risks/side effects of this treatment?	Worsening disease to be expected; potential tooth loss	Gum may recede so that some of the tooth roots may be visible when smiling; some increase in tooth sensitivity but treatment is available	Gum may recede so that some of the tooth roots may be visible when smiling; some increase in tooth sensitivity but treatment is available	Rare possibility of local nerve injury with some types of injections	No known risks to stopping nicotine use; If medications are used, side effects are possible; consult with your physician to learn more about options for nicotine cessation	Requires your commitment to frequent visits to dental office for professional care
How will this treatment impact my ability to work?	No benefit	Short office visit for instruction; instruction can be combined with other care	Multiple 1-hour appointments or several longer appointments; Most people return to work the same day or the day after treatment	Possible numbness of lips or tongue for a short while	Short office visit for counseling; counseling session can be combined with other treatment	1-hour follow-up appointment at frequent intervals
Are there other treatment options?		No reasonable alternative for most patients	Possible addition of antibiotics, gum surgery, or use of lasers	Possible use of oral or IV sedation in selected patients	No reasonable alternative for most patients	No reasonable alternative for most patients

B

Figure 11-7B. Patient Decision Aid for Diagnosis of Stage I, Grade A Periodontitis. Page two of a sample patient decision aid.

Section 4
Guidelines Related to Consent for Periodontal Treatment

According to the American Dental Hygienists' Association (ADHA) Code of Ethics, a patient has a right to informed consent prior to treatment, and they have the right to full disclosure of all relevant information so that they can make informed choices about their care.[1] This makes the patient a critical and willing participant in any plan involving periodontal therapy. As such, communication between the patient and dental practitioner is vital as the treatment plan develops.

Studies demonstrate that patients who believe that they have been well informed regarding their condition and who have had their questions answered by members of the dental team, are more compliant with treatment recommendations, have a higher trust in their health care providers, and are more satisfied with their care. These factors lead to better treatment outcomes and reduced malpractice risk.

1. **Informed Consent for Periodontal Treatment.** Informed consent is a patient's voluntary agreement to proposed treatment. A patient can only give informed consent to treatment after achieving an understanding of the relevant facts, benefits, and risks involved.[2]
   A. **What Constitutes Informed Consent?**
      1. Informed consent is not the same thing as a consent form that a patient is asked to sign. Rather, informed consent is the process of *communication* between a patient and a health care provider. It is a process that allows the patient to make a knowledgeable decision about his or her own dental care.
      2. An individual's consent is informed only if the recommended treatment, alternate treatment options, and the benefits and risks of treatment have been thoroughly described to the person in language understood by the patient.[3]
      3. Informed consent must be voluntary, and this informed consent originates from (1) a person's legal right to direct what happens to his or her body and (2) the ethical duty of the dental health care provider to involve the individual in his or her own dental care.
2. **The Reasonable Patient and Informed Consent**
   A. **Legal Claims.** Legal claims against dental health care providers usually consist of three parts: the clinician did not perform the treatment as s/he should have done; the clinician did not inform the patient properly about the risks involved with treatment; the clinician did not keep complete and accurate records.[28]
      1. When speaking about risks, judges tend to look at what a "reasonable patient" would want to know.[28]
      2. The Reasonable Patient Standard says a health care provider must disclose all information that a rational patient would want before making a choice to pursue or reject a treatment or procedure.
      3. Box 11-8 provides an example of the information a reasonable patient would need regarding local anesthesia prior to periodontal surgery.
   B. **Who Is Responsible for Informing the Patient?** The standard is that the health care provider who performs the treatment is ultimately responsible to informing the patient and obtaining consent.

Box 11-8. What Would a Reasonable Patient Need to Know?

Hypothetical Scenario: A clinician plans periodontal treatment in the mandible. What information should he provide to the patient about the risks of local anesthesia?

What are the risks? There is a possibility of injuring a nerve in the jaw. Nerve injury is not a life-threatening risk, but it can be annoying. The risk of injuring the lingual nerve while giving local anesthesia is very low. A recent study found that injuring the lingual nerve while giving local anesthesia occurred in 1 out of 2,667 cases.[29]

Are there alternative options? The anesthesia could be given around the teeth or gum (directly into the periodontal ligament or gingiva). The risk of nerve damage is much lower and the quality of anesthesia will be good. However, this technique does not provide profound local anesthesia and may be of shorter duration compared to a conventional mandibular block. Furthermore, this technique may require multiple injections in several papillae to adequately anesthetize the periodontal tissues in the mandible.

What if no anesthesia is used? Periodontal treatment may be painful without anesthesia. Without periodontal treatment, the likely outcome is unfavorable and tooth loss is probable.

C. **What Are the Goals of Informed Consent?** The most important goal of informed consent is to provide an individual an opportunity to be an informed participant in health care decisions, and it is generally accepted that a thorough informed consent includes a discussion of the following elements:

1. The diagnosis and an explanation of the periodontal condition that warrants the proposed treatment.
2. An explanation of the purpose of the proposed periodontal treatment.
3. A description of the proposed treatment and the individual patient's role and responsibilities during and after periodontal treatment.
4. A discussion of the known risks and benefits of the proposed periodontal treatment.
5. An assessment of the likelihood that the proposed treatment will accomplish the desired objectives.
   a. *Note that when discussing treatment outcomes, it is important not to appear to guarantee treatment outcomes to the patient.*
   b. Dental health care providers should remember that individual patients may respond differently to similar treatments.
6. A presentation of alternative treatment options, if any, and the known risks and benefits of these options.
7. The risks and benefits of not receiving the proposed periodontal treatment.
8. A discussion of the prognosis (or outcomes expected) if no treatment is provided.
9. A discussion of the actual costs associated with the proposed treatment.
10. Reinforcement of the individual's right to refuse consent to the proposed treatment.
    a. Keep in mind that patients often feel powerless when dealing with health care providers.
    b. To encourage the patient's voluntary consent, the dental health care provider should make it clear to the patient that she or he is participating in a decision, not merely signing a consent form.

3. **Informed Refusal for Periodontal Treatment.** Informed refusal is an individual's right to refuse all or a portion of the proposed treatment. Informed refusal requires that recommended treatment, alternate treatment options, and the likely consequences of declining treatment have been explained in language understood by the patient. A patient always has a legal right to refuse proposed periodontal care.

4. **Obtaining Informed Consent From Patients.** The doctrine of informed consent reminds dental health care providers to respect patients by fully and accurately providing information relevant to their health care decisions. The following are some guidelines to use when obtaining informed consent from a patient.

   A. **Use Understandable Language.** Information should be provided in language that is easily understood by the patient.
   1. Use simple, straightforward sentences.
   2. Use commonly recognizable terms.
   3. Avoid the use of professional jargon or technical terms, and explain any terms that may not be readily understood.
   4. Use a translator if the patient does not speak English or speaks English with little understanding.

   B. **Provide Opportunities for Patient Questions.** An opportunity should be provided for the patient to ask questions. Foster an open exchange of information and encourage the patient to ask questions. Using open-ended and nondirective questions such as those below can simplify this process.
   1. "What more would you like to know?"
   2. "What are your concerns?"
   3. "What is your next question?"

   C. **Assess Patient Understanding.** An assessment should be made of the patient's understanding of information provided.
   1. A simple strategy to assess understanding is to let patient know that, "Many people have difficulty understanding the information that I give them or have questions that they need answered. So, please let's discuss anything you do not understand."
   2. Another strategy is to make a comment such as, "Most of my patients want to explain my treatment suggestions to another family member. What additional information can I give you to help you explain this treatment to your spouse?"

5. **Legal Responsibility Related to the Consent Process**

   A. **The Dental Practitioner's Legal Responsibility Related to Consent**
   1. The dental hygienist has a legal responsibility for the services that he or she provides. Failure to obtain consent from the patient for services can have serious legal consequences.
   2. A patient could claim "battery" (i.e., unconsented touching) for dental services provided without the patient's consent.
   3. Patients also can claim "negligence" (i.e., lack of reasonable and prudent care resulting in harm) for failure to provide sufficient information for the patient to make an informed decision. This type of negligence also is called malpractice.

B. **Basic Legal Requirement to Demonstrate Informed Consent.** Basic requirements for demonstrating that informed consent has been obtained are listed below. If any element were missing, it would indicate that informed consent is not complete.
- Patient's periodontal diagnosis presented in language that is easily understood by the patient
- Discussion of proposed periodontal treatment and benefits presented in language that is easily understood by the patient
- Discussion of the risks and likelihood of success of the proposed periodontal therapy
- Discussion of alternative treatments
- Documentation that the patient was encouraged to ask questions and that answers were provided in language that is easily understood by the patient
- Patient's signature on the consent form

C. **Legal Requirements Necessary for a Patient to Give Informed Consent.** There are certain legal requirements necessary for a patient to give informed consent. These legal requirements are listed below.
- The patient is fully informed (as discussed in point "B" above).
- The patient is of legal age. Legal age is determined by state law—not federal law—and so may vary from state to state. Dental health care providers should know the legal age for the state in which they practice.
- The patient is mentally competent (understands information presented and can decide about the proposed treatment).
- The patient can give voluntary consent (without coercion from care providers, family members, or others).

6. **Format for the Consent Process.** The format for the consent process may be either verbal or written. Some states have statutes or regulations requiring dental professionals to secure written informed consent from patients.[1,30] Dental team members should ensure that they are familiar with and in compliance with the informed consent laws in their states.

A. **Written Consent.** Most dental health care providers prefer that the patient sign and date a written consent form for documentation of the consent process. Figure 11-8A,B shows an example of a written informed consent/informed refusal form.
1. In addition, the written consent document should be signed and dated by the dentist and a witness (generally, another staff member).
2. Once signed, a written consent document becomes part of the individual's permanent dental record.

B. **Verbal Consent.** If a written consent document is not used, the patient's verbal consent should be documented in the patient chart. An example of documentation of verbal consent would be a written entry in the patient's chart that says, "Discussed the diagnosis; purpose, description, benefits, and risks of the proposed treatment; alternative treatment options; the prognosis of no treatment; and costs. The patient asked questions and demonstrates that he understands all information presented during the discussion. Informed consent was obtained for the attached treatment plan."

SAMPLE INFORMED CONSENT TO NONSURGICAL PERIODONTAL THERAPY

I _____ (name), agree to the following treatment and/or surgery by_____

_____ (name of doctor) and _____ (name of hygienist).

Diagnosis: Disease of the gum tissues and supporting bone—Stage II Grade B periodontitis—that could lead to the loss of certain teeth.

Recommended Treatment Procedures: I have been advised that the proposed therapy is intended to extend the life expectancy of my teeth and involves a series of six 1-hour appointments for:
- Instruction in daily self-care/disease prevention measures
- Instrumentation of teeth (periodontal instrumentation)
- Polishing (air polishing for supra and subgingival biofilm control)
- Chemical gum (pocket) irrigation and/or placement medication (subgingival medication)
- The administration of numbing (anesthetic agents topically and by injection)
- Bite adjustment (occlusal adjustment)
- Treatment for sensitive teeth (root desensitization therapy)
- Professional recall appointments (periodontal maintenance therapy)

Treatment Alternatives: Further, I have been informed that possible alternatives to the above treatment include:

- No treatment
- Extraction(s)
- Other _____

We have discussed, however, that the procedures first recommended should be performed due to improved life expectancy of the teeth.

Non-Treatment Risks: I further understand that if no treatment is rendered, the risks to my dental health include, but are not limited to, the following:
- Premature loss of teeth
- Gum recession
- Bad breath
- Abscesses (gum boils)
- Tooth drifting, flaring, or other tooth movement
- Further loss of bone support to the teeth resulting in loosening of the teeth or tooth loss

Treatment Risks: Risks of the treatment include, but are not limited to:
- Allergic or other reactions to medications and anesthesia
- Temporary discomfort/ swelling/ pain
- Root sensitivity to hot or cold foods
- Roots of teeth visible in the mouth when smiling or talking
- Infection
- Spaces between teeth
- Other _____

A

Figure 11-8A. Sample Consent for Treatment Form. Page one of a sample consent for nonsurgical periodontal treatment.

No Warranty: No guarantee or assurance has been given to me that the proposed treatment will cure my gum (periodontal) problems and/or that the recommended treatment will be successful to my complete satisfaction. Due to individual patient differences, I understand that a risk of worsening of my present gum (periodontal) condition may result despite treatment and may require retreatment and/or extraction of teeth. However, it is doctor's opinion that therapy will be helpful and extend the life expectancy of my teeth.

I understand that the long-term success of treatment requires my cooperation and performance of daily removal of bacterial deposits (plaque) from my teeth, as well as routine professional recall appointments (periodic periodontal maintenance therapy) after the proposed treatment at a dental office.

CONSENT TO TREATMENT:
I AM CONSENTING TO THE ABOVE RECOMMENDED TREATMENT. I CERTIFY THAT I HAVE READ FULLY THE ABOVE CONSENT TO TREATMENT AND HAVE HAD ALL MY QUESTIONS ANSWERED.

SIGNED: _____

DATE: _____

WITNESS: _____

REFUSAL OF TREATMENT:
I AM REFUSING THE PROPOSED PERIODONTAL TREATMENT. I UNDERSTAND THE POSSIBLE CONSEQUENCES OF REFUSAL OF THE PROPOSED PERIODONTAL TREATMENT.

SIGNED: _____

DATE: _____

WITNESS: _____

B

Figure 11-8B. Sample Consent for Treatment Form. Page two of a sample consent for nonsurgical periodontal treatment.

Chapter Summary Statement

Shared decision-making is a communication approach that seeks to balance clinicians' expertise with patients' expectations and preferences. This process involves providing the patient with evidence-based information about options, outcomes, and uncertainties. When patients are given decision aids to help them make choices, they are more knowledgeable and satisfied with their periodontal care options. Through this interactive process, the clinician and patient reach a mutual decision about the subsequent periodontal care. A patient always has a legal right to refuse proposed periodontal care. Dental health care providers have a legal responsibility for the services that they provide. Failure to obtain informed consent from a patient can have serious legal ramifications.

Section 5
Focus on Patients

Ethical Scenario 1

Mrs. Emmerich lives in a rural area and drives 2 hours for dental care. Several years ago (Dental Office A), she was diagnosed with generalized periodontitis. Her general dentist recommended that she see a periodontist. Mrs. Emmerich—who did not want to make the long drive for a consultation with a periodontist—told her general dentist that she would just continue to keep her regular 6 month appointments with the hygienist. Neither the general dentist nor the hygienist pursued the discussion any further with Mrs. Emmerich.

Several years later, Mrs. Emmerich moved to the city to be nearer her adult daughter. She is a new patient in your general dentistry practice (Dental Office B) and a comprehensive periodontal examination reveals attachment loss and mobility of the molar teeth. You carefully explain the findings to Mrs. Emmerich using clear, easily understood words. Once Mrs. Emmerich fully understands the periodontal diagnosis, you begin the process of shared decision-making with her.

Mrs. Emmerich expresses her regret to you that no one at the previous dental office explained her periodontal condition or her treatment options. She believes that if she had understood the diagnosis that she would have sought a consultation with a periodontist. She feels that her condition is much worse now than it might have been.

- How do the approaches to care planning in the two dental offices differ?
- How do you think that shared decision-making at the time of the initial diagnosis (Dental Office A) might have affected the patient's choices?
- How do you think that shared decision-making at the time of the initial diagnosis (Dental Office A) might have affected the long-term prognosis of Mrs. Emmerich's dentition?
- Why do you think Mrs. Emmerich was willing to accept a referral to a periodontist (from Dental Office B)? Was it just that she now lives in a city?

Ethical Scenario 2

Mrs. Nguyen is the first patient of the afternoon in your periodontal office. She is new to the practice. She is a 50-year-old lady who has only lived in the United States for the last 3 years. Her English skills are minimal, but she works as a medical researcher, so you assume that she understands medical terminology.

Mrs. Nguyen has Stage II, Grade B periodontitis with generalized horizontal bone loss on her posterior teeth. You determine that periodontal instrumentation using local anesthesia is indicated. The next phase of treatment will be based on the findings at the time of the reevaluation, and will be determined by Dr. Evans, one of the periodontists in the office.

You review the proposed periodontal treatment plan with her. She asks no questions and signs at the bottom of the consent for treatment form, on the signature line. You tell her that you will begin the recommended treatment at today's appointment. You prepare the anesthesia syringe and as you approach Mrs. Nguyen, she becomes very agitated, screaming and covering her mouth with her hands. She refuses to allow any further treatment today. She gets up abruptly, and leaves the office.

1. What could the hygienist have done differently to avoid the above situation?
2. What ethical principles are in conflict in this dilemma?

3. Now that Mrs. Nguyen's experience has been a negative one for her; what is the best way to handle this ethical dilemma?
4. What changes might the hygienist make when explaining the proposed treatment to future patients?

References

1. Elwyn G, Laitner S, Coulter A, Walker E, Watson P, Thomson R. Implementing shared decision making in the NHS. *BMJ*. 2010;341:c5146.
2. O'Connor AM, Wennberg JE, Legare F, et al. Toward the 'tipping point': decision aids and informed patient choice. *Health Aff (Millwood)*. 2007;26(3):716–725.
3. Consent form—Contents—Prima facie evidence—Shared decision making—Patient decision aid—Failure to use. Title 7. Chapter 7.70, Section 7.70.060., Accessed March 2017.
4. H.R.3590—Patient Protection and Affordable Care Act, Stat. H.R.3590 (2009, 2009).
5. Equity and Excellence: Liberating the NHS, (July 2010, 2010).
6. Godolphin W. Shared decision-making. *Healthc Q*. 2009;12 Spec No Patient:e186–e190.
7. Sackett DL. *Evidence-Based Medicine: How to Practice and Teach EBM*. 2nd ed. Edinburgh: Churchill Livingstone; 2000.
8. Godolphin W. The role of risk communication in shared decision making. *BMJ*. 2003;327(7417):692–693.
9. Makoul G, Clayman ML. An integrative model of shared decision making in medical encounters. *Patient Educ Couns*. 2006;60(3):301–312.
10. Towle A, Godolphin W. Framework for teaching and learning informed shared decision making. *BMJ*. 1999;319(7212):766–771.
11. Wennberg JE. *Tracking Medicine: A Researcher's Quest to Understand Health Care*. 1st ed. Oxford, England: Oxford University Press; 2010.
12. Stacey D, Legare F, Col NF, et al. Decision aids for people facing health treatment or screening decisions. *Cochrane Database Syst Rev*. 2014;(1):CD001431.
13. McCannon JB, O'Donnell WJ, Thompson BT, et al. Augmenting communication and decision making in the intensive care unit with a cardiopulmonary resuscitation video decision support tool: a temporal intervention study. *J Palliat Med*. 2012;15(12):1382–1387.
14. Ubel PA, Angott AM, Zikmund-Fisher BJ. Physicians recommend different treatments for patients than they would choose for themselves. *Arch Intern Med*. 2011;171(7):630–634.
15. Volandes AE, Levin TT, Slovin S, et al. Augmenting advance care planning in poor prognosis cancer with a video decision aid: a preintervention-postintervention study. *Cancer*. 2012;118(17):4331–4338.
16. Volandes AE, Paasche-Orlow MK, Barry MJ, et al. Video decision support tool for advance care planning in dementia: randomised controlled trial. *BMJ*. 2009;338:b2159.
17. Council NR. *Crossing the Quality Chasm: A New Health System for the 21st Century*. Washington, DC: National Academies Press; 2001.
18. Guadagnoli E, Ward P. Patient participation in decision-making. *Soc Sci Med*. 1998;47(3):329–339.
19. Legare F, Ratte S, Gravel K, Graham ID. Barriers and facilitators to implementing shared decision-making in clinical practice: update of a systematic review of health professionals' perceptions. *Patient Educ Couns*. 2008;73(3):526–535.
20. Levinson W, Kao A, Kuby A, Thisted RA. Not all patients want to participate in decision making. A national study of public preferences. *J Gen Intern Med*. 2005;20(6):531–535.
21. Little P, Everitt H, Williamson I, et al. Preferences of patients for patient centred approach to consultation in primary care: observational study. *BMJ*. 2001;322(7284):468–472.
22. AHRQ. *The SHARE Approach*. Rockville, MD: U.S. Department of Health and Human Services; 2017 [updated February 2017May 2017]. Available from: https://www.ahrq.gov/professionals/education/curriculum-tools/shareddecisionmaking/index.html
23. Mulley AG, Trimble C, Elwyn G. *Patient's Preferences Matter: Stop the Silent Misdiagnosis*. London, England: The King's Fund; 2012:11–13. Available from: www.kingsfund.org.uk.
24. Murray E, Charles C, Gafni A. Shared decision-making in primary care: tailoring the Charles et al. Model to fit the context of general practice. *Patient Educ Couns*. 2006;62(2):205–211.
25. Stacey D, Bennett CL, Barry MJ, et al. Decision aids for people facing health treatment or screening decisions. *Cochrane Database Syst Rev*. 2011(10):CD001431.
26. Chewning B, Bylund CL, Shah B, Arora NK, Gueguen JA, Makoul G. Patient preferences for shared decisions: a systematic review. *Patient Educ Couns*. 2012;86(1):9–18.
27. Edwards A, Elwyn G. *Shared Decision-Making in Health Care: Achieving Evidence-Based Patient Choice*. 2nd ed. Oxford: Oxford University Press; 2009.
28. Brands WG. The standard for the duty to inform patients about risks: from the responsible dentist to the reasonable patient. *Br Dent J*. 2006;201(4):207–210.
29. Dam B, van Bruers J. Langdurige sensbiltetsstoorni ssen bij patienten. *Nederlands Tandartsenbiad*. 2004;59:36–37.
30. Sfikas PM. A duty to disclose. Issues to consider in securing informed consent. *J Am Dent Assoc*. 2003;134(10):1329–1333.

STUDENT ANCILLARY RESOURCES

A wide variety of resources to enhance your learning is available online:

- Audio Glossary
- Book Pages
- Chapter Review Questions and Answers

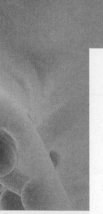

12 Etiologic Factors: Risk for Periodontal Disease

Clinical Application.
It is always a challenge to explain why periodontal disease affects some patients while others seem so resistant to its development. This chapter discusses the risk factors for periodontal disease, information about the biologic equilibrium involved with this disease, and the possible alterations to this equilibrium that can help clarify this perplexing issue. This information is useful when developing recommendations for a course of treatment for patients with periodontal diseases, as well as, when explaining the nature of these diseases to patients and other health care providers.

Learning Objectives

- Define and give examples of the term "risk factors."

- Define the term biologic equilibrium and discuss factors that can disrupt the balance between health and disease in the periodontium.

- Discuss the importance of a periodontal risk assessment in periodontal treatment planning.

- In a clinical setting—for a patient in your care with periodontitis—explain to your clinical instructor the factors that may have contributed to your patient's disease progression.

Key Terms

Oral health
Multifactorial etiology
Risk factors

Biologic equilibrium
Homeostasis
Risk assessment

Section 1
What Is Oral Health?

In recent years, oral health researchers have made significant advances in the understanding of the underlying biological etiologic mechanisms of oral diseases and the development of effective dental therapies. There has also been a heightened interest on the concept of oral health and how it is defined, rather than a focus solely on oral disease and its treatment. A broader biological-psychosocial model of oral health has evolved in recent years that has implications for clinical practice and research.

Recognizing the limitations of the disease model of oral health, the FDI World Dental Federation published a new definition of oral health.[1] An editorial by Glick and colleagues summarizes the new FDI definition of oral health[2]:

> Oral health is multifaceted and includes the ability to speak, smile, taste, touch, chew, swallow, and convey a range of emotions through facial expressions with confidence and without pain, discomfort, and disease of the craniofacial complex. Further, attributes include that it [oral health] is a fundamental component of health and physical well-being. It [oral health] exists along a continuum influenced by the values and attitudes of individuals and communities; [oral health] reflects the physiologic, social, and psychological attributes that are essential to quality of life; [oral health] is influenced by the individual's changing experiences, perceptions, expectations, and the ability to adapt to circumstances.

The FDI definition treats oral health as a changeable state of well-being, considering the physical, mental, and social aspects while addressing the demands of life and daily function (Fig. 12-1).

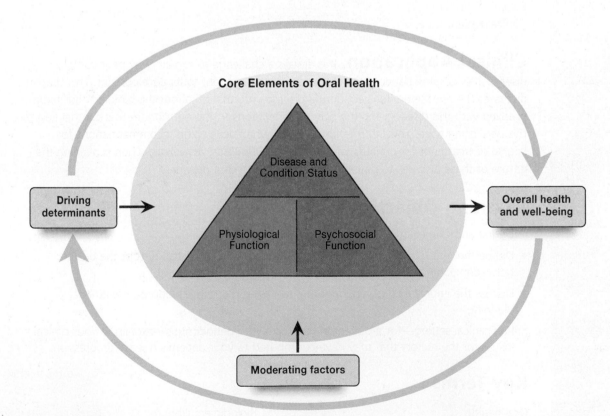

Figure 12-1. FDI Definition of Oral Health. The FDI definition describes the interactions among the three core elements of oral health: disease and condition status, physiological function, and psychosocial function.

Section 2
Risk Factors for Periodontal Disease

Research studies have clearly demonstrated that periodontal disease is a bacterial infection of the periodontium and that bacteria are the primary etiologic agents in the initiation of periodontal disease.[3-6] The presence of pathogenic bacteria, however, does not necessarily mean that an individual will experience periodontitis.

Periodontitis has a **multifactorial etiology**, that is, periodontitis is a disease that results from the interaction of many factors (Fig. 12-2). Some persons with abundant biofilm exhibit only mild disease, while others with sparse amounts of biofilm suffer severe disease. Untreated gingivitis does not always lead to periodontitis and everyone infected with periodontal pathogens does not experience periodontitis.

These findings suggest that additional factors, other than the mere presence of bacteria, must play a significant role in determining why some individuals are more susceptible to periodontal disease than others.[7-17] Many contributing factors help to determine the initiation and progression of periodontal disease. **Risk factors** are those variables that increase the likelihood of periodontitis developing in an individual. Risk factors are either *modifiable*, meaning that measures can be taken to change them, or *nonmodifiable*, which means these factors cannot be changed (Fig. 12-3). Risk factors are discussed in detail in Chapters 12 to 17.

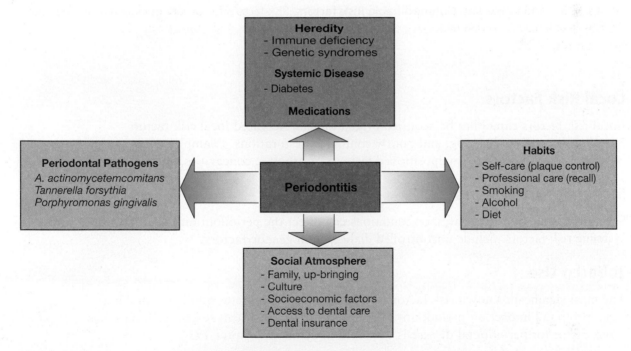

Figure 12-2. Risk Factors for Periodontal Disease. Periodontitis has a multifactorial etiology. Additional factors—other than the presence of bacteria—play a significant role in determining why some individuals are more susceptible to periodontal disease than others.

RISK FACTORS		
Modifiable Factors		**Non-modifiable Factors**

Local Factors

Acquired:

- Plaque and calculus
- Partial dentures
- Open contacts
- Overhanging and poorly contoured restorations

Anatomical:

- Malpositioned teeth
- Furcations
- Root grooves and concavities
- Enamel pearls

Systemic Factors

- Smoking
- Diabetes
- Poor diet
- Certain medications
- Stress

Emerging Evidence:

- Nutrition
- Alcohol
- Obesity/overweight

- Socioeconomic status
- Genetics
- Adolescence
- Pregnancy
- Age
- Leukemia

Figure 12-3. Modifiable and Nonmodifiable Risk factors. Risk factors for periodontal disease divided into modifiable and nonmodifiable factors.

Local Risk Factors

Local risk factors can either be acquired or anatomical. Acquired local risk factors include calculus, overhanging, and poorly contoured restorations. Examples of anatomical risk factors are malpositioned teeth, root grooves, concavities, and furcation.

Systemic Risk Factors

Several systemic diseases, states, or conditions can affect the periodontium. Examples of systemic risk factors include uncontrolled diabetes and genetic factors.

Tobacco Use

The most significant known risk factor for periodontitis is cigarette smoking. Smoking has a profound impact on periodontitis development and treatment response. Tobacco as a risk factor for periodontal disease is discussed in detail in Chapter 19.

Medications

Certain medications are known to cause overgrowth of the gingival tissues.

Other Risk Factors

Hormonal changes are known to affect the gingival tissues. Stress is known to affect both the general and periodontal health of patients.

Section 3
Balance Between Periodontal Health and Disease

1. **Biologic Equilibrium.** The human body is continually working to maintain a state of balance in the internal environment of the body, known as **biologic equilibrium** or **homeostasis.**
   A. **Periodontal Health**
      1. In the oral cavity, most of the time, things are in a state of balance between the biofilm bacteria and the host.
      2. For the periodontium to remain healthy, the bacterial challenge must be contained at a level that can be tolerated by the host.[4]
      3. The situation can be thought of as a balance scale, with the disease-promoting factors on one side of the scale and the health-promoting factors on the other (Fig. 12-4). As long as the two sides of the scale are in balance, there will be no disease progression.
   B. **Periodontal Disease**
      1. The intermittent pattern of disease activity seen in periodontitis is believed to result from the changing balance between the pathogenic bacteria and the host's inflammatory and immune responses.
      2. This balance also can be affected by other risk factors, such as local or systemic variables.
2. **The Delicate Balance Between Health and Disease.** When active periodontal disease sites are present in the mouth, the goal is to return the oral cavity to a state of biologic equilibrium.

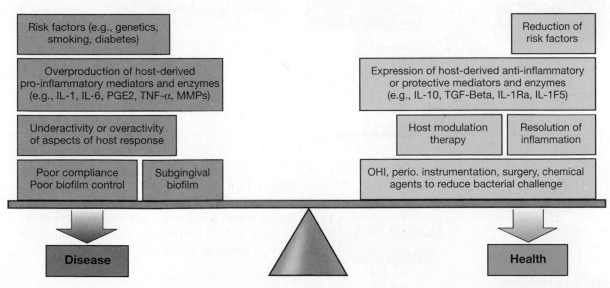

Figure 12-4. Periodontal Equilibrium. Equilibrium occurs when there is a balance between disease-promoting factors and health-promoting factors.

A. **Periodontal Equilibrium and Dental Plaque Biofilm**
   1. Experienced dental hygienists will attest to the fact that major differences exist in the way that individuals respond to the plaque biofilm.
      a. Many patients return to the dental office year after year with generalized plaque biofilm. These patients exhibit gingivitis and yet, year after year, show no clinical signs of progression to periodontitis. For some reason, in these individuals, gingivitis never progresses to periodontitis. Perhaps these individuals have no systemic or acquired risk factors that disrupt the biologic equilibrium. Basically, if an individual's immune system can effectively deal with a mouthful of periodontal pathogens, there will be no destructive periodontal disease (Fig. 12-5).
      b. In a few individuals, gingivitis progresses to periodontitis. It is theorized that in these individuals, the body's immune response (host response) is responsible for the tissue destruction seen in periodontitis. In addition, some individuals possess systemic risk factors (such as genetic variables or systemic disease) that significantly increase their susceptibility to periodontitis.
   2. There are many patients who are unable or unwilling to perform the thorough self-care necessary to control plaque biofilm. For these patients, it is necessary to increase the frequency of professional care to compensate for the inadequate level of self-care. Professional care at frequent intervals can be effective in restoring the balance between health and disease (Fig. 12-6).

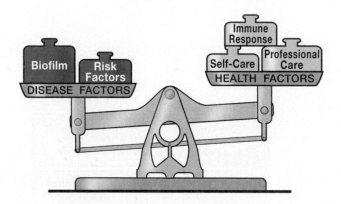

Figure 12-5. Gingivitis in the Presence of Plaque Biofilms. In individuals with a low susceptibility to periodontitis, gingivitis may never progress to periodontitis.

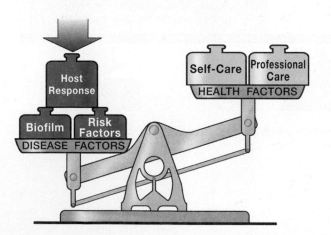

Figure 12-6. Periodontitis in the Presence of Plaque Biofilm. In susceptible individuals, the body's immune response (host response) results in damage to the periodontal tissues and progression from gingivitis to periodontitis.

B. **Local Contributing Factors**
1. It is possible to eliminate a local risk factor in many cases. A faulty restoration is a good example of a local factor that can be corrected, restoring the balance between local disease-promoting and health-promoting factors at the site.
2. In other cases, it is possible to compensate for a local risk factor by improving the patient's self-care and/or increasing the frequency of professional care. For example, the patient may need to use tufted dental floss to clean around the abutment teeth of a fixed bridge. This situation can be compared to adding more weight on the health-side of the balance scale to equal or exceed the weight on the disease-side of the scale.

C. **Systemic or Genetic Contributing Factors**
1. Certain systemic or acquired risk factors are possible to control or eliminate if the patient is willing to do so. For example, the individual can work with a physician to keep diabetes well controlled. A smoker may decide to stop smoking. In both cases, the individual has made a change that is health promoting, both systemically and for the periodontium (Fig. 12-7).
2. In the case of a contributing risk factor that cannot be controlled, it is necessary to add weight to the health-side of the scale. For example, some individuals have a genetic risk factor—such as abnormal neutrophil function—that causes them to be susceptible to severe periodontitis. At the present time, we are unable to eliminate or control genetic risk factors. It is possible, however, to assist the patient in maintaining health by increasing the extent of professional care. Frequent professional care will increase the weight on the health-side of the scale (Fig. 12-8).

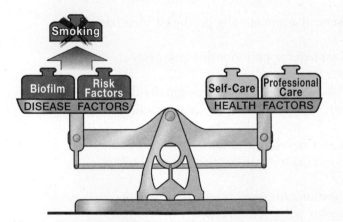

Figure 12-7. Eliminating a Systemic Risk Factor. Smoking cessation, combined with adequate self-care and professional care, restores the balance.

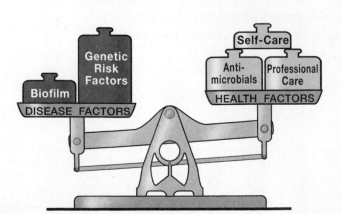

Figure 12-8. Management of a Genetic Risk Factor. Currently, there are some risk factors that cannot be eliminated or controlled. Professional care can help slow disease progression.

Section 4
Periodontal Risk Assessment

Dental healthcare providers are interested not only in diagnosing and treating periodontal disease, but also in predicting which individuals are more likely to develop periodontitis. The process of identifying risk factors that increase an individual's probability of disease is called risk assessment.[4,9–12,16,18–20] The American Academy of Periodontology (AAP) describes the risk assessment process as "increasingly important in periodontal treatment planning and should be part of every comprehensive dental and periodontal evaluation."[18]

1. **Assessing the Individual**
   A. **An Individual's Risk Factors**
      1. It is becoming possible to consider an individual's risk factors for periodontal disease (systemic disease, genetic information, personal habits, and characteristics) and to classify patients into high- or low-risk groups.
      2. For example, individuals who smoke have a higher risk of periodontitis than nonsmokers.
   B. **Disease Prevention for the Individual**
      1. Clinicians also use the risk assessment process to prevent disease (such as, identifying smokers and offering smoking cessation counseling).
      2. Information concerning individual risk for developing periodontal disease is obtained through careful evaluation of the individual's demographic data, medical history, dental history, and comprehensive periodontal clinical examination (Table 12-1).
2. **Risk Assessment Systems**
   A. **Web-Based Tools.** Currently, there are several commercially produced Web-based risk calculation tools.
      1. DentoRisk is a two-stage Web-based system for periodontitis risk assessment based on data collected on 20 separate factors.[21,22]
      2. Another system is the Periodontal Risk Assessment system, originally developed by Lang and Tonetti,[23] has been shown to be of practical value in clinical practice.
      3. The PreViser Periodontal Risk Calculator developed in 2002 is a Web-based system that aims to provide dental clinicians with an easy-to-use method to determine patients' periodontitis risk.[24–26]
   B. **Risk Questionnaires.** Risk assessment questionnaires are practical tools that can be helpful in identifying individuals who are at a high risk for periodontal disease. Figures 12-9A,B show an example of a simple two-page periodontal risk questionnaire that can elicit the presence of common periodontal risk factors. Dental hygienists can use risk questionnaires to initiate discussion with patients about periodontal risk factors.

TABLE 12-1	CLINICAL RISK ASSESSMENT FOR PERIODONTAL DISEASE
Demographic Data	Age
	Duration of exposure to contributing risk factors
	Self-care (plaque biofilm control)
	Frequency of professional care
	Male gender
	Dental awareness
	Socioeconomic status
Medical History	Tobacco use
	Diabetes
	Osteoporosis
	HIV/AIDS
	Genetic predisposition to aggressive disease
Dental History	Frequency of professional care
	Family history of early tooth loss
	Previous history of periodontal disease
Clinical Examination	Plaque biofilm accumulation and microbial composition
	Calculus deposits
	Bleeding on probing
	Loss of attachment
	Plaque retentive areas
	Anatomic contributing factors
	Restorative contributing factors

PERIODONTAL ASSESSMENT QUESTIONAIRE FOR _____

TOBACCO USE

Tobacco use is the most significant risk factor for gum disease.

Do you now or have you ever used the following?

	Amount per day?	How many years?	If you quit, what year?
☐ Cigarette	_____	_____	_____
☐ Cigar	_____	_____	_____
☐ Pipe	_____	_____	_____
☐ Chew	_____	_____	_____
☐ Snuff	_____	_____	_____

HEART ATTACK AND STROKE

Untreated gum disease can increase your risk for heart attack and stroke.

Do you have any other risk factors for heart disease or stroke?

☐ Family history of heart disease   ☐ Tobacco use
☐ High cholesterol   ☐ High blood pressure

If you have any of these other risk factors it is especially important for you to always keep your gums as healthy and inflammation free as possible to reduce your overall risk for heart attack and stroke.

MEDICATIONS

A side effect of some medications can cause changes in your gums.

Have you ever taken any of the following medications?

☐ Dilantin anti-seizure medication

☐ Calcium channel blocker blood pressure medicine
(such as Procardia, Cardizem, Norvasc, Verapamil, etc.)

☐ Cyclosporin immunosuppresant therapy

GENETIC

The tendency for gum disease to develop can be inherited.

Has anyone on your side of the family had gum problems? (e.g., your mother, father, or siblings)

☐ Yes

☐ No

CONTAGIOUS

The bacteria which cause gum disease may be spread to other family members.

Has anyone in your immediate family been tested or treated for gum problems? If so, whom?

☐ Spouse

☐ Children

FEMALES

Females can be at increased risk for gum disease at different points in their life.

The following can adversely affect your gums. Please check all that apply

☐ Pregnant   ☐ Nursing   ☐ Osteoporosis
☐ Taking birth control pills
☐ Taking hormone supplements
☐ Infrequent care during previous pregnancies

over

A

Figure 12-9A. Side 1 of Periodontal Risk Questionnaire. Risk assessment questionnaires are practical tools that can be helpful in identifying individuals who have a high susceptibility to periodontitis. Side 1 of a risk assessment questionnaire is shown here. See Figure 12-9B for side 2 of this questionnaire. (Courtesy of Timothy G. Donley, DDS, MSD, Bowling Green, KY.)

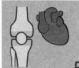

DIABETES

Gum disease is a common complication of diabetes. Untreated gum disease makes it more difficult for individuals with diabetes to control their blood sugar.

If you *ARE* diabetic...

For how many years? _____

Is your diabetes well controlled? ☐ Yes ☐ No

Who is your physician for diabetes? _____

If you *ARE NOT* diabetic...

Any family history of diabetes? ☐ Yes ☐ No

Have you had any of these warning signs of diabetes?

☐ Frequent urination   ☐ Excessive thirst
☐ Excessive hunger   ☐ Tingling or numbness in extremities
☐ Weakness and fatigue   ☐ Slow healing of cuts
☐ Unexplained weight loss   ☐ Any change of vision

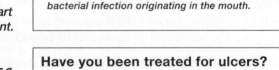

HEART MURMUR, ARTIFICIAL JOINT PROSTHESIS

With the slightest amount of gum inflammation, bacteria from the mouth can enter the bloodstream and cause a serious infection of the heart muscle or your artificial joint.

Do you have a heart murmur or artificial joint?
☐ Yes ☐ No

If so, does your physician recommend antibiotics prior to dental visits? ☐ Yes ☐ No

Name of physician: _____

It is especially important in your case to always keep your gums as healthy and inflammation-free as possible to reduce the chance of bacterial infection originating in the mouth.

GASTRIC ULCERS

When your gums are inflamed, bacteria from the mouth can travel to the gut and cause ulcers to become active.

Have you been treated for ulcers?
☐ Yes ☐ No

Is the ulcer active now?
☐ Yes ☐ No

Ulcers are caused by bacteria. If you have been treated for ulcers you should make sure your gums are as inflammation-free as possible.

ALL PATIENTS PLEASE COMPLETE THE FOLLOWING:

Have you noticed any of the following signs of gum disease?

☐ Bleeding gums during toothbrushing   ☐ Pus between the teeth and gums
☐ Red, swollen, or tender gums   ☐ Loose or separating teeth
☐ Gums that have pulled away from the teeth   ☐ Change in the way your teeth fit together
☐ Persistent bad breath   ☐ Food catching between teeth

Is it important to you to keep your teeth as long as possible? ☐ Yes ☐ No

Any particular reason why missing teeth have not been replaced?

_____

Do you like the appearance of your smile? ☐ Yes ☐ No
Do you like the color of your teeth? ☐ Yes ☐ No
Do your teeth keep you from eating any specific food? ☐ Yes ☐ No

B

Figure 12-9B. Side 2 of Periodontal Risk Questionnaire. Side 2 of a two-page risk assessment questionnaire. (Courtesy of Timothy G. Donley, DDS, MSD, Bowling Green, KY.)

Chapter Summary Statement

In the oral cavity, most of the time, things are in a state of balance between the bacteria in plaque biofilms and the host.

- For the periodontium to remain healthy, the bacterial challenge must be contained at a level that can be tolerated by the host.
- The situation can be thought of as a balance scale, with the disease-promoting factors on one side of the scale and the health-promoting factors on the other.
- As long as the two sides of the scale are in balance, there will be no disease progression.
- The intermittent pattern of disease activity seen in periodontitis is believed to result from the changing balance between the pathogenic bacteria and the host's inflammatory and immune responses.

Periodontal disease is a bacterial infection of the periodontium. The presence of pathogenic bacteria, however, does not necessarily mean that an individual will experience periodontitis.

- Additional factors play a role in determining why some individuals are more susceptible to periodontitis than others.
- Contributing factors are factors that increase an individual's susceptibility to periodontitis by modifying the host response to bacterial infection.
- Contributing factors such as systemic disease, smoking, and genetic factors can play a significant role in determining the onset and progression of periodontitis.

Thorough daily self-care (plaque control) by the patient and routine professional care are the best methods for prevention of periodontal disease. Other risk factors must be evaluated, however, to develop the best treatment plan for each individual.

Section 5
Focus on Patients

Evidence in Action

Mr. and Mrs. Merkel are patients in the general dental practice where you have been the dental hygienist for 10 years. Mrs. Merkel has been diagnosed with generalized Stage III, Grade C periodontitis and receives treatment in your office and at a periodontal practice. Mrs. Merkel is very compliant with her self-care and frequent professional care. Despite her best efforts, her periodontal disease is progressing.

During today's appointment, Mrs. Merkel breaks into tears. She tells you that she is so conscientious about her daily self-care and keeping all her dental appointments, yet her dental health continues to worsen. She cannot understand why her husband gives his teeth a quick brush and never flosses, yet he has good dental health (no gingivitis or periodontitis). She asks, "how this can be"?

Based on current dental research, how would you answer Mrs. Merkel's question?

Ethical Dilemma

Your first patient on Monday morning is Joyce Robbins. She is new to your practice. She has filled out a Periodontal Assessment Questionnaire to assist you in determining her risk assessment. She states that she has never filled one out before, and is concerned that she has received poor-quality dental work as a result. Her medical history and Periodontal Assessment Questionnaire reveal the following:

Joyce is a 58-year-old college professor. She has stage-1 hypertension, and takes 20 mg of Lisinopril daily as a result. She reports a family history of cardiac disease and her father developed Type II diabetes at age 50. She takes Simvastatin for high cholesterol. She is a borderline diabetic, and her blood sugar levels have been rising at each primary care visit. She suffers from osteoporosis of the spine and hip. She is presently a nonsmoker, but did smoke while she was in college.

Her oral exam and radiographs reveal periodontitis. She flosses daily, but hasn't had her teeth cleaned in 5 years. She frequently gets food stuck between her teeth, and is increasingly becoming concerned about "the way her teeth look and feel."

She wants to know what she can do to maintain her "pretty smile," and why no other office was as thorough with her care.

What do you think may be the cause of the patient's generalized recession?

What factors may have contributed to the patient's disease progression?

How will you discuss the balance between periodontal health and disease?

Is there an ethical dilemma involved?

Clinical Patient Care

CASE 1

Mr. Archie Newcomer is a new patient in your dental office. Mr. Newcomer is 35 years of age and reports that this is his first dental check-up in 5 or 6 years. *Mr. Newcomer's completed Periodontal Assessment Questionnaire is shown in Figures 12-10A,B on the next two pages of this module.* Review Mr. Newcomer's questionnaire, make a list of periodontal risk factors, and suggest strategies for managing these risk factors.

PERIODONTAL ASSESSMENT QUESTIONAIRE FOR *Mr. Newcomer*

TOBACCO USE

Tobacco use is the most significant risk factor for gum disease.

Do you now or have you ever used the following?

	Amount per day?	How many years?	If you quit, what year?
☒ Cigarette	*2 packs*	*15 yrs.*	
☐ Cigar			
☐ Pipe			
☐ Chew			
☐ Snuff			

HEART ATTACK AND STROKE

Untreated gum disease can increase your risk for heart attack and stroke.

Do you have any other risk factors for heart disease or stroke?

☐ Family history of heart disease   ☒ Tobacco use
☐ High cholesterol   ☐ High blood pressure

If you have any of these other risk factors it is especially important for you to always keep your gums as healthy and inflammation free as possible to reduce your overall risk for heart attack and stroke.

MEDICATIONS

A side effect of some medications can cause changes in your gums.

Have you ever taken any of the following medications?

☐ Dilantin anti-seizure medication

☐ Calcium channel blocker blood pressure medicine
   (such as Procardia, Cardizem, Norvasc, Verapamil, etc.)

☐ Cyclosporin immunosuppresant therapy

GENETIC

The tendency for gum disease to develop can be inherited.

Has anyone on your side of the family had gum problems? (e.g., your mother, father, or siblings)

☒ Yes

☐ No

CONTAGIOUS

The bacteria which cause gum disease may be spread to other family members.

Has anyone in your immediate family been tested or treated for gum problems? If so, whom?

☒ Spouse

☐ Children

FEMALES

Females can be at increased risk for gum disease at different points in their life.

The following can adversely affect your gums. Please check all that apply

☐ Pregnant   ☐ Nursing   ☐ Osteoporosis
☐ Taking birth control pills
☐ Taking hormone supplements
☐ Infrequent care during previous pregnancies

over

A

Figure 12-10A. Page 1 of Mr. Newcomer's Risk Questionnaire.

DIABETES

Gum disease is a common complication of diabetes. Untreated gum disease makes it more difficult for individuals with diabetes to control their blood sugar.

If you ARE diabetic...
For how many years? _20 yrs._
Is your diabetes well controlled? ☒ Yes ☐ No
Who is your physician for diabetes? _Dr. Samuel Burlington_

If you ARE NOT diabetic...
Any family history of diabetes? ☐ Yes ☐ No

Have you had any of these warning signs of diabetes?

- ☐ Frequent urination
- ☐ Excessive hunger
- ☐ Weakness and fatigue
- ☐ Unexplained weight loss
- ☐ Excessive thirst
- ☐ Tingling or numbness in extremities
- ☐ Slow healing of cuts
- ☐ Any change of vision

HEART MURMUR, ARTIFICIAL JOINT PROSTHESIS

With the slightest amount of gum inflammation, bacteria from the mouth can enter the bloodstream and cause a serious infection of the heart muscle or your artificial joint.

Do you have a heart murmur or artificial joint?
☐ Yes ☒ No

If so, does your physician recommend antibiotics prior to dental visits? ☐ Yes ☐ No

Name of physician: _____

It is especially important in your case to always keep your gums as healthy and inflammation-free as possible to reduce the chance of bacterial infection originating in the mouth.

GASTRIC ULCERS

When your gums are inflamed, bacteria from the mouth can travel to the gut and cause ulcers to become active.

Have you been treated for ulcers?
☐ Yes ☒ No

Is the ulcer active now?
☐ Yes ☐ No

Ulcers are caused by bacteria. If you have been treated for ulcers you should make sure your gums are as inflammation-free as possible.

ALL PATIENTS PLEASE COMPLETE THE FOLLOWING:

Have you noticed any of the following signs of gum disease?

- ☒ Bleeding gums during toothbrushing
- ☐ Red, swollen, or tender gums
- ☐ Gums that have pulled away from the teeth
- ☐ Persistent bad breath
- ☐ Pus between the teeth and gums
- ☐ Loose or separating teeth
- ☐ Change in the way your teeth fit together
- ☒ Food catching between teeth

Is it important to you to keep your teeth as long as possible? ☐ Yes ☐ No
Any particular reason why missing teeth have not been replaced?

_____

Do you like the appearance of your smile? ☒ Yes ☐ No
Do you like the color of your teeth? ☒ Yes ☐ No
Do your teeth keep you from eating any specific food? ☐ Yes ☒ No

B

Figure 12-10B. Page 2 of Mr. Newcomer's Risk Questionnaire.

References

1. Glick M, Williams DM, Kleinman DV, Vujicic M, Watt RG, Weyant RJ. Reprint of: a new definition for oral health supported by FDI opens the door to a universal definition of oral health. *J Dent*. 2017;57:1–3.

2. Glick M, Williams DM, Kleinman DV, Vujicic M, Watt RG, Weyant RJ. A new definition for oral health developed by the FDI World Dental Federation opens the door to a universal definition of oral health. *J Am Dent Assoc*. 2016;147(12):915–917.

3. Armitage GC. Learned and unlearned concepts in periodontal diagnostics: a 50-year perspective. *Periodontol 2000*. 2013;62(1):20–36.

4. Bartold PM, Van Dyke TE. Periodontitis: a host-mediated disruption of microbial homeostasis. Unlearning learned concepts. *Periodontol 2000*. 2013;62(1):203–217.

5. Dick DS, Shaw JR. The infectious and transmissible nature of the periodontal syndrome of the rice rat. *Arch Oral Biol*. 1966;11(11):1095–1108.

6. Wade WG. The oral microbiome in health and disease. *Pharmacol Res*. 2013;69(1):137–143.

7. Bouchard P, Carra MC, Boillot A, Mora F, Range H. Risk factors in periodontology: a conceptual framework. *J Clin Periodontol*. 2017;44(2):125–131.

8. Cullinan MP, Seymour GJ. Understanding risk for periodontal disease. *Ann R Australas Coll Dent Surg*. 2010;20:86–87.

9. Douglass CW. Risk assessment and management of periodontal disease. *J Am Dent Assoc*. 2006;137 Suppl:27S–32S.

10. Garcia RI, Compton R, Dietrich T. Risk assessment and periodontal prevention in primary care. *Periodontol 2000*. 2016;71(1):10–21.

11. Genco RJ, Borgnakke WS. Risk factors for periodontal disease. *Periodontol 2000*. 2013;62(1):59–94.

12. Koshi E, Rajesh S, Koshi P, Arunima PR. Risk assessment for periodontal disease. *J Indian Soc Periodontol*. 2012;16(3):324–328.

13. Matthews JB, Chen FM, Milward MR, et al. Effect of nicotine, cotinine and cigarette smoke extract on the neutrophil respiratory burst. *J Clin Periodontol*. 2011;38(3):208–218.

14. Mealey BL, Ocampo GL. Diabetes mellitus and periodontal disease. *Periodontol 2000*. 2007;44:127–153.

15. Michalowicz BS, Diehl SR, Gunsolley JC, et al. Evidence of a substantial genetic basis for risk of adult periodontitis. *J Periodontol*. 2000;71(11):1699–1707.

16. Peruzzo DC, Benatti BB, Ambrosano GM, et al. A systematic review of stress and psychological factors as possible risk factors for periodontal disease. *J Periodontol*. 2007;78(8):1491–1504.

17. Ziukaite L, Slot DE, Loos BG, Coucke W, Van der Weijden GA. Family history of periodontal disease and prevalence of smoking status among adult periodontitis patients: a cross-sectional study. *Int J Dent Hyg*. 2017;15(4):e28–e34.

18. American Academy of Periodontology. American Academy of Periodontology statement on risk assessment. *J Periodontol*. 2008;79(2):202.

19. Thyvalikakath TP, Padman R, Gupta S. An integrated risk assessment tool for team-based periodontal disease management. *Stud Health Technol Inform*. 2013;192:1150.

20. Trombelli L, Minenna L, Toselli L, et al. Prognostic value of a simplified method for periodontal risk assessment during supportive periodontal therapy. *J Clin Periodontol*. 2017;44(1):51–57.

21. Lindskog S, Blomlof J, Persson I, et al. Validation of an algorithm for chronic periodontitis risk assessment and prognostication: analysis of an inflammatory reactivity test and selected risk predictors. *J Periodontol*. 2010;81(6):837–847.

22. Lindskog S, Blomlof J, Persson I, et al. Validation of an algorithm for chronic periodontitis risk assessment and prognostication: risk predictors, explanatory values, measures of quality, and clinical use. *J Periodontol*. 2010;81(4):584–593.

23. Lang NP, Tonetti MS. Periodontal risk assessment (PRA) for patients in supportive periodontal therapy (SPT). *Oral Health Prev Dent*. 2003;1(1):7–16.

24. Page RC. Overview of efficacy outcome variables for the evaluation of periodontal disease treatment. *J Int Acad Periodontol*. 2005;7(4 Suppl):139–146.

25. Page RC, Krall EA, Martin J, Mancl L, Garcia RI. Validity and accuracy of a risk calculator in predicting periodontal disease. *J Am Dent Assoc*. 2002;133(5):569–576.

26. Page RC, Martin J, Krall EA, Mancl L, Garcia R. Longitudinal validation of a risk calculator for periodontal disease. *J Clin Periodontol*. 2003;30(9):819–827.

STUDENT ANCILLARY RESOURCES

A wide variety of resources to enhance your learning is available online:

- Audio Glossary
- Book Pages
- Chapter Review Questions and Answers

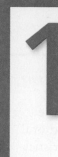

CHAPTER

13 Oral Biofilms

Clinical Application.
Caring for patients with periodontal diseases requires a comprehensive understanding of the concept of oral biofilms and how individual microbes interact as residents in these biofilm communities. This chapter discusses what is currently known about oral biofilms and sets the stage for the inevitable expansion of our knowledge about these biofilms as the results of additional research become available.

Learning Objectives
- Explain the difference in the cell envelope of a gram-positive versus a gram-negative bacterium.
- Define the term biofilm and explain the advantages to a bacterium of living in a biofilm.
- Describe the life cycle of a biofilm.
- Explain the significance of the extracellular protective matrix and fluid channels to a biofilm.
- Define coaggregation and explain its significance in bacterial colonization of the tooth surface.
- Define quorum sensing and explain its significance in coordinating and regulating microbial behavior and growth.
- Explain why systemic antibiotics and antimicrobial agents are not effective in eliminating dental plaque biofilms.
- State the most effective ways to control dental plaque biofilms.
- Name several reasons why newer microbe detection methods have brought Socransky's microbial complexes and the Specific Plaque Hypothesis model into question.
- Discuss the evolution of hypotheses to explain the role of bacteria in periodontal disease and how current hypotheses are distinct from the *Nonspecific Plaque Hypothesis* and the *Specific Plaque Hypothesis*.
- Discuss the hypothesis that plaque biofilm is necessary *but not sufficient* to cause destruction of the tissues of the periodontium and the implications for the treatment of individuals with periodontitis.

Key Terms
Microbe
Bacterium/Bacteria
Cell envelope
Gram staining
Gram-positive bacteria
Gram-negative bacteria
Polymicrobial Biofilm
Oral biofilm
Commensal bacteria
Dysbiosis
Symbiosis
Acquired pellicle
Coaggregation
Extracellular protective matrix
Extracellular polymeric substance
Microbial blooms
Mushroom-shaped microcolonies
Fluid channels
Quorum sensing
Tooth-associated plaque biofilms
Tissue-associated plaque biofilms
Unattached bacteria
Transmission
Nonspecific Plaque Hypothesis
Specific Plaque Hypothesis
Ecological Plaque Hypothesis
Microbial Homeostasis–Host Response Hypothesis
Keystone Pathogen–Host Response Hypothesis

Section 1
Microbial Biofilms

Bacteria are everywhere in nature. *One human mouth is home to more microorganisms than there are people on the planet Earth.* It is currently estimated that some 650 to 1,000 unique bacterial species reside in the oral cavity.[1-5] These microorganisms have evolved to survive in the environment of the tooth surface, gingival epithelium, and oral cavity. Though this is not a microbiology textbook, knowledge of several characteristics of bacteria is fundamental to understanding many of the ideas presented in this chapter.

The term microbe was coined to refer collectively to the microscopic organisms, including bacteria, fungi, protozoa, and viruses. However, the term is used commonly to denote any bacteria that are harmful and pathogenic. The bacterial characteristics discussed in this section include cell envelope structure, Gram staining of bacteria, and the role of the biofilm in microbiology and microbial ecology.

CHARACTERISTICS OF BACTERIA

1. **Characteristics of Bacteria**
   A. **Description**
      1. Bacterium (plural, bacteria). Bacteria are the simplest organisms and can be seen only through a microscope.
      2. There are thousands of kinds of bacteria, most of which are harmless to humans.
      3. Bacteria have existed on Earth for longer than any other organisms and are still the most abundant type of cell.
      4. Bacteria can replicate quickly. This ability to divide quickly enables populations of bacteria to adapt rapidly even to sudden changes in their environment.
   B. **Structure of the Bacterial Cell Envelope.** The bacterial cell envelope is a complex, multilayered structure that serves to protect the microorganism from the unpredictable and inhospitable external environment. One can imagine the bacterial cell envelope as being the "skin" of the microorganism. The physical structure of the cell envelope is the fundamental basis for a laboratory method known as Gram staining. Gram staining classifies bacteria into either one of the two groups based on the structure of their cell envelope: gram-positive microorganisms or gram-negative microorganisms.
      1. In 1884, Hans Christian Gram devised a staining technique to identify microorganisms under light microscopy. Today, it is known as Gram staining. Gram staining is a widely used diagnostic laboratory staining method that identifies bacteria based on the fundamental structural characteristics of the bacterial cell envelope. Depending on the permeability of the stain through the bacterial cell envelope, bacteria will appear either purple (gram-positive) or red (gram-negative) in color under a light microscope (Fig. 13-1).
      2. The defining features of each type of bacteria is listed below:
         a. Gram-positive bacteria (purple stain)
            1) This type of bacteria has a single, thick multilayered, mesh-like cell wall composed of peptidoglycan (a biological polymer composed of sugars and amino acids). This thick layer lies above the cytoplasmic (plasma) membrane which faces the interior of the cell.

2) It is this thick cell wall that permits the gram-positive bacteria to retain the purple color when stained with a dye known as crystal violet. Therefore, under a light microscope, gram-positive bacteria appear purple.

  b. Gram-negative bacteria (red stain)

    1) This type of bacteria has two membranes:

      a) The outer membrane faces the external environment. The outer membrane is highly composed of proteins and lipopolysaccharides (endotoxin). Lipopolysaccharides are important because they play a major role in the pathogenesis of gram-negative bacterial infections.

      b) There is also an inner cytoplasmic (plasma) membrane that faces the interior of the cell.

    2) Sandwiched in between the outer membrane and inner cytoplasmic membrane is a thin, single-layered cell wall layer composed of peptidoglycan. The thin cell wall does not allow for the retention of the purple stain. Therefore, the gram-negative microbe appears red or pink under light microscope.

C. Bacteria Are "Social Creatures"

  1. For years, microbes were thought of as being dormant "bags" of enzymes. Current research shows, however, that bacteria are "social creatures" that can live together in complex microbial communities.

  2. In a similar manner to human cities, "microbial cities" contain different species of microbes (they are multicultural) and spatially organized (well-engineered).

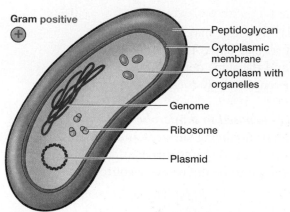

Gram positive

Peptidoglycan
Cytoplasmic membrane
Cytoplasm with organelles
Genome
Ribosome
Plasmid

Outer membrane
Periplasmatic space
Peptidoglycan
Cytoplasmic membrane

Attachment pili
Cytoplasm with organelles
Flagella
Fimbriae

Gram negative

Figure 13-1. Gram-Positive and Gram-Negative Bacterial Cell Envelopes. Gram-positive bacteria have a thick peptidoglycan cell wall that retains the purple color when stained with crystal violet dye. Gram-negative bacteria have a thin peptidoglycan layer which cannot retain the crystal violet dye. As a result, gram-negative bacteria appear red with the Gram staining method. Gram-negative bacteria are believed to play an important role in periodontal disease.

MICROBIAL COMMUNITIES

In the past, microbes were studied as they grew on culture plates in a laboratory. Recent advances in research technology have allowed researchers to study microbes in their natural environment. These studies reveal that under natural conditions, most microorganisms tend to live in complex communities attached to surfaces.

1. **Where Microbes Live.** Microbes rarely exist as planktonic (free-floating) forms. The majority live in complex polymicrobial biofilm communities attached to living surfaces (such as the root of a tooth) or nonliving surfaces (such as a prosthetic heart valve or a dental implant).
2. **Biofilms and Where They Form**
   A. **What Are Biofilms?**
      1. A biofilm is a complex and dynamic microbial community—containing a diverse array of many types of microbial species (bacteria, fungi, and viruses)—embedded within a self-protective matrix that adheres to a living or nonliving surface. Polymicrobial biofilm communities are characterized by the presence of several species of microorganisms.[6]
      2. The microbes in the biofilm synthesize and secrete the protective matrix. A very simplified description of this protective matrix is that the microbes are "embedded in a thick, slimy barrier of sugars and proteins that protects them from external threats."
      3. By some estimates 65% of all diseases may be biofilm-induced. Biofilm-induced diseases include tuberculosis, cystic fibrosis, subacute bacterial endocarditis, and periodontal disease.
   B. **Where Do Biofilms Form?**
      1. Biofilms are everywhere in nature (Fig. 13-2). "Biofilm" may seem like a new term, but everyone encounters biofilms on a regular basis. The plaque biofilm that forms on teeth, the slime in fish tanks, and the slime deposit that clogs the sink drain are all examples of biofilms. Even the slimy rocks in a stream of water are biofilm-coated.
      2. *Biofilms can exist on any solid surface that is exposed to a microbe-containing fluid.* Biofilms may form on living or nonliving surfaces and can be prevalent in natural, industrial, and hospital settings. Biofilms thrive in dental unit water and suction lines and have been shown to be the primary source of contaminated water delivered by dental units.

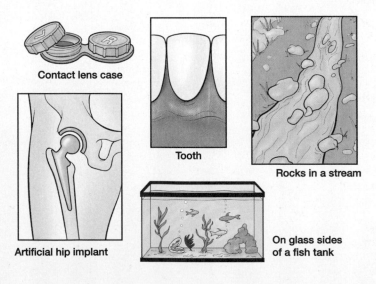

Contact lens case

Tooth

Rocks in a stream

Artificial hip implant

On glass sides of a fish tank

Figure 13-2. Biofilm Environments. Biofilms are found nearly everywhere in nature. They have a major impact on human health.

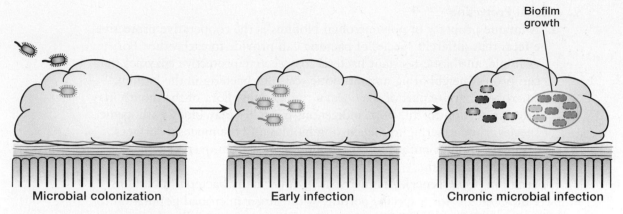

Biofilm
growth

Microbial colonization   Early infection   Chronic microbial infection

Figure 13-3. Biofilm Formation. Once microbes attach to the tooth surface, biofilms form quickly. Periodontitis is characterized by mature biofilms on tooth surfaces.

C. **How Quickly Do Biofilms Form?** Experimental laboratory studies show that free-floating bacteria—for example, *Staphylococci, Streptococci, Pseudomonas,* and *Escherichia coli*—typically form biofilms quickly.[7,8] A typical timeline for formation is that:

1. Within minutes: Free-floating microbes attach to a surface
2. Within 2 to 4 hours: Microbes form strongly attached microcolonies
3. Within 6 to 12 hours: Microbes produce an initial extracellular protective matrix and become increasingly resistant to antiseptics and antibiotics
4. Within 2 to 4 days: The biofilm evolves into fully mature biofilm colonies that are extremely resistant to antibiotics; can rapidly recover from mechanical disruption and reform a mature biofilm with 24 hours

D. **How Do Biofilms Mature?** As depicted in Figure 13-3, the first step is colonization of the tooth surface. Next, additional microbes join with the early colonizers and finally, a complex microbial community develops that is characteristic of chronic infection.

E. **How Do Mature Biofilms Protect Bacteria?** Biofilms greatly enhance the ability of inhabiting microbes to withstand the host's immune system, antimicrobials, and environmental stresses. Microbes in a biofilm can resist factors that would easily kill these same microbes when in a free-floating state.[9] The biofilm offers three inherent features that enable inhabiting microbes to tolerate various external stresses.

1. **Blocking.** The extracellular protective matrix protects microbes by preventing large molecules (e.g., antibodies) and inflammatory cells from penetrating deeply into the biofilm matrix. Mature biofilms may even block small molecules like antimicrobial agents.[10]

2. **Mutual Protection**

   a. A unique property of polymicrobial biofilms is the cooperative protective effects that different species of bacteria can provide to each other. For example, antibiotic resistant bacteria may secrete protective enzymes that can protect neighboring nonantibiotic resistant bacteria in the biofilm.[11]

   b. Microbes that are part of the normal (indigenous) flora of the mouth may offer protection for the host. Indigenous microbes may block pathogenic species from adhering to the existing biofilm and the mucosal surfaces. Thus, the biofilm can protect itself and the host from overgrowth of pathogenic bacteria.[12]

3. **Hibernation (Quiescence).** Another strategy that many bacteria in biofilms have developed is for a specific portion of the larger microbial population to hibernate. Since some antibiotics are only effective on metabolically active bacteria, hibernating bacteria in biofilms are unaffected by these types of antibiotics.[13,14] Research shows that standard oral doses of antibiotics—which effectively kill free-floating bacteria—may have little or no antimicrobial effect on the same type of bacteria in biofilm form.

ORAL BIOFILMS

An oral biofilm is a polymicrobial, three-dimensional community of numerous microbial species, embedded in a protective matrix that consists of microbial metabolic products and/or host components, such as salivary glycoproteins.[15] In health, the bacteria in the biofilm maintain a harmonious balance by keeping each other in check so that no one specific bacterial strain can dominate the biofilm community. If the biofilm is not disrupted frequently and allowed to accumulate, an imbalance occurs in the biofilm community where certain pathogenic species become dominant while other species become weaker. Figure 13-4 shows an artist's representation of a mature oral biofilm.

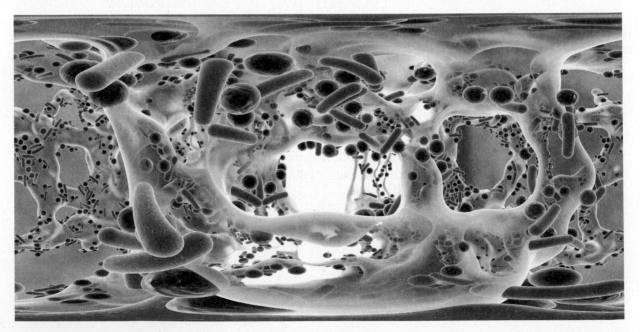

Figure 13-4. A Polymicrobial Biofilm. This three-dimensional illustration depicts a 360-degree spherical panorama view inside of antibiotic-resistant mature biofilm.

ORAL BIOFILMS: SYMBIOSIS VERSUS DYSBIOSIS

1. **Resident Microbes of the Oral Cavity.** A multitude of bacterial, viral, and fungal species inhabit the oral cavity. Many of these can associate to form biofilms, which are resistant to mechanical stress or antibiotic treatment.
   A. The oral cavity is inhabited by indigenous, resident bacteria (**commensal bacteria**). These commensal bacteria are part of the normal flora in the mouth, living in the oral cavity all the time and causing no problems.
   B. In a healthy state, all epithelial-lined surfaces (including the oral cavity) are colonized by a polymicrobial biofilm that is predominantly composed of commensal microorganisms.
2. **A Mutually Beneficial Relationship.** In health, there is a symbiotic (mutually beneficial) relationship between the host and commensal microorganisms.
   A. The commensal microorganisms contribute to host nutrition, maintenance of a robust immune system, and provide a cover over the mucous membranes (preventing the invasion and an overgrowth of pathogenic bacteria).[16]
   B. Conversely, the host provides the bacteria with nutrients and a stable environment in which to survive (Fig. 13-5).[17]
   C. **Symbiosis** translates to living in harmony. In health, commensal microbes in the oral biofilm have a symbiotic relationship with the host (human body).[18]

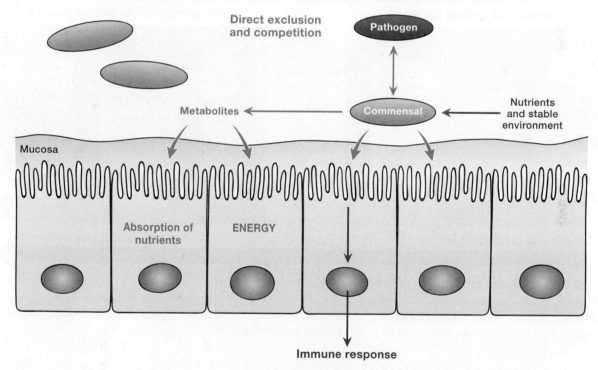

Figure 13-5. Commensal Bacteria Cross Talk With the Host. Commensal bacteria supply the host with essential nutrients and defend the host against opportunistic pathogens. In return, the host provides the bacteria with nutrients and a stable environment.

3. **Microbial Imbalance: The "Bad Guys" Take Over the Biofilm**
   A. **Early Dysbiosis**
      1. Dysbiosis is the opposite of symbiosis. **Dysbiosis** is a term for a microbial imbalance on or inside the body.
         a. It essentially means there is an imbalance of microbial colonies. The bacteria maintain a harmonious balance in a healthy biofilm by keeping each other in check so no one specific strain can dominate.

b. Dysbiosis can result if certain species of microbes become dominant while other species become weaker.

c. *If the oral biofilm is not disrupted frequently and is allowed to mature, the conditions within in it start to favor bacterial species that elicit a stronger host response.* In turn, the stronger host response leads to the development of gingival inflammation.

d. This state is known as initial dysbiosis or incipient dysbiosis because in most individuals, this gingivitis does not progress to periodontitis (Fig. 13-6).

B. Established Dysbiosis

1. Recent research has indicated that dysbiosis in the oral cavity can lead to periodontitis. The development of oral dysbiosis is likely to occur over an extended period of time, gradually changing the symbiotic host–microbe relationship to a pathogenic one.[18]

2. In susceptible patients, dysbiosis triggers an inappropriate and excessive host response (to the unhealthy change in the oral biofilm) which results in periodontal tissue damage (progression from gingivitis to periodontitis).[19]

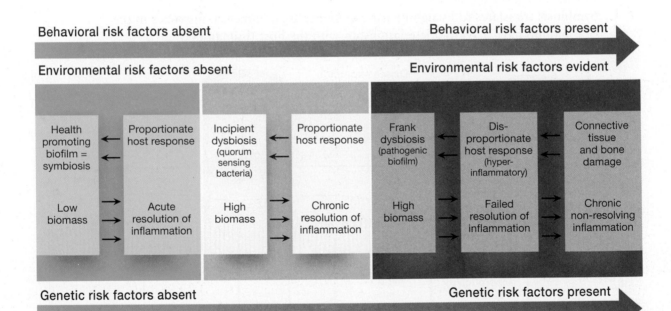

Figure 13-6. Model of Host–Microbe Interactions. If the oral biofilm is not disrupted frequently and is allowed to accumulate, the conditions within in it start to favor bacterial species that elicit a stronger host response, leading to the development of gingival inflammation. In susceptible individuals, dysbiosis triggers an exaggerated host response which results in progression from gingivitis to periodontitis.

4. Control of Microbial Growth Within a Mature Oral Biofilm

A. Biofilm Bacteria Are Resistant to Antibiotics and Antimicrobial Agents

1. Bacteria living in a biofilm are unusually resistant to systemic antibiotics (in dentistry, usually administered in pill form) and antimicrobials (placed locally in the oral cavity or taken as an oral rinse).[20]

2. *Antibiotic doses that kill free-floating bacteria, for example, need to be increased as much as 1,500 times to kill plaque biofilm bacteria* (and at these high doses, the antibiotic would kill the patient before the biofilm bacteria!).[21]

3. Antimicrobial agents work best when used in conjunction with mechanical cleaning that removes or disrupts the structural integrity of the dental plaque biofilm.[22]

B. **Physical Removal of Dental Plaque Biofilms Is Essential**
1. *Control of bacteria in dental plaque biofilms is best achieved by the physical disruption (such as brushing, flossing, and periodontal instrumentation) of the biofilm structure.*
   a. It takes some time for the complex structure of a mature plaque biofilm to form.
   b. Mechanical cleaning forces the bacteria to start over with initial attachment, initial colonization, secondary colonization and finally, to become a mature biofilm.
   c. In areas that are cleaned regularly, a mature biofilm will not be able to develop. The cleaner the tooth surface, the less complex the bacterial formation.
2. Toothbrushes and floss cannot reach the subgingival plaque biofilm located within pockets. For this reason, frequent periodontal instrumentation of subgingival root surfaces by a dental hygienist or dentist is an essential component in the treatment of periodontal disease.

5. **Transmission of Biofilm Bacteria**
A. Molecular epidemiology techniques that isolate DNA provide evidence that bacteria in the biofilm are transmissible.[23] Transmission is the transfer of bacteria from the oral cavity of one person to another.
B. The term transmissible refers to a disease that may be passed from one person to another by direct contact, such as the transfer of saliva through kissing, or indirect contact via salivary substances on inanimate objects.
C. Studies demonstrate that *Aggregatibacter actinomycetemcomitans* and *Porphyromonas gingivalis* strains isolated from parents and children within the same family exhibited identical restriction endonuclease DNA fragment patterns.[24–27] Kissing is the primary means by which saliva and its bacterial contents are transmitted.[26,28,29]
D. Table 13-1 provides a pronunciation guide to bacteria commonly associated with plaque biofilms.

TABLE 13-1	**PRONUNCIATION GUIDE TO BACTERIAL TONGUE TWISTERS**
Name	**Pronunciation Guide**
Aggregatibacter actinomycetemcomitans	ag-gre-gat-eee-bac-ter act-tin-oh-my-see-tem-comb-ah-tans
Tannerella forsythia	tann-er-ella fawr-**sith**-ee-uh
Fusobacterium nucleatum	fuse-so-back-tier-EEE-um nu-klee-ah-tum
Porphyromonas gingivalis	pour-fy-roh-mo-nas ging-jih-val-lis

SPECIES CAPABLE OF COLONIZING THE MOUTH

Many different species and subspecies can colonize the mouth. Figure 13-7 provides a few examples of the over 600 cultivable species.

	Gram positive ⊕		Gram negative ⊖	
	Facultative anaerobes	**Obligate anaerobes**	**Facultative anaerobes**	**Obligate anaerobes**
Cocci	**Streptococcus** –*S. anginosus* (*S. milleri*) –*S. mutans* –*S. sanguis* • **Ss** –*S. oralis* –*S. mitis* –*S. intermedius*	**Peptostreptococcus** –*P. micros* • **Pm** **Peptococcus**	**Neisseria** **Branhamella**	**Veillonella** –*V. parvula*
Rods	**Actinomyces** –*A. naeslundii* • **An** –*A. viscosus* • **Av** –*A. odontolyticus* –*A. israelii* **Propionibacterium** **Rothia** –*R. dentocariosa* **Lactobacillus** –*L. oris* –*L. acidophilus* –*L. salivarius* –*L. buccalis*	**Eubacterium** –*E. nodatum* • **En** –*E. saburreum* –*E. timidum* –*E. brachy* –*E. alactolyticum* **Bifidobacterium** –*B. dentium*	**Aggregatibacter** –*A. actinomycetem-comitans* • **Aa** **Capnocytophaga** –*C. ochracea* –*C. gingivalis* –*C. sputigena* **Campylobacter** –*C. rectus* • **Cr** –*C. curvus* –*C. showae* **Eikenella** –*E. corrodens* • **Ec** **Haemophilus** –*H. aphrophilus* –*H. segnis*	**Porphyromonas** –*P. gingivalis* • **Pg** –*P. endodontalis* **Prevotella** –*P. intermedia* • **Pi** –*P. nigrescens* –*P. denticola* –*P. loescheii* –*P. oris* –*P. oralis* **Tannerella** –*T. forsythia* • **Tf** **Fusobacterium** –*F. nucleatum* • **Fn** –*F. periodonticum* **Selenemonas** –*S. sputigena* –*S. noxia*
Spirochetes and mycoplasms	**Mycoplasm** –*M. orale* –*M. salivarium* –*M. hominis*		**Spirochetes of ANUG** **Treponema sp.** –*T. denticola* • **Td** –*T. socranskii* –*T. pectinovorum* –*T. vincentii*	
Eukaryotes	**Candida** –*C. albicans*	**Entamoeba**		**Trichomonas**

Figure 13-7. Examples of Microorganisms Capable of Colonizing the Mouth.

Section 2
The Structure and Colonization of Oral Biofilms

It can be very helpful for clinicians to develop an awareness of how biofilms form and mature on a tooth surface. The description below follows biofilm development starting with a recently cleaned tooth surface and progresses to a fully developed biofilm on that tooth surface.

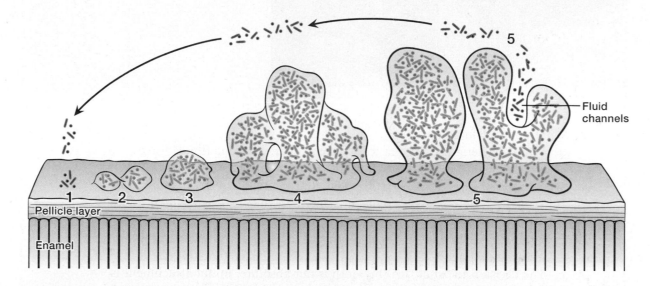

Figure 13-8. Five Phases in the Formation of a Biofilm. The five stages of biofilm development: (1) initial attachment, (2) irreversible attachment, (3) maturation I, (4) maturation II, and (5) dispersion.

STAGES OF POLYMICROBIAL BIOFILM FORMATION

Formation of the plaque biofilm begins with the attachment of free-floating microbes to the outer surface of the tooth pellicle. There are five stages of biofilm development: initial attachment, irreversible attachment, maturation I, maturation II, and dispersion.[30–33] These five stages are depicted in Figure 13-8.

1. The Five Stages of Plaque Biofilm Development in the Oral Cavity
    A. Stage 1—Initial Attachment of Microbes to Pellicle
        1. Formation
            a. Within minutes after cleaning, a film forms over the tooth surface. This film, the acquired pellicle, is composed of a variety of salivary glycoproteins (mucins) and antibodies. The purpose of the acquired pellicle is to protect the enamel from acidic activity.
            b. Within a few hours after pellicle formation, free-floating (planktonic) microbes begin to attach to the outer surface of the pellicle. Under natural conditions, most bacteria are not free-floating, but tend to attach to surfaces. Figure 13-9 shows a scanning electron micrograph of plaque-forming bacteria.

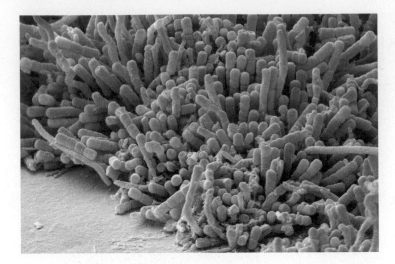

Figure 13-9. Plaque-Forming Bacteria. Scanning electron micrograph of plaque-forming bacteria growing on top of the outer surface of an acquired pellicle.

2. **What does it take to stick?**
   a. Motile bacteria use flagella to overcome hydrodynamic (fluid) forces within the oral cavity. One can think of the flagella as being the tail of the microorganism that gives it the capability to "swim" in fluid.
   b. Some bacteria possess attachment structures, such as extracellular adhesive substances or extracellular hair-like structures that enable them to attach rapidly upon contact with the tooth surface. The hair-like structures are termed fimbriae.
   c. The decision to "stick" to the tooth is not absolute; initial attachment is dynamic and reversible, during which the microbes can detach and rejoin the free-floating population if disturbed by hydrodynamic forces or in response to nutrient availability.

B. **Stage 2—Permanent Attachment**
   1. Permanent attachment is attained by microbes that can weather hydrodynamic (fluid) forces and maintain a steadfast grip on the tooth surface.
   2. At this stage, the microbes begin producing substances that stimulate other free-floating bacteria to join the community. Thus, the attachment of initial species becomes the scaffolding to which other species may adhere.
   3. This process by which genetically distinct bacteria become attached to one another is commonly referred to as coaggregation. As a result, the composition of early colonizers determines which microbes colonize at later time points, consequently, influencing the development of the biofilm.[34]

C. **Stage 3—Maturation Phase I: Self-Protective Matrix Formation**
   1. Once firmly attached, the bacteria begin to secrete a surrounding protective substance, known as an extracellular protective matrix (or an extracellular polymeric substance). Figure 13-10 shows an example of microbes in an oral biofilm surrounded by an extracellular protective matrix.
   2. The exact composition of the extracellular protective matrix varies according to the microorganisms in the biofilm, but generally consists of proteins, glycolipids, and bacterial DNA.[11]
   3. Thus, the microbes are cocooned in a self-protective matrix. Inside the host, the matrix protects biofilm microbes from exposure to host immune defenses (such as phagocytosis) and antibiotic treatments. As a result, the biofilm persists, eventually establishing a chronic disease state (periodontitis).

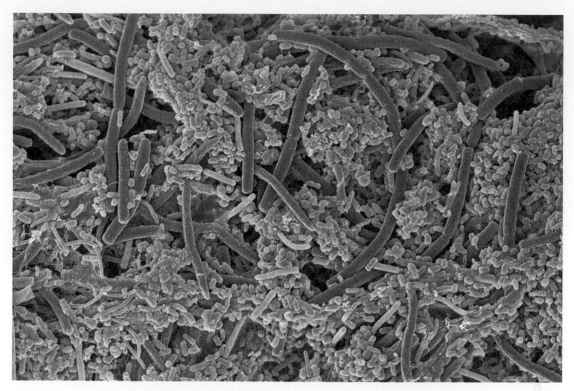

Figure 13-10. Protective Extracellular Matrix. Scanning electron micrograph of dental plaque biofilm showing bacteria (*red and yellow stain*) and the protective matrix (*orange stain*). (Courtesy of Getty Images.)

D. **Stage 4—Maturation Phase II: Mushroom-Shaped Microcolonies**
  1. **Microcolony Formation.** At this stage, the biofilm continues to grow through a combination of cell division and recruitment. Microbial blooms are periods when specific species or groups of species grow at rapidly accelerated rates. The proliferating microbes begin to grow away from the tooth.
     a. The microbes cluster together to form mushroom-shaped microcolonies that are attached to the tooth surface at a narrow base. The result is the formation of complex collections of different microbes linked to one another.
     b. Each microcolony is a bustling community of microbes that actively exchanges and shares products that play a pivotal role in providing a favorable living environment for the resident microbes.
        1) Environmental conditions within each microcolony vary radically. The environmental conditions among several microcolonies may include differences in oxygen concentration, pH, and temperature.
        2) The differing environmental conditions within a biofilm mean that the microbial population is very diverse—with each different species preferring a certain environment within the biofilm.
           a) This diversity helps to ensure the survivability of the plaque biofilm in widely varying oral conditions.
           b) If the plaque biofilm had only one microbial species, it would be much more likely that a toxic agent or condition would destroy the biofilm.

2. Internal Organization of Mature Biofilm
   a. **Layers and Layers of Microbes.** The biofilm develops by stacking one microbial species on top of another. A mature dental biofilm does not consist of only one species of microbe, rather it is polymicrobial.
   b. **Fluid Channels**
      1) As the plaque biofilm develops, a series of **fluid channels** are formed that penetrate the extracellular protective matrix.
      2) These fluid channels direct fluids in and around the biofilm bringing nutrients and oxygen to the microbes and carrying waste products away.
      3) The fluids include everything from saliva to any beverages consumed.
   c. **Cell-to-Cell Communication System**
      1) Direct cell-to-cell interaction occurs among the microbes in the biofilm.
      2) The microcolonies use chemical signals to communicate with each other.
      3) This cell-to-cell communication also results in the transfer of genes among microbes.
   d. **Bacterial Signaling**
      1) Bacterial communication occurs when microbes within the biofilm release and sense small proteins (signaling molecules). This type of communication among microbes is termed **quorum sensing**.
      2) Microbes in the biofilm use quorum sensing to trigger events such as adhesion of additional microbes to the biofilm and formation of the extracellular protective matrix.
      3) In quorum sensing, individual bacteria "talk" with other bacteria to share information that is critical for their growth and survivability. In the oral environment, this is especially important since bacteria need to adapt rapidly to any sudden adverse change in environmental conditions, such as a sudden change in oral pH or in oxygen concentration. Continual back-and-forth communication permits microbes to coordinate their behavior collectively in order to adapt to changes in the local environment. This ensures survivability of all microorganisms living within the biofilm.
      4) Quorum sensing is not limited to bacteria from a single species communicating with bacteria from the same species. Rather, bacteria from one species can communicate with those from other species (interspecies communication) through the same process. The capacity for interspecies communication is critical for the growth, coordination, and development of the polymicrobial community residing within the oral biofilm.
      5) Current research in microbiology is investigating mechanisms that could interfere with the quorum sensing system. In other words, if there is a way to block the communication between microorganisms, there may be a means of inhibiting the growth of the biofilm.
E. **Stage 5—Dispersion: Escape From the Matrix**
   1. Dispersal of microbes from the biofilm colony is an essential stage of the biofilm life cycle. Dispersal enables biofilms to spread and colonize new tooth surfaces.

BACTERIAL COLONIZATION AND SUCCESSION OF ORAL BIOFILMS

1. Colonization
   A. Sequence of Bacterial Colonization
      1. Early bacterial colonizers of the tooth surface include many streptococcal species, such as *Streptococcus mitis* and *S. oralis* that can attach to the tooth pellicle, as well as, to each other.[35,36]
      2. The early bacterial colonizers release chemical signals that indicate to the next group of bacteria that conditions are favorable for them to join the biofilm. This best characterizes quorum sensing which is essential in the coordination and regulation of the activities of a polymicrobial biofilm community.
      3. Free-floating microbes cannot join the biofilm until the conditions are favorable. The succession of bacteria joining the biofilm is comparable to elementary school students who are asked to line up in alphabetical order as their teacher calls out their names. Students whose last names start with the letter "O" cannot get in line until all the students whose last names start with "M and N" have taken their place in line.
      4. A mature plaque biofilm is a very complex collection of multiple microbial species. Figure 13-11 illustrates the complex structure of a mature biofilm.

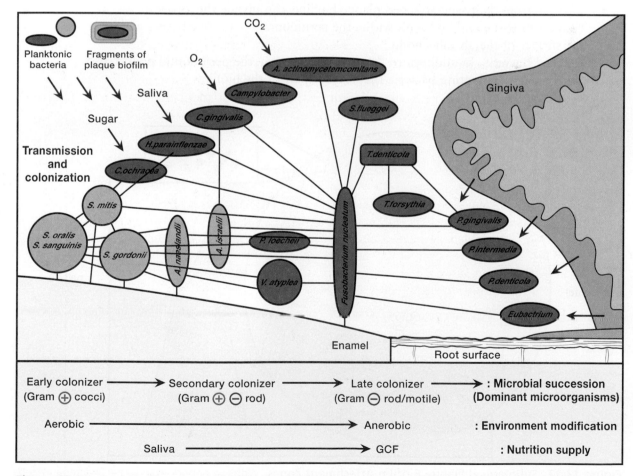

Figure 13-11. Oral Biofilm. An oral biofilm is an organized, structural collective of different, genetically distinct microorganisms adhering to the tooth surface and/or attaching to each other (coaggregation).

BACTERIAL ATTACHMENT ZONES

The zones of *sub*gingival bacterial attachment (Fig. 13-12) are the tooth surface and the epithelial lining of the periodontal pocket. Bacteria also may attach to other bacteria that are attached to one of these surfaces. In addition to the attached bacteria, some bacteria remain free-floating in the gingival sulcus or pocket.

1. Tooth-Associated Plaque Biofilms—bacteria that are attached to the tooth surface.
   A. Bacteria attach to an area of the tooth surface that extends from the gingival margin almost to the junctional epithelium at the base of the pocket.
   B. Subgingival bacteria appear to have the ability to invade the dentinal tubules of the cementum.
   C. Filamentous microorganisms, cocci, and rods—including *S. mitis*, *S. sanguis*, and *Actinomyces viscosus*—dominate the tooth-associated plaque biofilms.
2. Tissue-Associated Plaque Biofilms—bacteria that adhere to the epithelium.
   A. The bacteria that adhere loosely to the epithelium of the pocket wall are distinctly different from those of the tooth-associated plaque biofilms.
   B. The layers closest to the soft tissue wall contain large numbers of spirochetes and flagellated bacteria. Gram-negative cocci and rods also are present. There is a predominance of species such as *S. oralis*, *S. intermedius*, *P. gingivalis*, *Prevotella intermedia*, *Tannerella forsythia*, and *Fusobacterium nucleatum*.
   C. Bacteria from the tissue-attached plaque biofilms can invade the gingival connective tissue and be found within the periodontal connective tissues and on the surface of the alveolar bone.
3. Unattached Bacteria. In addition to the attached bacteria, the periodontal pocket also contains many free-floating bacteria that are not part of the biofilm.

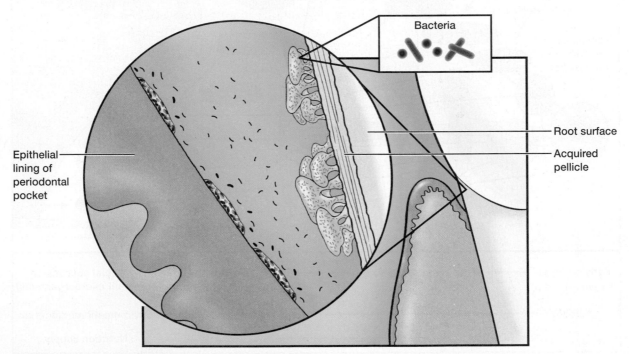

Figure 13-12. Subgingival Plaque Biofilm Attachment Zones. Within a periodontal pocket, bacteria attach to the tooth surface or the epithelial lining of the periodontal pocket.

Section 3
The Role of Bacteria in Periodontal Disease

CHANGING EVIDENCE FOR THE ROLE OF BACTERIA

In 1683, Antonie van Leeuwenhoek used a homemade microscope to first describe oral microorganisms. Since then, over 700 bacterial species have been identified in the human oral cavity. Yet, despite over 330 years of scientific investigation in the field of oral microbiology, microbiologists have yet to identify specific bacterial pathogens that cause periodontitis.[37] Over the years, five different and distinct hypotheses have emerged to explain the role of bacteria in periodontal disease: (1) Nonspecific Plaque Hypothesis, (2) Specific Plaque Hypothesis, (3) Ecological Plaque Hypothesis, (4) Microbial Homeostasis–Host Response Hypothesis, and (5) Keystone Pathogen–Host Response Hypothesis.

HISTORICAL PERSPECTIVES ON THE ROLE OF BACTERIA

Two hypotheses from the recent past focused on the role of the numbers of bacteria and the specific bacteria present in oral biofilms. The Nonspecific Plaque Hypothesis postulated that the accumulation of bacterial biofilms leads to periodontal disease. A later theory, the Specific Plaque Hypothesis postulated that specific pathogenic bacteria and their products in the biofilm lead to periodontal disease. Although these hypotheses are now considered to be too simplistic, these hypotheses served as important stepping stones to our current understanding of the role of bacteria in the development of periodontal disease.

1. Historical Perspective: Nonspecific Plaque Hypothesis
    A. **Hypothesis.** This theory proposed that the accumulation of plaque biofilm—an abundance of bacteria in the biofilm—adjacent to the gingival margin led to gingival inflammation and the subsequent tissue destruction seen in periodontitis.[37–39]
    B. **Problems With the Nonspecific Plaque Hypothesis**
        1. There is now a consensus among researchers that this hypothesis is too simplistic.[19]
        2. A serious criticism of this hypothesis is that it fails to explain why most cases of gingivitis never progress to periodontitis. Some individuals with heavy amounts of plaque biofilm fail to develop periodontitis. Yet, puzzlingly other individuals with very light amounts of biofilm suffer from aggressive forms of periodontitis.[40]
        3. This hypothesis cannot clarify why some sites in an individual's periodontium experience considerable periodontal destruction while other sites are unaffected.
2. Historical Perspective: Specific Plaque/Microbial Shift Hypothesis
    A. **Hypothesis.** This long-standing paradigm suggests that as periodontitis develops, the oral microbiota shifts from one consisting primarily of beneficial microbes to one consisting of pathogens.[38,39,41] In the Specific Plaque Hypothesis, the microbial composition of the oral biofilm—rather than the amount—is the deciding factor in the development of periodontal disease.
        1. An increase in the number of specific pathogens was thought to be associated with periodontitis.
        2. This model postulates that a microbial shift occurs in which the bacteria in the biofilm change from a predominantly gram-positive aerobic community to one consisting mainly of groups of gram-negative anaerobes.[41]

B. **Socransky's Microbial Complexes.** Research efforts, over many years, focused on the hypothesis that specific microorganisms are the cause of various periodontal diseases and conditions.

1. These studies identified specific groups of bacteria—*T. forsythia*, *P. gingivalis*, and *Treponema denticola*—that were significantly associated with periodontitis. It was noted that these bacteria were interdependent and often could not exist without the presence of the others.[42,43]

2. Using advanced checkerboard DNA-DNA hybridization techniques, Socransky grouped microorganisms into "complexes" and assigned each complex a color.[43] Figure 13-13 depicts Socransky's color designations for microbial groups.

   a. Microorganisms assigned to the orange and red complexes are the species that were thought to be the major etiologic agents of periodontal disease.

   b. Microbes designated as the yellow, green, blue, and purple complexes were thought to be compatible with gingival health.

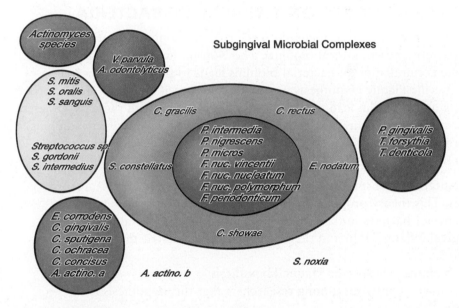

Figure 13-13. Socransky's Microbial Complexes. Socransky organized bacteria into complexes and assigned each complex a color. (Data from Socransky SS, Haffajee AD, Cugini MA, Smith C, Kent RL, Jr. Microbial complexes in subgingival plaque. *J Clin Periodontol.* 1998;25(2):134–144.)

3. The theory that microbes could be divided into nonpathogenic and pathogenic groups had a great deal of appeal. ***The theory was widely accepted until newer molecular-based approaches to microbe detection brought its validity into question.***

C. **Problems With the Specific Plaque Hypothesis.** The appeal of the Specific Plaque Hypothesis resides in its fundamental concept that a single group of select pathogens (red complex microorganisms) are the major cause in the tissue destruction seen in periodontitis. However, as noted above, the Specific Plaque Hypothesis has several weaknesses:

1. It is established that red complex organisms can be found in the absence of periodontal disease.[44,45] The fact that *P. gingivalis* and *T. forsythia* frequently are found in healthy periodontal sites brings into question whether these bacteria are the direct cause of periodontal breakdown.[46–48]

2. The periodontal microbe population is more heterogeneous and diverse than previously thought.[49–51] Over 700 organisms are recognized as possible oral inhabitants, of which around 200 can be present in any one individual.[1] Many of these newly recognized organisms show good or better correlation with periodontal disease than the classical red complex microorganisms.[46,52,53] The identification of so many more bacterial species in the oral cavity makes the concept of specific bacteria causing periodontitis even more unlikely.[12]

3. *Contrary to the doctrine that gram-negative bacteria dominate disease sites in periodontitis, numbers of gram-positive anaerobic bacteria species are shown to exhibit a significant increase in deep periodontal pockets relative to healthy sites and can be detected in greater numbers than gram-negative species in some studies.*[53]

4. It is evident that the concept of a three-species red complex as a primary causative factor in periodontitis requires refinement.[54]

CONTEMPORARY PERSPECTIVES ON THE ROLE OF BACTERIA

Rapid advances in the fields of microbiology and immunology have reshaped our previous notions about the role of bacteria in the pathogenesis of periodontal disease. *We now recognize that (1) a pathogenic microbial biofilm is a prerequisite for periodontitis to develop, but the presence of a pathogenic oral biofilm alone is insufficient to cause the disease, and (2) while red complex microorganisms are strongly associated with an inflammatory disease, there is no current evidence to support the argument that the red complex bacteria are potent initiators of the disease.* As such, three relatively recent hypotheses have been proposed to reconcile the limitations of the Nonspecific Plaque Hypothesis and the Specific Plaque Hypothesis. These theories are the (1) Ecological Plaque Hypothesis, (2) Microbial Homeostasis–Host Response Hypothesis, and (3) Keystone Pathogen–Host Response Hypothesis.

1. Current Perspective #1: Ecological Plaque Hypothesis

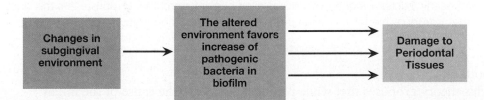

Figure 13-14. Ecological Plaque Hypothesis. This theory postulates that it is a shift in the local environment that drives the changes in microbial composition that lead to periodontal disease.

A. Hypothesis. This theory combines the key points from the Specific Plaque Hypothesis and the Nonspecific Plaque Hypothesis.[41]

1. The Ecological Plaque Hypothesis postulates that the accumulation of nonspecific bacteria triggers the host inflammatory response. In turn, the host inflammatory response alters the local environment within the gingival sulcus (higher GCF flow, increased bleeding, raised pH, decreased oxygen concentration). Figure 13-14 depicts the events postulated by the Ecological Plaque Hypothesis.

2. As the local environment changes, the environment, itself, becomes more conducive to the growth of specific pathogenic bacteria which leads to further changes in the environment, greater tissue destruction, and a growing predominance of specific periodontal pathogens.

3. Homeostasis is dependent on a balanced local environment. If there is a disruption in ecological homeostasis, it will change the environment that is favorable for specific microorganisms (Fig. 13-14). *Thus, according to this hypothesis, it is a shift in the local environment that drives the changes in microbial composition which result in pathologic disease, and not vice versa.*[55]

B. Support for This Hypothesis
   1. Sites with bleeding upon probing and deeper probing depths are strongly associated with a higher gingival crevicular flow (GCF flow). In turn, the higher GCF flow alters the microbial ecology by favoring the growth of pathogenic microorganisms. This suggests that environmental factors—such as GCF flow, pH, temperature, oxygen tension—are forces that drive dysbiosis in the oral cavity.[15]

   2. Subgingival periodontal instrumentation alters the subgingival ecosystem. This, in turn, reduces the number of pathogens. By reducing the inflammatory status of the gingiva, it is suggested that the flow of gingival crevicular fluid decreases, thereby blocking a rich source of nutrients that is necessary for the growth of pathogenic bacteria.[56,57]

2. **Current Perspective #2: Microbial Homeostasis–Host Response Hypothesis**

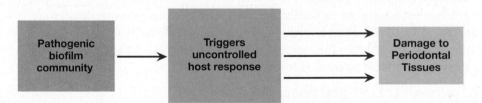

Figure 13-15. Microbial Homeostasis–Host Response Hypothesis. This theory postulates that a shift from beneficial to pathogenic bacteria triggers an uncontrolled host inflammatory response. It is this uncontrolled host response that is responsible for the tissue destruction seen in periodontitis.

A. Hypothesis
   1. This theory proposes that while plaque biofilms are the cause of the initial inflammatory response leading to gingivitis, the pathogenic bacteria are not the direct cause of the destruction of tissues seen in periodontitis.[58] Figure 13-15 depicts the events postulated by the microbial homeostasis–host response hypothesis.

   2. The findings that bacteria are not the direct cause of tissue destruction led researchers to focus on the individual host and the complexities of the immune response rather than the bacteria.

   3. *Host-related factors, such as genetic variations and the inflammatory immune response, and environmental factors, including smoking, stress, and systemic health, are all now recognized as major factors that contribute to the initiation and progression of periodontal disease.*[59]
      a. Evidence for the role of host response in periodontal destruction first emerged in the landmark paper by Page and Schroeder.[60] Host immune response is discussed in detail in Chapters 14 and 15.

    b. *Page and Schroeder noted that established gingivitis would not progress to periodontitis unless some other unknown factor tipped the delicate biofilm-host balance toward further tissue destruction.*

    c. Thus, it is proposed that the shift from beneficial microbes to a pathogenic community triggers a potent host inflammatory response which contributes to the tissue destruction and alveolar bone loss characteristic of periodontitis.[61]

B. Support for This Hypothesis

1. The biofilm microbe population associated with *periodontal health* appears to remain stable over time and exists in a state of biologic equilibrium or homeostasis.

2. While researchers have identified 6 to 17 *potential periodontal pathogens*,[62] decades of research have failed to provide evidence that bacterial pathogens are directly and solely responsible for the tissue destruction seen in periodontitis.

3. *Overwhelming evidence demonstrates that it is the uncontrolled host inflammatory and immune response—rather than pathogenic bacteria—that cause the tissue destruction seen in periodontitis.*[63] (The shift to a pathogenic biofilm community triggers the host response; the host response causes the tissue destruction.)

3. Current Perspective #3: Keystone Pathogen–Host Response Hypothesis

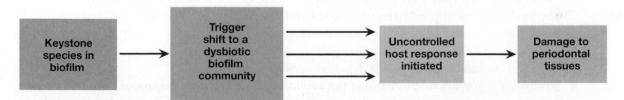

Figure 13-16. Keystone Pathogen Hypothesis. The presence of certain microbial pathogens—even in low numbers—can cause a shift from beneficial to pathogenic microbes in the biofilm community. The key concept of this theory is that even at low levels, keystone pathogens can have a significant impact on the oral biofilm that initiates an uncontrolled host immune response.

A. Hypothesis. This hypothesis builds upon the Microbial Homeostasis–Host Response Hypothesis. As stated above, the microbial homeostasis–host response hypothesis theorizes that a shift from beneficial to pathogenic microbes triggers the host response responsible for the tissue destruction seen in periodontitis. The Keystone Pathogen Hypothesis postulates that a *specific bacterial species* is the key in creating the shift from symbiotic microbes to dysbiotic microbes in the biofilm community. In turn, the dysbiotic biofilm community triggers the uncontrolled host response that results in damage to the periodontal tissues.[54] Figure 13-16 depicts the events postulated by the Keystone Pathogen Hypothesis.

1. According to Hajishengallis et al.,[54] *P. gingivalis* is the "keystone species" in initiating this change in the biofilm community. Keystone species is an ecological term to describe a species that has a disproportionately large effect on its community relative to its abundance. In other words, *although present in small numbers*, a keystone species can exert a profound effect on the plaque biofilm.

2. Thus, this hypothesis postulates that a keystone species—*P. gingivalis*—initiates a shift from beneficial to pathogenic microbes in the biofilm community that in turn, triggers the host inflammatory response responsible for the tissue destruction seen in periodontitis. In other words, the transition to periodontitis requires both a polymicrobial dysbiotic biofilm community and a susceptible host.

B. **Support for This Hypothesis**
1. Decades of research have failed to provide evidence that specific bacterial pathogens are the direct cause of the tissue destruction seen in periodontitis.
2. Current evidence indicates that *the uncontrolled host inflammatory and immune responses cause the tissue destruction seen in periodontitis.*[63]

C. **Summation of Periodontal Disease Hypotheses.** Currently, each hypothesis falls short in fully unraveling the mechanisms that govern the change from periodontal health to disease. Nevertheless, current periodontal microbiology research is continuing to further investigate the diverse, polymicrobial ecosystem of the oral biofilm, and the factors that drive the host inflammatory response. Table 13-2 summarizes the evolution of periodontal disease hypotheses.

1. Despite the difficulty in defining the precise etiology of periodontitis, one thing that is certain is the striking difference in the immune status of periodontal tissue between healthy and diseased patients. Details of the many immunological differences were recently discussed in a review by Darveau.[61]
   a. Clinically healthy periodontal tissue maintains a highly ordered, mild state of subclinical inflammation.[61,64,65]
   b. Clinically diseased periodontal tissue exhibits a marked histopathologic change characterized by a disordered state of severe inflammation.[61,66,67]
2. It is proposed that the shift from beneficial microbes to a pathogenic community triggers a potent host inflammatory response which contributes to the tissue destruction and alveolar bone loss characteristic of periodontitis.[61]
3. Regardless of which disease hypothesis one subscribes to, one must fully appreciate the concept that *plaque biofilm, itself, is necessary, but not sufficient to cause the tissue destruction seen in periodontitis.*
4. Instead, it is *the uncontrolled host inflammatory and immune responses which cause periodontal tissue destruction.*[63]

TABLE 13-2	EVOLUTION OF PERIODONTAL DISEASE THEORIES	
Hypothesis	**Status**	**Theory in Brief**
Nonspecific Plaque	Historical	An *abundance* of biofilm bacteria causes the tissue destruction seen in periodontitis.
Specific Plaque	Historical	The presence of *specific* bacteria in the biofilm directly causes the tissue destruction seen in periodontitis.
Ecological Plaque Hypothesis	Current	*Changes in the subgingival environment* can dictate or select the specific microbial composition of the biofilm; the pathogenic biofilm community causes the tissue destruction seen in periodontitis.
Microbial Homeostasis–Host Response Hypothesis	Current	A shift from beneficial to pathogenic microbes triggers the host inflammatory response; *the host response* causes the tissue destruction seen in periodontitis.
Keystone Pathogen Hypothesis	Current	A *keystone species* initiates a shift from beneficial to dysbiotic microbes in the biofilm community that in turn, trigger the host inflammatory response responsible for the tissue destruction seen in periodontitis.

Chapter Summary Statement

An oral biofilm is a polymicrobial, three-dimensional community of numerous microbial species, embedded in a matrix that consists of microbial metabolic products and/or host components, such as salivary glycoproteins. The protective biofilm matrix makes microbes extremely resistant to systemic antibiotics, antimicrobial agents, and the body's immune system. Mechanical removal is the most effective treatment for the control of dental plaque biofilms.

To date, there is no definitive evidence that specific bacteria are directly responsible for the progression of periodontal disease. *Plaque biofilm, itself, is necessary, but not sufficient to cause the tissue destruction seen in periodontitis. Considerable evidence indicates that it is more likely to be the host inflammatory and immune response to the plaque biofilm that leads to the tissue destruction seen in periodontitis.* It is proposed that a shift from beneficial microbes to a dysbiotic biofilm community triggers a potent host inflammatory response which leads to the tissue destruction and alveolar bone loss characteristic of periodontitis.

In addition, it should be noted that there is emerging evidence indicating that genetics, stress, smoking, diet, and general health play a major role in modulating the host response. These additional factors become more important to take into consideration as newer treatment regimens emerge which are more geared toward controlling and redirecting the host-mediated inflammatory response, rather than the mechanical disruption of the plaque biofilm alone.

Section 4
Focus on Patients

Clinical Patient Care

CASE 1

You have just completed periodontal instrumentation of a tooth surface. Describe the sequence of plaque biofilm formation that will occur on the tooth over the next few days if the patient does absolutely no further self-care of the tooth surface.

CASE 2

Imagine that you are holding an "interview" with the bacteria living in an oral biofilm. How might the bacteria respond to your question about advantages of living in a biofilm?

Evidence in Action

Mr. Smirnov is a new patient. His employer just began to offer dental insurance and so Mr. Smirnov decided to take advantage of his dental insurance after not seeking dental care for 10 years.

A thorough periodontal assessment shows that Mr. Smirnov has generalized Stage II, Grade B periodontitis. The dental team explains the findings and treatment options to him. Mr. Smirnov asks *"Why can't I just take something to kill off all the bacteria in my mouth once and for all rather than me going to all the bother to remove them every single day from my teeth?"*. How would you respond to Mr. Smirnov?

References

1. Aas JA, Paster BJ, Stokes LN, Olsen I, Dewhirst FE. Defining the normal bacterial flora of the oral cavity. *J Clin Microbiol.* 2005;43(11):5721–5732.

2. Jenkinson HF, Lamont RJ. Oral microbial communities in sickness and in health. *Trends Microbiol.* 2005;13(12):589–595.

3. Manson JM, Rauch M, Gilmore MS. The commensal microbiology of the gastrointestinal tract. *Adv Exp Med Biol.* 2008;635:15–28.

4. Paster BJ, Olsen I, Aas JA, Dewhirst FE. The breadth of bacterial diversity in the human periodontal pocket and other oral sites. *Periodontol 2000.* 2006;42:80–87.

5. Wade WG. The oral microbiome in health and disease. *Pharmacol Res.* 2013;69(1):137–143.

6. Brogden KA. Polymicrobial diseases of animals and humans. In: Brogden KA, Guthmiller JM, eds. *Polymicrobial Diseases.* Washington, DC: ASM Press; 2002.

7. Bester E, Kroukamp O, Wolfaardt GM, Boonzaaier L, Liss SN. Metabolic differentiation in biofilms as indicated by carbon dioxide production rates. *Appl Environ Microbiol.* 2010;76(4):1189–1197.

8. Costerton JW. The etiology and persistence of cryptic bacterial infections: a hypothesis. *Rev Infect Dis.* 1984;6 Suppl 3:S608–S616.

9. Flemming HC, Neu TR, Wozniak DJ. The EPS matrix: the "house of biofilm cells". *J Bacteriol.* 2007;189(22):7945–7947.

10. Gulot E, Georges P, Brun A, Fontaine-Aupart MP, Bellon-Fontaine MN, Briandet R. Heterogeneity of diffusion inside microbial biofilms determined by fluorescence correlation spectroscopy under two-photon excitation. *Photochem Photobiol.* 2002;75(6):570–578.

11. Hall-Stoodley L, Stoodley P. Evolving concepts in biofilm infections. *Cell Microbiol.* 2009;11(7):1034–1043.

12. Avila M, Ojcius DM, Yilmaz O. The oral microbiota: living with a permanent guest. *DNA Cell Biol.* 2009;28(8):405–411.

13. Conley J, Olson ME, Cook LS, Ceri H, Phan V, Davies HD. Biofilm formation by group a streptococci: is there a relationship with treatment failure?. *J Clin Microbiol.* 2003;41(9):4043–4048.

14. Olson ME, Ceri H, Morck DW, Buret AG, Read RR. Biofilm bacteria: formation and comparative susceptibility to antibiotics. *Can J Vet Res.* 2002;66(2):86–92.

15. Teles R, Teles F, Frias-Lopez J, Paster B, Haffajee A. Lessons learned and unlearned in periodontal microbiology. *Periodontol 2000.* 2013;62(1):95–162.

16. Mazmanian SK, Liu CH, Tzianabos AO, Kasper DL. An immunomodulatory molecule of symbiotic bacteria directs maturation of the host immune system. *Cell.* 2005;122(1):107–118.

17. Mandar R, Mikelsaar M. Transmission of mother's microflora to the newborn at birth. *Biol Neonate.* 1996;69(1):30–35.

18. Roberts FA, Darveau RP. Microbial protection and virulence in periodontal tissue as a function of polymicrobial communities: symbiosis and dysbiosis. *Periodontol 2000.* 2015;69(1):18–27.

19. Meyle J, Chapple I. Molecular aspects of the pathogenesis of periodontitis. *Periodontol 2000.* 2015;69(1):7–17.

20. Kouidhi B, Al Qurashi YM, Chaieb K. Drug resistance of bacterial dental biofilm and the potential use of natural compounds as alternative for prevention and treatment. *Microb Pathog.* 2015;80:39–49.

21. Elder MJ, Stapleton F, Evans E, Dart JK. Biofilm-related infections in ophthalmology. *Eye (Lond).* 1995;9(Pt 1):102–109.

22. Costerton JW, Lewandowski Z, Caldwell DE, Korber DR, Lappin-Scott HM. Microbial biofilms. *Annu Rev Microbiol.* 1995;49:711–745.

23. da Silva Bastos Vde A, Freitas-Fernandes LB, Fidalgo TK, et al. Mother-to-child transmission of Streptococcus mutans: a systematic review and meta-analysis. *J Dent.* 2015;43(2):181–191.

24. Alaluusua S, Saarela M, Jousimies-Somer H, Asikainen S. Ribotyping shows intrafamilial similarity in Actinobacillus actinomycetemcomitans isolates. *Oral Microbiol Immunol.* 1993;8(4):225–229.

25. DiRienzo JM, Slots J. Genetic approach to the study of epidemiology and pathogenesis of Actinobacillus actinomycetemcomitans in localized juvenile periodontitis. *Arch Oral Biol.* 1990;35 Suppl:79S–84S.

26. Petit MD, van Steenbergen TJ, Scholte LM, van der Velden U, de Graaff J. Epidemiology and transmission of Porphyromonas gingivalis and Actinobacillus actinomycetemcomitans among children and their family members. A report of 4 surveys. *J Clin Periodontol.* 1993;20(9):641–650.

27. Slots J, Feik D, Rams TE. Actinobacillus actinomycetemcomitans and Bacteroides intermedius in human periodontitis: age relationship and mutual association. *J Clin Periodontol.* 1990;17(9):659–662.

28. Petit MD, van Steenbergen TJ, Timmerman MF, de Graaff J, van der Velden U. Prevalence of periodontitis and suspected periodontal pathogens in families of adult periodontitis patients. *J Clin Periodontol.* 1994;21(2):76–85.

29. Petit MD, van Winkelhoff AJ, van Steenbergen TJ, de Graaff J. Porphyromonas endodontalis: prevalence and distribution of restriction enzyme patterns in families. *Oral Microbiol Immunol.* 1993;8(4):219–224.

30. Berezow AB, Darveau RP. Microbial shift and periodontitis. *Periodontol 2000.* 2011;55(1):36–47.

31. Kostakioti M, Hadjifrangiskou M, Hultgren SJ. Bacterial biofilms: development, dispersal, and therapeutic strategies in the dawn of the postantibiotic era. *Cold Spring Harb Perspect Med.* 2013;3(4):a010306.

32. Peters BM, Jabra-Rizk MA, O'May GA, Costerton JW, Shirtliff ME. Polymicrobial interactions: impact on pathogenesis and human disease. *Clin Microbiol Rev.* 2012;25(1):193–213.

33. Willems HM, Xu Z, Peters BM. Polymicrobial biofilm studies: from basic science to biofilm control. *Curr Oral Health Rep.* 2016;3(1):36–44.

34. Rickard AH, Gilbert P, High NJ, Kolenbrander PE, Handley PS. Bacterial coaggregation: an integral process in the development of multi-species biofilms. *Trends Microbiol.* 2003;11(2):94–100.

35. Bradshaw DJ, Marsh PD, Watson GK, Allison C. Role of Fusobacterium nucleatum and coaggregation in anaerobe survival in planktonic and biofilm oral microbial communities during aeration. *Infect Immun.* 1998;66(10):4729–4732.

36. Li J, Helmerhorst EJ, Leone CW, et al. Identification of early microbial colonizers in human dental biofilm. *J Appl Microbiol.* 2004;97(6):1311–1318.

37. Loe H, Theilade E, Jensen SB. Experimental gingivitis in man. *J Periodontol.* 1965;36:177–187.

38. Loesche WJ. Chemotherapy of dental plaque infections. *Oral Sci Rev.* 1976;9:65–107.

39. Theilade E. The non-specific theory in microbial etiology of inflammatory periodontal diseases. *J Clin Periodontol.* 1986;13(10):905–911.

40. Socransky SS, Haffajee AD. Evidence of bacterial etiology: a historical perspective. *Periodontol 2000.* 1994;5:7–25.

41. Marsh PD. Microbial ecology of dental plaque and its significance in health and disease. *Adv Dent Res.* 1994;8(2):263–271.

42. Socransky SS, Haffajee AD. Dental biofilms: difficult therapeutic targets. *Periodontol 2000*. 2002;28:12–55.

43. Socransky SS, Haffajee AD, Cugini MA, Smith C, Kent RL, Jr. Microbial complexes in subgingival plaque. *J Clin Periodontol*. 1998;25(2):134–144.

44. Mayanagi G, Sato T, Shimauchi H, Takahashi N. Detection frequency of periodontitis-associated bacteria by polymerase chain reaction in subgingival and supragingival plaque of periodontitis and healthy subjects. *Oral Microbiol Immunol*. 2004;19(6):379–385.

45. Ximenez-Fyvie LA, Haffajee AD, Socransky SS. Comparison of the microbiota of supra- and subgingival plaque in health and periodontitis. *J Clin Periodontol*. 2000;27(9):648–657.

46. Kumar PS, Leys EJ, Bryk JM, Martinez FJ, Moeschberger ML, Griffen AL. Changes in periodontal health status are associated with bacterial community shifts as assessed by quantitative 16S cloning and sequencing. *J Clin Microbiol*. 2006;44(10): 3665–3673.

47. Papapanou PN. Population studies of microbial ecology in periodontal health and disease. *Ann Periodontol*. 2002;7(1):54–61.

48. Riep B, Edesi-Neuss L, Claessen F, et al. Are putative periodontal pathogens reliable diagnostic markers? *J Clin Microbiol*. 2009;47(6):1705–1711.

49. Curtis MA, Zenobia C, Darveau RP. The relationship of the oral microbiota to periodontal health and disease. *Cell Host Microbe*. 2011;10(4):302–306.

50. Dewhirst FE, Chen T, Izard J, et al. The human oral microbiome. *J Bacteriol*. 2010;192(19):5002–5017.

51. Griffen AL, Beall CJ, Firestone ND, et al. CORE: a phylogenetically-curated 16S rDNA database of the core oral microbiome. *PLoS One*. 2011;6(4):e19051.

52. Griffen AL, Beall CJ, Campbell JH, et al. Distinct and complex bacterial profiles in human periodontitis and health revealed by 16S pyrosequencing. *ISME J*. 2012;6(6):1176–1185.

53. Kumar PS, Griffen AL, Moeschberger ML, Leys EJ. Identification of candidate periodontal pathogens and beneficial species by quantitative 16S clonal analysis. *J Clin Microbiol*. 2005;43(8):3944–3955.

54. Hajishengallis G, Lamont RJ. Beyond the red complex and into more complexity: the polymicrobial synergy and dysbiosis (PSD) model of periodontal disease etiology. *Mol Oral Microbiol*. 2012;27(6):409–419.

55. Bartold PM, Van Dyke TE. Periodontitis: a host-mediated disruption of microbial homeostasis. Unlearning learned concepts. *Periodontol 2000*. 2013;62(1):203–217.

56. Socransky SS, Haffajee AD, Smith C, et al. Use of checkerboard DNA-DNA hybridization to study complex microbial ecosystems. *Oral Microbiol Immunol*. 2004;19(6):352–362.

57. Teles FR, Teles RP, Sachdeo A, et al. Comparison of microbial changes in early redeveloping biofilms on natural teeth and dentures. *J Periodontol*. 2012;83(9):1139–1148.

58. Page RC, Kornman KS. The pathogenesis of human periodontitis: an introduction. *Periodontol 2000*. 1997;14:9–11.

59. Hasturk H, Kantarci A. Activation and resolution of periodontal inflammation and its systemic impact. *Periodontol 2000*. 2015;69(1):255–273.

60. Page RC, Schroeder HE. Pathogenesis of inflammatory periodontal disease. A summary of current work. *Lab Invest*. 1976;34(3):235–249.

61. Darveau RP. The oral microbial consortium's interaction with the periodontal innate defense system. *DNA Cell Biol*. 2009;28(8):389–395.

62. Perez-Chaparro PJ, Goncalves C, Figueiredo LC, et al. Newly identified pathogens associated with periodontitis: a systematic review. *J Dent Res*. 2014;93(9):846–858.

63. Page RC, Offenbacher S, Schroeder HE, Seymour GJ, Kornman KS. Advances in the pathogenesis of periodontitis: summary of developments, clinical implications and future directions. *Periodontol 2000*. 1997;14:216–248.

64. Moughal NA, Adonogianaki E, Thornhill MH, Kinane DF. Endothelial cell leukocyte adhesion molecule-1 (ELAM-1) and intercellular adhesion molecule-1 (ICAM-1) expression in gingival tissue during health and experimentally-induced gingivitis. *J Periodontal Res*. 1992;27(6):623–630.

65. Tonetti MS, Imboden MA, Lang NP. Neutrophil migration into the gingival sulcus is associated with transepithelial gradients of interleukin-8 and ICAM-1. *J Periodontol*. 1998;69(10):1139–1147.

66. Ren L, Leung WK, Darveau RP, Jin L. The expression profile of lipopolysaccharide-binding protein, membrane-bound CD14, and toll-like receptors 2 and 4 in chronic periodontitis. *J Periodontol*. 2005;76(11):1950–1959.

67. Tonetti MS, Imboden MA, Gerber L, Lang NP, Laissue J, Mueller C. Localized expression of mRNA for phagocyte-specific chemotactic cytokines in human periodontal infections. *Infect Immun*. 1994;62(9):4005–4014.

 ## STUDENT ANCILLARY RESOURCES

A wide variety of resources to enhance your learning is available online:

- Audio Glossary
- Book Pages
- Chapter Review Questions and Answers

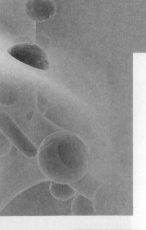

14 Basic Concepts of Immunity and Inflammation

Clinical Application. Periodontal diseases are due, in part, to the body's reaction to a bacterial challenge in the oral cavity. It is critical for health care providers caring for patients with periodontal disease to have a basic understanding of immunity and inflammation. This chapter presents a brief outline of this complex topic that can prove invaluable during further study of periodontal diseases and in understanding the fundamental behavior of these diseases.

Learning Objectives

- Define the term immune system and describe its function.
- Describe the role of polymorphonuclear leukocytes, macrophages, B-lymphocytes, and T-lymphocytes in the immune system.
- Contrast the terms macrophage and monocyte.
- Describe the three ways that antibodies participate in the host defense.
- Define the complement system and explain its principle functions in the immune response.
- Describe the steps in the process of phagocytosis.
- Give an example of a type of injury or infection that would result in inflammation in an individual's arm. Describe and contrast the symptoms of inflammation that the individual would experience due to acute inflammation versus chronic inflammation.
- Define the term inflammatory mediator and give several examples of inflammatory mediators of importance in periodontitis.

Key Terms

Immune system
Host
Host response
Leukocyte
Polymorphonuclear leukocytes (PMNs)
Neutrophil
Chemotaxis

Lysosome
Neutropenia
Macrophage
Monocyte
Lymphocyte
B-lymphocyte
Antibody
Immunoglobulin
T-lymphocyte

Cytokine
Complement system
Membrane attack complex
Opsonization
Endothelium
Transendothelial migration

Phagocytosis
Phagosome
Phagolysosome
Inflammation
Inflammatory biochemical mediator
Chemokines
Acute inflammation

C-reactive protein (CRP)
Homeostasis
Resolution process
Chronic inflammation

Section 1
The Body's Defense System

Humans are surrounded by millions of microorganisms, many of which may prove to be deadly. Our hands, alone, harbor up to two million microorganisms. The only reason that the human body survives is that it has a multi-layered defense system that is remarkably effective in recognizing and fighting disease-causing microorganisms. The immune system is a complex system that is responsible for defending the body against millions of bacteria, viruses, fungi, toxins, and parasites.

INTRODUCTION TO THE IMMUNE SYSTEM

1. Description
    A. A Complex System of Responses
        1. The immune system is a collection of responses that protects the body against infections by bacteria, viruses, fungi, toxins, and parasites.
        2. Bacteria, viruses, and other disease-causing microorganisms attack the human body over 100 million times a day. For this reason, the human immune system attempts to control quickly the spread of invading microorganisms.
        3. The immune system is composed of two major subdivisions—the innate and adaptive immune systems (Table 14-1).[1]
            a. The innate immune system—which humans are born with—is the first line of defense against invading organisms while the adaptive immune system acts as a second line of defense and affords protection against re-exposure to the same pathogen.
            b. The adaptive immune system—which develops throughout life—requires some time to react to an invading organism, whereas the innate immune system includes defenses that, for the most part, are present and ready to be mobilized immediately upon infection.
            c. The adaptive immune system demonstrates immunological memory. It "remembers" that it has encountered an invading organism and reacts more rapidly on subsequent exposure to the same organism. In contrast, the innate immune system does not demonstrate immunological memory.

TABLE 14-1	INNATE AND ADAPTIVE IMMUNITY
Innate Immunity	**Adaptive Immunity**
Present at birth	Develops throughout life
Not antigen-specific (exposure results in no immunologic memory)	Antigen-specific (exposure results in immunologic memory)
Present always (immediate response to infection)	Lag time between infection and response (develops in response to infection)
Does not improve with repeated exposure to an infectious agent	Memory develops which may provide lifelong immunity to reinfection to the same infectious agent

B. **Self versus Nonself.** When the immune system encounters cells or molecules, it must determine whether these are *self* (part of the body) or foreign substances. Molecules might be harmless substances, such as pollen, or constitute part of a microorganism. Microorganisms, in turn, might be innocuous or pathogenic.

2. **Function**
   A. **Prime Purpose**
      1. The prime purpose of the human immune system is to defend the life of the individual (host) by identifying foreign substances in the body (bacteria, viruses, fungi, or parasites) and developing a defense against them (Fig. 14-1).[1,2]
      2. The body recognizes bacteria, viruses, fungi, and parasites as something foreign to itself and *responds by (1) sending certain types of cells to the infection site and (2) producing biochemical substances to counteract the foreign invaders.*
   B. The way that an individual's body responds to an infection is known as the host response.

3. **Consequences of Loss of Immune Function.** Loss of immune function is deadly to the body. An example is the human immunodeficiency virus (HIV), the virus that causes acquired immune deficiency syndrome (AIDS). HIV disables a specific group of immune system cells responsible for coordinating immune responses. People infected with HIV may develop infections from microorganisms that rarely cause infection in individuals with normal, healthy immune systems.

4. **Consequences of an Overzealous Immune Response.** The immune system can sometimes become confused or so intense in its response *that it begins to harm the body that it is trying to protect.* Rheumatic heart disease is an example of a confused immune response to infection. The problem begins as an infection of the skin or pharynx with streptococcal bacteria. Unfortunately, there are similarities between certain molecules of the streptococcal bacteria and molecules of human heart tissue. Because of this molecular similarity, immune responses against the streptococcal bacteria also attack and damage the heart tissue of the infected individual.

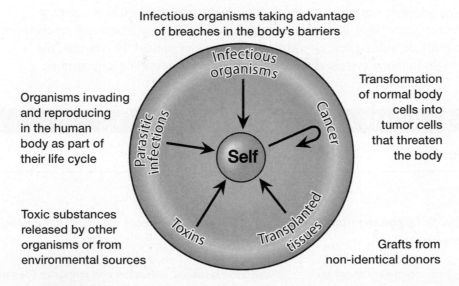

Figure 14-1. The Immune Defense System. The immune system defends the body against invading microorganisms, as well as toxins in the environment. This includes protection against infectious organisms, parasitic infections, toxins, and cancerous cells. Unfortunately, cells of transplanted tissues are recognized as "nonself" or invaders. For this reason, immunosuppressants are needed to keep the body's immune system from rejecting a transplant.

COMPONENTS OF THE IMMUNE SYSTEM

Components of the immune system that play an important role in combating periodontal disease are the (1) cellular defenders (phagocytes, lymphocytes), and (2) complement system (Table 14-2).[1,2]

TABLE 14-2	SUMMARY: COMPONENTS OF THE IMMUNE SYSTEM
Component	**Function**
Polymorphonuclear leukocyte (PMN) 	• Phagocytosis • Release of lysosomes • Release of powerful regulatory proteins (cytokines) that signal the immune system to send additional phagocytic cells to the site of an infection
Macrophage 	• Phagocytosis • Release of lysosomes • Release of powerful regulatory proteins (cytokines) that signal the immune system to send additional phagocytic cells to the site of an infection
B-lymphocyte/ Plasma cell 	• Production of immunoglobulins
T-lymphocytes 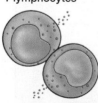	• Further stimulate the immune response
Immunoglobulins IgG, IgM, IgA, IgD, IgE	• Neutralize bacteria or bacterial toxins • Coat bacteria to facilitate phagocytosis • Activate the complement system
Complement System	• Lysis of cell membranes of certain bacteria • Phagocytosis • Recruitment of additional phagocytic cells to the infection site and clearance of immune complexes from circulation

CELLS OF THE IMMUNE SYSTEM

1. **Leukocytes.** Leukocytes are white blood cells that act much like independent single-cell organisms able to move and capture microorganisms on their own (Fig. 14-2).

   A. **Polymorphonuclear Leukocytes.** Polymorphonuclear leukocytes (PMNs) are phagocytes that play a vital role in combating the bacteria in plaque biofilms (Fig. 14-3).

      1. PMNs, also known as neutrophils, are phagocytic cells that actively engulf and destroy microorganisms.
      2. These cells are the *rapid responders*. They provide the first line of defense against many common microorganisms and are essential for the control of bacterial infections.
      3. Once in the blood stream, PMNs can move through capillary walls and into the tissue. PMNs are attracted to bacteria by a process called chemotaxis.
      4. The cytoplasm of a PMN contains many granules filled with strong bactericidal and digestive enzymes. These granules (called lysosomes) can kill and digest bacterial cells after phagocytosis.
      5. PMNs are *short-lived cells* that die when they become engorged with the bacteria they phagocytize. The pus formed at sites of inflammation contains many dead and dying PMNs. PMNs have a short life span, generally less than 1 day.
      6. The bacteria associated with periodontal disease are most effectively phagocytized by PMNs.
      7. Normally, each milliliter of blood contains between 3,000 to 6,000 PMNs. A PMN count of less than 1,000 cells/mL is called neutropenia and indicates an increased risk of infection.

   B. **Monocytes/Macrophages.** Macrophages are large phagocytes with a single kidney-shaped nucleus and some granules (Figs. 14-4 and 14-5).

      1. These leukocytes are called monocytes when found in the bloodstream and macrophages when they are in the tissues.

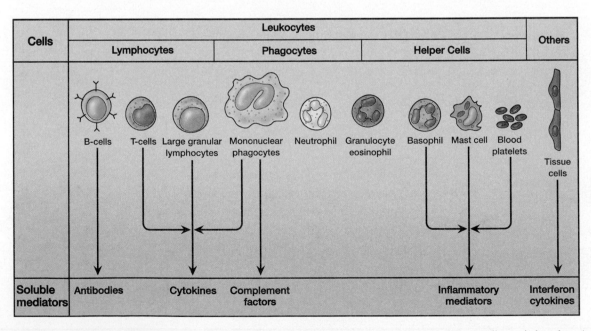

Figure 14-2. Cells and Chemical Mediators of the Immune System. Immune system cells and the chemical mediators are closely related since the cells produce most of the mediators.

2. Macrophages are highly phagocytic cells that actively engulf and destroy microorganisms. Macrophages contain a few lysosomes that are filled with bactericidal and digestive enzymes.
3. Macrophages are slower to arrive at the infection site than PMNs. The slower, long-lived macrophages are often the most numerous cells in chronic inflammation.
4. Macrophages present antigen to T-cells. Together, macrophages and T-lymphocytes play an important role in chronic inflammation.

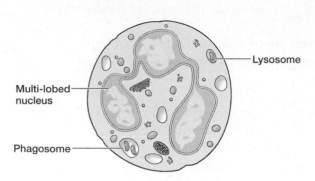

Figure 14-3. Morphology of a Polymorphonuclear Leukocyte. PMNs contain granules called lysosomes that are used to digest bacteria.

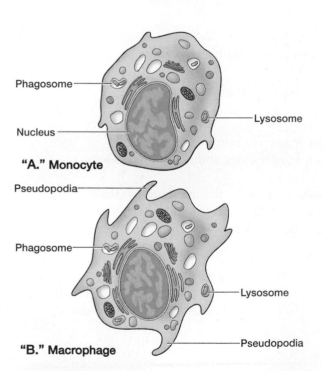

Figure 14-4. Morphology of a Monocyte and a Macrophage. These phagocytic leukocytes are called monocytes **(A)** when found in the bloodstream and macrophages **(B)** when they are in the tissues. Of the immune cells, macrophages are the largest—thus, the name "macro." Macrophages are five- to tenfold larger than monocytes and contain more lysosomes.

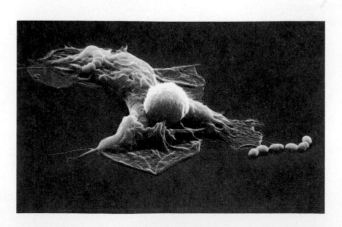

Figure 14-5. SEM of Macrophage. A scanning electron micrograph (SEM) of a human macrophage (*gray*) approaches a chain of *Streptococcus pyogenes* (*orange*). Riding atop, the macrophage is a spherical lymphocyte. Both macrophages and lymphocytes are important in eliminating infection. (SEM courtesy of Cells Alive.)

2. **Lymphocytes.** Lymphocytes are small white blood cells that play an important role in recognizing and controlling foreign invaders. The two main types of lymphocytes that are important in defense against the bacteria in plaque biofilm are B-lymphocytes (B-cells) and T-lymphocytes (T-cells).
   A. **B-Lymphocytes**
      1. **Description**
         a. B-lymphocytes are small leukocytes that help in the defense against bacteria, viruses, and fungi.
         b. B-lymphocytes can further differentiate into one of the two types of B-cells: plasma B-cells and memory B-cells.
         c. The principal functions of B-lymphocytes are to **make antibodies**. Once a B-cell has been activated, it manufactures millions of antibodies and releases them into the bloodstream (Fig. 14-6).
      2. **Antibodies**
         a. Antibodies are Y-shaped proteins. One end of the Y binds to the outside of the B-cell. The other end binds to a microorganism and helps to kill it.
         b. Antibodies are known collectively as **immunoglobulins**. The five major classes of immunoglobulin are immunoglobulin M (IgM), immunoglobulin D (IgD), immunoglobulin G (IgG), immunoglobulin A (IgA), and immunoglobulin E (IgE).
         c. Antibodies participate in host defense in three main ways:
            1. Neutralize bacteria or bacterial toxins to prevent bacteria from destroying host cells.
            2. Coat bacteria making them more susceptible to phagocytosis.
            3. Activate the complement system.
   B. **T-Lymphocytes**
      1. T-lymphocytes are small leukocytes whose main function is to intensify the response of other immune cells—such as B-lymphocytes and macrophages—to the bacterial invasion.
      2. T-cells can produce substances called cytokines, such as the interleukins (ILs), that further stimulate the immune response. Cytokine is a general name for any protein that is secreted by cells and affects the behavior of nearby cells.

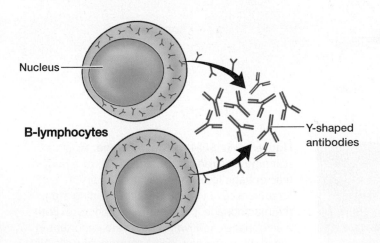

Figure 14-6. B-Lymphocytes. Diagram of a B-cell showing the Y-shaped antibody protein attached to the cell wall.

Nucleus

B-lymphocytes

Y-shaped antibodies

THE COMPLEMENT SYSTEM

In addition to the cellular defenders, the other major component of the immune response is the Complement System. The cellular defenders only respond after they encounter a microorganism. Pathogens, however, can avoid contact with the immune cells. If this happens, the complement system provides a second layer of defense.

1. **Definition.** The Complement System is a complex series of proteins circulating in the blood that works to facilitate phagocytosis or kill bacteria directly by puncturing bacterial cell membranes. The complement proteins are activated by and work with (complement) the antibodies, hence the name.

2. **Three Principal Functions of Complement.** After activation, the complement proteins interact, in a highly-regulated cascade, to carry out several defensive functions (Fig. 14-7):

   A. **Destruction of Pathogens.** Components of complement can destroy certain microorganisms directly by forming pores in their cell membranes. To accomplish this task, the complement system creates a protein unit called the membrane attack complex that can puncture the cell membranes of certain bacteria (lysis).

   B. **Opsonization of Pathogens.** The complement system facilitates the engulfment and destruction of microorganisms by phagocytes. This process, known as opsonization of pathogens, is the most important action of the complement system. Complement components coat the surface of the bacterium allowing the phagocytes to recognize, engulf, and destroy the bacterium.

   C. **Recruitment of Phagocytes.** The complement system recruits additional phagocytic cells to the site of the infection.

   D. **Immune Clearance.** Finally, the complement system performs a "housekeeping" function, the removal of immune complexes from circulation.

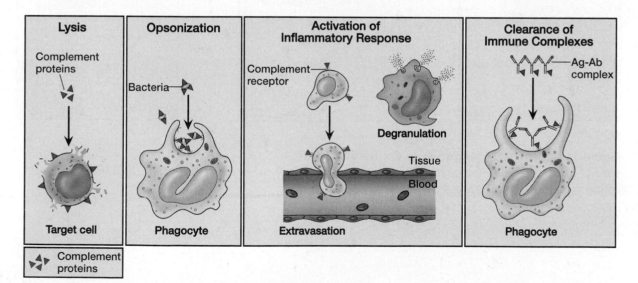

Figure 14-7. Activities of the Complement System. In this diagram, complement proteins are represented by small red triangles. Complement proteins facilitate several immune activities: puncturing the cell membranes of certain bacteria (lysis), phagocytosis of bacteria (opsonization), further activation of the inflammatory response by recruitment of additional phagocytic cells to the infection site, and clearance of immune complexes from circulation.

Section 2
Leukocyte Migration, Chemotaxis, and Phagocytosis

1. **Leukocyte Migration from the Blood Vessels**
   A. **Transendothelial Migration**
      1. To fight an infection, the cells of the immune system travel through the bloodstream and into the tissues (Fig. 14-8).
         a. Near the infection site, the immune cells push their way between the endothelial cells lining the blood vessels (extravasation) and enter the connective tissue.[3]
         b. The thin layer of epithelial cells that line the interior surface of the blood vessels is called the endothelium. For this reason, the process of immune cells exiting the vessels and entering the tissues is called transendothelial migration.
      2. Defects in transendothelial migration are associated with severe forms of periodontitis underscoring the importance of this process in the defense against the bacteria found in plaque biofilms.
   B. **Leukocyte Migration to the Infection Site**
      1. Once the leukocytes enter the connective tissue, the cells must migrate to the site of the infection.
      2. Chemotaxis is the process whereby leukocytes are attracted to the infection site in response to biochemical compounds released by the invading microorganisms.

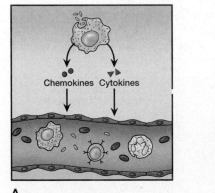
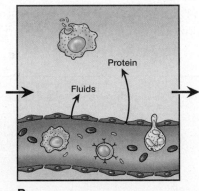
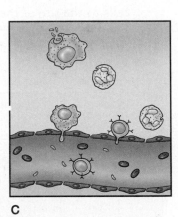

A   B   C

Figure 14-8. Leukocyte Migration to Connective Tissue. A. Leukocytes travel through the blood stream to the site of infection. **B.** Leukocytes squeeze between the cells of the blood vessel wall. **C.** Leukocytes enter the connective tissue and are attracted to the invading bacteria.

2. Phagocytosis
   A. **Description.** Phagocytosis is the process by which leukocytes engulf and digest microorganisms.[4]
   1. **Steps in Phagocytosis**
      a. First, the external cell wall of a phagocytic cell (such as a neutrophil or macrophage) adheres to the bacterium (Fig. 14-9). The phagocytic cell extends finger-like projections (pseudopodia) that surround the bacterium.
      b. Next, a phagocytic vesicle called a phagosome surrounds the ingested bacterium.
      c. Lysosome granules fuse with the vesicle to form a phagolysosome.
      d. The bacterium is digested within the phagolysosome.
      e. Finally, the phagocytic cell discharges the contents of the phagolysosome into the surrounding tissue.
   2. **Local Tissue Destruction from Phagocytosis**
      a. Lysosomal enzymes and other microbial products are released from a leukocyte after phagocytosis or when the leukocyte dies.
      b. Once released, the lysosomal enzymes cause damage to tissue cells in the same manner that they destroy bacteria.

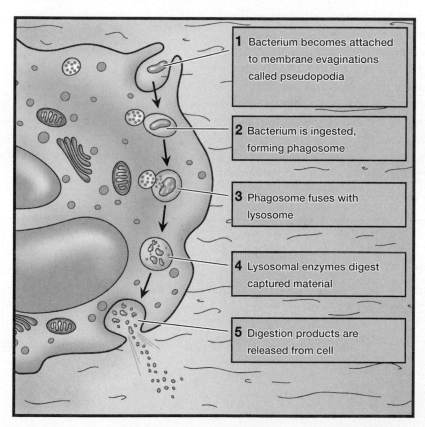

Figure 14-9. Phagocytosis. The steps involved in phagocytosis, the process by which leukocytes engulf and digest microorganisms.

Section 3
The Inflammatory Process

Inflammation is the body's protective response to pathogens, foreign bodies, or an injury. The inflammatory response concentrates host defense components at the site of an infection or injury to eliminate microorganisms and heal damaged tissue. Inflammation is characterized by dilation of the blood vessels, enhanced permeability of the blood capillaries, increased blood flow and leukocyte movement into tissues.[1,2,5]

MAJOR EVENTS IN THE INFLAMMATORY RESPONSE

1. The inflammatory response is triggered by the invasion of pathogens or tissue injury.
2. Immediately, mast cells (located in the connective tissues near to blood vessels) release chemicals that dilate the capillaries and increase vascular permeability (Fig. 14-10).
3. Minutes after tissue injury, there is an increase in blood flow to the area. Higher blood volume heats the tissue and causes it to redden. This increased blood flow is needed to deliver immune "cellular defenders" to the site.
4. Within hours, leukocytes pass through the walls of capillaries into the connective tissue. Plasma proteins leak from the capillaries and accumulate in the tissues.
5. The leukocytes phagocytose invading pathogens and release inflammatory mediators that contribute to the inflammatory response.
   A. **Inflammatory biochemical mediators** are biologically active compounds secreted by cells that activate the body's inflammatory response.
   B. Inflammatory mediators of importance in periodontitis are the cytokines, prostaglandins, and matrix metalloproteinases.
      1. Leukocytes secrete cytokines that play a major role in regulating the behavior of immune cells.
      2. **Chemokines**, a major subgroup of cytokines, cause additional immune cells to be attracted to the site of infection or injury.[4]

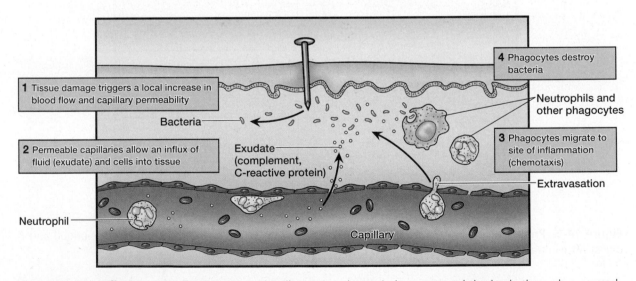

Figure 14-10. Inflammatory Response. In this illustration, bacteria have entered the body through a wound created by a nail puncture. The entry of bacteria initiates an inflammatory response that begins with the release of chemical substances that attract phagocytic cells to the site of the bacterial invasion.

TWO STAGES OF INFLAMMATION

1. Acute Inflammation
   A. Description
      1. Acute inflammation is a short-term, normal process that protects and heals the body following physical injury or infection (Fig. 14-11).
      2. In the absence of inflammation, wounds and infections would never heal and the progressive tissue destruction would threaten the life of the individual.
      3. The acute inflammatory process is achieved by the increased movement of plasma and leukocytes from the blood into the injured tissues.

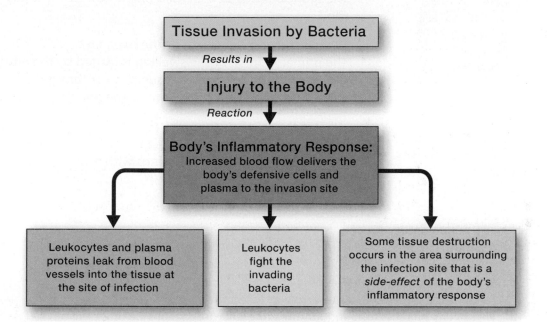

Figure 14-11. Major Events in the Body's Inflammatory Response. Inflammation is the body's response to injury or invasion by disease-producing organisms. This response focuses the body's defense mechanisms at the site of an injury or infection.

   B. **Five Classic Symptoms of Acute Inflammation.** To inflame means "to set on fire," which makes us think of red, heat, and pain. Clinically, there are five classic symptoms of acute inflammation (Box 14-1) at the site of infection or injury:
      1. **Heat**—a localized rise in temperature due to an increased amount of blood at the site.
      2. **Redness**—the result of increased blood in the area.
      3. **Swelling**—the result of the accumulation of fluid at the site. The leukocytes and plasma that collect at the site cause the swelling (edema) associated with inflammation.
      4. **Pain**—the result of pressure from edema in the tissue. The excess fluid in the tissues puts pressure on sensitive nerve endings, causing pain.
      5. **Loss of function**—the result of swelling and pain. For example, inflammation of a finger (swelling and pain) would cause you to favor that finger and not use it in a normal manner.

Box 14-1. Everyday Example of Acute Inflammation

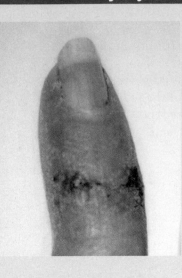

Callie L. sustained a deep cut to her little finger. She applied an antiseptic cream and covered the wound with an adhesive bandage. A few hours later, the injured finger is quite painful. When Callie applies pressure to the area near the wound, it feels warm and the pressure of her touch is quite painful. The finger looks red and swollen.

What is the source of the redness?
The redness is due to increased blood flow at the injury site.

What is the primary source of the swelling?
The primary source of the swelling is caused by the entry of fluid into the connective tissue. Cells entering the connective tissue also contribute to the swelling.

What is the cause of the warmth?
The warmth of an inflamed area results from increased blood flow to the area that brings with it the warmth.

C. **The Acute Inflammatory Process**
1. **Description.** The process of acute inflammation is initiated by the blood vessels near the injured tissue, which alter to allow the release of plasma proteins and leukocytes into the surrounding tissue.
2. PMNs are the first leukocytes to arrive at the injured site.
   a. These cells phagocytose and kill invading microorganisms through the release of nonspecific toxins. These nonspecific toxins kill pathogens as well as adjacent host cells, sick and healthy alike.
   b. The PMNs release cytokines, including IL and tumor necrosis factor (TNF).
   c. Such inflammatory cytokines, in turn, induce the liver to synthesize various plasma proteins called acute phase reactant proteins.
      1) The liver produces C-reactive protein (CRP), a type of acute phase reactant protein, during episodes of acute inflammation. The levels of CRP increase up to 50,000-fold in acute inflammation.
      2) Periodontitis, as well as other systemic diseases—diabetes, hypertension, and cardiovascular disease—are associated with elevated levels of CRP.[6,7]
      3) *A study published in the Journal of Periodontology, reports that the inflammatory effects from periodontal disease cause oral bacterial byproducts to enter the bloodstream and trigger the liver to make CRP that inflames the arteries and promotes blood clot formation.*[8]
3. PMNs are short-lived and so are primarily involved in the early stages of inflammation.
4. If the body succeeds in eliminating all microorganisms, the tissue will heal and the inflammation will cease. The goal at this stage of the inflammatory process is to establish tissue homeostasis (the process of the body's tissue maintaining its optimal state of being). Immune cells leave the area, tissue structures return to normal, and blood flow is reduced with no damage to the tissues. In most

cases of infection within the body, the acute inflammatory process eliminates the disease-producing organisms.

5. Resolution of the acute inflammatory process is a coordinated process. The **resolution process** uses cells to provide "stop signals" that lead to shut down and clearance of immune cells.[9]
   a. Thus, the body attempts to eliminate bacterial invaders and, once this is accomplished, actively shuts down the inflammatory response to limit self-damage to host tissues.
   b. The process of shutting down the inflammatory response prevents tissue injury and progression of acute inflammation into chronic inflammation.

6. Inflammation is the body's first line of defense against injury and infection, but it's a double-edged sword. If the acute inflammatory responses are not effective in eliminating the invading microorganisms or due to a defective/aggravated immune response, the inflammatory response does not shut down and becomes chronic (Fig. 14-12).

7. *Periodontal diseases are characterized by the dysfunction of the resolution pathways that shut down the acute inflammatory process. The result is a failure of the periodontal tissues to heal and a chronic, progressive, and destructive, nonresolving inflammation.*[10,11]

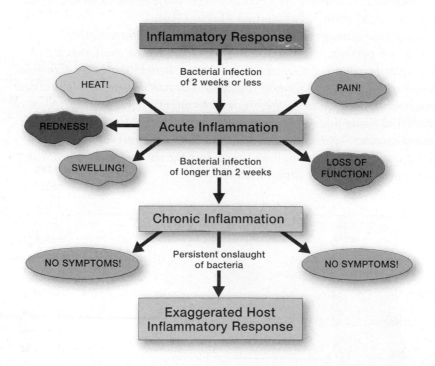

Figure 14-12. Two Stages of Inflammation. Acute inflammation is of short duration, whereas chronic inflammation is a long-lived inflammatory response.

2. **Chronic Inflammation**
   A. **Description**
      1. Chronic inflammation is a long-lived, *out-of-control* inflammatory response that continues for more than a few weeks and results in varying degrees of tissue injury.[12]
         a. It is a pathological condition characterized by active inflammation, host tissue destruction, and attempts at repair.

b. *The warning signs of acute inflammation are absent in chronic inflammation—such as periodontitis—and the problem may go unnoticed by the host (patient). Clinically, pain often is absent.*

2. The inflammatory response has one all-important goal: respond immediately to destroy infectious microorganisms in the damaged tissue before they can spread to other areas of the body.

    a. Chronic inflammation occurs when the body is unable to eliminate the infection. In this stage, the invading microorganisms are persistent and stimulate an exaggerated response by the host's immune system.

    b. *In cases where inflammation becomes chronic, the inflammation can become so intense that it inflicts permanent damage to the body tissues.* This is the case in periodontitis.

B. **The Chronic Inflammatory Process**

1. The accumulation of macrophages characterizes chronic inflammation.

2. Macrophages engulf and digest microorganisms.

3. Leukocytes release several different inflammatory mediators, including IL-1, TNF-α, and prostaglandins that perpetuate the inflammatory response (Fig. 14-13).

    a. One of the principal cytokines secreted by macrophages is TNF-α.[13] Evidence indicates that TNF-α contributes to the tissue destruction that characterizes chronic inflammation (Table 14-3).

    b. In fact, *tissue damage is the hallmark of chronic inflammation.*

4. If the infection persists, inflammation can last months or even years.

5. Chronic inflammation is abnormal and does not benefit the body. *Chronic inflammation is an out-of-control response that can destroy healthy tissue and cause more damage than the original problem.* As with other forms of host-mediated tissue injury—such as asthma, rheumatoid arthritis, diabetes, and atherosclerosis—periodontitis is characterized by unresolved, chronic inflammation that leads to ongoing tissue damage through continuous and recurring episodes of acute inflammation.[10,14]

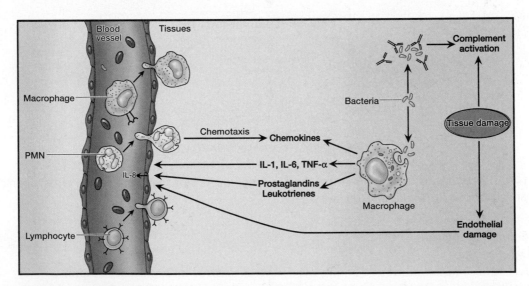

Figure 14-13. Cellular Defenders and Mediators in Inflammatory Response. The three primary cells involved in the inflammatory response are the polymorphonuclear leukocytes (PMNs), macrophages, and lymphocytes. The first of these cells to migrate into the tissues are the PMNs, followed by macrophages, and then the lymphocytes. In addition, this illustration shows some of the many chemical mediators that play a part in the inflammatory response. These include chemokines, IL-1, IL-6, TNF-α, prostaglandins, and leukotrienes.

TABLE 14-3 | INFLAMMATORY BIOCHEMICAL MEDIATORS

Name	Effects
IL-1	Increased vascular permeability T-cell and B-cell activation Fever Synthesis of proteins, such as C-reactive protein, by liver
IL-6	Increased vascular permeability T-cell and B-cell activation Increased immunoglobulin synthesis Fever Synthesis of proteins, such as C-reactive protein, by liver
IL-8	Attraction of PMNs to infection site
Leukotrienes	Allow leukocytes to exit the blood vessel and move into the connective tissue
Prostaglandins	Cause vasodilatation, fever, and pain
TNF-alpha	Increased vascular permeability Chemotaxis T-cell and B-cell activation Fever Synthesis of proteins, such as C-reactive protein, by liver Systemic effects of inflammation such as loss of appetite and increased heart rate

Chapter Summary Statement

The immune system is a collection of responses that is responsible for defending the body against millions of bacteria, viruses, fungi, toxins, and parasites. The prime purpose of the human immune system is to defend the life of the individual (host) by identifying foreign substances and developing a defense against them. The way that an individual's body responds to infection is known as the host response. Without an effective immune system, human beings would not survive.

Components of the immune system that play an important role in combating periodontal disease are the cellular defenders and the complement system. To fight an infection, immune cells travel through the blood stream and into the tissues (transendothelial migration). The process whereby leukocytes are attracted to the infection site in response to the invading microorganisms is known as chemotaxis. Phagocytosis is the process by which leukocytes engulf and digest microorganisms.

Inflammation is the body's reaction to injury or invasion by disease-producing organisms. The inflammatory response concentrates host immune components at the site of an infection to eliminate microorganisms and heal damaged tissue. It relies on both the physical actions of leukocytes and the biochemical compounds that these cells produce. Acute inflammation is a short-term, normal process that protects and heals the body. Chronic inflammation is a long-lived, out-of-control response that continues for more than a few weeks. In chronic inflammation, the immune system response can sometimes become so intense that it begins to harm the body that it is trying to protect. Tissue damage is the hallmark of chronic inflammation.

Periodontal disease is a bacterial infection that induces an inflammatory response in the periodontal tissues. Chapter 15 focuses on the host immune response to periodontal disease.

Section 4
Focus on Patients

Evidence in Action

CASE 1

You injure your arm by accidentally stabbing it with an ice pick. Within minutes following the injury, you note some changes in the tissues around the injury. What changes in the tissues should you expect if your body responds with a typical inflammatory response?

CASE 2

A new patient in your office reports a history of rheumatic heart disease at a very early age on her health questionnaire. The patient explains that her physician at the time thought that the rheumatic heart disease was a result of a streptococcal skin infection that she developed a few months prior to the discovery of the heart disease, but that the physician did not explain any of the details of these conditions to her. Explain how an infection of the skin could result in damage to the heart tissue.

References

1. Murphy K, Weaver C, *Janeway's Immunobiology*. 9th ed. New York, NY: Garland Science/Taylor & Francis Group, LLC; 2017.
2. Paul WE. *Fundamental Immunology*. Philadelphia, PA: Wolters Kluwer Health/Lippincott Williams & Wilkins; 2013. Available from: http://libproxy.lib.unc.edu/login?url=http://www.UNC.eblib.com/EBLWeb/patron/?target=patron&extendedid=P_2031826_0.
3. Marshall D, Haskard DO. Clinical overview of leukocyte adhesion and migration: where are we now? *Semin Immunol*. 2002;14(2):133–140.
4. Van Haastert PJ, Devreotes PN. Chemotaxis: signalling the way forward. *Nat Rev Mol Cell Biol*. 2004;5(8):626–634.
5. Kumar V, Abbas AK, Aster JC. *Robbins and Cotran Pathologic Basis of Disease*. 9th ed. Philadelphia, PA: Elsevier/Saunders; 2015:1391.
6. Fitzsimmons TR, Sanders AE, Bartold PM, Slade GD. Local and systemic biomarkers in gingival crevicular fluid increase odds of periodontitis. *J Clin Periodontol*. 2010;37(1):30–36.
7. Megson E, Fitzsimmons T, Dharmapatni K, Bartold PM. C-reactive protein in gingival crevicular fluid may be indicative of systemic inflammation. *J Clin Periodontol*. 2010;37(9):797–804.
8. Noack B, Genco RJ, Trevisan M, Grossi S, Zambon JJ, De Nardin E. Periodontal infections contribute to elevated systemic C-reactive protein level. *J Periodontol*. 2001;72(9):1221–1227.
9. Serhan CN, Chiang N. Novel endogenous small molecules as the checkpoint controllers in inflammation and resolution: entree for resoleomics. *Rheum Dis Clin North Am*. 2004;30(1):69–95.
10. Hasturk H, Kantarci A. Activation and resolution of periodontal inflammation and its systemic impact. *Periodontol 2000*. 2015;69(1):255–273.
11. Van Dyke TE, Serhan CN. Resolution of inflammation: a new paradigm for the pathogenesis of periodontal diseases. *J Dent Res*. 2003;82(2):82–90.
12. Gilroy DW, Lawrence T, Perretti M, Rossi AG. Inflammatory resolution: new opportunities for drug discovery. *Nat Rev Drug Discov*. 2004;3(5):401–416.
13. Tieri P, Valensin S, Latora V, et al. Quantifying the relevance of different mediators in the human immune cell network. *Bioinformatics*. 2005;21(8):1639–1643.
14. Kornman KS, Page RC, Tonetti MS. The host response to the microbial challenge in periodontitis: assembling the players. *Periodontol 2000*. 1997;14:33–53.

STUDENT ANCILLARY RESOURCES

A wide variety of resources to enhance your learning is available online:

- Audio Glossary
- Book Pages
- Chapter Review Questions and Answers

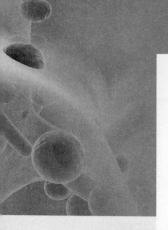

CHAPTER

15 Host Immune Response to Plaque Biofilm

Clinical Application.
Members of the dental team will encounter many patients with gingivitis and periodontitis. Recognizing the clinical features of these conditions will become second nature to all clinicians. However, understanding the underlying body defense mechanisms that serve to protect the host but can also do damage to the periodontium will not always be so straightforward. This chapter focuses on the host responses to plaque biofilm and the tissue destruction that ensues when bacteria, present in plaque biofilm, elicit a response in the host.

Learning Objectives

- Define the term host response and explain its primary function.
- Name factors that can enhance the microbial challenge to the periodontium.
- Define the term biochemical mediator and name three types of mediators.
- Describe the role of cytokines in the pathogenesis of periodontitis.
- Describe the role of prostaglandins in the pathogenesis of periodontitis.
- Describe the effect of matrix metalloproteinases (MMPs) on periodontal tissues.
- Explain the phases of the bone remodeling cycle.
- Explain the significance of a balanced OPG-to-RANKL ratio.
- Describe the link between periodontitis and RANKL-mediated bone resorption.
- For each of the histologic stages of gingivitis and periodontitis listed below, name one change in the host immune response likely to be encountered:

  ✓ Bacterial Accumulation   ✓ Established Gingivitis
  ✓ Early Gingivitis   ✓ Periodontitis

Key Terms

Host response	Biochemical mediators	TIMP	RANKL
Virulence factor	Cytokines	Pathogenesis	OPG
Catabasis	Prostaglandins	Bone remodeling	Homeostatic condition
Pro-resolving lipid mediators	PGE	Osteoblasts	Bone resorption
	MMP	Osteoclasts	

Section 1
The Host Response in Periodontal Disease

Periodontal disease is a bacterial infection that induces an inflammatory response in the periodontal tissues.[1-3] Research findings indicate that although bacteria are essential for disease to occur, the presence of suspected periodontal pathogens alone is insufficient to cause the tissue destruction seen in periodontitis. Rather, it appears to be the body's response to the bacteria present in plaque biofilm that is the cause of nearly all the destruction seen in periodontal disease.[1-4]

The body's response to bacteria is referred to as the host response. In the instance of periodontal disease, the immune system strives to defend the body against bacteria present in plaque biofilm. The body's defenses are activated to eliminate the potential pathogens and limit the spread of infection, not actually to preserve the tooth or its supporting periodontal tissues. Figure 15-1 depicts the chain of events that is theorized to lead to periodontitis.

FACTORS ENHANCING THE MICROBIAL CHALLENGE

The presence of bacteria is essential for the initiation and progression of periodontal disease. Certain bacteria can activate the human immune and inflammatory system, which subsequently can lead to damage of the periodontium.[1,2]

The term virulence factor refers to the mechanisms that enable biofilm bacteria to colonize and damage the tissues of the periodontium. Virulence factors may be either structural characteristics of the bacteria themselves or substances that are produced by the bacteria. The primary bacterial virulence factors that can enhance damage to the periodontium are:

1. **Presence of lipopolysaccharide (LPS):** Gram-negative bacteria are a component of mature plaque biofilm. Gram-negative bacteria are virulent because of lipopolysaccharide (LPS), an endotoxin present on the outer membrane of the bacteria. LPS can be responsible for initiating inflammation in periodontal tissues.
2. **Ability to invade tissues:** There is good evidence that several subgingival bacteria can invade epithelial cells.[5] Some of the periodontal bacteria—such as *Porphyromonas gingivalis (P.g)* and *Aggregatibacter actinomycetemcomitans (A.a)*—can invade host tissues. Penetration of tissues can to some degree allow the bacteria to escape host defense mechanisms.
3. **Ability to produce enzymes:** Several periodontal bacteria produce enzymes such as collagenases and proteases that can directly degrade host proteins that are a basic part of the structure of the periodontium.

FACTORS AFFECTING THE HOST IMMUNE RESPONSE

Certain factors may influence the host's susceptibility to periodontal disease by modifying the host response or tissue metabolism.[6,7] These factors include genetic factors, environmental factors, and acquired factors—all of which can play important roles in periodontal disease pathogenesis.

1. **Genetic Factors.** Genetic factors appear to contribute to periodontal disease. Studies in twins and families indicate an association between periodontal disease and genetic factors.[8] Diseases with genetic origin such as Papillon–Lefèvre syndrome and leukocyte adhesion deficiency (LAD) are associated with aggressive type of

periodontal diseases. Also, variations in genes controlling formation of biochemical mediators can modify the immune response to plaque biofilm, increasing the susceptibility to periodontal disease.[9–12]

2. **Environmental Factors.** Tobacco smoking is a known risk factor for periodontal diseases. It has a significant effect on the immune and inflammatory system. Smoking has been shown to decrease polymorphonuclear neutrophil (PMN) phagocytic capacity, decrease vascularity of gingival tissues, and affect both T- and B-lymphocyte response to periodontal pathogens.[13–17]

3. **Acquired Factors.** Diabetes mellitus is a known risk factor for periodontal diseases and its progression.[18–22] Abnormal blood glucose levels seen in diabetes mellitus affects the host response by reducing PMN function, increasing interleukin (IL)-1, tumor necrosis factor-α (TNF-α), and prostaglandin E_2 (PGE$_2$) levels in gingival crevicular fluid and reducing growth and proliferation of periodontal ligament fibroblasts and osteoblasts in periodontium.[7]

INFLAMMATION: A PROTECTIVE HOST RESPONSE THAT CAN TURN HARMFUL

1. **Acute Inflammation**
   A. **Host Response to Microbes.** When pathogenic bacteria successfully infect the periodontium, the body responds by mobilizing defensive immune cells and releasing a series of biochemical mediators to combat the bacteria.
      1. Cells involved in immune and inflammatory processes include inflammatory cells, PMNs, antigen-presenting cells (macrophages and Langerhans cells), T- and B-lymphocytes, fibroblasts, and epithelial cells. These cellular components of the immune and inflammatory processes are discussed in Chapter 14.
      2. *Acute inflammation has a host-protective effect.* It serves as the body's first line of defense against microbial invasion, eliminates the harmful stimuli, replaces injurious host cells, and creates an environment favorable to tissue repair.
      3. After the microbial challenge has been eliminated, however, the host must be able to dampen (shutdown) the acute inflammatory response.
   B. **Resolution of Acute Inflammation Following Removal of Microbial Challenge**
      1. *To maintain a healthy status, both the activation of acute inflammation and its resolution must be efficient.*
         a. It is not the extent of an acute inflammatory response, but rather how effectively the acute inflammation resolves that determines whether the inflammation is favorable or detrimental to the periodontium.
         b. *Periodontitis is associated with unresolved inflammation.* Indeed, uncontrolled or unresolved inflammation is now recognized as a major driver of human pathologies, including arthritis, asthma, cancers, cardiovascular diseases, and periodontitis.[23–25]
      2. Traditionally, resolution of inflammation was thought to be a passive process resulting from the reduction of biochemical mediators, the eventual disappearance of the inflammatory response, and a return to a state of tissue health. However, recent studies indicate that resolution of inflammation and return to a noninflammatory state is an actively regulated biologic process. This return to homeostasis is referred to as catabasis.
      3. Catabasis is thought to be a complicated biologic process that is just as complicated as the onset of inflammation.[1,24,25]

a. **Proinflammation Mediators**
   1) In periodontitis, the lipid mediators of inflammation include prostaglandins, thromboxanes, prostacyclins, and leukotrienes.
   2) The mediators are associated with recruitment of PMNs, destruction of the connective tissue matrix, and resorption of alveolar bone. The overrecruitment or overactivity of PMNs can amplify the inflammatory process and result in tissue damage.

b. **Inflammation-Resolving Mediators**
   1) The resolution of inflammation is regulated by the activity of chemical mediators known as specialized **pro-resolving lipid mediators**.[1,26]
   2) Specialized pro-resolving lipid mediators are actively produced by the body during the resolution phase of acute inflammation. Specialized pro-resolving lipid mediators work in a programmed systematic process to (1) terminate PMN recruitment to the site, (2) stimulate macrophages to remove dead cells, (3) promote antibacterial activities, and (4) promote tissue repair and regeneration to achieve homeostasis.[25]
   3) Future research is focused on understanding the key steps that control the resolution phase of acute inflammation—rather than solely focusing on controlling the bacterial infection or suppressing the activity of pro-inflammatory mediators. This may lead to new treatment protocols.[1]

2. **Chronic Inflammation.** If the host is unable to tamp down the inflammation soon after removal of the microbial challenge, the acute inflammation will progress to uncontrolled and unresolved chronic inflammation which can have pathologic effects on host tissue. Figure 15-1 depicts the possible events in the inflammatory response and resolution of acute inflammation.

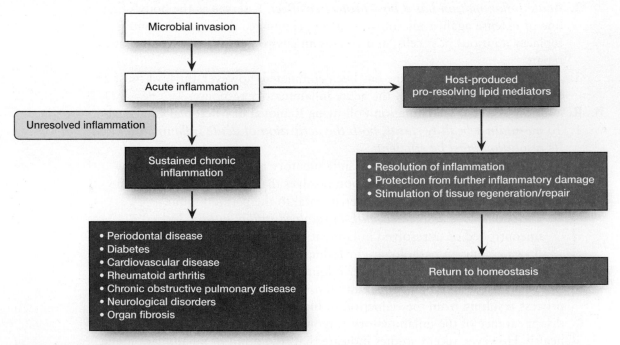

Figure 15-1. Inflammatory Response and Resolution. This flow chart outlines the possible cascade of events following an acute inflammatory response to an event of bacterial invasion in a host. Note that there are two possible body responses: (1) resolution of the acute inflammation and return to a state of homeostasis or (2) lack of resolution to the acute inflammation and conversion to a chronic inflammatory response that can in turn lead to damage to the host.

INFLAMMATORY BIOCHEMICAL MEDIATORS OF THE HOST RESPONSE

In response to a microbial challenge, host immune cells secrete biologically active compounds called biochemical mediators. These biochemical mediators are the "middlemen" sent by the host cells to activate the inflammatory response. Biochemical mediators of importance in periodontitis are cytokines, prostaglandins, and matrix metalloproteinases (MMPs) (Table 15-1).

1. **Cytokines.** Cytokines are powerful regulatory proteins released by host immune cells that influence the behavior of other cells. The cytokine (literally "cell protein") is a molecule that transmits information or signals from one cell to another. When released by host cells, cytokines act as signaling molecules that alert and activate the immune system for help—that is, to send additional phagocytic cells to the site of an infection.

   A. **Sources of Cytokines.** Many different cells including PMNs, macrophages, B-lymphocytes, epithelial cells, gingival fibroblasts, and osteoblasts can produce cytokines in response to the bacterial challenge or tissue injury.

   B. **Functions of Cytokines**
      1. Cytokines bind to specific cell surface receptors expressed on the target cell. This is a necessary step for a cytokine to recruit immune cells, such as PMNs and macrophages, to the infection site.
      2. Paradoxically, cytokines have diametrically opposed roles—they can be tissue protective on the one hand, but tissue destructive on the other hand. Cytokines increase vascular permeability allowing immune cells and complement to move into the tissues at the infection site. However, cytokines have the potential to initiate tissue destruction and bone loss in chronic inflammatory diseases, such as periodontitis.

   C. **Key Cytokines.** Cytokines that play an important role in periodontitis include IL-1, IL-6, IL-8, and TNF-α.[5-9]

2. **Prostaglandins.** Prostaglandins are a group of powerful biochemical mediators derived from fatty acids expressed on the cell surface of most cells. Biologically important prostaglandins are prostaglandin D, E, F, G, H, and I. Prostaglandins of the E series (PGE) play an important role in the bone destruction seen in periodontitis.

   A. **Sources of Prostaglandins.** The major source of PGE in inflamed periodontal tissues is the macrophage, although PMNs and gingival fibroblasts also produce them.

   B. **Functions of Prostaglandins**
      1. Prostaglandins increase the permeability and dilation of the blood vessels which facilitates the rapid influx of PMNs and monocytes to the infected site.
      2. Prostaglandins can trigger osteoclasts to destroy alveolar bone. *Prostaglandins initiate most of the alveolar bone destruction in periodontitis.*
      3. Prostaglandins can promote the overproduction of destructive MMP enzymes.

3. **Matrix Metalloproteinases.** MMPs are a family of at least 12 different proteolytic enzymes produced by various cells of the body. These enzymes act together to break down the connective tissue matrix.

   A. **Sources of MMPs.** PMNs, macrophages, gingival fibroblasts, and junctional epithelial cells can produce MMPs. The cells providing the major source of MMPs in periodontitis are PMNs and gingival fibroblasts.

   B. **Functions of MMPs**
      1. **MMPs Effects in Health.** In the absence of disease, MMPs facilitate the normal turnover of the periodontal connective tissue matrix. The overactivity

of MMPs is tightly suppressed by host-derived tissue inhibitors of matrix metalloproteinases (TIMP). The MMP–TIMP balance is critical in maintaining the integrity and the health of the connective tissue. The balance also plays an important role in regulating normal turnover of the extracellular matrix. Any disruption in the MMP–TIMP balance will result in excessive, uncontrolled pathologic breakdown of the connective tissue matrix.

2. **MMPs Effects in Chronic Infection and Inflammation**
   a. In the presence of chronic bacterial infection, the host immune system responds by releasing elevated levels of cytokines and prostaglandins. These mediators, in turn, stimulate leukocytes and fibroblasts to release MMPs.
   b. As the inflammation becomes more intense, leukocytes and fibroblasts produce excessive amounts of MMPs. The elevated MMP levels soon overwhelm the capacity of TIMPs to regulate the activity of MMP.
   c. *In the presence of increased MMP levels, extensive collagen destruction occurs in the periodontal tissues.* It should be noted that collagen provides the structural framework of all periodontal tissues. Without collagen, the tissues of the gingiva, periodontal ligament, and supporting alveolar bone degrade. This degradation results in gingival recession, pocket formation, periodontal attachment loss, root exposure, and tooth mobility.
   d. Periostat (20-mg doxycycline). A subantimicrobial dose of doxycycline is an oral medication that can be prescribed to patients with periodontitis. Its low dose of doxycycline does not provide it with any antimicrobial effect. Rather, it functions by inhibiting the activity of MMPs. When prescribed, it should be used as an adjunct to periodontal instrumentation.

TABLE 15-1 TISSUE DESTRUCTION BY BIOCHEMICAL MEDIATORS IN PERIODONTITIS

Mediators	Local Effects
Cytokine IL-1	Stimulates osteoclast activity resulting in bone resorption[27–30] Induces breakdown of collagen matrix in gingiva, periodontal ligament, and alveolar bone[28,31]
Cytokine IL-6	Stimulates bone resorption[27,32] Inhibits bone formation[27,33]
Cytokine IL-8	Stimulates connective tissue destruction[27,34] Stimulates bone resorption[27,29,35,36]
Cytokine TNF-α	Stimulates bone resorption[27,30,37] Induces breakdown of collagen matrix in gingiva, periodontal ligament, and alveolar bone[27,30,37]
Prostaglandin E$_2$ (PGE$_2$)	Stimulates MMP secretion[4,38] Stimulates bone resorption[30,39–41]
MMP enzymes	Induce breakdown of the collagen matrix in gingiva, periodontal ligament, and alveolar bone[30,40]
RANK	The receptor found on the surface of osteoclasts. When bound by its ligand (RANKL), osteoclasts become activated.[42]

CURRENT THEORY OF PATHOGENESIS

In summary, the chain of events—pathogenesis—that leads from health to gingivitis to periodontitis is complex and multilayered. For example, the microbial infection activates the host response. Genetic and environmental factors modify the immunoinflammatory response. Mediators, such as cytokines and antibodies, are produced by the cells of the immunoinflammatory response. Finally, advances in knowledge about resolution of inflammation have influenced our thinking about the pathogenesis of periodontitis. Figure 15-2 depicts the interaction of the various factors involved in the pathogenesis of periodontal disease.

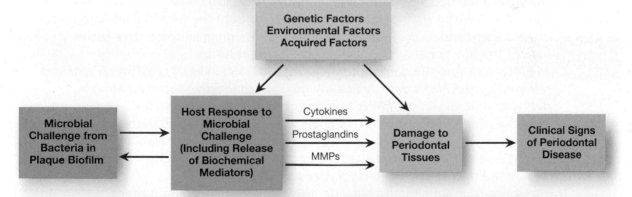

Any disease-modifying risk factor can alter the host immunoinflammatory response, and ultimately, render an individual more susceptible to developing periodontitis. Examples of disease-modifying risk factors include genetic factors (such as a genetic deficiency in PMN function), environmental factors (such as smoking), and acquired factors (such as diabetes). It is now well-established that the presence of microbial biofilm alone is not sufficient to result in periodontitis; instead disease-modifying risk factors must be present to make an individual susceptible to the disease. On the other hand, in the absence of disease-modifying factors, the host immune response should be able to readily eliminate the pathogenic invasion and restrict irreversible periodontal tissue destruction

Genetic Factors
Environmental Factors
Acquired Factors

Microbial Challenge from Bacteria in Plaque Biofilm

Host Response to Microbial Challenge (Including Release of Biochemical Mediators)

Cytokines
Prostaglandins
MMPs

Damage to Periodontal Tissues

Clinical Signs of Periodontal Disease

Periodontal disease is the result of an imbalance between the microbial biofilm challenge and the resulting host response. Microbial pathogens in the biofilm produce virulence factors such as antigens or lipopolysaccharides. In response, the host immune system fights back by deploying immune cells, such as PMNs, to the site of the infection and stimulating leukocytes to produce antibodies. If the host immune response is able to successfully eliminate the microbial challenge (i.e., plaque biofilm), the inflammation will resolve and the host tissues will be able to repair the damage. This part of the pathogenesis pathway represents the "initial, early, and established lesions" of periodontal disease.

If the modifying factors are present and if bacteria continue to challenge the host immune response, the following occurs:

-The host immune response deploys more PMNs, which produce cytokines, prostaglandins, and MMPs to target the pathogenic bacteria. However, these factors also cause collateral damage by mediating the destruction of connective tissue and alveolar bone.

-Clinical signs of periodontitis become evident.

-This part of the pathogenesis pathway represents the "advanced lesion" (periodontitis).

Figure 15-2. Theory of Pathogenesis. It is well accepted that the development of periodontitis is a multifactorial process through which a bacterial-induced inflammation, modified by environmental, genetic, and biological mechanisms leads to an excessive host response and associated tissue destruction.

Section 2
Histologic Stages in the Development of Periodontal Disease

Researchers Page and Schroeder conducted the classic, landmark research on the histologic development of gingivitis and periodontitis.[4,43,44] They described four distinct histologic stages in the development of periodontal disease: *initial lesion, early lesion, established lesion*, and *advanced lesion*. For clarity, these terms appear in the discussion below, but more is understood today about the host immune response related to these stages than when they initially published their descriptions (Boxes 15-1 to 15-4 and Figs. 15-3 to 15-6).

Box 15-1. Bacterial Accumulation (*Initial Lesion*)

1. **Bacterial Features.** Bacteria colonize the tooth surface near the gingival margin (Fig. 15-3).
2. **Cellular Features.** The presence of gram-negative bacteria and their metabolic products initiates the host immune response.
   A. In response to the bacterial pathogens, the junctional epithelial cells release various biochemical mediators, including *cytokines, PGE$_2$, MMPs, and TNFα.*
   B. These mediators stimulate the immune response, recruiting polymorphonuclear leukocytes (PMNs) to the site.
   C. PMNs pass from blood vessels into the gingival connective tissue.
      1. The PMNs need to reach the sulcus into order to fight the bacterial infection located there and so they must travel through the gingival connective tissue toward the junctional epithelium and the gingival sulcus.
      2. As PMNs pass into the gingival connective tissue they release cytokines. *Cytokines released by the PMNs destroy healthy gingival connective tissue creating a pathway that allows the PMNs to move quickly through the tissue*.
      3. The goal of the PMNs is to reach the bacteria in the sulcus and destroy them. The damage to the healthy connective tissue is not normally a concern. In a healthy body, tissue will be repaired after the bacterial infection is brought under control.
   D. PMNs migrate into sulcus and phagocytize bacteria.
   E. The presence of gram-negative bacteria activates the complement system.
3. **Tissue Level Features**
   A. Initial location of the plaque biofilm is supragingival.
   B. There is vascular dilatation of arterioles, capillaries, and venules in the dentogingival complex.
   C. Gingival crevicular fluid increases in volume.
4. **Clinical Features**
   A. *At this stage, the gingiva looks healthy clinically.*
   B. This initial lesion phase develops 2 to 4 days following plaque biofilm accumulation.
5. **Outcome of Host Response**
   A. The host response is successful, if most of the bacteria are destroyed.
   B. If the bacterial infection is brought under control—through the efforts of the immune system and effective plaque biofilm control—the body can repair the destruction caused by the immune response.
   C. If the bacterial pathogens are not controlled, however, early gingivitis develops.

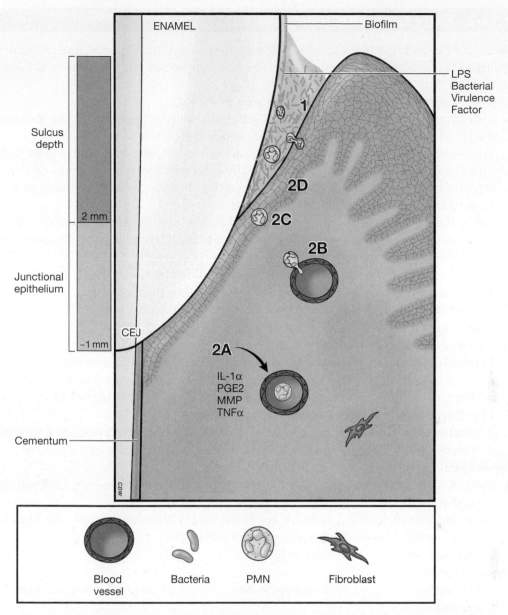

Figure 15-3. Bacterial Accumulation (*Initial Lesion*). This first phase is characterized by bacterial colonization near the gingival margin, increased vascular dilatation, and PMN migration into the gingival sulcus. Although the host immune and inflammatory responses are activated, the gingival tissue looks clinically healthy in this phase.

Box 15-2. Early Gingivitis (*Early Lesion*)

1. **Bacterial Features.** Bacterial accumulation continues and biofilm maturation occurs. This results in the production of bacterial toxins and byproducts that penetrate the junctional epithelium (Fig. 15-4).
2. **Cellular Features: Migration and Chemotaxis of PMNs**
   A. *Cytokines*—released by the junctional epithelial cells in response to the increased bacterial challenge—attract additional cellular defenders to the site.
   B. Increased permeability of the blood vessels allows larger numbers of PMNs to move into the gingival connective tissue near the infection site. On their way to the infection site, PMNs destroy additional healthy gingival connective tissue as they rush toward the bacterial invaders in the sulcus.
   C. PMNs then migrate through the junctional epithelium to form a "wall of cells" between the biofilm and the sulcus wall. These PMNs comprise the most important component of the local defense against bacteria.
   D. *Cytokines* released by the PMNs cause localized destruction of the connective tissue. This tissue destruction allows more PMNs to migrate through the connective tissue toward the sulcus. PMNs phagocytize bacteria in the sulcus in an effort to protect the host tissues from the bacterial challenge.
3. **Migration of Additional Cellular Defenders**
   A. Macrophages are recruited to the connective tissue. These cells release biochemical mediators including cytokines, PGE_2, and MMPs. These biochemical mediators recruit additional immune cells to the infection site. MMP is responsible for the excessive loss of collagen in the affected connected tissue zone.
   B. T-lymphocytes migrate to the connective tissue and produce *cytokines* and antibodies. The early lesion is predominantly a T-cell lesion.
4. **Tissue Level Features**
   A. Sulcular epithelium and the adjacent connective tissue are affected the most: **collagen loss of 60% to 70% is noted at this stage.**
   B. Sulcular epithelium starts forming epithelial ridges (epithelial extensions that protrude into connective tissue) due to inflammatory changes.
   C. Junctional epithelial cells start to proliferate.
5. **Clinical Features**
   A. *Inflammatory changes such as edema and redness of gingival marginal tissue can be observed clinically.*
   B. Early lesion phase develops 4 to 7 days following plaque biofilm accumulation. Duration of early gingivitis can vary between individuals.
6. **Outcome of Host Response at the Stage**
   A. The large number of PMNs, macrophages, and T-lymphocytes may control the bacterial pathogens.
   B. Initiation of good patient self-care can disrupt the plaque biofilm and result in a return to health. If the bacterial infection is brought under control—through the efforts of the immune system and effective plaque biofilm control—the body can repair the destruction caused by the immune response.
   C. If the host immune response fails to "hold the line," the early lesion will progress to the "*established gingivitis*"—the next phase of disease progression.

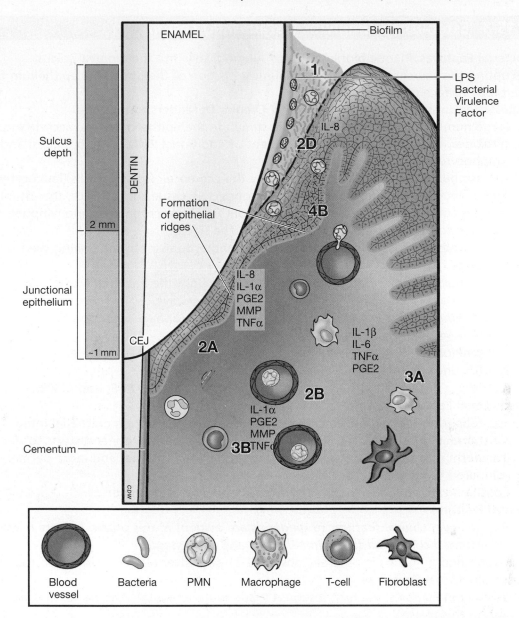

Figure 15-4. Early Gingivitis (*Early Lesion*). The Biofilm Overgrowth Phase is characterized by subgingival plaque biofilm formation and intensified immune and inflammatory response compared to plaque biofilm accumulation phase. Early inflammatory changes are observed clinically as redness and swelling of the marginal gingiva.

Box 15-3. Established Gingivitis (*Established Lesion*)

1. **Bacterial Features.** Plaque biofilm extends subgingivally into the gingival sulcus, disrupting the attachment of the coronal-most portion of the junctional epithelium from the tooth surface (Fig. 15-5).
2. **Cellular Features: Migration of Additional Cellular Defenders to the Site.**
   A. Large numbers of subgingival bacteria stimulate the epithelial cells to secrete more *cytokines*, resulting in greater recruitment of additional PMNs, macrophages, and lymphocytes.
   B. The established lesion is predominated by the presence of plasma cells (leukocytes that produce antibodies) in the affected connective tissue zone. Hence, the established lesion is considered to be a plasma cell lesion. *PMNs*, macrophages, and lymphocytes continue to assist in fighting the bacteria in the sulcus.
   C. Plasma cells produce large quantities of antibodies to assist in controlling the bacterial challenge.
   D. The immune system sends more immune cells to fight the bacteria. More toxic chemicals are released and additional healthy connective tissue is destroyed.
      1. *Cytokines*, *PGE$_2$*, and *MMPs* are produced by macrophages exposed to gram-negative bacteria.
      2. *Cytokines* recruit additional macrophages and lymphocytes to the area.
      3. *PGE$_2$* and the *MMPs* initiate collagen destruction.
      4. Gingival fibroblasts are stimulated to produce additional *PGE$_2$* and *MMPs*.
3. **Tissue Level Features**
   A. Epithelial ridges extend deeper in connective tissue to maintain epithelial integrity.
   B. Junctional epithelium loosens its attachment to the root surface and starts to transform into pocket epithelium. Pocket epithelium is thinner and more permeable compared to junctional epithelium.
   C. Continued collagen loss in the infiltrated connective tissue zone.
4. **Clinical Features**
   A. *All the usual clinical features of gingivitis are evident in this phase, but are more accentuated compared to the initial stage and early stage.*
   B. Established gingivitis is generally observed 21 days after plaque biofilm accumulation.
5. **Outcome of Host Response**
   A. In many individuals, the host response is adequate to contain the bacterial challenge during this phase.
   B. Periodontal instrumentation and patient education, at this point, can be helpful in controlling the bacterial challenge. The combination of professional treatment and good patient self-care can stop the bacterial challenge and return the periodontium to health.
   C. In certain susceptible individuals if the bacterial infection is not controlled, established gingivitis progresses to periodontitis. Unfortunately, no one can predict when and if established gingivitis will progress to periodontitis. Current research is directed to trying to determine which individuals are at risk for developing periodontitis.

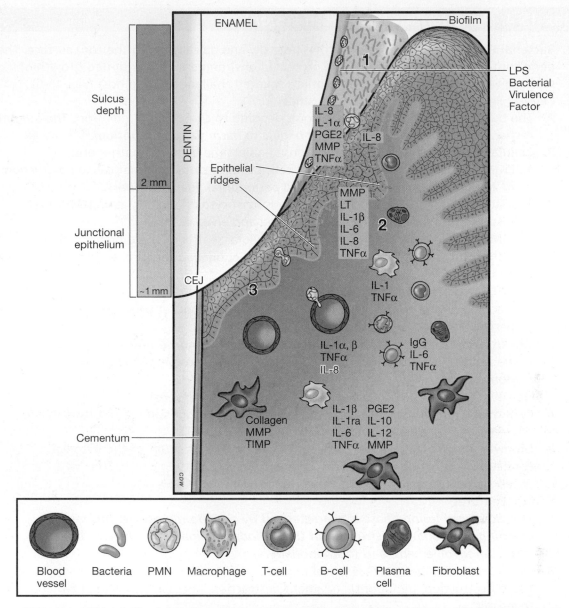

Figure 15-5. Established Gingivitis (*Established Lesion*): The Subgingival Plaque Phase. Subgingival plaque biofilm extends to junctional epithelium. Increased cellular infiltrate and collagen breakdown in connective tissue is observed. All clinical characteristics of gingivitis are evident in this phase.

Box 15-4. Periodontitis (*Advanced Lesion*)

1. **Bacterial Features.** Plaque biofilm grows laterally and apically along the root surface. The periodontal pocket provides an ideal protected environment for continued growth of subgingival bacteria presenting a chronic, repeated challenge to the host (Fig. 15-6).

2. **Cellular Features: Host Response Intensifies**
   A. The bacterial infection becomes chronic, leading to chronic inflammation. *The immune response becomes so intense that it begins to harm the periodontium.*[27,40]
   B. Cellular defenders intensify their defense against the bacterial pathogens.
      1. PMNs, macrophages, and epithelial cells produce *cytokines* that *cause destruction of the gingival connective tissue and periodontal ligament fibers.*
      2. Macrophages produce high concentrations of *cytokines, PGE$_2$, and MMPs* that **result in** *destruction of connective tissue and alveolar bone.*[30,40]
      3. MMPs mediate destruction of the extracellular matrix of the gingiva, collagen fibers attached at the apical edge of the junctional epithelium, and the periodontal ligament.
      4. *PGE$_2$* mediates bone destruction by stimulating large numbers osteoclasts to resorb the crest of the alveolar bone. The gingival pocket progresses to become a periodontal pocket.
   C. *The tissue destruction caused by the host immune response now overwhelms any tissue repair. Tissue destruction becomes the main outcome of the immune system response.*

3. **Tissue Level Features (Destruction of Periodontal Tissues Ensues)**
   A. Cells of the junctional epithelium migrate apically on root surface resulting in the development of a *periodontal pocket.*
   B. Gingival fibroblasts shift to a state that favors the *destruction of the gingival connective tissue and periodontal ligament fibers* (Fig. 15-5).
   C. Osteoclasts *destroy the crest of the alveolar bone* (Fig. 15-5).

4. **Clinical Features**
   A. *This advanced lesion phase is characterized by periodontal pocket formation, bleeding on probing, destruction of the periodontal ligament, alveolar bone loss, furcation involvement, and tooth mobility.*
   B. These tissue changes (such as apical migration of junctional epithelium, connective tissue destruction, periodontal ligament destruction, and alveolar bone loss) are not reversible.

5. **Outcome of Host Response**
   A. Chronic infection by the periodontal pathogens induces a chronic inflammatory response. *The chronic inflammation destroys periodontal tissues and causes more damage to the periodontium than the bacterial infection. Irreversible tissue damage is the hallmark of periodontitis.*
   B. Factors influencing the host's failure to control the bacterial challenge may include:
      1. Abnormal PMN function.
      2. Persistence and virulence of bacteria in the biofilm.
      3. Acquired and environmental factors such as smoking and stress.
      4. Systemic factors such as uncontrolled diabetes mellitus or genetic factors.

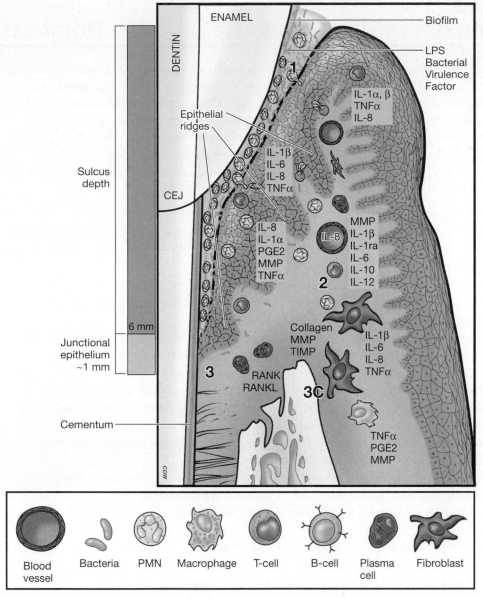

Figure 15-6. Periodontitis (*Advanced Lesion*). This phase is characterized by periodontal pocket formation, bleeding on probing, alveolar bone loss, furcation involvement, and tooth mobility.

Section 3
The Impact of Host Response on Bone Homeostasis

Despite its solid appearance, bone is in a constant state of remodeling. Bone remodeling is the breakdown of old bone and the subsequent creation (deposition) of new bone. Remodeling occurs constantly, for example: (1) when bones grow, remodeling maintains the shape and structure of the bone and (2) in response to new stresses applied to a bone, remodeling increases bone strength by adding new bone tissue where appropriate. The remodeling cycle is repeated throughout the course of an individual's life. In the periodontium, remodeling means that at all times some parts of the jaw bone are being resorbed, while other parts are growing by formation of new bone.

1. **The Bone Remodeling Cycle**
   A. The bone remodeling cycle is tightly coordinated by the concerted interactions of two principal cells: the osteoblasts (bone-building cells) and the osteoclasts (bone-resorbing cells).
      1. Osteoclasts are specialized multinucleated cells. Functionally, an osteoclast breaks down (resorbs) existing bone matrix. This function is critical in the maintenance, repair, and remodeling of bone.
      2. Osteoblasts are specialized bone forming cells that synthesize collagen and other bone proteins and are involved in mineralization of the bone matrix.
   B. The normal bone remodeling cycle is an ongoing process that results from the continuous resorption of bone followed by the subsequent deposition of new bone. Figure 15-7 depicts the sequential phases of the bone remodeling cycle.
      1. **Resorption phase:** Remodeling is initiated by the attraction of osteoclasts to the bone surface. The *osteoclasts* break down the bone mineral and matrix, creating erosion cavities in the bone.
      2. **Reversal phase:** In this phase, the osteoclasts cease the process of bone resorption and detach from the erosion cavity. Mononuclear cells then adhere to the erosion cavity and release signals that attract osteoblasts to the eroded area.
      3. **Formation phase:** *Osteoblasts* line the erosion cavity and form a matrix to replace resorbed bone with new bone. Under normal conditions, the amount of new mineralized bone is equal to the amount of bone resorbed by the osteoclasts.
      4. **Resting phase:** A lengthy resting period follows the formation phase. The resting phase is maintained until the next bone remodeling cycle.
2. **Regulation of the Bone Remodeling Cycle.** Control of the normal bone remodeling cycle is governed by an intricate signaling mechanism that occurs between the immature osteoclasts and osteoblasts.
   A. **The "Main Players" in Bone Metabolism**
      1. Receptor activator of nuclear factor-κB—abbreviated as RANKL—is a cell membrane–bound protein that regulates osteoclast differentiation (maturation) and activation. It is associated with bone remodeling and repair.
         a. Bone resorption occurs when osteoclasts are stimulated by RANKL to resorb the alveolar bone.
         b. In addition to osteoclasts, RANKL is also expressed on stromal cells, lymphocytes, chondrocytes, and other mesenchymal cells.

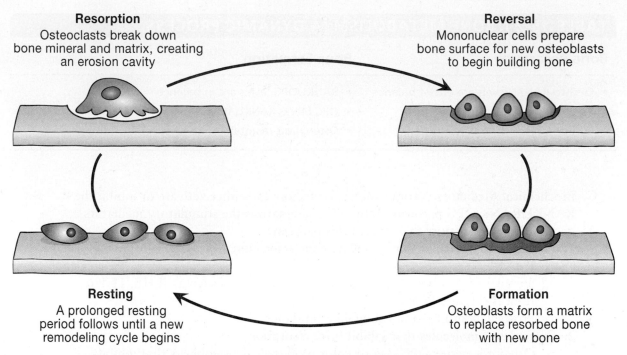

Resorption
Osteoclasts break down
bone mineral and matrix, creating
an erosion cavity

Reversal
Mononuclear cells prepare
bone surface for new osteoblasts
to begin building bone

Resting
A prolonged resting
period follows until a new
remodeling cycle begins

Formation
Osteoblasts form a matrix
to replace resorbed bone
with new bone

Figure 15-7. The Bone Remodeling Cycle. Normal bone remodeling is an ongoing process that results from the continuous resorption of bone with the subsequent replacement of lost bone. The four stages of this cycle are the resorption phase, reversal phase, formation phase, and the resting phase.

2. Osteoprotegerin (OPG) is secreted by osteoblasts and protects bone from excessive resorption by binding to RANKL. Thus, by binding to RANKL, OPG suppresses resorption of alveolar bone, thus bone levels remain stable.

B. Mechanism of Bone Metabolism. *Bone metabolism is a dynamic process that balances bone formation and bone resorption.* The RANKL/OPG balance is an important factor in regulating alveolar bone resorption.

1. A homeostatic condition occurs when the body is able to maintain stable levels of alveolar bone.

   a. *Homeostatic conditions are thought to exist when the levels of RANKL and OPG are in* balance in the periodontal tissues.

   b. When the RANKL/OPG levels are in balance, OPG blocks RANKL, thus inhibiting the activation of osteoclasts. Bone resorption is inhibited, thus alveolar bone levels remain stable.

2. Bone resorption occurs when osteoclasts are stimulated by RANKL to resorb alveolar bone.

   a. When the periodontium is inflamed, levels of OPG decrease.

   b. When the OPG-to-RANKL levels are out of balance in the periodontal tissues, osteoclast activity stimulates resorption of alveolar bone.

TABLE 15-2	BONE METABOLISM: A DYNAMIC PROCESS

Bone Resorption	Bone Formation
• OPG-to-RANKL levels are out of balance	• RANKL/OPG levels are in balance
• RANKL stimulate osteoclasts	• OPG blocks RANKL, thus inhibiting activation of osteoclasts
• Osteoclasts cause bone resorption	• Osteoblasts maintain bone levels

C. **Biochemical Mediators.** Various molecular factors can either activate or inhibit the RANKL/RANK/OPG pathway. Table 15-2 summarizes the stimulatory mediators and inhibitory mediators that govern this pathway.
1. **Examples of molecules that stimulate bone resorption**
   a. RANKL
   b. Stimulatory cytokines—pro-inflammatory mediators such as IL-1β, TNF-α, IL-6, IL-11, and IL-17.
   c. Prostaglandin E2—a hormone-like substance.
2. **Examples of molecules that inhibit bone resorption**
   a. Osteoprotegerin (OPG)—a receptor produced by osteoblasts that inhibits osteoclastic differentiation.
   b. Inhibitory cytokines—anti-inflammatory mediators such as IL-4, IL-10, IL-12, IL-13, IFN-γ.
3. **The Link Between Periodontitis and RANKL-Mediated Bone Resorption.** As discussed, the normal bone remodeling process is dependent on a delicate balance between the activities of the osteoclast and the osteoblast.
   A. In periodontal disease, however, the invading pathogens and inflammatory host response tips the balance which ultimately results in bone loss. Figure 15-8 depicts the process of alveolar bone destruction.
      1. In response to microbial invasion, the body deploys a wide array of different types of immune cells to participate in the counterattack.
      2. These immune cells include PMNs, macrophages, dendritic cells, B lymphocytes, T lymphocytes, and monocytes/macrophages.
      3. When reaching the infection site, the immune cells release their full arsenal of proinflammatory mediators, such as IL-1β, TNF-α, IL-6, IL-11, IL-17, PGE$_2$ to combat the microbial invasion.
   B. While these same proinflammatory mediators protect the host from the microbial attack, they also stimulate the osteoblasts, fibroblasts, T lymphocytes, and B lymphocytes to produce RANKL, which, in turn, activates osteoclasts. If left unabated, the host inflammatory response leads to irreversible destruction of alveolar bone (45).

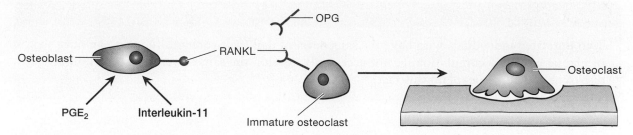

Figure 15-8. Destruction of Alveolar Bone. Cascade of events postulated to result in destruction of alveolar bone. Various factors can stimulate osteoblasts to produce RANKL, which in turn activates osteoclasts and leads to bone resorption. On the other hand, various factors, such as OPG, can inhibit bone resorption by blocking RANKL.

Chapter Summary Statement

The immune system provides the body with a strong defense against invading periodontal pathogens. In many cases, PMNs attracted to the site can contain the bacterial challenge and no tissue damage occurs. If the bacterial challenge is not contained, the plaque biofilm extends subgingivally and develops into a highly organized anaerobic biofilm. In many cases, the host response still can contain the bacterial pathogens. In some individuals, however, host resistance is insufficient to contain the bacterial challenge. *Biochemical mediators produced by immune cells are largely responsible for the tissue destruction seen in periodontitis. High levels of cytokines, RANKL, MMPs, and PGE$_2$ characterize periodontitis. The unrelenting, chronic bacterial infection triggers immune responses that (1) destroy the connective tissue of the gingiva, (2) destroy the periodontal ligament, and (3) resorb the alveolar bone. Therefore, while the host immune response has an important protective role, it has also been implicated in playing a significant role in the pathologic destruction of the periodontium.*

Section 4
Focus on Patients

Clinical Patient Care

CASE 1

Mrs. Smith is a new patient in the dental office. Mrs. Smith is 45 years of age and has not received regular dental care in the past. Her new employer provides dental insurance and she comes to your office for oral health care. Mrs. Smith has chronic periodontitis. How will you explain inflammatory periodontal disease to Mrs. Smith?

CASE 2

Two unrelated individuals who have the same level of daily self-care and the same amount of plaque biofilm accumulation do not necessarily develop the same severity of periodontal disease. How do you explain this fact?

Evidence in Action

CASE 1

In reading a dental journal you find an article that describes a new medication that is reported to stop collagen destruction by one of the matrix metalloproteinases (MMPs). If this new medication indeed blocks such collagen destruction, what effect might this medication have on a patient with periodontitis? Can you think of another biochemical mediator target that could be inhibited that would benefit a patient with periodontitis?

Ethical Dilemma

CASE 1

The next two patients, Mary and Katherine, are identical twin sisters who are new to your practice. They request that you review their health histories together. You learn that they are 68 years old, both widowed, and live together. They have received routine dental care from their longtime friend and dentist, Dr. Lipmann, who just retired at 80, so they have decided to become patients in your dental office. They inform you that their mother is still alive at 90, but is edentulous, as she lost all her teeth due to "gum disease." They both state that they are in good health, however Mary was diagnosed with type II diabetes a few years back. She states that she hasn't paid much attention to it.

Your examination and radiographs of Katherine reveal that she has generally good oral health, with localized gingivitis on the mandibular anterior region. Her self-care appears to be more than adequate, and you compliment her on it.

Mary's examination is quite the opposite. She presents with generalized periodontitis, and vertical bone loss on her mandibular posterior teeth. She exhibits attachment loss in the 4 to 5 mm range, with localized posterior readings of 6 to 7 mm. Some of her mandibular posterior teeth are mobile. She too has good self-care, but becomes very agitated when you present your findings to her. She states that she and Katherine "always" went to Dr. Lipmann together, and received the same treatments. She questions why her outcome is so different than that of her sister, and asks if you think Dr. Lipmann provided substandard dental care.

1. What factors may have contributed to the different disease presentation seen in these two sisters?
2. How will you discuss with Katherine the host immune response regarding her periodontal disease presentation?
3. What potential ethical dilemmas are involved in this situation?

References

1. Bartold PM, Van Dyke TE. Periodontitis: a host-mediated disruption of microbial homeostasis. Unlearning learned concepts. *Periodontol 2000.* 2013;62(1):203–217.
2. Darveau RP. Periodontitis: a polymicrobial disruption of host homeostasis. *Nat Rev Microbiol.* 2010;8(7):481–490.
3. Ebersole JL, Dawson DR, 3rd, Morford LA, Peyyala R, Miller CS, Gonzalez OA. Periodontal disease immunology: 'double indemnity' in protecting the host. *Periodontol 2000.* 2013;62(1):163–202.
4. Page RC, Offenbacher S, Schroeder HE, Seymour GJ, Kornman KS. Advances in the pathogenesis of periodontitis: summary of developments, clinical implications and future directions. *Periodontol 2000.* 1997;14:216–248.
5. Colombo AV, da Silva CM, Haffajee A, Colombo AP. Identification of intracellular oral species within human crevicular epithelial cells from subjects with chronic periodontitis by fluorescence in situ hybridization. *J Periodontal Res.* 2007;42(3):236–243.
6. Albandar JM. Global risk factors and risk indicators for periodontal diseases. *Periodontol 2000.* 2002;29:177–206.
7. Salvi GE, Lawrence HP, Offenbacher S, Beck JD. Influence of risk factors on the pathogenesis of periodontitis. *Periodontol 2000.* 1997;14:173–201.
8. Cagli NA, Hakki SS, Dursun R, et al. Clinical, genetic, and biochemical findings in two siblings with Papillon-Lefèvre Syndrome. *J Periodontol.* 2005;76(12):2322–2329.
9. Baker PJ. Genetic control of the immune response in pathogenesis. *J Periodontol.* 2005;76(Suppl 11):2042–2046.
10. Hart TC, Kornman KS. Genetic factors in the pathogenesis of periodontitis. *Periodontol 2000.* 1997;14:202–215.
11. Michalowicz BS. Genetic and heritable risk factors in periodontal disease. *J Periodontol.* 1994;65(Suppl 5):479–488.
12. Nibali L, O'Dea M, Bouma G, et al. Genetic variants associated with neutrophil function in aggressive periodontitis and healthy controls. *J Periodontol.* 2010;81(4):527–534.
13. Barbour SE, Nakashima K, Zhang JB, et al. Tobacco and smoking: environmental factors that modify the host response (immune system) and have an impact on periodontal health. *Crit Rev Oral Biol Med.* 1997;8(4):437–460.
14. Johnson GK, Guthmiller JM. The impact of cigarette smoking on periodontal disease and treatment. *Periodontol 2000.* 2007;44:178–194.
15. Kenney EB, Kraal JH, Saxe SR, Jones J. The effect of cigarette smoke on human oral polymorphonuclear leukocytes. *J Periodontal Res.* 1977;12(4):227–234.
16. Rezavandi K, Palmer RM, Odell EW, Scott DA, Wilson RF. Expression of ICAM-1 and E-selectin in gingival tissues of smokers and non-smokers with periodontitis. *J Oral Pathol Med.* 2002;31(1):59–64.
17. Tomar SL, Asma S. Smoking-attributable periodontitis in the United States: findings from NHANES III. National Health and Nutrition Examination Survey. *J Periodontol.* 2000;71(5):743–751.
18. Diabetes and periodontal diseases. Committee on Research, Science and Therapy. American Academy of Periodontology. *J Periodontol.* 2000;71(4):664–678.
19. Botero JE, Yepes FL, Roldan N, et al. Tooth and periodontal clinical attachment loss are associated with hyperglycemia in patients with diabetes. *J Periodontol.* 2012;83(10):1245–1250.
20. Deshpande K, Jain A, Sharma R, Prashar S, Jain R. Diabetes and periodontitis. *J Indian Soc Periodontol.* 2010;14(4): 207–212.
21. Mealey BL, Oates TW; American Academy of Periodontology. Diabetes mellitus and periodontal diseases. *J Periodontol.* 2006;77(8):1289–1303.
22. Preshaw PM, Bissett SM. Periodontitis: oral complication of diabetes. *Endocrinol Metab Clin North Am.* 2013;42(4): 849–867.
23. Nathan C, Ding A. Nonresolving inflammation. *Cell.* 2010;140(6):871–882.
24. Serhan CN. Resolution phase of inflammation: novel endogenous anti-inflammatory and proresolving lipid mediators and pathways. *Annu Rev Immunol.* 2007;25:101–137.
25. Serhan CN, Gotlinger K, Hong S, et al. Anti-inflammatory actions of neuroprotectin D1/protectin D1 and its natural stereoisomers: assignments of dihydroxy-containing docosatrienes. *J Immunol.* 2006;176(3):1848–1859.
26. Serhan CN. Controlling the resolution of acute inflammation: a new genus of dual anti-inflammatory and proresolving mediators. *J Periodontol.* 2008;79(Suppl 8):1520–1526.
27. Graves D. Cytokines that promote periodontal tissue destruction. *J Periodontol.* 2008;79(Suppl 8):1585–1591.
28. McDevitt MJ, Wang HY, Knobelman C, et al. Interleukin-1 genetic association with periodontitis in clinical practice. *J Periodontol.* 2000;71(2):156–163.
29. Qwarnstrom EE, MacFarlane SA, Page RC. Effects of interleukin-1 on fibroblast extracellular matrix, using a 3-dimensional culture system. *J Cell Physiol.* 1989;139(3):501–508.
30. Schwartz Z, Goultschin J, Dean DD, Boyan BD. Mechanisms of alveolar bone destruction in periodontitis. *Periodontol 2000.* 1997;14:158–172.
31. Reynolds JJ, Meikle MC. Mechanisms of connective tissue matrix destruction in periodontitis. *Periodontol 2000.* 1997;14:144–157.
32. Roodman GD. Interleukin-6: an osteotropic factor? *J Bone Miner Res.* 1992;7(5):475–478.
33. Hughes FJ, Howells GL. Interleukin-6 inhibits bone formation in vitro. *Bone Miner.* 1993;21(1):21–28.
34. Meikle MC, Atkinson SJ, Ward RV, Murphy G, Reynolds JJ. Gingival fibroblasts degrade type I collagen films when stimulated with tumor necrosis factor and interleukin 1: evidence that breakdown is mediated by metalloproteinases. *J Periodontal Res.* 1989;24(3):207–213.
35. Bertolini DR, Nedwin GE, Bringman TS, Smith DD, Mundy GR. Stimulation of bone resorption and inhibition of bone formation in vitro by human tumour necrosis factors. *Nature.* 1986;319(6053):516–518.
36. Thomson BM, Mundy GR, Chambers TJ. Tumor necrosis factors alpha and beta induce osteoblastic cells to stimulate osteoclastic bone resorption. *J Immunol.* 1987;138(3):775–779.
37. Kinane DF. Regulators of tissue destruction and homeostasis as diagnostic aids in periodontology. *Periodontol 2000.* 2000;24:215–225.
38. Gemmell E, Marshall RI, Seymour GJ. Cytokines and prostaglandins in immune homeostasis and tissue destruction in periodontal disease. *Periodontol 2000.* 1997;14:112–143.

39. Dietrich JW, Goodson JM, Raisz LG. Stimulation of bone resorption by various prostaglandins in organ culture. *Prostaglandins*. 1975;10(2):231–240.

40. Giannobile WV. Host-response therapeutics for periodontal diseases. *J Periodontol*. 2008;79(Suppl 8):1592–1600.

41. Zubery Y, Dunstan CR, Story BM, et al. Bone resorption caused by three periodontal pathogens in vivo in mice is mediated in part by prostaglandin. *Infect Immun*. 1998;66(9):4158–4162.

42. Giannopoulou C, Martinelli-Klay CP, Lombardi T. Immunohistochemical expression of RANKL, RANK and OPG in gingival tissue of patients with periodontitis. *Acta Odontol Scand*. 2012;70(6):629–634.

43. Page RC. The etiology and pathogenesis of periodontitis. *Compend Contin Educ Dent*. 2002;23(Suppl 5):11–14.

44. Page RC, Schroeder HE. Pathogenesis of inflammatory periodontal disease. A summary of current work. *Lab Invest*. 1976;34(3):235–249.

45. McCauley LK, Nohutcu RM. Mediators of periodontal osseous destruction and remodeling: principles and implications for diagnosis and therapy. *J Periodontol*. 2002;73(11):1377–1391.

 STUDENT ANCILLARY RESOURCES

A wide variety of resources to enhance your learning is available online:

- Audio Glossary
- Book Pages
- Chapter Review Questions and Answers

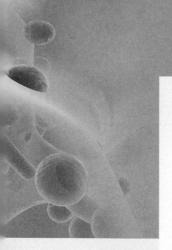

16 Systemic Risk Factors That Amplify Susceptibility to Periodontal Disease

Clinical Application.
Plaque biofilm is the fundamental etiology for periodontal disease, but evaluating patients with periodontal disease often can be quite confusing. Frequently, patients with minimal plaque biofilm challenge will have advanced disease for no clear reason. Some of these patients will have systemic conditions that can amplify their susceptibility to the periodontal disease, presenting a confusing clinical presentation. All members of the dental team must be alert for the possibility of systemic risk factors when evaluating patients with the signs of periodontal disease. This chapter focuses on how common modifying factors, such as diabetes, metabolic syndrome, hormonal changes, stress, and HIV/AIDS influence the risk for periodontal disease.

Learning Objectives

- Name several systemic diseases/conditions that may modify the host response to periodontal pathogens.
- Engage other health professionals—appropriate to the specific care situation—in shared patient-centered problem-solving.
- Place the interests of patients at the center of interprofessional health care delivery.
- Recognize the importance of educating patients about the relationship between oral health and systemic diseases, states, or conditions (such as the link between diabetes mellitus and periodontitis).
- Discuss the potential implications of these systemic conditions on the periodontium: uncontrolled diabetes, leukemia, and acquired immunodeficiency syndrome.
- Describe the significance of the AGE–RAGE interactions and its role in amplifying periodontal inflammation.
- Discuss how hormone alterations may affect the periodontium.
- Define the term osteoporosis and discuss the link between skeletal osteoporosis and alveolar bone loss in the jaw.
- Discuss the implications of Down syndrome on the periodontium.
- Name three medications that can cause gingival enlargement.
- For a patient in your care with periodontal disease that is amplified by a systemic condition, explain to your clinical instructor the risk factors that may have contributed to the severity of your patient's periodontal disease.

Key Terms

Systemic risk factors
Diabetes mellitus
Well-controlled (diabetes)
Interprofessional collaborative practice
Pregnancy gingivitis

Pregnancy-associated pyogenic granuloma
Menopausal gingivostomatitis
Metabolic syndrome
Acquired immunodeficiency syndrome

Human immunodeficiency virus
Linear gingival erythema
Osteoporosis
Drug-induced gingival enlargement
Medication-related osteonecrosis of the jaw

Neutropenia
Down syndrome
Leukemia
Oral mucositis
Phenytoin
Cyclosporine
Nifedipine

Section 1
Systemic Conditions as Risk Factors for Periodontitis

Additional factors, other than the presence of plaque biofilms, play a significant role in determining why some individuals are more susceptible to periodontal disease than others. A number of systemic diseases, states, or conditions can affect the periodontium in a generalized manner. Systemic risk factors are conditions or diseases that increase an individual's susceptibility to periodontal infection by modifying or amplifying the host response to microbial infection. Systemic risk factors can be modifiable, such as smoking, or nonmodifiable, such as genetic factors, age, or gender.

Many systemic conditions predispose patients to development of more severe and progressive forms of periodontal disease. Proven systemic conditions that are risk factors for periodontitis include diabetes mellitus, osteoporosis, hormone alteration, certain medications, tobacco use, and genetic influences. *The most important known risk factor for periodontitis is cigarette smoking. Tobacco use as a risk factor for periodontal disease is discussed in Chapter 19.*

The relationship between periodontal disease and systemic disease is bidirectional—like a two-way street. On one hand, certain systemic diseases/conditions are risk factors for more severe periodontal disease. On the other hand, periodontal inflammation may play a role in the etiology of some systemic conditions and diseases. *The role of periodontal inflammation in systemic health is discussed in Chapter 34.*

DIABETES MELLITUS

Despite advances in the prevention and medical management, diabetes mellitus continues to be an alarming public health problem in the United States. Recent analysis has estimated that the number of Americans living with diabetes has tripled while the number of new cases has doubled from 1990 to 2010.[1] Moreover, in a recent analysis assessing the mortality rate of diabetic adults versus nondiabetic adults, the mortality rate for adults above the age of 18 years was 1.5 times higher for individuals diagnosed with diabetes compared to individuals not diagnosed with diabetes.[2]

Figures obtained by extrapolating the National Health and Nutrition Examination Survey (NHANES) data to the United States' population indicate that approximately 8.1 million people in the United States have *undiagnosed* diabetes mellitus while 21 million Americans have *diagnosed* diabetes mellitus.[2] The negative impact of diabetes and its complications are not only confined to the United States. The World Health Organization (WHO) projects that that number of diabetic adults worldwide will rise to 366 million and will become the seventh leading cause of death by the year 2030.[3]

Among the various risk factors for periodontitis, diabetes mellitus has been confirmed as a major risk factor.[4,5] Diabetic individuals tend to show a greater prevalence and greater severity of periodontitis compared to nondiabetics. Furthermore, the prevalence of periodontitis is higher and its symptoms are more severe in individuals with diabetes mellitus compared with nondiabetics.[4,6,7] The link between diabetes and periodontal diseases has been the subject of study for many years. Findings from many studies corroborate that diabetes mellitus leads to a hyperinflammatory response to oral microbial biofilms, and impairs resolution of inflammation and repair, which leads to accelerated periodontal destruction.

1. **Characteristics of Diabetes Mellitus.** Diabetes mellitus is a chronic, lifelong metabolic disorder in which the body does not produce and/or properly use insulin. Insulin is a hormone that is needed to convert sugar, starches, and other food into energy that the body uses to sustain life.

2. **Diabetes as a Risk Factor for Periodontitis**

   A. **Well-Controlled Diabetes and Periodontal Disease**

      1. Patients with *well-controlled diabetes* are not any more susceptible to periodontal disease compared to nondiabetic patients. Diabetes is well-controlled if the blood glucose levels are stabilized within the recommended range.

      2. The response of individuals with *controlled diabetes* to nonsurgical periodontal therapy is like that of nondiabetic persons, with similar trends in improved probing depth and attachment gain.[8]

   B. **Undiagnosed or Poorly Controlled Diabetes and Periodontal Disease**

      1. *Diabetes mellitus is currently considered as an established risk factor for periodontitis and contributes to increased prevalence, severity, and progression of periodontitis.*[4,7,9]

      2. Periodontal disease is considered a complication of uncontrolled diabetes. Many epidemiologic studies demonstrate that periodontitis is more prevalent and severe in individuals with uncontrolled diabetes mellitus versus well-controlled or nondiabetic individuals (Figs. 16-1 to 16-3). *People with uncontrolled or undiagnosed diabetes are approximately three times more likely to develop periodontitis.*[8–15]

         a. Individuals with undiagnosed or poorly controlled diabetes have high blood glucose levels. There is a clear relationship between the degree of high blood sugar and the severity of periodontitis.[11,12] As glucose levels increase, individuals with undiagnosed or poorly controlled diabetes experience a dramatic decline in periodontal health.[12,16–18]

         b. Periodontal attachment loss (connective tissue destruction and bone loss) occurs more frequently in individuals with poorly controlled diabetes than in individuals with well-controlled diabetes.[16,18–21]

         c. A person with diabetes who smokes, and who is age 45 or older, is 20 times more likely than a nondiabetic, nonsmoking individual to experience severe periodontitis.

         d. The composition of subgingival periodontal microbiota in a diabetic patient is no different to that found in a nondiabetic patient.[10] In a study comparing diabetic children and their nondiabetic siblings, no differences in the subgingival microflora were found.[22] It can be concluded, then, that diabetes does not favor or influence the growth of a specific periodontal pathogen. Instead, the periodontal destruction seen in diabetic patients may be attributed to the host immunoinflammatory response to nonspecific periodontal pathogens.

         e. Wound healing is adversely affected by diabetes, especially if poorly controlled. An unfavorable treatment outcome may occur in long-term maintenance therapy of individuals with poorly controlled diabetes.[23] Individuals with *poorly controlled* diabetes have a poorer response to nonsurgical and surgical periodontal therapy, more rapid recurrence of deep pockets, and a less favorable long-term response to treatment.

   C. **Other Oral Complications of Poorly Controlled Diabetes Mellitus**

      1. Reduced salivary flow, multiple episodes of abscess formation, cheilosis (painful inflammation at the corners of the lip), and burning mouth or tongue are common complaints of patients with uncontrolled diabetes.[22,24,25] Dental health

care professionals should suspect an underlying undiagnosed diabetes if a patient presents with these symptoms. Referral of the patient to a physician for medical evaluation is strongly recommended.

2. Reduced salivary flow and xerostomia can encourage the growth of *Candida albicans* and the development of oral candidiasis.[26] It can also create an environment that is conducive to cariogenic bacterial growth, thereby predisposing the oral cavity to a higher risk of caries.

3. Individuals with undiagnosed or poorly controlled diabetes frequently present with multiple periodontal abscesses, leading to rapid destruction of periodontal bone support.

4. While these complications are seen in poorly controlled diabetic patients, well-controlled diabetic patients do not typically present with these conditions as they have a normal immune defense against bacterial invasion and normal tissue response.

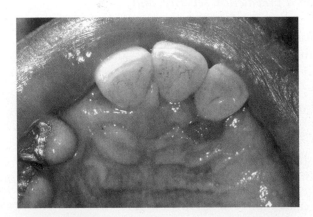

Figure 16-1. Inflammatory Reaction. Note the localized inflammatory swelling of the gingiva on the palatal surface of the maxillary lateral incisor. The patient has uncontrolled diabetes mellitus. This intense inflammatory reaction is typical for individuals with uncontrolled diabetes. (Courtesy of Dr. Ralph Arnold, San Antonio, TX.)

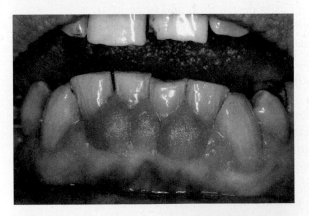

Figure 16-2. Periodontitis Associated With Poorly Controlled Diabetes. Marked tissue changes are evident in this individual with poorly controlled diabetes. (Courtesy of Dr. Richard Foster, Guilford Technical Community College, Jamestown, NC.)

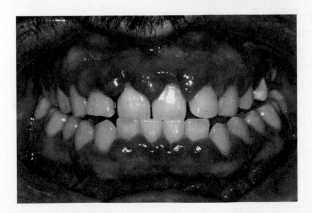

Figure 16-3. Periodontitis Associated With Uncontrolled Diabetes. Examination of this patient revealed pronounced tissue changes and loss of attachment. The patient stated that he has been diagnosed with diabetes but that he is not seeing a physician or taking any medications for diabetes. (Courtesy of Dr. Richard Foster, Guilford Technical Community College, Jamestown, NC.)

3. **Effects of Uncontrolled/Poorly Controlled Diabetes on the Periodontium.** An association between diabetes mellitus and destructive periodontal diseases has been reported in the literature since the 1960s. A combination of several mechanisms is postulated to explain the link between diabetes mellitus and periodontitis including a hyperinflammatory response to infection, the uncoupling of bone destruction and repair, and the role of RAGE.[27] Box 16-1 summarizes key points of the association of diabetes mellitus and periodontal disease.

   A. **Altered Inflammatory Response to Infection.** As mentioned previously, it was hypothesized that individuals with diabetes mellitus might have different oral microbial profiles than individuals without diabetes mellitus.

      1. Researchers studying the subgingival bacterial profiles of individuals with diabetes and individuals without diabetes, however, find that both groups have similar bacterial profiles.[28]

      2. Individuals with diabetes mellitus developed accelerated and exaggerated gingival inflammation compared with those without the disorder, despite a similar bacterial challenge.[29] These study results indicate that it is the host immune response to the oral microbial challenge that primarily drives the intensity of periodontal destruction seen in patients with diabetes mellitus.

         a. **Defective neutrophilic function** in the diabetic patient impairs the initial immune response to infection. Hence, the diabetic patient is more susceptible to infection.

         b. **Hyperresponsive monocytes/macrophages** in diabetic patients results in significant elevated production of proinflammatory cytokines in response to pathogenic invasion. In the presence of periodontal pathogens, the oral cavity is flooded with elevated proinflammatory mediators. These proinflammatory cytokines, such as tumor necrosis factor (TNF)-α, may initiate or worsen the diabetic-related complication or spread to other organ systems and contribute to the worsening of other types of chronic inflammatory conditions, such as cardiovascular disease.

      3. Diabetes mellitus may increase the inflammatory response to bacteria both locally (in the oral cavity) and systemically.

Box 16-1. Key Points: The Diabetes Mellitus—Periodontal Disease Association

- Diabetes mellitus is an established risk factor for periodontitis.
- Diabetes mellitus leads to a hyperinflammatory response to the microbial challenge in periodontitis and impaired repair; these effects are at least partly mediated by the signaling mechanisms of the AGE–RAGE interaction.

   B. **Imbalanced Bone Destruction and Repair.** Research indicates several mechanisms to explain the enhanced alveolar bone destruction seen in individuals with diabetes mellitus.

      1. Alveolar bone is a dynamic, living tissue that is continuously remodeling itself. Bone remodeling serves to maintain the integrity of the bony architecture to meet changing mechanical needs and helps to repair microdamages in the bone matrix. For example, the mandibular condyle is continuously undergoing bone remodeling to respond to everyday mechanical stress that is being applied to it.

         a. The process of bone remodeling is a lifelong process that occurs through the coordinated actions of osteoclasts and osteoblasts.[30]

         b. Osteoclasts are cells that remove old bone (bone resorption). Osteoblasts are cells that then refill the bone cavities with new bone and aid in its mineralization.

    c. In the bone remodeling process, the act of bone formation is tightly coordinated with bone resorption. This coordinated, balanced activity between osteoblasts and osteoclasts is referred to as coupling.

  2. While some of the tissue damage associated with periodontitis likely results from the direct actions of bacteria and infiltrating leukocytes, the rapid alveolar bone loss seen in individuals with diabetes mellitus may result from an uncoupling of the activities of osteoblasts and osteoclasts. Two recent studies indicate that diabetes mellitus could contribute to the net loss of alveolar bone in periodontitis via prolonged osteoclastic formation and activity and increased programmed cell death (apoptosis) of osteoblasts, which impairs bone formation following bone resorption.[31,32]

C. The Role of RAGE

  1. AGE and RAGE

    a. Glycation is a natural metabolic process in which the glucose in the bloodstream (from carbohydrates and sugars) irreversibly attaches to proteins and lipids, forming harmful new molecules called *advanced glycation end products* or AGEs.

      1) In homeostasis, AGEs can be found at such low levels that they do not have any demonstrable pathologic effect.

      2) Under certain pathologic conditions, such as hyperglycemia in patients with diabetes, AGE formation is increased beyond normal physiologic levels.

    b. AGE-modified proteins have been found in the gingival tissues of diabetic patients with periodontitis and in the saliva of diabetic patients.[33,34]

    c. Excessive accumulation of AGE proteins has been implicated in altering the physiologic properties and normal function of collagen which is the major protein found in the human body.

      1) AGEs allegedly degrade collagen and elastin, causing these fibers to harden and lose elasticity.

      2) This process is of particular concern for diabetics, who already suffer from the effects of poor glucose control. In fact, elevated levels of AGEs contribute to a number of diabetes-related complications, including neuropathy, retinal disease, and kidney failure.

    d. Direct interaction of AGE to a cell surface receptor known as RAGE triggers pathologic tissue destruction. Cell surface receptors are important proteins in the membranes of cells that mediate communication between the cell and the outside world. They act by binding to extracellular molecules.

      1) A receptor, nicknamed RAGE, from *receptor for advanced glycation end products*, is found on the cell membrane surface of many cells, such as endothelial cells, neurons, monocytes/macrophages, and even cells of the periodontium.

      2) The interaction of AGE–RAGE stimulates the release of proinflammatory cytokines, such as TNF-α and interleukin (IL)-1β. Over time, if diabetes is left uncontrolled, the continuous activation of the AGE–RAGE interaction leads to a massive release of proinflammatory mediators. Thus, the AGE–RAGE interaction is one of the major factors that contribute to the **exaggerated periodontal and systemic inflammation, insulin resistance,** and **impaired tissue repair** seen in diabetic patients with periodontitis.

    e. Increased RAGE expression is reported in gingival tissues of individuals with diabetes mellitus and periodontitis.[35–37]

2. Thus, it is believed that the bacterial challenge in an environment of enhanced RAGE expression in the periodontium of an individual with diabetes mellitus leads to exaggerated inflammation and impaired repair, which then results in accelerated and severe periodontal destruction.[27] Figure 16-4 depicts the postulated effects of uncontrolled diabetes mellitus on the periodontium.

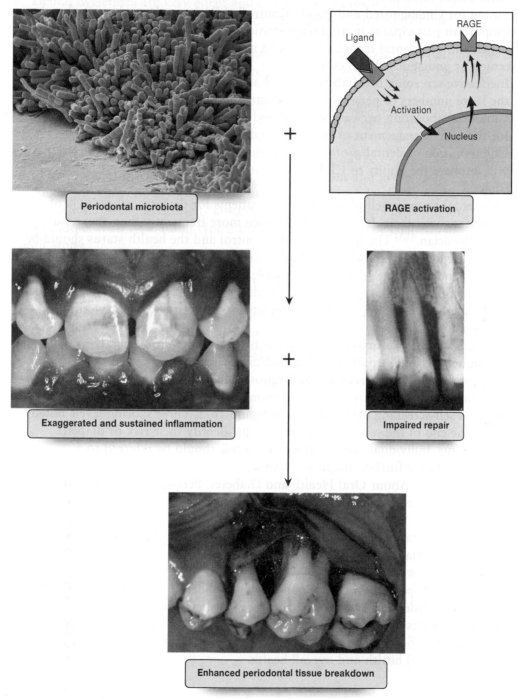

Figure 16-4. Postulated Effects of Uncontrolled Diabetes Mellitus on the Periodontium. A model for the role of diabetes mellitus in the accelerated periodontal destruction in individuals with uncontrolled or poorly controlled diabetes mellitus. The microbial challenge combined with an environment of enhanced RAGE expression leads to exaggerated inflammation and impaired repair, which in turn, causes accelerated and severe periodontal destruction. RAGE, receptor for advanced glycation end products.

Did you know that:

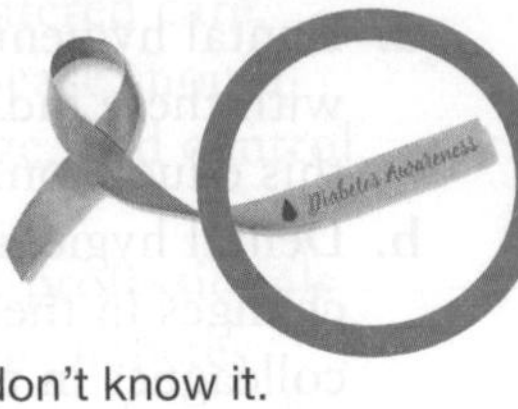

- Diabetes causes destruction of your eyesight, kidneys, nerves and heart.
- Diabetes increases your risk for gum disease which leads to tooth loss.
- Diabetes slows your ability to heal from injury and infections sometimes resulting in amputation.
- 115 million adults in the US have either diabetes or pre-diabetes and 1/3 don't know it.

Assess Your Diabetes Risk

1. Are you more than 10% above ideal body weight?

○ Yes   ○ No

2. Is your waist size over 35" (for women) or 40" (for men)?

○ Yes   ○ No

3. Do you have any biologic family members with a history of diabetes?

○ Yes   ○ No

4. Are you African American, Alaskan Native, American Indian, Hispanic, or of Arabic descent??

○ Yes   ○ No

5. Do you have a history of, or take medication for high blood pressure?

○ Yes   ○ No

6. Do you have or take medications for high cholesterol or abnormal good/bad cholesterol ratio?

○ Yes   ○ No

7. Do you experience tingling, pain, or numbness in your hands or feet?

○ Yes   ○ No

8. Do you experience unexplainable hunger, thirst, or frequent urination?

○ Yes   ○ No

9. Have you experienced blurred vision, cataracts or glaucoma?

○ Yes   ○ No

10. Do your gums bleed when you brush your teeth?

○ Yes   ○ No

11. Are you over 35 years old?

○ Yes   ○ No

12. If you are over 35, are you also over 65?

○ Yes   ○ No

Scoring Key.
Low risk = 2 or less yes answers; Moderate risk = 3 to 5 yes answers;
High risk = 6 or more yes answers.

Figure 16-5. Diabetes Self-Screening Tool. This 14-point self-screening tool is based on (1) known risk factors for metabolic syndrome, diabetes, insulin resistance; (2) symptoms of hyperglycemia; and (3) diabetic complications. (Used by permission of Dr. Susan Maples, Holt, MI.)

STRESS

1. Characteristics of Stress
   A. A stress response, such as a fight-or-flight response, is one of the body's survival mechanisms. An acute stress response prepares the cardiovascular, musculoskeletal, and neuroendocrine systems to respond to a fight-or-flight situation.
   B. While *acute* stress can be immunoenhancing, ***chronic*** stress has been shown to impair the physiological regulatory mechanism that governs the immune response. The regulatory mechanism is mediated by elevated levels of cortisol. Cortisol is a steroid hormone made in the cortex of the adrenal glands and then released into the blood. Cortisol has anti-inflammatory and immunosuppressive properties, and whose levels in the blood may become elevated in response to physical or psychological stress. Figure 16-6 depicts the relationship of chronic stress to systemic conditions and periodontal disease.
   C. The potential effects of chronic stress can be manifested as anxiety, depression, impaired cognition, or altered self-esteem.

2. Stress as a Risk Factor for Periodontitis
   A. Numerous clinical studies have investigated the correlation between chronic periodontal disease and stress.[49–52]
      1. The majority of studies included in a recent systematic review showed a positive relationship between stress and periodontal disease.[53]
      2. High financial stress and depression are significant risk factors for periodontal disease after adjusting for age, gender, smoking, diabetes, and periodontal microorganisms.[52,54]
   B. Stress-induced behavioral changes may explain the detrimental effect of stress on periodontal health. These behavioral changes include poor self-care,[55] changed dietary habits,[56] increased smoking,[51] increased alcohol consumption,[57] and nonadherence to periodontal maintenance regimens.[58]
      1. The relationship between stress and neglected self-care is demonstrated in medical students undertaking medical exams. Exam students reported a reduction in thoroughness of oral hygiene behavior and had higher plaque scores than the control group of students not taking exams.[59] The authors of this study conclude that stress may induce neglect of self-care routines and increase biofilm accumulation.
      2. Stress-induced eating behaviors—such as excessive consumption of refined carbohydrates—may increase accumulation of plaque biofilm.[60]
   C. Stress: Implications for the Dental Hygienist
      1. Prolonged or intense periods of stress can cause suppression of the immune system which might tip the host-microbial interaction in favor of bacteria causing increased attachment loss. Stress also effects how people look after themselves and might lead to less effective daily plaque biofilm removal, increased tobacco use, and poor nutrition.
      2. Managing periodontal health in people undergoing significant stress requires recognition of stress as a risk factor for periodontal disease.
      3. Making patients aware of the potential effects of stress on their general and oral health is a method for the hygienist in guiding patients to think about strategies for stress management. In this context, the dental team may need to work in cooperation with the patient's physician and a mental health care expert to achieve optimal treatment outcomes.
      4. It may be necessary to recommend shorter intervals between professional care appointments to compensate for the patient's behavioral changes.

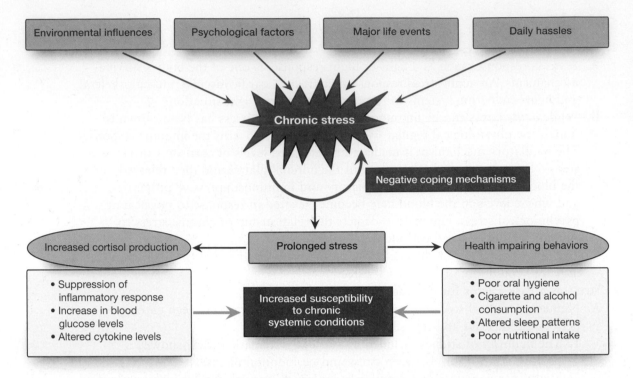

Figure 16-6. Relationship of Chronic Stress to Systemic Conditions and Periodontal Disease.

HORMONAL FLUCTUATIONS DURING PUBERTY, PREGNANCY, AND MENOPAUSE

Changes in sex hormones occurring in puberty, pregnancy, and following menopause can influence the periodontal tissues.

1. **Puberty**
   A. **Impact of Puberty on the Periodontium**
      1. During puberty, there are increased levels of estradiol in females and testosterone in males. Increased levels of sex hormones during puberty cause increased blood circulation to the gingival tissues and may cause an increased sensitivity to local irritants, such as plaque biofilms, resulting in pubertal gingivitis.
      2. The period around puberty is associated with increased gingival inflammation in both sexes, despite constant plaque biofilm levels.[61–64]
         a. Changes in the composition of the subgingival microbiota, rather than in the amount of plaque biofilm, are the most likely contributing factors.[65]
         b. The increased secretion of steroid hormones during puberty may have a direct association with the prevalence of certain periodontal pathogens.
      3. Pubertal gingivitis occurs equally in girls and boys. The tendency for plaque-induced gingivitis usually decreases as the young person progresses through puberty.
      4. Clinical features of pubertal gingivitis include:
         • An accumulation of plaque biofilm
         • Red, inflamed, swollen gingival tissue; bleeding upon probing
         • Inflammation that is reversible with meticulous daily self-care; reversible following puberty
   B. **Implications for the Dental Hygienist**
      1. Dental hygienists should stress that daily attention to biofilm control (self-care) and frequent professional care are very important for gingival health during puberty.[66]

2. Since early diagnosis ensures the greatest chance for successful treatment, it is important that children and adolescents receive a periodontal examination as part of their routine dental visits.

3. Depending on the patient's level of self-care, the frequency of professional care may need to be increased.

2. **Pregnancy**

A. **Impact of Hormonal Fluctuations in Pregnancy on the Periodontium**

1. Studies show that no pregnancy-related changes occur if the gingiva is clinically healthy.[67,68] However, under the influence of increased sex hormones, the severity and extent of *existing* gingival inflammation is dramatically exaggerated during pregnancy.[69–73]

2. Increased levels of estrogen have been shown to alter the microbial profile of subgingival plaque.

   a. In a classic study conducted by Kornman and Loesche examining the subgingival microbial profile in pregnancy, it was found that the second trimester was associated with increased gingival inflammation and increased levels of *Prevotella intermedia*.[74]

   b. It was surmised that the increased growth of *P. intermedia* was due to this specific microorganism's ability to exploit estrogen as a substitute for its natural growth factor, menadione. This finding would suggest that elevated levels of *P. intermedia* is associated with pregnancy-induced gingivitis.

3. Inflammation of the gingiva increases in pregnant women in the presence of even small amounts of plaque biofilm. Pregnant women tend to exhibit more gingival inflammation than do women 6 months postpartum, despite similar plaque scores.

   a. The likelihood of gingival inflammation increases in the second and third trimesters when elevated estrogen levels in the blood exaggerate the host response to plaque biofilm and other local irritants.[75] Pregnant women, near or at term, produce high levels of estradiol, estriol, and progesterone.

   b. Elevated progesterone levels in pregnancy enhance capillary permeability and dilation, resulting in increased gingival exudate and edema.[76]

   c. During pregnancy, profound changes in immune response impact the periodontal tissues.[77] High levels of progesterone and estrogen associated with pregnancy have been shown to suppress the immune response to dental plaque biofilm. polymorphonuclear neutrophil (PMN) chemotaxis and phagocytosis have been reported to be depressed in response to high levels of gestational hormones.[78]

4. Gingival inflammation initiated by plaque biofilms, and exacerbated by hormonal changes in the second and third trimesters of pregnancy, is referred to as **pregnancy gingivitis**.

   a. The gingival tissue may be edematous and dark red, with bulbous interdental papillae (Figs. 16-7 and 16-8).

   b. In some cases, a gingival papilla can react so strongly to plaque biofilm that a large, localized overgrowth of gingival tissue called a **pregnancy-associated pyogenic granuloma** (pregnancy tumor), may form on the interdental gingiva or on the gingival margin (Fig. 16-9).

      1) These growths are benign and are generally not painful.

      2) If the growth persists after delivery, it can be surgically removed.

   c. Probing depths, bleeding on probing, and crevicular fluid flow are increased in pregnancy gingivitis.

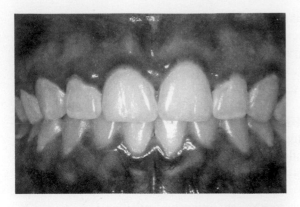

Figure 16-7. Pregnancy Gingivitis. Clinical appearance of reddened, swollen tissues of pregnancy gingivitis. (Courtesy of Dr. Richard Foster, Guilford Technical Community College, Jamestown, NC.)

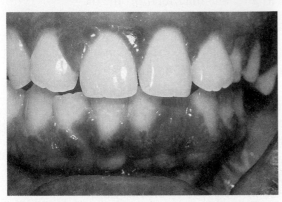

Figure 16-8. Hormonal Gingivitis. Hormonal gingivitis is evident 3 weeks postpartum (after giving birth) in this female patient. (Used with permission from Langlais RP. *Color Atlas of Common Oral Diseases*. Philadelphia, PA: Wolters Kluwer; 2003.)

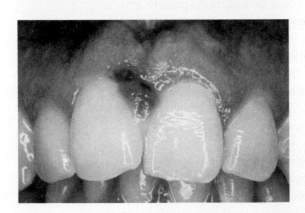

Figure 16-9. Pregnancy-Associated Pyogenic Granuloma. The clinical appearance of a pyogenic granuloma (pregnancy tumor).

B. **Expectant Patient: Implications for the Dental Hygienist**
1. Dental professionals and gynecologists should educate pregnant patients about the importance of oral health. The perinatal period is an ideal time to educate and perform dental treatment on expectant mothers.[74,79] Pregnancy provides an opportunity to educate women regarding oral health self-care and future child-care.[80]
   a. The dental hygienist should ask the expectant woman if she has any concerns about getting dental care while pregnant and be ready to address her concerns.
   b. Expectant women should be advised that prevention, diagnosis, and treatment of oral diseases—including needed dental x-ray and use of local anesthesia—is safe, beneficial, and can be undertaken any time during pregnancy.[81,82] Also, acute/emergency care may be provided at any time during pregnancy.

    c. Hygienists should encourage behaviors that support good oral health:
       1) Meticulous daily self-care for biofilm control.
       2) Prenatal vitamins, including folic acid to reduce the risk of birth defects such as cleft lip and palate.
       3) Chewing xylitol-containing gum to decrease caries risk.

  2. Expectant women experiencing frequent nausea and vomiting should be advised that erosion of tooth surfaces might be reduced by:
    a. Eating more frequent, smaller meals consisting of nutritious foods.
    b. A rinse comprised of one-teaspoon baking soda in a cup of water should be used to rinse and spit out after vomiting. Caution the patient to avoid tooth brushing directly after vomiting as the effect of erosion can be exacerbated.

  3. A comprehensive periodontal treatment plan should be developed for preventive, treatment, and maintenance care throughout pregnancy. In addition, the importance of regular dental care during the postpartum period and thereafter should be emphasized.

  4. Dental care should be coordinated with the expectant woman's medical care professional to ascertain whether other risk factors—such as gestational diabetes—are present and to advise the medical professional of the periodontal status of the patient and any proposed treatment.[82]

3. Menopause

  A. Impact of Menopause on the Periodontium

    1. Menopause typically occurs in the fourth-to-fifth decade of a woman's life.
      a. Menopause is a natural condition that all women experience as they age.
        1) Unlike the pubertal stage and the pregnancy stage, menopause is characterized by a *decreased* production of estrogen by the ovaries (Fig. 16-10).
        2) This decreased estrogen production has wide-spread systemic effects since estrogen is a key hormone that regulates the function of many parts of the body, such as the brain, heart, blood vessels, skin, reproductive organs, and bones.
      b. In menopause, many physical and behavioral changes occur. Several of these changes may adversely affect the oral cavity and make some women more susceptible to periodontal disease.
        1) Dental health care providers often are the first professionals to notice changes that occur during menopause. The periodontium is extremely susceptible to hormonal changes that take place just before and during menopause.
        2) A literature review by Dutt and colleagues compiled data on the major orodental complications observed during menopause. This review observed that the health of the periodontium is most severely affected, followed by dry mouth and burning mouth, which in turn, may increase the occurrence of oral mucosal and dental diseases, such as candidiasis.[83]

    2. If menopause does affect the gingiva, it is called **menopausal gingivostomatitis**. Menopausal gingivostomatitis is characterized by gingivae that bleed readily, with an abnormally pale, dry, shiny erythematous appearance.[84]

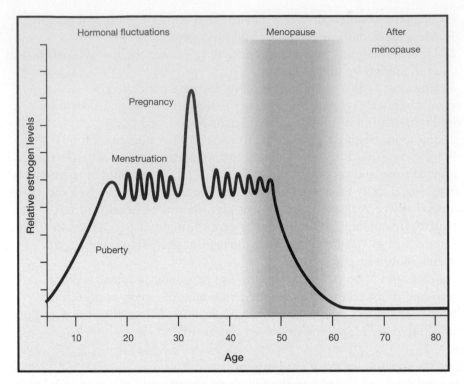

Figure 16-10. Fluctuation in Estrogen Levels Throughout a Woman's Life.

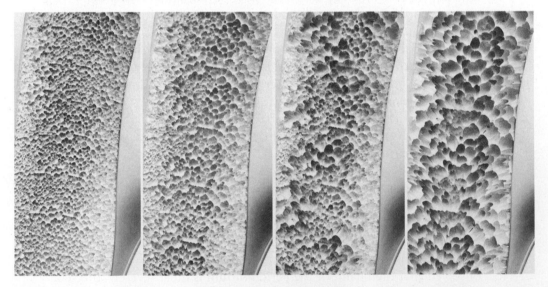

Figure 16-11. Healthy Bone Versus Bone With Osteoporosis. The first illustration on the left depicts the structure of healthy bone. The center two illustrations show progressive reduction in bone mass. The illustration on the far right depicts the significant reduction in bone mass commonly seen in osteoporosis.

3. During menopause, there is a decline in hormonal levels, most notably, a rapid decline in estrogen levels.
   a. Lack of estrogen during and after menopause may cause the loss of bone density (Fig. 16-11). The rapid decline in estrogen can lead to systemic bone loss. Osteoporosis is a reduction in bone mass that causes an increased susceptibility to fractures (Fig. 16-11). Osteopenia is a condition in which there is a lower than average bone density but not necessarily an increase in the risk or incidence of fracture.
   b. Decreased estrogen levels in women with osteopenia were found to be associated with loss of crestal density of alveolar bone.[85]
4. Bisphosphonates are the most commonly prescribed medications to inhibit the bone resorption of systemic osteoporosis. In dentistry, there is concern about medication-related osteonecrosis of the jaw.[86] Medication-related osteonecrosis of the jaw is a rare disorder characterized by painful areas of exposed bone in the mouth that fail to heal after an extraction or oral surgery procedure. Bisphosphonates and osteonecrosis are discussed in Chapter 28, Host Modulation Therapy.
5. The same processes that lead to loss of bone in the spine and hips can also lead to loss of alveolar bone.
   a. There may be a link between skeletal osteoporosis, alveolar bone loss in the jaw, and tooth loss.[87–91] Preliminary studies report significant correlations between mandibular bone mineral density and hipbone mineral bone density.[89,90]
   b. A vast number of studies show a positive association between osteoporosis and periodontal destruction.[90,92,93–96]
   c. However, there are also studies which show no association between osteoporosis and periodontal disease.[97,98] Thus, ongoing research is being performed to improve our understanding of the link between bone metabolic disorders and periodontal destruction. The relationship between alveolar bone loss and systemic bone loss, however, is not yet fully understood.[99]

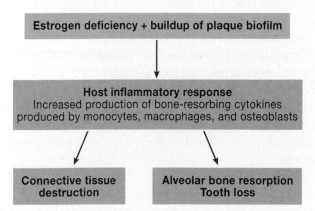

Figure 16-12. Postulated Effects of Estrogen Deficiency on the Periodontium. Estrogen deficiency leads to a decrease in bone mineral density in the alveolar bone. Together with the oral biofilm infection and the host inflammatory response, the affected site will exhibit accelerated bone loss and more exaggerated connective tissue destruction.

     d. Estrogen replacement therapy improves bone density in postmenopausal women. In a 3-year study, hormone/estrogen replacement therapy significantly increased alveolar bone alveolar bone mass compared with placebo and tended to improve alveolar crest.[100]

   6. Genco and Grossi[93] have proposed a model for estrogen deficiency as a risk factor for periodontal disease (Fig. 16-12).

   7. Postmenopausal female smokers were more likely to lose alveolar bone height and density than nonsmokers with a similar periodontitis, plaque, and gingival bleeding experience. In addition, both smoking and osteoporosis/osteopenia provided a negative influence on alveolar bone.[94]

B. Menopause: Implications for the Dental Hygienist

   1. Dental hygienists and gynecologists should educate postmenopausal women about osteoporosis and interventions such as calcium supplements and weight-bearing exercise.

   2. Meticulous daily self-care, combined with regular professional care, decreases the likelihood of periodontal problems during menopause.

   3. Dental hygienists need to advise patients of the common risk factors, such as smoking, for both osteoporosis and periodontal disease.[94]

   4. Dental hygienists should be aware of the possible oral side effects associated with bisphosphonates, antiresorptive agents, and antiangiogenic medications and should be able recognize the signs and symptoms of MRONJ.

   5. As newer classes of osteoporotic medications are being approved and introduced to the public, dental hygienists should be aware of how they work and what possible oral side-effects these agents may possess.

METABOLIC SYNDROME

1. Characteristics of Metabolic Syndrome

   A. Metabolic syndrome refers to a combination of closely related metabolic disturbances—increased blood pressure, high blood sugar, excess body fat around the waist, abnormal cholesterol or triglyceride levels, a proinflammatory state, and an increased tendency toward thrombosis (blood clots in blood vessels)—that occur together, increasing the risk of heart disease, stroke, and diabetes.[95]

   B. The benefit in defining metabolic syndrome is that it helps to identify individuals at high risk for developing type 2 diabetes mellitus and cardiovascular disease–related conditions.[96]

     1. A diagnosis of metabolic syndrome is made based on a patient having abdominal obesity with any two of the four following factors: hypertension, hyperglycemia, high cholesterol, and raised triglyceride levels.[101]

     2. Metabolic syndrome has a greater prevalence reported among older populations.[97] However, recent reports show that metabolic syndrome affects a significant portion of children and adolescents in many ethnic groups.[98,102,103] In the United States alone, one out of every three adults are estimated to have metabolic syndrome.[104]

2. Metabolic Syndrome and Periodontitis

   A. Impact of Metabolic Syndrome on the Periodontium

     1. Metabolic syndrome and abdominal obesity are considered to be risk factors for periodontitis.[5,105–112] Having three or more components of metabolic syndrome is significantly associated with a higher prevalence of periodontitis.[113]

2. The apparent association between metabolic syndrome and periodontitis may be explained by shared common risk factors, such as obesity, diet, and inadequate self-care.[110] Obesity is associated with increased levels and proportions of periodontal pathogens, especially in patients with periodontitis.[114]

3. Metabolic syndrome may influence the progression of periodontitis by contributing to chronic low-grade inflammation of prolonged duration.[115,116]
   a. Low-grade chronic inflammation is postulated to be due to the sustained actions of the adipocytes (fat cells). Previously, adipocytes were thought to be dormant, inactive cells.
   b. However, recent research has shed light that adipocytes are very active cells that produce various types of adipokines (cytokines secreted by adipose tissue).
   c. In obese patients, the increased numbers of adipocytes lead to greater release of adipokines which causes a sustained inflammatory state, insulin resistance, and increased susceptibility to periodontal disease[117] (Fig. 16-13).

4. Hypertension associated with metabolic syndrome may exacerbate periodontitis due to impaired blood flow to the periodontium.[118]

B. **Metabolic Syndrome: Implications for the Dental Hygienist**
   1. Results from a recent randomized controlled trial indicate that periodontal therapy in individuals with metabolic syndrome leads to a significant improvement in periodontal health.[119]
   2. Management of metabolic syndrome is based on lifestyle modifications, including increased physical activity and dietary modifications. Dental hygienists are well positioned to provide nutritional counseling for individuals exhibiting signs of metabolic syndrome.

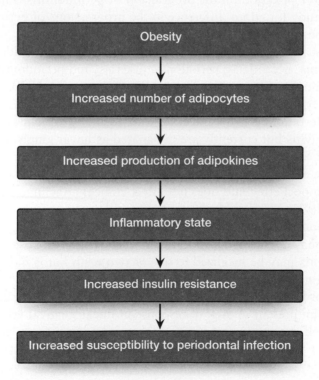

Figure 16-13. Relationship of Metabolic Syndrome and Periodontal Disease. In obese patients, the increased numbers of adipocytes lead to greater release of adipokines which causes a sustained inflammatory state, insulin resistance, and increased susceptibility to periodontal disease.

HIV/AIDS

1. Characteristics of HIV Infection
   A. Acquired immunodeficiency syndrome (AIDS) is a communicable disease caused by human immunodeficiency virus (HIV). People with acquired immunodeficiency syndrome are at an increased risk for developing certain cancers and for infections that usually occur only in individuals with a weak immune system.
      1. In most developed countries, the death rate from AIDS among adults has declined largely because of newer antiretroviral therapies and improved access to these therapies.[120,121]
      2. Nevertheless, because of the large numbers of numbers of existing plus new cases of HIV infection, dental and medical practitioners will still be required to treat oral and periodontal conditions in HIV-infected adults and children.[122]
   B. HIV infection has a profound effect on cellular immunity (T-lymphocytes, B-cells, monocyte/macrophage function). Decreased monocyte chemotaxis and phagocytosis, together with increased production of TNF-α and IL-1, and diminished capacity to present antigen to T-cells explain the increased periodontal attachment loss found in HIV-infected individuals.[123–126]
   C. Studies of healing following tooth extraction in HIV-positive patients indicate that there is a delayed healing response in both the hard and soft tissues.[117,127]
2. Periodontal and Oral Manifestations of HIV Infection
   A. HIV-related oral manifestations include hairy leukoplakia, candidiasis, herpes labialis, recurrent intraoral herpes simplex, herpes zoster, recurrent aphthous ulcers, and Kaposi sarcoma.
   B. Studies suggest that gingival recession and alveolar bone loss are more frequent in HIV-positive patients.[128–130]
      1. The effect of HIV infection on the progression of periodontitis is not clear. A recent 7-year study found no difference in the progressions of periodontitis between HIV-positive and HIV-negative women.[132]
      2. Periodontal diseases strongly associated with HIV-infection include linear gingival erythema, necrotizing periodontal diseases, and periodontitis.[120,133]
   C. Necrotizing periodontal diseases are discussed in Chapters 9 and 30.
   D. Linear Gingival Erythema
      1. Gingival manifestations of HIV infection were formerly known as HIV-associated gingivitis but currently are designated as linear gingival erythema. Linear gingival erythema (LGE) is characterized by a 2- to 3-mm marginal band of intense erythema (redness) in the free gingiva (Fig. 16-14). LGE is not associated with pocketing and does not affect clinical attachment levels or alveolar bone levels.
      2. The band of gingival erythema may extend into the attached gingiva and/or extend beyond the mucogingival line into the alveolar mucosa.[134] Linear gingival erythema may be localized to one or two teeth but is more commonly a generalized gingival condition.
      3. The intensity of LGE inflammation is exaggerated in relation to the amount of plaque biofilm present. A lack of response of linear gingival erythema to conventional self-care and periodontal therapy is an important criterion in its diagnosis.[135]

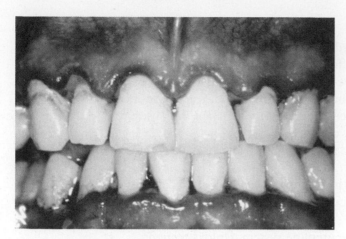

Figure 16-14. Linear Gingival Erythema. Gingival changes associated with linear gingival erythema. Note the marginal band of intense erythema in the free gingiva.

4. The etiology of linear gingival erythema is not well understood. Research suggests that organisms not generally associated with gingivitis, such as *Candida* species, are associated with linear gingival erythema.[134,136]
5. With the advent of antiretroviral therapy for HIV-positive patients, the prevalence of HIV-specific lesions has been dramatically reduced.[11,108,137,138]

3. **HIV-Infected Individuals: Implications for the Dental Hygienist**
   A. Evidence suggests that it is safe to perform periodontal therapy in HIV-infected patients. Even surgical therapy is permitted as long as the individual's immune system is competent.[139]
      1. The initial treatment for linear gingival erythema should be standard periodontal therapy plus the use of 0.12% chlorhexidine gluconate as a mouth rinse. Consideration may be given to the use of antibiotics.[135]
      2. HIV-infected individuals should be monitored to prevent irreversible periodontal damage.
      3. The need for early periodontal therapy and more frequent maintenance visits should be stressed. Continuity of dental care remains important for HIV+ patients even when they are being treated with antiretroviral therapies.[137,140,141]
      4. Dental health care providers should emphasize the importance of careful self-care at home and frequent professional care visits.[140]
   B. Care should be coordinated with other health professionals. Interprofessional collaboration among professionals such as physicians, dental professionals, social workers, dieticians, and case managers is an essential component of patient-centered care.[142,143] To assess for a patient's HIV status, consultation with the patient's physician (or nurse practitioner) requesting the most up-to-date CD4+ count (the number of functioning T-helper cells) and viral level count should be performed.
   C. Despite the beneficial effects of antiretroviral therapies, drug interactions with other medications have been observed. For instance, fluconazole, ketoconazole, itraconazole, metronidazole, ciprofloxacin, midazolam, and triazolam can interact with some antiretroviral medications, such as zidovudine, nevirapine, and ritonavir. Dental professionals need an understanding of possible drug interactions in HIV-infected individuals that can occur during the course and duration of dental treatment.[120]
   D. Strict adherence to infection control is strongly recommended by the ADA and the CDC. This will minimize the risk to both dental staff and immunocompromised patients who are not only at risk of transmitting the disease, but also at risk of acquiring an infection from a health care setting.

NEUTROPENIA

1. **Characteristics of Neutropenia.** As discussed in previous chapters, PMNs are a type of white blood cell important to fighting off infections—particularly those caused by bacteria. Neutropenia (noo-troe-PEE-nee-uh) is a disorder characterized by the presence of abnormally few numbers of neutrophils in the blood, leading to increased susceptibility to infection. A diagnosis of neutropenia is made when the absolute neutrophil count falls below 1,500 cells/μL of blood.

   A. Neutropenias may be the result of bone marrow failure and/or accelerated destruction of PMNs.

   B. Neutropenias may be congenital—such as cyclic neutropenia—associated with leukemia, drug-induced, radiation-induced, or idiopathic (of unknown cause).

2. **Neutropenia and Periodontitis**

   A. Since PMNs are the first responders, the immune system deploys to fight off microbial invasion, individuals with neutropenia are more susceptible to periodontal diseases compared to nonneutropenic, healthy individuals.[142]

   B. Higher plaque scores, gingival bleeding, gingival inflammation, and alveolar bone loss are reported in individuals with neutropenia.[144–147] Figure 16-15 shows a patient with cyclic neutropenia who exhibits pronounced gingival inflammation.

3. **Neutropenia: Implications for the Dental Hygienist**

   A. Prevention of oral infections is important in reducing the risk of systemic bacteremia and septicemia, as well as, maintaining the patient's dentition for quality of life.[145,148,149]

      1. Periodontal infections may induce fever and systemic dissemination of microorganisms. Hygienists should educate patients with neutropenia about the importance of meticulous self-care and frequent professional care for the maintenance of systemic and oral health.

      2. Chlorhexidine gluconate mouthwash (0.12%) has been shown to reduce the severity of oral mucosal inflammation and decrease plaque scores.[150–153]

   B. Acute periodontal exacerbations should be treated by removal of local causative factors by gentle periodontal instrumentation, chlorhexidine mouthwash rinse, and/or irrigation.[154]

   C. Patients with neutropenia are considered to be immunocompromised. Therefore, strict adherence to infection control is strongly recommended to reduce the risk of neutropenic patients acquiring a disease from a health care setting.

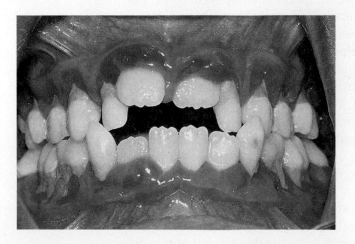

Figure 16-15. Cyclic Neutropenia. This individual with cyclic neutropenia exhibits pronounced gingival erythema. (Used with permission from Langlais RP. *Color Atlas of Common Oral Diseases*. Philadelphia, PA: Wolters Kluwer; 2003.)

DOWN SYNDROME

1. **Characteristics of Down Syndrome.** Down syndrome is a genetic disorder caused by a gene problem that happens before birth. Down syndrome is a lifelong condition, which varies in severity, causing intellectual disability and developmental delays, and in some people, health problems.
    A. **Genetic Changes in Down Syndrome**
        1. Normally, the nucleus of each cell contains 46 chromosomes. In Down syndrome, however, the nucleus contains 47 chromosomes. Most cases of Down syndrome occur because there are three copies of the 21st chromosome. For this reason, Down syndrome is also referred to as trisomy 21.
        2. Due to advances in medical treatment, individuals with Down syndrome are living longer. As the mortality rate associated with Down syndrome decreases, the prevalence of adults with Down syndrome in our society will increase. More and more dental health care providers will interact with individuals with this condition, increasing the need for education and acceptance.
    B. **Orofacial Features Characteristic of People With Down Syndrome.** Among the most common orofacial traits of individuals with Down syndrome are:
        1. An underdeveloped midfacial region, affecting the appearance of the lips, tongue, and palate.
            a. The maxilla, the bridge of the nose, and the bones of the midface region are smaller than in the general population, creating a prognathic occlusal relationship. Mouth breathing may occur because of smaller nasal passages, and the tongue may protrude because of a smaller midface region. People with Down syndrome often have a strong gag reflex due to placement of the tongue, as well as anxiety associated with any oral stimulation.
            b. The palate, although normal sized, may appear highly vaulted and narrow. This deceiving appearance is due to the unusual thickness of the sides of the hard palate. This thickness restricts the amount of space the tongue can occupy in the mouth and affects the ability to speak and chew.
            c. The lips may grow large and thick. Fissured lips may result from chronic mouth breathing. Additionally, decreased muscle tone may cause the mouth to droop and the lower lip to protrude. Increased drooling, compounded by a chronically open mouth, contributes to angular cheilitis.
            d. The tongue also develops cracks and fissures with age; this condition can contribute to halitosis.
        2. Malocclusion is found in most people with Down syndrome because of the delayed eruption of permanent teeth and underdevelopment of the maxilla. A smaller maxilla contributes to an open bite, leading to poor positioning of teeth and increasing the likelihood of periodontal disease and dental caries.
    C. **Medical and Developmental Problems of Patients With Down Syndrome**
        1. Children are at increased risk for congenital heart defects, susceptibility to infection, respiratory problems, gastrointestinal abnormalities, and childhood leukemia.
        2. Abnormal PMN function is seen in about half of all patients with Down syndrome.
        3. Most individuals with Down syndrome have IQs in the mild to moderate range of mental retardation. Those who receive good medical care and experience a supportive social environment can attend school, hold jobs, and participate in decisions that affect them (Fig. 16-16).

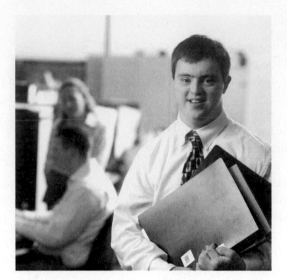

Figure 16-16. Individuals With Down Syndrome in the Workforce. With appropriate training and support people with Down Syndrome can and do make a huge contribution to their workplace. (Courtesy of Getty Images.)

2. **Down Syndrome and Periodontitis.** Down syndrome is one of the most common birth defects. Though rare genetic syndromes are unlikely to be encountered by the dental hygienist outside a hospital setting, *persons with Down syndrome are frequently treated by members of the dental team in general and periodontal dental offices.*
    A. It is widely known that individuals with Down syndrome often exhibit severe and rapid periodontal breakdown.
        1. The prevalence of periodontal disease ranges from 58 to 96 percent of young adults under 35 years of age with Down syndrome.[155]
        2. Substantial plaque biofilm formation, deep periodontal pockets, and extensive gingival inflammation characterize periodontal disease in Down syndrome (Figs. 16-17 and 16-18).[156]
    B. Children experience rapid, destructive periodontal disease. Consequently, large numbers of them lose their permanent anterior teeth in their early teens.
        1. At least some children with Down syndrome are congenitally missing at least one salivary gland.[157]
        2. Studies indicate that various periodontal pathogens colonize the gingival tissues in the very early childhood years of children with Down syndrome.[158]
    C. The etiology of periodontal disease in persons with Down syndrome is complex. The prevalence of periodontal disease cannot simply be attributed to poor daily self-care. In recent years, much focus has been placed on the altered immune response resulting from the underlying genetic disorder.[155,159]
        1. Impaired PMN chemotaxis and phagocytosis most likely explain the high prevalence and increased severity of periodontitis associated with Down syndrome.
        2. Impaired cellular motility of gingival fibroblasts that prevents wound healing and regeneration of periodontal tissues may be involved in the etiology of Down syndrome periodontitis.[160]
3. **Down Syndrome: Implications for the Dental Hygienist**
    A. Early and frequent professional treatment and meticulous daily care at home can mitigate the severity of periodontal disease in individuals with Down syndrome.
        1. Some people with Down syndrome can brush and floss independently, but many need help from caregivers.
        2. Encourage independence in daily self-care in those individuals who are capable on their own. Involve patients in hands-on demonstrations of brushing and interdental cleaning aids.

B. Hygienists should educate caregivers about daily self-care. The dental health care provider should demonstrate proper home care techniques to both the patient and the caregiver. A power toothbrush and power water flossing device can simplify oral care.

1. The hygienist can demonstrate techniques to caregivers on techniques to access the oral cavity, such as having the person close slightly for improved access to the posterior teeth and where to sit or stand to gain easier access to different areas of the dentition.

2. The hygienist should emphasize to the caregiver the importance of establishing a daily routine for oral care.

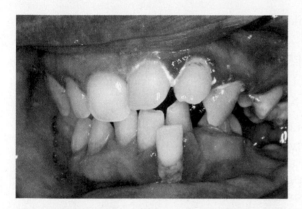

Figure 16-17. Periodontitis and Down Syndrome. A 25-year-old patient with Down syndrome exhibits severe periodontal destruction. (Courtesy of Dr. Richard Foster, Guilford Technical Community College, Jamestown, NC.)

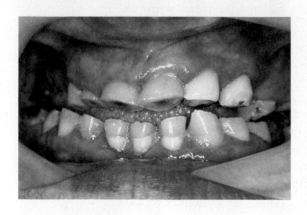

Figure 16-18. Periodontitis and Down Syndrome. This patient with Down syndrome exhibits pronounced attrition and localized loss of attachment. (Courtesy of Dr. Richard Foster, Guilford Technical Community College, Jamestown, NC.)

LEUKEMIA

1. **Characteristics of Leukemia**
   A. Leukemia is cancer of the blood cells that usually begins in the bone marrow.
      1. Most often, it is a cancer of white blood cells, but it can be a cancer of other types of cells, such as red blood cells and platelets.
      2. In people with leukemia, the bone marrow produces many abnormally functioning cells.
         a. At first, leukemia cells function almost normally. In time, however, they may spread throughout the body (such as the lymph nodes, liver, and spleen) and crowd out normal functioning white blood cells, red blood cells, and platelets.
         b. The increase in number of leukemic cells in the blood circulation leads to several serious systemic disorders: leukopenia (a decrease in the number of normal functioning white blood cells), thrombocytopenia (a decrease in

the number of normal functioning platelets), and anemia (a decrease in the number of normal functioning red blood cells).

3. Leukemia is a disease of both children and adults and is more common in men and boys than girls and women.

B. **Types of Leukemia**

1. Leukemia is classified on the duration (acute or chronic) and the type of cell involved (myeloid or lymphoid).

    a. Leukemia is either *chronic* (gets worse slowly) or *acute* (gets worse quickly and is rapidly fatal).

    b. Leukemia that affects the lymphocytes is called *lymphocytic*. Leukemia that affects the myeloid cells (such as red blood cells, platelets, and neutrophils) is called *myelogenous* leukemia.

2. Leukemia is the most common cancer in children younger than 15 years old.[161]

C. **Medical Treatment of Leukemia**

1. Treatment for leukemia is complex and is not the same for all patients. Treatment varies with the type of leukemia, extent of the disease, and on the patient's age, symptoms, and general health. The physician tailors the treatment to fit each individual patient's needs.

2. Most patients with leukemia are treated with chemotherapy. Some also may have radiation therapy and/or bone marrow transplantation or biological therapy.

3. Chemotherapy causes patients to suffer from severe suppression of the immune system. Chemotherapy functions by suppressing the growth and spread of malignant cells; unfortunately, normal cells are also adversely affected. Normal cells with the highest rate of cell turnover (proliferation)—such as those of the periodontium—are affected because chemotherapy interferes with cell production, maturation, and replacement.

4. Dental care is a vital component of treatment. Anticancer treatments for leukemia can make the mouth sensitive, easily infected, and likely to bleed.[149,153,161–164]

2. **Oral Complications of Leukemia**

A. **Leukemia-Associated Gingivitis**

1. **Inflammation of the Gingiva.** Signs of gingival inflammation in the leukemic patient include swollen, glazed, and spongy tissues that are red to deep purple in appearance (Fig. 16-19) and bleed with the slightest provocation or even spontaneously. Leukemic patients exhibit profuse gingival bleeding because of a reduction in the number of normal functioning platelets (thrombocytopenia).

    a. In a study of 1,093 adult in-patients undergoing chemotherapy treatment for leukemia, 14.9% of patients manifested gross bleeding from the mouth during the course of chemotherapy.[165,166] The most common oral bleeding sites were the lips, tongue, and gingiva.

    b. In children, the prevalence of gingival inflammation is highest in the maintenance phase of chemotherapy followed by the induction phase with radiotherapy.[162]

2. **Gingival Enlargement.** Gingival enlargement is a common characteristic, initially beginning at the interdental papilla followed by marginal and attached gingiva. This enlargement is due to increased infiltration of immature leukemic cells in the gingiva. Additionally, as the gingiva enlarges, a periodontal pocket is created which will harbor more pathogenic microorganisms and worsen the inflammation.

3. **Oral Infection.** Compared to healthy, nonleukemic individuals, leukemic patients are more susceptible to oral infection due to a reduction in the number of normal functioning white blood cells (leukopenia). As a result, leukemic patients have an impaired immune system.

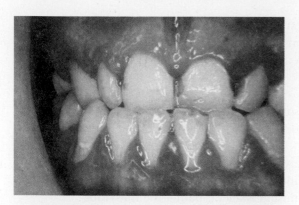

Figure 16-19. Leukemia-Associated Gingivitis. Note the swollen, red gingival tissues in this patient with leukemia. (Courtesy of Dr. Ralph Arnold, San Antonio, TX.)

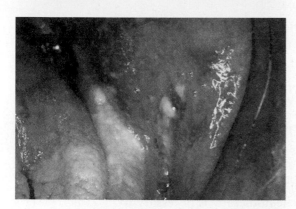

Figure 16-20. Mucositis Associated With Chemotherapy. Oral mucositis directly attributable to antileukemia chemotherapy occurs in almost 20% of adults undergoing such treatment. The associated extreme discomfort may produce physical and psychological obstructions to continued anticancer treatment.

B. **Oral Mucositis as an Oral Complications of Leukemia Therapy**
1. Oral mucositis is an inflammation of the oral mucous membranes caused when chemotherapy attacks and kills the rapidly dividing cells of the mucous membranes. Cells of the oral mucosa have a lifespan of only 10 to 14 days. Therefore, during chemotherapy, mucosal cells are dying at a faster rate than new cells can be produced.
2. Sloughing of mucosal surfaces can be localized or generalized involving the buccal mucosa, palate, floor of the mouth, gingiva, lips, and/or tongue (Fig. 16-20). Ulcerations of the oral cavity also are a common complication of chemotherapy.
3. While oral mucositis is an undesired side effect of leukemic therapy, this is not a reason for a leukemic patient to avoid chemotherapy. Instead, while on chemotherapy, the oral condition of the leukemic patient should be closely monitored by a dental professional for signs of oral mucositis. Early detection and management of oral mucositis in a leukemic patient is critical in reducing the severity of the tissue sloughing and relieving the pain associated with this complication.
C. **Xerostomia as an Oral Complications of Leukemia Therapy**
1. Xerostomia may occur due to damage of the salivary glands during radiation therapy. A reduction in salivary flow alters the self-cleaning mechanisms of the oral cavity resulting in rapid biofilm accumulation and the development of dental caries.
2. Lack of saliva also can result in diminished taste perception and/or difficulty in swallowing and talking.
3. Reduced salivary flow and xerostomia can encourage the growth of C. *albicans* and the development of oral candidiasis.[167]
4. While xerostomia is an undesired side effect of leukemic therapy, this should also not be a reason for a leukemic patient to undergo avoid therapy. Instead,

while on radiation therapy, the oral condition of the leukemic patient should be closely monitored by a dental professional for signs of xerostomia. Early detection and management of xerostomia in a leukemic patient is critical in reducing the severity of this complication.

3. **Leukemia: Implications for the Dental Hygienist**

A. The dental team can act as an important point of contact for early screening and diagnosis of undiagnosed leukemia. In some individuals, the first signs of leukemia show up in the oral cavity.[161,168]

1. When a dental patient has spontaneous gingival bleeding and/or gingival enlargement for no apparent reason—combined with symptoms such as facial swelling, tiredness, poor appetite, lethargy, musculoskeletal pain—the individual should be referred to a medical specialist.[161,168]

2. The fact that leukemia frequently presents with early oral manifestations emphasizes the need for dental professionals to be aware of the early oral signs of leukemia and can provide a timely referral. Timely referral to a medical specialist is critical.

B. Frequent unfavorable oral conditions of individuals undergoing anticancer therapy for leukemia highlights the responsibility of the otolaryngologist and oncologist to refer these patients to the dental office.[162,169,170] The planning of anticancer therapy for leukemia should include dental professionals in the multidisciplinary oncology team.

1. Immune suppression during chemotherapy may cause serious oral infections.

2. Adequate oral care before, during and after chemotherapy is necessary to prevent oral diseases and systemic complications of oral origin. Frequent dental care is essential for improvement in oral conditions that may diminish patient suffering and prevent the spread of serious infections from the oral cavity to other parts of the body.[162]

3. Chemotherapy can cause a sore and sensitive mouth that bleeds easily. Soft toothbrushes with gentle brushing should be recommended. If the mouth is too sensitive to tolerate tooth brushing, soft dental sponges (available from a pharmacy) can be recommended.

C. Pain from oral mucositis afflicts from 40% to 70% of patients receiving chemotherapy or radiation therapy.

1. Current methods of clinical pain management (e.g., topical anesthetics, systemic analgesics) have limited success.[171] Oral mucositis is common in children undergoing chemotherapy.

2. In 2011, a study by Soares suggests that the prophylactic use of 0.12% chlorhexidine gluconate reduces the frequency of oral mucositis and oral pathogens in children with leukemia.[153]

D. Care should be coordinated with other health professionals. Interprofessional collaboration among professionals such as physicians, dental professionals, dieticians, and case managers is an essential component of patient-centered care.[142]

Section 2
Systemic Medications With Periodontal Side Effects

Many medications used to treat systemic diseases can cause oral complications. Effects of medications can modify oral hygiene habits, plaque biofilm composition, size of gingival tissues, level of bone, and salivary flow. Educating patients about potential oral side effects is critical to reducing the medication-related risks of periodontal disease. Commonly prescribed medications that can affect the periodontium are summarized in Table 16-1.

TABLE 16-1	HARMFUL EFFECTS OF COMMONLY PRESCRIBED MEDICATIONS ON PERIODONTIUM	
Medication Class	**Generic Name (Brand Name)**	**Effect on Periodontium**
Anticonvulsant	Phenytoin (Dilantin)	Gingival overgrowth
Antianxiety agents	Alprazolam (Xanax)	Increased biofilm formation
Antihypertensive	Enalapril (Vasotec)	Increased gingival inflammation
Calcium blocker	Nifedipine (Procardia)	Gingival overgrowth
Immunosuppressive	Cyclosporine (Sandimmune)	Gingival overgrowth

1. **Medications That Alter Plaque Biofilm Composition, pH, or Salivary Flow**
   A. **Plaque Biofilm Composition or pH**
      1. Many oral medications alter plaque biofilm composition and pH in ways that are harmful to the periodontium.
      2. Sugar is a major component of some cough drops, liquid medications, cough syrups, tonics, chewable vitamins, antacid tablets, and other medications. Medications that contain sugar add significantly to the alteration of pH and composition of the biofilm.
      3. Sugar is metabolized by bacteria to form acid, causing enamel to demineralize. The demineralized areas are rough and act as attachment sites for bacteria, keeping bacterial plaque biofilm against tissues and eventually resulting in inflammation of the gingiva.
      4. Some over-the-counter (OTC) preparations contain sugar and vitamin C (ascorbic acid). This combination delivers sugar and may lower the pH.
      5. Products that alter the plaque biofilm pH significantly can cause root-surface caries in older adults and influence the metabolism of periodontal pathogens.[172,173]
   B. **Salivary Flow and pH**
      1. Adequate saliva flow is necessary for the maintenance of healthy oral tissues. The ability of saliva to limit the growth of pathogens is a major determinant of systemic and oral health.
         a. The physical flow of the saliva helps to dislodge microbes from the teeth and mucosa surfaces. Saliva can also cause bacteria to clump together so that they can be swallowed before they become firmly attached.

    b. Saliva is rich in antimicrobial components. Certain molecules in saliva can directly kill or inhibit a variety of microbes.

  2. Patients with xerostomia suffer from an increase in the incidence of oral candidiasis, coronal and root-surface caries, as well as excess plaque biofilm formation.

  3. More than 400 OTC and prescription drugs have xerostomia as a possible side effect.[174]

  4. Some of the more common groups of medications that cause xerostomia are cardiovascular medications (blood pressure, diuretics, calcium channel blockers); antidepressants; sedatives; antiparkinsonism medications; allergy medications; and antacids.[175]

2. Drug-Induced Gingival Enlargement

  A. Introduction

    1. Drug-induced gingival enlargement is an esthetically disfiguring overgrowth of the gingiva that is a side effect associated with certain medications.

    2. *Drugs associated with gingival enlargement can be broadly divided into three categories: anticonvulsants, calcium channel blockers, and immunosuppressants.* These three classes of medications influence gingival fibroblasts to overproduce collagen matrix when stimulated by plaque-induced inflammation.[176]

      a. More than 20 medications have been shown to have the potential to induce gingival enlargement.

      b. The anticonvulsant phenytoin accounts for the highest prevalence rate (>50%) of drug-associated gingival enlargement. Calcium channel blockers account for 6% to 15% of drug-associated gingival enlargements while immunosuppressants account for 25% to 30% of drug-associated gingival enlargements seen in adults.[177]

    3. The clinical characteristics of drug-induced gingival enlargement include painless enlargement of the keratinized gingiva with a tendency to occur more often in the anterior gingiva, a prevalence in younger age groups, an increased tendency to bleed, and an onset within 3 months of use.[165] Drug-induced gingival enlargement rarely affects the mucosal tissue and never appears in edentulous areas.

    4. Drug-induced gingival enlargement may make effective self-care more difficult due to the size and mass of enlarged gingival tissue. As a result, this may contribute to the retention of pathogenic microorganisms around the enlarged gingiva. Thus, reinforcement of good oral hygiene is critical in controlling plaque biofilm levels and reducing inflammation. However, good oral hygiene will not do anything to eliminate or lessen the gingival overgrowth that is induced by the medication.

  B. Anticonvulsants

    1. Phenytoin (FEN-i-toyn) is one of the most commonly prescribed anticonvulsant medications used to control convulsions or seizures in the treatment of epilepsy. Phenytoin is marketed worldwide under various trade names including Dilantin, Phenytek, Cerebyx, and Phenytoin. Phenytoin is among the 20 most-prescribed drugs in the world.

    2. Overgrowth of the gingiva is one of the most common side effects of phenytoin. It has been estimated that 40% to 50% of the millions of individuals who take phenytoin will develop gingival overgrowth to some extent.[177] Overgrowths appear to be more common in children and young adults.

3. Gingival overgrowth begins with enlargement of the interdental papillae.
   a. The interdental papillae overgrow, forming firm triangular tissue masses that protrude from the interdental area.
   b. Gradually, the enlarged papilla from one interdental area may unite with the adjacent enlarged papilla to partially cover the anatomical crown with marginal gingiva (Fig. 16-21). Overgrowths are most commonly seen on the facial aspect of the maxillary and mandibular anterior teeth. The gingival overgrowth may serve as plaque-retentive areas.
   c. In the presence of good biofilm control, the enlarged tissue is pink in color and firm and rubbery in consistency. In the presence of poor biofilm control, the tissue appears red, edematous, and spongy.

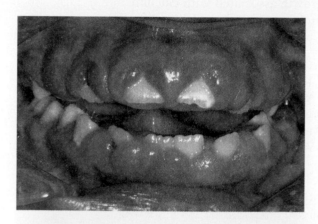

Figure 16-21. Phenytoin-Influenced Gingival Overgrowth. Severe enlargement of the gingiva associated with phenytoin (Dilantin) medication in an individual with epilepsy. (Courtesy of Dr. Ralph Arnold, San Antonio, TX.)

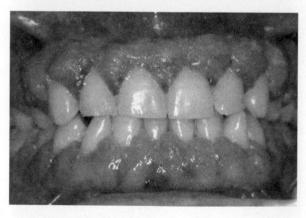

Figure 16-22. Cyclosporine-Influenced Gingival Overgrowth. The clinical appearance of cyclosporine-associated gingival overgrowth resembles that of phenytoin-associated gingival enlargement. (Courtesy of Dr. Ralph Arnold, San Antonio, TX.)

C. Immunosuppressants
   1. Cyclosporine (SIGH-kloe-spor-een) belongs to the group of medicines known as immunosuppressive agents used for prevention of transplant rejection as well as for management of several autoimmune conditions such as rheumatoid arthritis.
   2. The incidence of cyclosporine-associated gingival overgrowth affects approximately 25% to 30% of adult patients taking the medication. However, in children, the prevalence of cyclosporine-associated drug enlargement can be as much as 70%.
   3. The clinical appearance of cyclosporine-associated gingival overgrowth resembles that of phenytoin-associated gingival enlargement (Fig. 16-22).
D. Calcium Channel Blockers
   1. Antihypertensive drugs in the calcium channel blocker group are used extensively in elderly patients who have angina or peripheral vascular disease.

2. The use of calcium channel blockers is associated with an increased risk of gingival hyperplasia.[166,178]

   a. **Nifedipine** (nye-FED-I-peen), one type of calcium channel blocker, is used as a coronary vasodilator in the treatment of hypertension, angina, and cardiac arrhythmias. Calcium channel blockers are a class of drugs that block the influx of calcium ions through cardiac and vascular smooth muscle cell membranes. This results in the dilation of the main coronary and systemic arteries.

   b. Various other calcium channel blocking medications, such as diltiazem, felodipine, nitrendipine, and verapamil also may induce gingival enlargement.

3. The clinical appearance of gingival overgrowth associated with calcium channel blockers resembles that of phenytoin-associated gingival enlargement (Figs. 16-23 and 16-24).

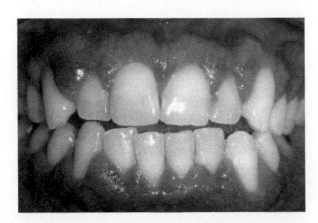

Figure 16-23. Gingival Overgrowth Associated With Nifedipine. Gingival overgrowth in a patient who takes Nifedipine for the treatment of cardiac arrhythmia. (Courtesy of Dr. Ralph Arnold, San Antonio, TX.)

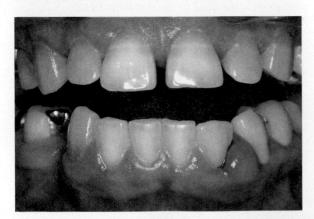
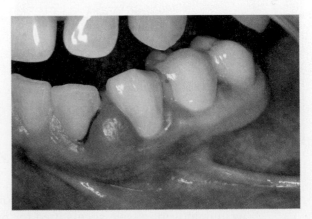

Figure 16-24. Gingival Enlargement Associated With Calcium Channel Blocking Drugs. Gingival enlargement of the papilla between the lateral incisor and canine induced by the calcium channel blocking medication Norvasc. (Courtesy of Dr. Richard Foster, Guilford Technical Community College, Jamestown, NC.)

E. **Systemic Medications: Implications for the Dental Hygienist**
  1. Dental hygienists should be alert for patient medications that can alter biofilm composition, pH, or salivary flow.
     a. Sugar-containing liquid or chewable medications are sometimes used in the treatment of children with chronic medical problems. Parents should be made aware of the oral health consequences of such medications. Giving the medications at mealtimes instead of between meals is helpful.
     b. Some OTC preparations contain sugar and vitamin C. This combination delivers sugar and the vitamins cause an acid pH. Examples of products containing sugar and vitamin C include chewable vitamin C tablets, certain cough drops, and certain liquid cough preparations.
  2. Closer collaboration between medical and dental clinical teams is necessary for the joint management of individuals being treated with anticonvulsants, calcium channel blockers, or immunosuppressants.[142] Patients receiving cyclosporine are usually medically compromised, requiring close consultation with the patient's physician to assure safe management of the patient's periodontal condition. In addition to professional and at-home plaque biofilm control, it has been shown that azithromycin induced a striking reduction in cyclosporine-induced gingival hyperplasia.[179]
  3. Treatment of gingival enlargement should include consultation with the physician, substitution of the current medication for another whenever possible, nonsurgical periodontal therapy, frequent periodontal maintenance, and surgical therapy, if needed.[179]
     a. The hygienist should emphasize the importance of meticulous daily self-care and involve patients in hands-on demonstrations of brushing and interdental cleaning aids.
     b. Surgical elimination of the tissue overgrowth is often required. If plaque biofilm control is inadequate, the re-growth will occur rapidly. The patient should be advised of the likelihood of the recurrence of the gingival overgrowth following surgery.

Chapter Summary Statement

The presence of dental plaque biofilm does not necessarily mean that an individual will experience periodontitis. Additional factors play a role in determining why some individuals are more susceptible to periodontitis than others. Significant systemic contributing factors include diabetes mellitus, leukemia, acquired immunodeficiency syndrome, hormonal fluctuations, genetic risk factors, and systemic medications. Contributing risk factors must be evaluated to develop the best treatment plan for each individual. Dental professionals should provide health promotion education that contributes to overall systemic and periodontal health and collaborate with medical team members for joint patient management.

Section 5
Focus on Patients

Clinical Patient Care

CASE 1

A patient, who has been previously treated for periodontitis and has been followed by your dental team for several years, calls your dental office with a concern. She is scheduled to undergo a liver transplant and has been warned by her physician that the medications she will need will make her more susceptible to infections. She asks if these medications might modify her continuing treatment for periodontitis. How might you respond to her concern?

CASE 2

The parents of a young patient currently being treated by your dental team inform you that following a lengthy illness, their daughter has recently been diagnosed by her physician with a neutrophil defect. Neutrophils are also known as polymorphonuclear leukocytes. They inquire about any dental implications of this diagnosis. How might you respond to this inquiry?

Evidence in Action

CASE 1

A new patient in your office reports that she has recently been diagnosed with diabetes mellitus and that her physician suggested that she should have a dental checkup. The patient confides in you that she feels like this disease is really changing her lifestyle. She laughingly says "I have always had such good reports from my previous dentist, and I just don't really see why I need to be worried about my teeth now." Based upon what is known about the relationship between diabetes and periodontal disease, how might you explain the need for the recommended dental exam to the patient?

CASE 2

James is a 10-year-old patient who is new to your dental office. James' family just relocated to your city for his father's new job. James' health history indicates a history of epilepsy. He takes phenytoin (Dilantin) for seizure control. You note gingival enlargement and bleeding on probing during the intraoral examination. Based on what you know about the relationship between phenytoin and gingival enlargement, what information would you provide to James and his parent? Would a consultation with James' physician be indicated?

Ethical Dilemma

You have just recently married and moved across the country to the city where your husband was raised. His parents helped you secure a full-time dental hygiene position with their family dentist, Dr. Ramos. You are quite happy working with the office staff, as well as meeting and getting to know many of your in-law's family and friends, who are patients of the practice as well.

Today your mother-in-law, June, is scheduled for her 6-month recall appointment. This is the first time you will be treating her. You review her medical history, and she states that lately she's been feeling tired, lethargic, and has a poor appetite. She assumed she was just overtired from all the wedding planning and festivities. She hasn't been able to work out regularly, as she has musculoskeletal aches and pains.

Your clinical examination reveals gingival enlargement and spontaneous gingival bleeding, despite excellent self-care. Her tissues are swollen, glazed, and spongy, and red to deep purple in appearance, and ooze blood intermittently. She also appears to have facial swelling. You review the notes from her last appointment, which was 6 months ago, and see that her tissues were classified as normal and healthy.

You become very concerned that June may have a serious medical condition, and you are not sure what to do. You feel that you need to discuss this with your husband before saying anything to June.

1. What systemic condition do you think could be causing June's signs/symptoms?
2. What ethical principles are in conflict in this dilemma?
3. What is the best way for you to handle this ethical dilemma?

References

1. Gregg EW, Li Y, Wang J, Burrows NR, Ali MK, Rolka D, et al. Changes in diabetes-related complications in the United States, 1990–2010. *N Engl J Med.* 2014;370(16):1514–1523.
2. Centers for Disease Control and Prevention (CDC). *National Diabetes Statistics Report, 2014: Estimates of Diabetes and its Burden in the United States.* Atlanta, GA: US Department of Health and Human Services; 2014.
3. Wild S, Roglic G, Green A, Sicree R, King H. Global prevalence of diabetes: estimates for the year 2000 and projections for 2030. *Diabetes Care.* 2004;27(5):1047–1053.
4. Chavarry NG, Vettore MV, Sansone C, Sheiham A. The relationship between diabetes mellitus and destructive periodontal disease: a meta-analysis. *Oral Health Prev Dent.* 2009;7(2):107–127.
5. Khader YS, Dauod AS, El-Qaderi SS, Alkafajei A, Batayha WQ. Periodontal status of diabetics compared with nondiabetics: a meta-analysis. *J Diabetes Complications.* 2006;20(1):59–68.
6. Marigo L, Cerreto R, Giuliani M, Somma F, Lajolo C, Cordaro M. Diabetes mellitus: biochemical, histological and microbiological aspects in periodontal disease. *Eur Rev Med Pharmacol Sci.* 2011;15(7):751–758.
7. Taylor GW, Borgnakke WS. Periodontal disease: associations with diabetes, glycemic control and complications. *Oral Dis.* 2008;14(3):191–203.
8. Christgau M, Palitzsch KD, Schmalz G, Kreiner U, Frenzel S. Healing response to non-surgical periodontal therapy in patients with diabetes mellitus: clinical, microbiological, and immunologic results. *J Clin Periodontol.* 1998;25(2):112–124.
9. Mealey BL, Oates TW; American Academy of Periodontology. Diabetes mellitus and periodontal diseases. *J Periodontol.* 2006;77(8):1289–1303.
10. Diabetes and periodontal diseases. Committee on Research, Science and Therapy. American Academy of Periodontology. *J Periodontol.* 2000;71(4):664–678.
11. Deshpande K, Jain A, Sharma R, Prashar S, Jain R. Diabetes and periodontitis. *J Indian Soc Periodontol.* 2010;14(4): 207–212.
12. Preshaw PM, Alba AL, Herrera D, et al. Periodontitis and diabetes: a two-way relationship. *Diabetologia.* 2012;55(1): 21–31.
13. Preshaw PM, Bissett SM. Periodontitis: oral complication of diabetes. *Endocrinol Metab Clin North Am.* 2013;42(4): 849–867.
14. Salvi GE, Yalda B, Collins JG, et al. Inflammatory mediator response as a potential risk marker for periodontal diseases in insulin-dependent diabetes mellitus patients. *J Periodontol.* 1997;68(2):127–135.
15. Taylor JJ, Preshaw PM, Lalla E. A review of the evidence for pathogenic mechanisms that may link periodontitis and diabetes. *J Periodontol.* 2013;84(4 Suppl):S113–S134.
16. Botero JE, Yepes FL, Roldan N, et al. Tooth and periodontal clinical attachment loss are associated with hyperglycemia in patients with diabetes. *J Periodontol.* 2012;83(10):1245–1250.

17. Demmer RT, Holtfreter B, Desvarieux M, et al. The influence of type 1 and type 2 diabetes on periodontal disease progression: prospective results from the Study of Health in Pomerania (SHIP). *Diabetes Care.* 2012;35(10):2036–2042.

18. Haseeb M, Khawaja KI, Ataullah K, Munir MB, Fatima A. Periodontal disease in type 2 diabetes mellitus. *J Coll Physicians Surg Pak.* 2012;22(8):514–518.

19. Apoorva SM, Sridhar N, Suchetha A. Prevalence and severity of periodontal disease in type 2 diabetes mellitus (non-insulin-dependent diabetes mellitus) patients in Bangalore city: an epidemiological study. *J Indian Soc Periodontol.* 2013;17(1): 25–29.

20. Daniel R, Gokulanathan S, Shanmugasundaram N, Lakshmigandhan M, Kavin T. Diabetes and periodontal disease. *J Pharm Bioallied Sci.* 2012;4(Suppl 2):S280–S282.

21. Monea A, Mezei T, Monea M. The influence of diabetes mellitus on periodontal tissues: a histological study. *Rom J Morphol Embryol.* 2012;53(3):491–495.

22. Lin CC, Sun SS, Kao A, Lee CC. Impaired salivary function in patients with noninsulin-dependent diabetes mellitus with xerostomia. *J Diabetes Complications.* 2002;16(2):176–179.

23. Tervonen T, Karjalainen K. Periodontal disease related to diabetic status. A pilot study of the response to periodontal therapy in type 1 diabetes. *J Clin Periodontol.* 1997;24(7):505–510.

24. Busato IM, Ignacio SA, Brancher JA, Gregio AM, Machado MA, Azevedo-Alanis LR. Impact of xerostomia on the quality of life of adolescents with type 1 diabetes mellitus. *Oral Surg Oral Med Oral Pathol Oral Radiol Endod.* 2009;108(3): 376–382.

25. Moore PA, Guggenheimer J, Etzel KR, Weyant RJ, Orchard T. Type 1 diabetes mellitus, xerostomia, and salivary flow rates. *Oral Surg Oral Med Oral Pathol Oral Radiol Endod.* 2001;92(3):281–291.

26. Ueta E, Osaki T, Yoneda K, Yamamoto T. Prevalence of diabetes mellitus in odontogenic infections and oral candidiasis: an analysis of neutrophil suppression. *J Oral Pathol Med.* 1993;22(4):168–174.

27. Lalla E, Papapanou PN. Diabetes mellitus and periodontitis: a tale of two common interrelated diseases. *Nat Rev Endocrinol.* 2011;7(12):738–748.

28. Lalla E, Kaplan S, Chang SM, et al. Periodontal infection profiles in type 1 diabetes. *J Clin Periodontol.* 2006;33(12): 855–862.

29. Salvi GE, Kandylaki M, Troendle A, Persson GR, Lang NP. Experimental gingivitis in type 1 diabetics: a controlled clinical and microbiological study. *J Clin Periodontol.* 2005;32(3):310–316.

30. Crockett JC, Rogers MJ, Coxon FP, Hocking LJ, Helfrich MH. Bone remodelling at a glance. *J Cell Sci.* 2011;124 (Pt 7):991–998.

31. He H, Liu R, Desta T, Leone C, Gerstenfeld LC, Graves DT. Diabetes causes decreased osteoclastogenesis, reduced bone formation, and enhanced apoptosis of osteoblastic cells in bacteria stimulated bone loss. *Endocrinology.* 2004;145(1): 447–452.

32. Liu R, Bal HS, Desta T, et al. Diabetes enhances periodontal bone loss through enhanced resorption and diminished bone formation. *J Dent Res.* 2006;85(6):510–514.

33. Al-Khabbaz AK, Al-Shammari KF, Al-Saleh NA. Knowledge about the association between periodontal diseases and diabetes mellitus: contrasting dentists and physicians. *J Periodontol.* 2011;82(3):360–366.

34. Gossain VV, Aldasouqi S. The challenge of undiagnosed prediabetes, diabetes, and cardiovascular Disease. *Int J Diabetes Mellit.* 2010;2:43–46.

35. Katz J, Yoon TY, Mao S, Lamont RJ, Caudle RM. Expression of the receptor of advanced glycation end products in the gingival tissue of smokers with generalized periodontal disease and after nornicotine induction in primary gingival epithelial cells. *J Periodontol.* 2007;78(4):736–741.

36. Schmidt AM, Weidman E, Lalla E, et al. Advanced glycation endproducts (AGEs) induce oxidant stress in the gingiva: a potential mechanism underlying accelerated periodontal disease associated with diabetes. *J Periodontal Res.* 1996;31(7):508–515.

37. Takeda M, Ojima M, Yoshioka H, et al. Relationship of serum advanced glycation end products with deterioration of periodontitis in type 2 diabetes patients. *J Periodontol.* 2006;77(1):15–20.

38. Aldasouqi S, Gossain V, Llittle R. Undiagnosed diabetes equals undiagnosed CVD: a call for more effective diabetes screening. *Rev Endocrinol.* 2009;3:21–23.

39. Chapple IL, Genco R; Working group 2 of the joint EFP/AAP workshop. Diabetes and periodontal diseases: consensus report of the Joint EFP/AAP Workshop on Periodontitis and Systemic Diseases. *J Periodontol.* 2013;84(4 Suppl):S106–S112.

40. Lopes MH, Southerland JH, Buse JB, Malone RM, Wilder RS. Diabetes educators' knowledge, opinions and behaviors regarding periodontal disease and diabetes. *J Dent Hyg.* 2012;86(2):82–90.

41. Dye BA, Genco RJ. Tooth loss, pocket depth, and HbA1c information collected in a dental care setting may improve the identification of undiagnosed diabetes. *J Evid Based Dent Pract.* 2012;12(3 Suppl):12–14.

42. Lalla E, Kunzel C, Burkett S, Cheng B, Lamster IB. Identification of unrecognized diabetes and pre-diabetes in a dental setting. *J Dent Res.* 2011;90(7):855–860.

43. Maples S, Aldasouqi S, Little R, Baughman H, Joshi M, Salhi R. Detection of undiagnosed prediabetes and diabetes in dental patients: A proposal of a dental-office-friendly diabetes screening tool. *J Diabetes Mellitus.* 2016;6:25–37.

44. Sandberg GE, Sundberg HE, Wikblad KF. A controlled study of oral self-care and self-perceived oral health in type 2 diabetic patients. *Acta Odontol Scand.* 2001;59(1):28–33.

45. Kanjirath PP, Kim SE, Rohr Inglehart M. Diabetes and oral health: the importance of oral health-related behavior. *J Dent Hyg.* 2011;85(4):264–272.

46. Strauss SM, Singh G, Tuthill J, et al. Diabetes-related knowledge and sources of information among periodontal patients: is there a role for dental hygienists? *J Dent Hyg.* 2013;87(2):82–89.

47. Lalla E, Cheng B, Lal S, et al. Diabetes mellitus promotes periodontal destruction in children. *J Clin Periodontol.* 2007;34(4):294–298.

48. Nip A, Pihoker C, Mayer-Davies E, et al., eds. *Disordered Eating Behaviors in Youth and Young Adults with Type 1 and Type 2 Diabetes: The Search for Diabetes in Youth Study. American Diabetes Association 2017 Scientific Sessions, 2017 June 10,* San Diego, CA, June 9–13, 2017.

49. Genco RJ, Ho AW, Grossi SG, Dunford RG, Tedesco LA. Relationship of stress, distress and inadequate coping behaviors to periodontal disease. *J Periodontol.* 1999;70(7):711–723.

50. Marcenes WS, Sheiham A. The relationship between work stress and oral health status. *Soc Sci Med.* 1992;35(12):1511–1520.

51. Monteiro da Silva AM, Newman HN, Oakley DA, O'Leary R. Psychosocial factors, dental plaque levels and smoking in periodontitis patients. *J Clin Periodontol.* 1998;25(6):517–523.
52. Wimmer G, Janda M, Wieselmann-Penkner K, Jakse N, Polansky R, Pertl C. Coping with stress: its influence on periodontal disease. *J Periodontol.* 2002;73(11):1343–1351.
53. Peruzzo DC, Benatti BB, Ambrosano GM, et al. A systematic review of stress and psychological factors as possible risk factors for periodontal disease. *J Periodontol.* 2007;78(8):1491–1504.
54. Genco RJ, Ho AW, Kopman J, Grossi SG, Dunford RG, Tedesco LA. Models to evaluate the role of stress in periodontal disease. *Ann Periodontol.* 1998;3(1):288–302.
55. Kurer JR, Watts TL, Weinman J, Gower DB. Psychological mood of regular dental attenders in relation to oral hygiene behaviour and gingival health. *J Clin Periodontol.* 1995;22(1):52–55.
56. Wardle J, Steptoe A, Oliver G, Lipsey Z. Stress, dietary restraint and food intake. *J Psychosom Res.* 2000;48(2):195–202.
57. Lipton R. The relationship between alcohol, stress, and depression in Mexican Americans and non-Hispanic whites. *Behav Med.* 1997;23(3):101–111.
58. Cucalon A, 3rd, Smith RJ. Relationship between compliance by adolescent orthodontic patients and performance on psychological tests. *Angle Orthod.* 1990;60(2):107–114.
59. Deinzer R, Hilpert D, Bach K, Schawacht M, Herforth A. Effects of academic stress on oral hygiene–a potential link between stress and plaque-associated disease? *J Clin Periodontol.* 2001;28(5):459–464.
60. Newman HN. Diet, attrition, plaque and dental disease. *Dent Health (London).* 1975;14(2):3–11.
61. Mombelli A, Gusberti FA, van Oosten MA, Lang NP. Gingival health and gingivitis development during puberty. A 4-year longitudinal study. *J Clin Periodontol.* 1989;16(7):451–456.
62. Mombelli A, Rutar A, Lang NP. Correlation of the periodontal status 6 years after puberty with clinical and microbiological conditions during puberty. *J Clin Periodontol.* 1995;22(4):300–305.
63. Nakagawa S, Fujii H, Machida Y, Okuda K. A longitudinal study from prepuberty to puberty of gingivitis. Correlation between the occurrence of Prevotella intermedia and sex hormones. *J Clin Periodontol.* 1994;21(10):658–665.
64. Sutcliffe P. A longitudinal study of gingivitis and puberty. *J Periodontal Res.* 1972;7(1):52–58.
65. Knight ET, Liu J, Seymour GJ, Faggion CM, Jr., Cullinan MP. Risk factors that may modify the innate and adaptive immune responses in periodontal diseases. *Periodontol 2000.* 2016;71(1):22–51.
66. Kara C, Demir T, Tezel A. Effectiveness of periodontal therapies on the treatment of different aetiological factors induced gingival overgrowth in puberty. *Int J Dent Hyg.* 2007;5(4):211–217.
67. Holm-Pedersen P, Loe H. Flow of gingival exudate as related to menstruation and pregnancy. *J Periodontal Res.* 1967;2(1):13–20.
68. Silness J, Loe H. Periodontal disease in pregnancy. 3. Response to local treatment. *Acta Odontol Scand.* 1966;24(6):747–759.
69. Arafat AH. Periodontal status during pregnancy. *J Periodontol.* 1974;45(8):641–643.
70. Cohen DW, Friedman L, Shapiro J, Kyle GC. A longitudinal investigation of the periodontal changes during pregnancy. *J Periodontol.* 1969;40(10):563–570.
71. Cohen DW, Shapiro J, Friedman L, Kyle GC, Franklin S. A longitudinal investigation of the periodontal changes during pregnancy and fifteen months post-partum. II. *J Periodontol.* 1971;42(10):653–657.
72. Loe H, Silness J. Periodontal disease in pregnancy. I. Prevalence and severity. *Acta Odontol Scand.* 1963;21:533–551.
73. Silness J, Loe H. Periodontal disease in pregnancy. II. Correlation between oral hygiene and periodontal condition. *Acta Odontol Scand.* 1964;22:121–135.
74. Kornman K, W Loesche. The subgingival microbial flora during pregnancy. *J Periodontol Res.* 1980;15:111–122.
75. Gursoy M, Gursoy UK, Sorsa T, Pajukanta R, Kononen E. High salivary estrogen and risk of developing pregnancy gingivitis. *J Periodontol.* 2013;84(9):1281–1289.
76. Straka M. Pregnancy and periodontal tissues. *Neuro Endocrinol Lett.* 2011;32(1):34–38.
77. Armitage GC. Bi-directional relationship between pregnancy and periodontal disease. *Periodontol 2000.* 2013;61(1):160–176.
78. Lundgren D, Magnusson B, Lindhe J. Connective tissue alterations in gingivae of rats treated with estrogen and progesterone. A histologic and autoradiographic study. *Odontol Revy.* 1973;24(1):49–58.
79. Silk H, Douglass AB, Douglass JM, Silk L. Oral health during pregnancy. *Am Fam Physician.* 2008;77(8):1139–1144.
80. Boggess KA, Edelstein BL. Oral health in women during preconception and pregnancy: implications for birth outcomes and infant oral health. *Matern Child Health J.* 2006;10(5 Suppl):S169–S174.
81. American College of Obstetricians and Gynecologists Women's Health Care Physicians; Committee on Health Care for Underserved Women. Committee Opinion No. 569: oral health care during pregnancy and through the lifespan. *Obstet Gynecol.* 2013;122(2 Pt 1):417–422.
82. Hilgers KK, Douglass J, Mathieu GP. Adolescent pregnancy: a review of dental treatment guidelines. *Pediatr Dent.* 2003;25(5):459–467.
83. Dutt P, Chaudhary S, Kumar P. Oral health and menopause: a comprehensive review on current knowledge and associated dental management. *Ann Med Health Sci Res.* 2013;3(3):320–323.
84. Friedlander AH. The physiology, medical management and oral implications of menopause. *J Am Dent Assoc.* 2002;133(1):73–81.
85. Payne JB, Reinhardt RA, Nummikoski PV, Patil KD. Longitudinal alveolar bone loss in postmenopausal osteoporotic/osteopenic women. *Osteoporos Int.* 1999;10(1):34–40.
86. Carey JJ, Palomo L. Bisphosphonates and osteonecrosis of the jaw: innocent association or significant risk? *Cleve Clin J Med.* 2008;75(12):871–879.
87. Al Habashneh R, Alchalabi H, Khader YS, Hazza'a AM, Odat Z, Johnson GK. Association between periodontal disease and osteoporosis in postmenopausal women in Jordan. *J Periodontol.* 2010;81(11):1613–1621.
88. Bertulucci Ldc A, Pereira FM, de Oliveira AE, Brito LM, Lopes FF. Periodontal disease in women in post-menopause and its relationship with osteoporosis. *Rev Bras Ginecol Obstet.* 2012;34(12):563–567.
89. Vishwanath SB, Kumar V, Kumar S, Shashikumar P, Shashikumar Y, Patel PV. Correlation of periodontal status and bone mineral density in postmenopausal women: a digital radiographic and quantitative ultrasound study. *Indian J Dent Res.* 2011;22(2):270–276.
90. Jeffcoat M. The association between osteoporosis and oral bone loss. *J Periodontol.* 2005;76(11 Suppl):2125–2132.

91. Chang WP, Chang WC, Wu MS, et al. Population-based 5-year follow-up study in Taiwan of osteoporosis and risk of periodontitis. *J Periodontol*. 2014;85:e24–e30.

92. Esfahanian V, Shamami MS. Relationship between osteoporosis and periodontal disease: review of the literature. *J Dent (Tehran)*. 2012;9(4):256–264.

93. Genco RJ, Grossi SG. Is estrogen deficiency a risk factor for periodontal disease? *Compend Contin Educ Dent Suppl*. 1998(22):S23–S29.

94. Payne JB, Reinhardt RA, Nummikoski PV, Dunning DG, Patil KD. The association of cigarette smoking with alveolar bone loss in postmenopausal females. *J Clin Periodontol*. 2000;27(9):658–664.

95. Alberti KG, Zimmet P, Shaw J. Metabolic syndrome—a new world-wide definition. A Consensus Statement from the International Diabetes Federation. *Diabet Med*. 2006;23(5):469–480.

96. Sattar N, McConnachie A, Shaper AG, et al. Can metabolic syndrome usefully predict cardiovascular disease and diabetes? Outcome data from two prospective studies. *Lancet*. 2008;371(9628):1927–1935.

97. Ford ES, Giles WH, Dietz WH. Prevalence of the metabolic syndrome among US adults: findings from the third National Health and Nutrition Examination Survey. *JAMA*. 2002;287(3):356–359.

98. Sinha R, Fisch G, Teague B, et al. Prevalence of impaired glucose tolerance among children and adolescents with marked obesity. *N Engl J Med*. 2002;346(11):802–810.

99. Pilgram TK, Hildebolt CF, Yokoyama-Crothers N, et al. Relationships between longitudinal changes in radiographic alveolar bone height and probing depth measurements: data from postmenopausal women. *J Periodontol*. 1999;70(8):829–833.

100. Civitelli R, Pilgram TK, Dotson M, et al. Alveolar and postcranial bone density in postmenopausal women receiving hormone/estrogen replacement therapy: a randomized, double-blind, placebo-controlled trial. *Arch Intern Med*. 2002;162(12):1409–1415.

101. Alberti KG, Zimmet P, Shaw J; IDF Epidemiology Task Force Consensus Group. The metabolic syndrome—a new worldwide definition. *Lancet*. 2005;366(9491):1059–1062.

102. Valery PC, Moloney A, Cotterill A, Harris M, Sinha AK, Green AC. Prevalence of obesity and metabolic syndrome in Indigenous Australian youths. *Obes Rev*. 2009;10(3):255–261.

103. Weiss R, Dziura J, Burgert TS, et al. Obesity and the metabolic syndrome in children and adolescents. *N Engl J Med*. 2004;350(23):2362–2374.

104. Aguilar M, Bhuket T, Torres S, Liu B, Wong RJ. Prevalence of the metabolic syndrome in the United States, 2003–2012. *JAMA*. 2015;313(19):1973–1974.

105. Benguigui C, Bongard V, Ruidavets JB, et al. Metabolic syndrome, insulin resistance, and periodontitis: a cross-sectional study in a middle-aged French population. *J Clin Periodontol*. 2010;37(7):601–608.

106. D'Aiuto F, Nibali L, Parkar M, Patel K, Suvan J, Donos N. Oxidative stress, systemic inflammation, and severe periodontitis. *J Dent Res*. 2010;89(11):1241–1246.

107. Fukui N, Shimazaki Y, Shinagawa T, Yamashita Y. Periodontal status and metabolic syndrome in middle-aged Japanese. *J Periodontol*. 2012;83(11):1363–1371.

108. Khader YS, Albashaireh ZS, Hammad MM. Periodontal status of type 2 diabetics compared with nondiabetics in north Jordan. *East Mediterr Health J*. 2008;14(3):654–661.

109. Kushiyama M, Shimazaki Y, Yamashita Y. Relationship between metabolic syndrome and periodontal disease in Japanese adults. *J Periodontol*. 2009;80(10):1610–1615.

110. Li P, He L, Sha YQ, Luan QX. Relationship of metabolic syndrome to chronic periodontitis. *J Periodontol*. 2009;80(4):541–549.

111. Nibali L, D'Aiuto F, Griffiths G, Patel K, Suvan J, Tonetti MS. Severe periodontitis is associated with systemic inflammation and a dysmetabolic status: a case-control study. *J Clin Periodontol*. 2007;34(11):931–937.

112. Shimazaki Y, Saito T, Yonemoto K, Kiyohara Y, Iida M, Yamashita Y. Relationship of metabolic syndrome to periodontal disease in Japanese women: the Hisayama Study. *J Dent Res*. 2007;86(3):271–275.

113. Hasegawa T, Watase H. Multiple risk factors of periodontal disease: a study of 9260 Japanese non-smokers. *Geriatr Gerontol Int*. 2004;4:37–43.

114. Maciel SS, Feres M, Goncalves TE, et al. Does obesity influence the subgingival microbiota composition in periodontal health and disease? *J Clin Periodontol*. 2016;43(12):1003–1012.

115. Bullon P, Morillo JM, Ramirez-Tortosa MC, Quiles JL, Newman HN, Battino M. Metabolic syndrome and periodontitis: is oxidative stress a common link?. *J Dent Res*. 2009;88(6):503–518.

116. Festa A, D'Agostino R, Jr., Howard G, Mykkanen L, Tracy RP, Haffner SM. Chronic subclinical inflammation as part of the insulin resistance syndrome: the Insulin Resistance Atherosclerosis Study (IRAS). *Circulation*. 2000;102(1):42–47.

117. Porter SR, Scully C, Luker J. Complications of dental surgery in persons with HIV disease. *Oral Surg Oral Med Oral Pathol*. 1993;75(2):165–167.

118. Yu H, Rakugi H, Higaki J, Morishita R, Mikami H, Ogihara T. The role of activated vascular angiotensin II generation in vascular hypertrophy in one-kidney, one clip hypertensive rats. *J Hypertens*. 1993;11(12):1347–1355.

119. Lopez NJ, Quintero A, Casanova PA, Ibieta CI, Baelum V, Lopez R. Effects of periodontal therapy on systemic markers of inflammation in patients with metabolic syndrome: a controlled clinical trial. *J Periodontol*. 2012;83(3):267–278.

120. Goncalves LS, Goncalves BM, de Andrade MA, Alves FR, Junior AS. Drug interactions during periodontal therapy in HIV-infected subjects. *Mini Rev Med Chem*. 2010;10(8):766–772.

121. Ryder MI, Nittayananta W, Coogan M, Greenspan D, Greenspan JS. Periodontal disease in HIV/AIDS. *Periodontol 2000*. 2012;60(1):78–97.

122. Hirnschall G, Harries AD, Easterbrook PJ, Doherty MC, Ball A. The next generation of the World Health Organization's global antiretroviral guidance. *J Int AIDS Soc*. 2013;16:18757.

123. Mann DL, Gartner S, LeSane F, Blattner WA, Popovic M. Cell surface antigens and function of monocytes and a monocyte-like cell line before and after infection with HIV. *Clin Immunol Immunopathol*. 1990;54(2):174–183.

124. Petit AJ, Terpstra FG, Miedema F. Human immunodeficiency virus infection down-regulates HLA class II expression and induces differentiation in promonocytic U937 cells. *J Clin Invest*. 1987;79(6):1883–1889.

125. Pinching AJ, McManus TJ, Jeffries DJ, et al. Studies of cellular immunity in male homosexuals in London. *Lancet*. 1983;2(8342):126–130.

126. Roux-Lombard P, Modoux C, Cruchaud A, Dayer JM. Purified blood monocytes from HIV 1-infected patients produce high levels of TNF alpha and IL-1. *Clin Immunol Immunopathol*. 1989;50(3):374–384.

127. Dodson TB. HIV status and the risk of post-extraction complications. *J Dent Res*. 1997;76(10):1644–1652.

128. McKaig RG, Patton LL, Thomas JC, Strauss RP, Slade GD, Beck JD. Factors associated with periodontitis in an HIV-infected southeast USA study. *Oral Dis*. 2000;6(3):158–165.

129. McKaig RG, Thomas JC, Patton LL, Strauss RP, Slade GD, Beck JD. Prevalence of HIV-associated periodontitis and chronic periodontitis in a southeastern US study group. *J Public Health Dent*. 1998;58(4):294–300.

130. Robinson PG, Sheiham A, Challacombe SJ, Wren MW, Zakrzewska JM. Gingival ulceration in HIV infection. A case series and case control study. *J Clin Periodontol*. 1998;25(3):260–267.

131. Yeung SC, Stewart GJ, Cooper DA, Sindhusake D. Progression of periodontal disease in HIV seropositive patients. *J Periodontol*. 1993;64(7):651–657.

132. Alves M, Mulligan R, Passaro D, et al. Longitudinal evaluation of loss of attachment in HIV-infected women compared to HIV-uninfected women. *J Periodontol*. 2006;77(5):773–779.

133. Mataftsi M, Skoura L, Sakellari D. HIV infection and periodontal diseases: an overview of the post-HAART era. *Oral Dis*. 2011;17(1):13–25.

134. Armitage GC. Development of a classification system for periodontal diseases and conditions. *Ann Periodontol*. 1999;4(1):1–6.

135. Yin MT, Dobkin JF, Grbic JT. Epidemiology, pathogenesis, and management of human immunodeficiency virus infection in patients with periodontal disease. *Periodontol 2000*. 2007;44:55–81.

136. Velegraki A, Nicolatou O, Theodoridou M, Mostrou G, Legakis NJ. Paediatric AIDS–related linear gingival erythema: a form of erythematous candidiasis? *J Oral Pathol Med*. 1999;28(4):178–182.

137. Fricke U, Geurtsen W, Staufenbiel I, Rahman A. Periodontal status of HIV-infected patients undergoing antiretroviral therapy compared to HIV-therapy naive patients: a case control study. *Eur J Med Res*. 2012;17:2.

138. Kroidl A, Schaeben A, Oette M, Wettstein M, Herfordt A, Haussinger D. Prevalence of oral lesions and periodontal diseases in HIV-infected patients on antiretroviral therapy. *Eur J Med Res*. 2005;10(10):448–453.

139. Ryder MI. Periodontal management of HIV-infected patients. *Periodontol 2000*. 2000;23:85–93.

140. Lemos SS, Oliveira FA, Vencio EF. Periodontal disease and oral hygiene benefits in HIV seropositive and AIDS patients. *Med Oral Patol Oral Cir Bucal*. 2010;15(2):e417–e421.

141. Vernon LT, Demko CA, Whalen CC, et al. Characterizing traditionally defined periodontal disease in HIV+ adults. *Community Dent Oral Epidemiol*. 2009;37(5):427–437.

142. Bridges DR, Davidson RA, Odegard PS, Maki IV, Tomkowiak J. Interprofessional collaboration: three best practice models of interprofessional education. *Med Educ Online*. 2011;16.

143. Hein C. Translating evidence of oral-systemic relationships into models of interprofessional collaboration. *J Dent Hyg*. 2009;83(4):188–189.

144. Carlsson G, Fasth A. Infantile genetic agranulocytosis, morbus Kostmann: presentation of six cases from the original "Kostmann family" and a review. *Acta Paediatr*. 2001;90(7):757–764.

145. Hong CH, Napenas JJ, Hodgson BD, et al. A systematic review of dental disease in patients undergoing cancer therapy. *Support Care Cancer*. 2010;18(8):1007–1021.

146. Stabholz A, Soskolne V, Machtei E, Or R, Soskolne WA. Effect of benign familial neutropenia on the periodontium of Yemenite Jews. *J Periodontol*. 1990;61(1):51–54.

147. Stabholz A, Soskolne WA, Shapira L. Genetic and environmental risk factors for chronic periodontitis and aggressive periodontitis. *Periodontol 2000*. 2010;53:138–153.

148. De Beule F, Bercy P, Ferrant A. The effectiveness of a preventive regimen on the periodontal health of patients undergoing chemotherapy for leukemia and lymphoma. *J Clin Periodontol*. 1991;18(5):346–347.

149. Javed F, Utreja A, Bello Correa FO, et al. Oral health status in children with acute lymphoblastic leukemia. *Crit Rev Oncol Hematol*. 2012;83(3):303–309.

150. Ellepola AN, Samaranayake LP. The effect of brief exposure to sub-therapeutic concentrations of chlorhexidine gluconate on the germ tube formation of oral Candida albicans and its relationship to post-antifungal effect. *Oral Dis*. 2000;6(3): 166–171.

151. Meurman JH, Laine P, Murtomaa H, et al. Effect of antiseptic mouthwashes on some clinical and microbiological findings in the mouths of lymphoma patients receiving cytostatic drugs. *J Clin Periodontol*. 1991;18(8):587–591.

152. Pereira Pinto L, de Souza LB, Gordon-Nunez MA, et al. Prevention of oral lesions in children with acute lymphoblastic leukemia. *Int J Pediatr Otorhinolaryngol*. 2006;70(11):1847–1851.

153. Soares AF, Aquino AR, Carvalho CH, Nonaka CF, Almeida D, Pinto LP. Frequency of oral mucositis and microbiological analysis in children with acute lymphoblastic leukemia treated with 0.12% chlorhexidine gluconate. *Braz Dent J*. 2011;22(4):312–316.

154. Overholser CD, Peterson DE, Williams LT, Schimpff SC. Periodontal infection in patients with acute nonlymphocyte leukemia. Prevalence of acute exacerbations. *Arch Intern Med*. 1982;142(3):551–554.

155. Morgan J. Why is periodontal disease more prevalent and more severe in people with Down syndrome? *Spec Care Dentist*. 2007;27(5):196–201.

156. Barr-Agholme M, Dahllof G, Modeer T, Engstrom PE, Engstrom GN. Periodontal conditions and salivary immunoglobulins in individuals with Down syndrome. *J Periodontol*. 1998;69(10):1119–1123.

157. Odeh M, Hershkovits M, Bornstein J, Loberant N, Blumenthal M, Ophir E. Congenital absence of salivary glands in Down syndrome. *Arch Dis Child*. 2013;98(10):781–783.

158. Amano A, Kishima T, Kimura S, et al. Periodontopathic bacteria in children with Down syndrome. *J Periodontol*. 2000;71(2):249–255.

159. Cavalcante LB, Tanaka MH, Pires JR, et al. Expression of the interleukin-10 signaling pathway genes in individuals with Down syndrome and periodontitis. *J Periodontol*. 2012;83(7):926–935.

160. Murakami J, Kato T, Kawai S, Akiyama S, Amano A, Morisaki I. Cellular motility of Down syndrome gingival fibroblasts is susceptible to impairment by Porphyromonas gingivalis invasion. *J Periodontol*. 2008;79(4):721–727.

161. Sepulveda E, Brethauer U, Fernandez E, Cortes G, Mardones C. Oral manifestations as first clinical sign of acute myeloid leukemia: report of a case. *Pediatr Dent*. 2012;34(5):418–421.

162. Azher U, Shiggaon N. Oral health status of children with acute lymphoblastic leukemia undergoing chemotherapy. *Indian J Dent Res.* 2013;24(4):523.

163. Bektas-Kayhan K, Kucukhuseyin O, Karagoz G, et al. Is the MDR1 C3435T polymorphism responsible for oral mucositis in children with acute lymphoblastic leukemia? *Asian Pac J Cancer Prev.* 2012;13(10):5251–5255.

164. Mathur VP, Dhillon JK, Kalra G. Oral health in children with leukemia. *Indian J Palliat Care.* 2012;18(1):12–18.

165. Drug-induced gingival hyperplasia. *Prescrire Int.* 2011;20(122):293–294.

166. Parwani RN, Parwani SR. Management of phenytoin-induced gingival enlargement: a case report. *Gen Dent.* 2013;61(6):61–67.

167. Mikulska M, Calandra T, Sanguinetti M, Poulain D, Viscoli C; Third European Conference on Infections in Leukemia Group. The use of mannan antigen and anti mannan antibodies in the diagnosis of invasive candidiasis: recommendations from the Third European Conference on Infections in Leukemia. *Crit Care.* 2010;14(6):R222.

168. Silva BA, Siqueira CR, Castro PH, Araujo SS, Volpato LE. Oral manifestations leading to the diagnosis of acute lymphoblastic leukemia in a young girl. *J Indian Soc Pedod Prev Dent.* 2012;30(2):166–168.

169. Thomaz EB, Mouchrek JC, Jr., Silva AQ, et al. Longitudinal assessment of immunological and oral clinical conditions in patients undergoing anticancer treatment for leukemia. *Int J Pediatr Otorhinolaryngol.* 2013;77(7):1088–1093.

170. Dreizen S, McCredie KB, Keating MJ. Chemotherapy-associated oral hemorrhages in adults with acute leukemia. *Oral Surg Oral Med Oral Pathol.* 1984;57(5):494–498.

171. Berger A, Henderson M, Nadoolman W, et al. Oral capsaicin provides temporary relief for oral mucositis pain secondary to chemotherapy/radiation therapy. *J Pain Symptom Manage.* 1995;10(3):243–248.

172. Steele JG, Sheiham A, Marcenes W, Fay N, Walls AW. Clinical and behavioural risk indicators for root caries in older people. *Gerodontology.* 2001;18(2):95–101.

173. Touger-Decker R, van Loveren C. Sugars and dental caries. *Am J Clin Nutr.* 2003;78(4):881S–892S.

174. Ciancio SG. Medications' impact on oral health. *J Am Dent Assoc.* 2004;135(10):1440–1448; quiz 68–69.

175. Guggenheimer J, Moore PA. Xerostomia: etiology, recognition and treatment. *J Am Dent Assoc.* 2003;134(1):61–69; quiz 118–119.

176. Dongari-Bagtzoglou A; Research, Science and Therapy Committee, American Academy of Periodontology. Drug-associated gingival enlargement. *J Periodontol.* 2004;75(10):1424–1431.

177. Mohan RP, Rastogi K, Bhushan R, Verma S. Phenytoin-induced gingival enlargement: a dental awakening for patients with epilepsy. *BMJ Case Rep.* 2013;2013.

178. Sanz M. Current use of calcium channel blockers (CCBs) is associated with an increased risk of gingival hyperplasia. *J Evid Based Dent Pract.* 2012;12(3 Suppl):147–148.

179. Ramalho VL, Ramalho HJ, Cipullo JP, Azoubel R, Burdmann EA. Comparison of azithromycin and oral hygiene program in the treatment of cyclosporine-induced gingival hyperplasia. *Ren Fail.* 2007;29(3):265–270.

STUDENT ANCILLARY RESOURCES

A wide variety of resources to enhance your learning is available online:

- Audio Glossary
- Book Pages
- Chapter Review Questions and Answers

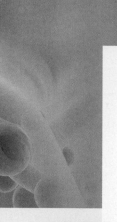

17 Local Factors Contributing to Periodontal Disease

Clinical Application. As discussed in other chapters of this book, periodontal diseases are inflammatory conditions that are initiated by bacterial pathogens. Additionally, individuals may possess local (intraoral) contributing factors that (1) make it more likely to develop periodontal disease, (2) affect the progress of existing periodontal disease, or (3) predispose a specific site of a tooth to periodontal disease. The dental team must be able to identify and eliminate local factors to minimize their impact on the periodontium. This chapter describes local contributing factors and explains how these factors can alter periodontal disease in patients.

Learning Objectives

- Describe local factors that contribute to the retention and accumulation of plaque biofilm.
- Explain what distinguishes a local contributing factor from a systemic contributing factor.
- Identify and differentiate the location, composition, modes of attachment, mechanisms of mineralization, and pathologic potential of supra- and subgingival calculus deposits.
- Describe local contributing factors that can lead to direct damage to the periodontium.
- Explain the role of trauma from occlusion as a possible contributing factor in periodontal disease.

Key Terms

Local contributing factors
Disease site
Dental calculus
Pellicle
Morphology
Cervical enamel projections
Enamel pearl
Iatrogenic factor
Overhanging restoration
Open margin
Embrasure space

Prosthesis
Biologic width
Supracrestal tissue
   attachment
Factitious injury
Malingering
Food impaction
Tongue thrust
Mouth breathing
Traumatic tooth brushing
Dehiscence

Fenestration
Trauma from occlusion
Primary trauma from
   occlusion
Secondary trauma from
   occlusion
Functional occlusal forces
Parafunctional occlusal forces
Clenching
Bruxism
Frenal pull

Section 1
Introduction to Local Contributing Factors

It is clear that the primary etiology of gingivitis and periodontitis is microbial plaque biofilm. There are, additionally, certain local contributing factors that can increase the risk of developing gingivitis and periodontitis or that can increase the severity of an already established gingivitis and periodontitis.[1-3] **Local contributing factors** for periodontal disease are intraoral conditions or habits that increase an individual's susceptibility to periodontal infection or that can damage the periodontium in specific sites within the dentition. *Local contributing factors do not actually initiate either gingivitis or periodontitis, but these factors can contribute to the progression of an already established disease that is previously initiated by bacterial plaque biofilm.*

It is critical for the dental team to search for local contributing factors during a comprehensive periodontal assessment and understand their impact on the periodontium. The dental team should always eliminate or at least minimize the impact of existing local contributing factors during all phases of periodontal treatment.

The conditions discussed in this chapter refer to circumstances that favor periodontal breakdown and can contribute to gingivitis or periodontitis in individual sites in the mouth. In the context of this discussion, a **disease site** is an individual tooth or specific surface of a tooth. For instance, a local contributing factor—such as a mesial root concavity—might predispose the mesial surface of a maxillary premolar tooth to periodontal breakdown, but not affect the periodontal support on the distal surface of the same tooth. Examples of potential local contributing factors can include dental calculus, faulty dental restorations, developmental factors in teeth, plaque retentive features of cavitated lesions, certain patient habits, and trauma from occlusion.

Local contributing factors can predispose an individual to developing gingivitis or periodontitis through several mechanisms or through combinations of these mechanisms. Table 17-1 summarizes mechanisms for increased disease risk in local sites, and each of these mechanisms is discussed in detail in the following sections of this chapter. There are three primary mechanisms by which local factors can increase the risk of developing periodontal disease or increase the severity of existing periodontal disease.

1. A local factor can increase plaque biofilm retention.
2. A local factor can increase plaque biofilm pathogenicity (disease-causing potential).
3. A local factor can cause direct damage to the periodontium.

TABLE 17-1	MECHANISMS FOR INCREASED DISEASE RISK IN LOCAL SITES
Mechanism	**Clinical Example**
Local factor that increases plaque biofilm retention	Rough edge on a restoration harbors plaque biofilm and makes it difficult to remove plaque biofilm with a brush and floss
Local factor that increases plaque biofilm pathogenicity (disease-causing potential)	Calculus deposits harbor plaque biofilm, allowing the biofilm community to grow uninhibited for an extended period
Local factor that can inflict damage to the periodontium	Ill-fitting dental appliance that puts excessive pressure on the gingiva History of traumatic toothbrushing Trauma from occlusion High frenal attachment

Section 2
Local Factors That Increase Biofilm Retention

This section discusses local factors that can increase plaque biofilm retention. Most often these local contributing factors have rough or irregular surfaces that decrease the effectiveness of a patient's self-care and lead to increased plaque biofilm retention.

1. **Dental Calculus.** Dental calculus is the most obvious example of a local contributing factor that can lead to increased plaque biofilm retention. **Dental calculus** is mineralized bacterial plaque biofilm, covered on its external surface by nonmineralized, living bacterial plaque biofilm. Mineralization of plaque biofilm can begin from 48 hours up to 2 weeks after plaque biofilm formation.
   A. **Effects of Calculus on the Periodontium**
      1. The surface of a calculus deposit at the microscopic level is quite irregular in contour and is always covered with disease-causing bacteria. Thus, even calculus that has not built up enough to result in a ledge or grossly altered tooth contour can lead to plaque biofilm retention at the site simply because of its roughened and porous surface and its tendency to harbor bacteria.
      2. As dental calculus deposits build up, they can lead to even more irregular surfaces, ledges on the teeth, and other alterations of the contours of the teeth (Fig. 17-1). As calculus deposits accumulate, they create more and more areas of plaque biofilm retention that are difficult or impossible for a patient to clean.
   B. **Pathologic Potential**
      1. Since a layer of living bacterial plaque biofilm always covers a calculus deposit, dental calculus plays a significant role as a local contributing factor in periodontal disease. Moreover, with its close proximity to the periodontal tissues, calculus serves as a fixed source for continual plaque accumulation which will perpetuate the gingival inflammation.
      2. It is difficult to bring either gingivitis or periodontitis under control in the presence of dental calculus on affected teeth, and the importance of removing these deposits in patients with gingivitis and periodontitis cannot be overemphasized.

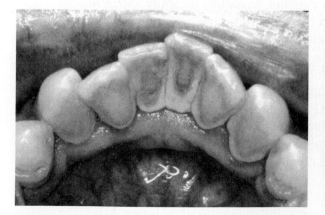
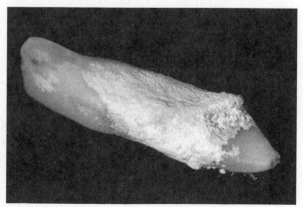

Figure 17-1. Irregular Surface of Calculus Deposits. The clinical photo on the left shows heavy calculus deposits on the lingual surfaces of the mandibular anterior teeth. These deposits are so large that they interfere with the patient's self-care efforts. In addition, calculus deposits harbor living bacteria that can be in constant contact with the gingival tissue. The photo on the right shows calculus on the crown and root surfaces of an extracted mandibular canine. (Photograph [right] courtesy of Dr. Don Rolfs, Wenatchee, WA.)

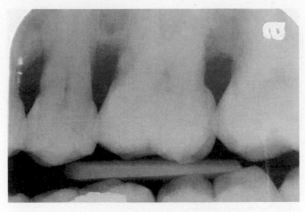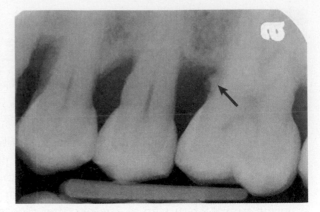

Figure 17-2. Significance of Radiographic Technique. Two radiographs of the same maxillary left posterior region with the x-ray tube oriented in different horizontal angulations. Both radiographs were taken in the same appointment. In the radiograph on the left, note the absence of radiographic calculus on the mesial surface of the maxillary first molar. However, in the right-hand radiograph, the calculus deposit is evident on the same surface.

C. **Composition of Dental Calculus.** Calculus is comprised of an inorganic (or mineralized) component and an organic component.
   1. Inorganic Portion of Calculus
      a. The inorganic part of calculus makes up 70% to 90% of the overall composition of calculus.
      b. This inorganic part of dental calculus is primarily calcium phosphate, but the dental calculus also contains some calcium carbonate and magnesium phosphate.
      c. The inorganic part of calculus is similar to the inorganic components of bone.
      d. Due to its high inorganic content, calculus may be detectable on a radiograph as a dense, radiopaque deposit attached to the tooth. Conventional radiographs can sometimes be a valuable means of detecting calculus.
      e. However, radiographs are not sensitive to detect calculus 100% of the time. This can be attributed to the degree of mineralization of the calculus deposit and the size of the deposit. In addition, since radiographs are only a two-dimensional image of a three-dimensional object, calculus located on the lingual or facial surfaces of teeth may not be radiographically apparent.
      f. It should be noted that differences in radiographic technique and procedures may also account for calculus deposits showing up on radiographs (Fig. 17-2).
   2. Organic Portion of Calculus
      a. The organic part of calculus makes up 10% to 30% of the overall composition of calculus.
      b. Components of the organic part include materials derived from plaque biofilm, dead epithelial cells, and dead white blood cells. It can also include living bacteria within the deposits of calculus.
D. **Types of Dental Calculus**
   1. Crystalline Forms of Dental Calculus. As calculus ages on a tooth surface, the inorganic component changes through several different crystalline forms. It is interesting to note that some of these crystalline forms of calculus are quite similar to the crystal forms in the tooth itself.
      a. Newly formed calculus deposits appear as a crystalline form called brushite.
      b. In calculus deposits that are a bit more mature, but less than 6 months old, the crystalline form is primarily octacalcium phosphate.

    c. In mature deposits that are more than 6 months old, the crystalline form is primarily hydroxyapatite.

  2. Location of Calculus Deposits

    a. Supragingival calculus deposits are calculus deposits located coronal to (above) the gingival margin. Other terms that have been used to refer to deposits coronal to the gingival margin are supramarginal calculus and salivary calculus. Because of its location relative to the gingival margin, supragingival calculus is visible during routine clinical examination.

      1) Though supragingival calculus deposits can be found on any tooth surface, they usually are found in localized areas of the dentition, such as lingual surfaces of mandibular anterior teeth, facial surfaces of maxillary molars, and on teeth that are crowded or in malocclusion. It is interesting to note that supragingival calculus is frequently found in areas adjacent to large salivary ducts (such as the lingual surfaces of mandibular anterior teeth and the facial surfaces of maxillary posterior teeth).

      2) Though supragingival calculus can form in most any shape, these deposits most often are irregular, large deposits.

    b. Subgingival deposits are calculus deposits located apical to (below) the gingival margin. Other terms that have been used for deposits apical to the gingival margin are submarginal calculus or serumal calculus. Subgingival calculus is not visible on routine clinical examination because it is apical to the gingival margin. Instead, subgingival calculus can only be detected by careful and delicate tactile perception with a fine-tipped explorer. Radiographs may be useful in confirming the presence of subgingival calculus, but should not be used as a substitute for clinical detection.

      1) The distribution of subgingival deposits may be localized in certain areas or generalized throughout the mouth.

      2) The shape of subgingival deposits is most often flattened. It is thought that the shape of the deposit may be guided by pressure of the pocket wall against the deposit.

      3) Generally, a deposit of calculus can be present supragingivally and extend subgingivally. However, sometimes the individual calculus deposit is present below the gingival margin, but absent supragingivally. This can occur if complete supragingival calculus removal is combined with ineffective subgingival instrumentation.

      4) It important to note that the classification of calculus is based on its location in relation to the gingival margin. If the gingiva recedes, then what was previously classified as subgingival calculus can be reclassified as supragingival calculus.

E. Modes of Attachment to Tooth Surfaces. Dental calculus attaches to tooth surfaces through several different modes, and different attachment mechanisms can even exist in the same calculus deposit.

  1. Attachment by Means of Pellicle

    a. Calculus can attach to the tooth surface by attaching to pellicle on the surface. The pellicle is a thin, bacteria-free membrane that forms on the surface of the tooth during the late stages of eruption.

    b. This mode of attachment occurs most commonly on enamel surfaces.

    c. Calculus deposits attached via the pellicle are usually removed easily because this attachment is on the surface of the pellicle (and not actually locked into the tooth surface).

2. **Attachment to Irregularities in the Tooth Surface**
    a. Calculus can also attach to irregularities in tooth surfaces. These irregularities include cracks in the teeth, tiny openings left where periodontal ligament (PDL) fibers are detached, and grooves in cemental surfaces created as the result of faulty instrumentation during previous calculus removal procedures.
    b. Complete calculus removal in areas of irregularities in tooth surfaces is usually difficult since the deposits can be sheltered in these tooth defects.

3. **Attachment by Direct Contact of the Calcified Component and the Tooth Surface**
    a. Calculus can also attach to tooth surfaces by attaching directly to the calcified component of the tooth. In this mode of attachment, the matrix of the calculus deposit is interlocked with the inorganic crystals of the tooth.
    b. Deposits, firmly interlocked in the tooth surface, are usually difficult to remove.

2. **Tooth Morphology.** Morphology is the study of the anatomic surface features of the teeth. There are a variety of local contributing factors that relate to tooth morphology.
   A. **Tooth Grooves or Concavities**
      1. Naturally occurring developmental grooves and concavities in tooth surfaces frequently lead to difficulty in self-care at the site and can also be a local contributing factor for gingivitis and periodontitis because of the increased plaque biofilm retention at the site.
      2. During the natural development of some incisor teeth, a groove forms on the palatal surface of the tooth. This groove is a developmental anomaly called a **palatogingival groove** and is most frequently seen on maxillary lateral incisors. Plaque biofilm retention is a common problem associated with a palatogingival groove since the groove is often difficult or impossible to clean effectively (Fig. 17-3).
      3. Some tooth root surfaces have naturally occurring **concavities** or depressions that can lead to plaque biofilm retention (Fig. 17-4). The mesial surface of maxillary first premolar teeth often has a pronounced concavity in the surface. This concavity is a natural contour for that tooth, but if exposed in the oral cavity, can make it extremely difficult for a patient to maintain effective self-care at the site.
   B. **Cervical Enamel Projections and Enamel Pearls**
      1. A **cervical enamel projection** is an apical deviation of the cementoenamel junction (CEJ) toward the direction of the furcation entrance (Fig. 17-5). It is a flat, triangular-shaped projection of enamel pointing in the direction of the furcation.
      2. An **enamel pearl** is a well-defined ectopic, spherical-shaped deposit of enamel found on the root surface (Fig. 17-6). Radiographically, enamel pearls appear as radiopaque, dense masses. Both cervical enamel projections and enamel pearls have a predilection to be found on the root surfaces of molar teeth.
      3. Both a cervical enamel projection and an enamel pearl act as areas that retain plaque biofilm. As a result, they are considered to be local factors that contribute to the development of furcation invasions. All effort should be made to identify these local factors through thorough clinical and radiographic methods. Following detection, these local factors should be surgically removed.

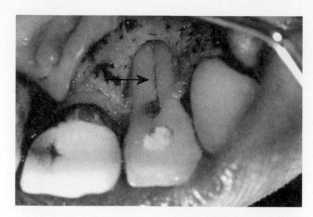

Figure 17-3. Palatogingival Groove. A palatogingival groove on the lingual surface of this maxillary lateral incisor is revealed during a periodontal surgical procedure. The gingiva has been lifted off the bone and tooth root. The palatogingival groove allowed plaque biofilm to mature undisturbed in the groove and contribute to the extensive alveolar bone loss localized to the lateral incisor.

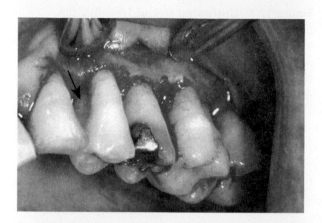

Figure 17-4. Root Concavity. The mesial root concavity on a maxillary first premolar. This photograph was taken during a periodontal surgical procedure designed to allow better visualization and treatment of the root concavity. (Courtesy of Dr. Ralph Arnold, San Antonio, TX.)

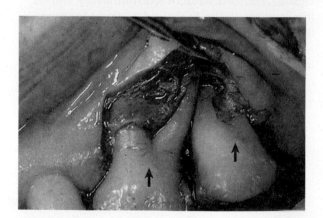

Figure 17-5. Cervical Enamel Projections. Note how the CEJ in the mid-buccal region of the maxillary first and second molars points apically toward the furcation entrance.

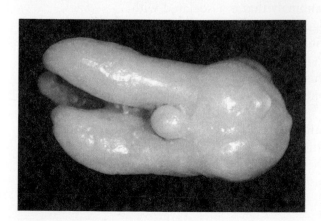

Figure 17-6. Enamel Pearl. Note, the spherical-shaped deposit of enamel on the root of this molar tooth. Enamel pearls act as areas that retain plaque biofilm.

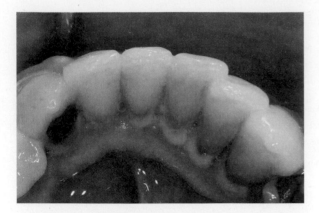

Figure 17-7. Plaque-Retentive Features of Malocclusion. Crowding of teeth results increased rendition of plaque biofilm that can hinder the best attempts by the patient to keep the area clean. (Courtesy of Dr. Ralph Arnold, San Antonio, TX.)

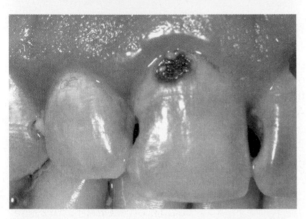

Figure 17-8. Untreated Decay. Note that this untreated tooth decay leaves an actual hole (cavity) in the tooth surface that can then harbor periodontal pathogens and can allow them to grow undisturbed by self-care efforts. (Courtesy of Dr. Ralph Arnold, San Antonio, TX.)

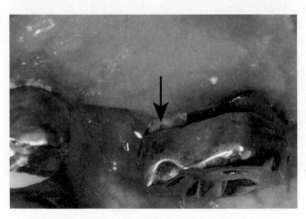

Figure 17-9. Untreated Recurrent Decay and Its Implications to the Surrounding Periodontium. Note the area of recurrent decay under the crown margin of the maxillary first molar. The cavitated lesion retains plaque well and handicaps self-care measures. Consequently, the gingival tissue is inflamed.

C. Malocclusion
1. Dental malocclusion is a developmental anomaly that is associated with irregular alignment of teeth. Teeth malalignment predisposes the area to biofilm retention and, as a result, gingival inflammation (Fig. 17-7).
2. The ideal treatment outcome would be to orthodontically realign the teeth to make the area less plaque retentive. This can only be accomplished by close interdisciplinary care involving all members of the dental team and the orthodontist.
D. **Dental Caries.** Untreated tooth decay is another example of a local contributing factor that can increase plaque biofilm retention. Since tooth decay can result in defects in tooth structure (dental cavities), these defects (cavities) can also act as protected environments for bacteria that cause gingivitis and periodontitis to live and grow undisturbed (Figs. 17-8 and 17-9).

E. **Orthodontic Appliances.** Orthodontic appliances, such as brackets and bonded retainers, favor plaque biofilm retention and are areas not easily accessible for the patient to keep clean. As a result, orthodontic appliances may lead to pathogenic bacterial colonization which causes gingival inflammation. Figure 17-10 shows a patient during orthodontic treatment with an orthodontic retainer in place on the lingual surfaces of the mandibular anterior teeth. Figure 17-11 shows the same patient, post-treatment, after removal of the retainer; note the calculus deposits on the lingual surfaces of the mandibular anterior teeth.

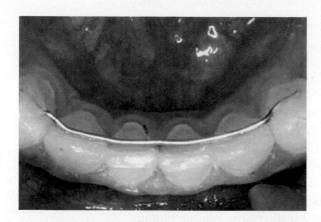

Figure 17-10. Orthodontic Appliance on Mandibular Anterior Teeth. Patient with orthodontic retainer bonded to the mandibular anterior teeth. Note mild gingival inflammation and marginal calculus deposits.

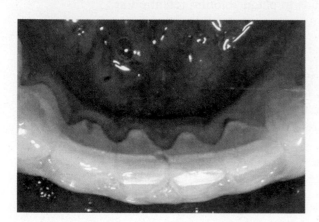

Figure 17-11. Calculus Deposits Evident on Same Patient. The same patient case (as in Fig. 17-10) after the bonded retainer was removed. Note the light rim of supragingival calculus on the lingual tooth surfaces. (Courtesy of Dr. Corrie VanWanzeele, Indiana University School of Dentistry, Indianapolis, IN.)

Section 3
Dental Restorations as Local Factors

Most dental procedures have a positive impact on oral health. In some cases, however, some dental treatment may contribute to the onset of oral diseases, such as tooth decay or periodontal disease. Treatment that results in an inadvertent, adverse outcome is known as an **iatrogenic factor**. Some well-known examples of iatrogenic factors that increase plaque retention are poorly contoured crowns, overhanging margins, open margins, open contacts, orthodontic appliances, or a poorly designed dental prosthesis.

1. **Damage due to Improperly Contoured Restorations**
   A. **Overhanging Margins on Restorations**
      1. Ideally, the restorative margin should blend smoothly with the natural contours of the restored tooth. However, in some cases, it is not always possible for the dentist to contour the restoration smoothly with the surrounding tooth. When excess restorative material extends over the cavity margin or normal contours of the tooth, this condition is referred to as an **overhanging restoration** or more simply an overhang (Figs. 17-12 and 17-13). One can think of an overhang as the excess part of the restoration that "hangs over" the normal contours of the tooth.
      2. Because of difficulty accessing the tooth surfaces apical to the overhanging restoration, it is often impossible for a patient to remove plaque biofilm effectively from the tooth surface. This leads to plaque biofilm retention at the site and can subsequently lead to increased severity of either gingivitis or periodontitis at the site.
   B. **Open Margins on Restorations**
      1. There should be a smooth transition and seal between a restoration and the surrounding tooth, without any gaps, spaces, grooves, or rough areas. Whenever there is a space or gap between the edge of a restoration and the natural, unprepared tooth structure, it is referred to as an **open margin** (Fig. 17-14).
      2. Open margins are a problem when plaque biofilm gets into this space. Thus, overhanging and open margins have a similar adverse effect on the periodontium.

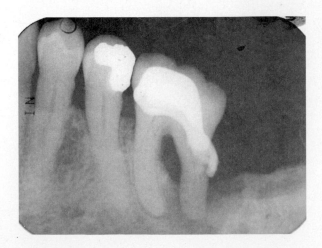

Figure 17-12. Radiographic Evidence of Poorly Contoured Restorations. Note that the restoration margins on the distal surfaces of the second premolar and first molar are not smoothly contoured with the actual tooth surfaces. This leads to increased biofilm retention these areas. (Courtesy of Dr. Richard Foster, Guilford Technical Community College, Jamestown, NC.)

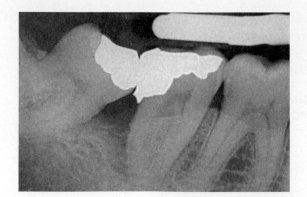

Figure 17-13. Radiographic Evidence of a Poorly Contoured Restoration. Note the large distal overhanging margin on the mandibular second molar. The distal overhanging margin on the second molar is a plaque biofilm retentive area that contributes to the formation of an angular defect in the alveolar bone.

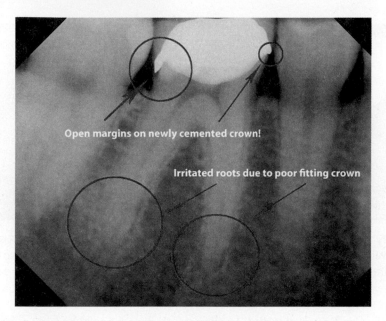

Figure 17-14. Radiographic Evidence of an Open Margin. Note the open margins on the mandibular first molar. (Courtesy of Dr. Christian W. Hahn, Prospect, Kentucky.)

C. Bulky or Overcontoured Crowns or Restorations

1. Bulky or overcontoured crowns or restorations can result in inadequate space between the teeth to accommodate the natural form of the interdental papilla.
   a. The space apical to the contact area of two adjacent teeth is referred to as an **embrasure space**. In health, the embrasure space is filled by an interdental papilla.
   b. Bulky crowns reduce the size of the embrasure space so that inadequate space exists between the teeth to accommodate the interdental papilla. In this situation, the bulky crowns are described as encroaching on the embrasure space (Fig. 17-15).

2. A restoration with a bulky contour acts as an area of biofilm accumulation and retention.
   a. The effectiveness of patient self-care is limited when a restoration is poorly contoured to the tooth surface. A poorly contoured restoration is a contributing factor to the development and spread of periodontal inflammation.
   b. It should be kept in mind that a poorly contoured restoration on a dental implant can have the same adverse effects as on a natural tooth (Fig. 17-16).

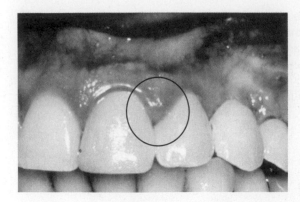

Figure 17-15. Bulky Crown Encroaching on Embrasure Space. The crowns shown here are so bulky in contour on their proximal surfaces that they fill the embrasure space leaving no room for the natural form of the papilla. Note the papilla between the central and lateral incisor appears enlarged because it is being pushed from between the teeth.

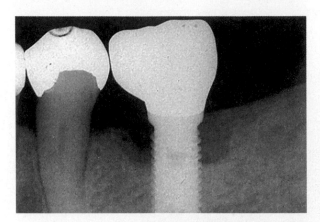
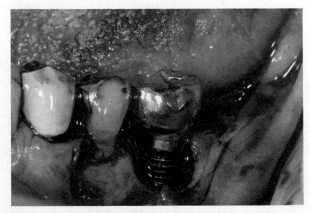

Figure 17-16. Poorly Contoured Crown on an Implant. This radiograph reveals a cup-like bony defect around the coronal third of a dental implant. Periodontal surgery (flap reflection) reveals an extensive defect in the alveolar around the implant. (Courtesy of Dr. Kazushi Yasumasu, Munakata, Fukuoka, Japan.)

2. **Damage due to Faulty Prosthetics and Appliances.** A dental prosthesis is an intraoral substitute—such as crown, fixed bridge, or removable denture—used to restore missing parts of teeth, missing teeth, and missing soft or hard tissues of the jaw and palate. The dental prosthesis, can be a challenging area for the patient to keep clean (Figs. 17-17 and 17-18). As a result, a dental prosthesis will be a plaque retentive area that could potentially trigger periodontal inflammation. A dental practitioner should be aware of the risk associated with a faulty designed prosthesis and should make every effort to design a prosthesis that has minimal plaque biofilm retentive features.

   A. **Inappropriate Crown Placement.** A crown is a metal, ceramic, or ceramic-bonded-to-metal covering for a badly damaged tooth. Placing a crown on a damaged tooth is a common way of restoring the form, function, and esthetics of the damaged tooth.

      1. A properly contoured crown with the edges of the crown (called margins) placed at least 2 mm *coronal* to the alveolar crest is paramount in maintaining gingival health and improving the prognosis of the previously damaged tooth.

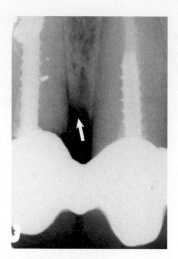

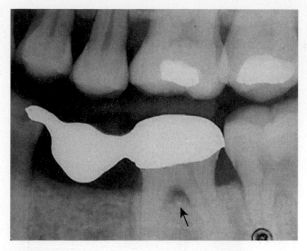

Figure 17-17. Splinted Crowns on the Maxillary Central Incisors. The incisor teeth have splinted crowns (the crowns are connected). This splinting makes interdental plaque removal difficult for the patient. As a result, an angular defect has formed in the alveolar bone between the two incisors.

Figure 17-18. The Design of the Dental Prosthesis Can Facilitate Plaque Biofilm Retention. The patient has difficulty in maintaining good oral hygiene around this bulky fixed bridge prosthesis. Note the furcation invasion on the abutment tooth (the mandibular left first molar).

2. A crown margin that is closer than 2 mm to the crest of the alveolar bone can result in resorption of alveolar bone. This is known as biologic width violation.
3. **Biologic width** refers to the zone of soft tissue occupied by the junctional epithelium and the connective tissue attachment fibers immediately apical to (below) the junctional epithelium (Fig. 17-19). One can think of the biologic width as the part of the periodontium that is *coronal* to the alveolar crest.
   a. This biologic width can be "violated" if the margin of a restoration encroaches upon this zone. If this occurs, the body will attempt to re-establish this zone by re-creating room between the alveolar crest and the restorative margin to allow space for the junctional epithelium and the connective tissue to reform.
   b. Unfortunately, by violating the biologic width, bone loss and gingival recession are unintended consequences. Figure 17-20 shows a restorative margin that violates the biologic width.

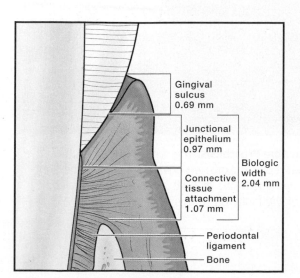

Gingival
sulcus
0.69 mm

Junctional
epithelium
0.97 mm

Biologic
width
2.04 mm

Connective
tissue
attachment
1.07 mm

Periodontal
ligament

Bone

Figure 17-19. Biologic Width in Health. Illustration showing the biologic width in health with average dimensions that have been reported in the literature. The 2017 AAP/EFP World Workshop recommends that the term "biologic width" be replaced by the more appropriate term "**supracrestal tissue attachment**" to reflect the zone of soft tissue coronal to the alveolar crest. For the purposes of this textbook, however, the term "biologic width" will be used throughout this chapter since this is the term that remains widely used in contemporary dental practice.

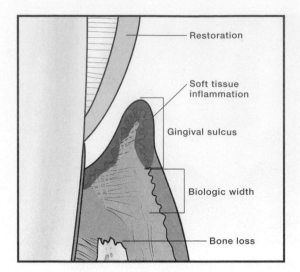

Figure 17-20. Consequences of a Restorative Margin that Violates the Biologic Width. If a restorative margin is placed too subgingival and violates the biologic width, two undesirable consequences may occur: unpredictable bone loss and/or gingival inflammation. Violating the biologic width will then lead to swelling, bleeding, and pain.

B. Faulty Removable Prosthesis

1. A removable prosthesis is one that the patient can remove for cleaning and before going to bed. A removable prosthesis that replaces a few teeth is commonly called a removable partial denture. A removable prosthesis that replaces an entire arch is referred to as a removable complete denture. A removable prosthesis that is attached to implants is known as an implant supported denture.

2. A removable prosthesis should be differentiated from a fixed prosthesis. A fixed prosthesis is permanently cemented to a single tooth (a crown), to several teeth (also known as a fixed bridge), or to an implant or several implants (known as implant-supported crown or bridge).

3. A damaged or poorly fitting removable prosthesis can impinge on gingival tissue and favor plaque biofilm accumulation. Eventually, this initiates periodontal inflammation (Fig. 17-21).

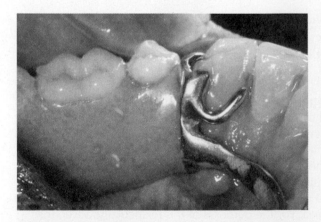
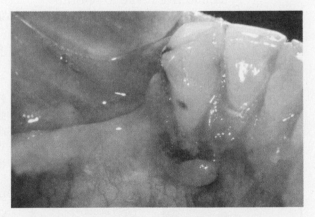

Figure 17-21. Tissue Damage by a Poorly Fitting Removable Prosthesis. The clinical photograph on the left shows a removable prosthesis (lower partial denture) that replaces extracted posterior teeth. In the right-hand photograph, the prosthesis is removed and the tissue damage to the mandibular canine is revealed. Gingival recession on the canine is due in part to the clasp of the faulty prosthesis impinging upon the gingival tissue. (Courtesy of Dr. Don Rolfs, Wenatchee, WA.)

Section 4
Local Factors That Cause Direct Damage

Section 4 discusses a few local contributing factors that may actually cause direct damage to the periodontium. These factors also may alter the progress of periodontal disease at individual sites. Some local contributing factors that can directly damage the periodontium include food impaction, patient habits, and faulty restorations or appliances.

In some patients, habits such as tongue thrusting, mouth breathing, or the improper use of toothbrushes, toothpicks, and other dental cleaning aids can also cause direct damage to the periodontium. This type of habit is known as a factitious injury (self-inflicted injury).

Most oral factitious injury is committed inadvertently without malingering intent. However, some patients may present with oral factitious injuries that are premediated with malingering intent. In the context of damage to the periodontium, malingering is defined as the intentional injury to the tissues by the patient to deliberately feign or exaggerate a physical or psychological symptom with the goal of receiving a reward. The motives for intentional trauma may include such incentives as insurance settlement, avoidance of work, or to seek sympathy from others. Malingering is difficult to diagnose because patients do not admit to causing their injury. In this case, proper consultation with a mental health care expert may be warranted.

1. **Direct Damage due to Food Impaction**
   A. **Definition.** Food impaction refers to forcing food (such as pieces of tough meat) between teeth during chewing, trapping the food in the interdental area (Fig. 17-22).
   B. **Effect of Food Impaction**
      1. Food forced into a tooth sulcus can strip the gingival tissues away from the tooth surface and contribute to periodontal breakdown in addition to the more obvious danger of serving as nutrients for tooth decaying bacteria.
      2. Food impaction not only damages the gingival tissues directly, but can also lead to alterations in gingival contour that result in interdental areas that are difficult for patients to clean.
2. **Direct Damage From Patient Habits and Oral Piercings**
   A. **Improper Use of Plaque Biofilm Control Aids.** Improper use of plaque biofilm control aids can result in direct damage to the gingival tissues causing alteration of the natural contours of the tissues (Fig. 17-23).
   B. **Tongue Thrusting.** Tongue thrusting is the application of forceful pressure against the anterior teeth with the tongue (Fig. 17-24).
      1. Tongue thrusting is often the result of an abnormal tongue positioning during the initial stage of swallowing.
      2. This oral habit exerts excessive lateral pressure against the teeth and may be traumatic to the periodontium.
   C. **Mouth Breathing.** Mouth breathing is the process of inhaling and exhaling air primarily through the mouth, rather than the nose, and often occurs while the patient is sleeping. Mouth breathing has a tendency to dry out the gingival tissues in the anterior region of the mouth.
   D. **Traumatic Toothbrushing.** Traumatic tooth brushing is the aggressive, forceful use of a toothbrush in a horizontal or rotary fashion (Fig. 17-25). This trauma may be a result of either improper toothbrushing habits or overzealous toothbrushing practices.
      1. The deleterious effect of traumatic toothbrushing may be exacerbated by the use of highly abrasive dentifrices. The dental clinician should make every effort to identify signs of traumatic toothbrushing and reinforce proper toothbrushing techniques to the patient.

2. If left unabated, traumatic toothbrushing will result in tissue abrasion, gingival recession with loss of alveolar bone on the labial side, and subsequently root exposure.

3. This type of bony defect is known as **dehiscence** (Fig. 17-26). A dehiscence should not be confused with a **fenestration** which is a "window" of bone loss bordered by alveolar bone on its coronal aspect. A fenestration is not commonly associated with gingival recession.

E. **Oral Jewelry.** Body piercing is the placement of a foreign object through tissue of the body. Figure 17-27 shows a pierced tongue.

1. Oral piercings, such as a tongue piercing or lip piercing, can cause direct damage by mechanically traumatizing the periodontal tissues. Common adverse events associated with oral piercing include gingival recession, infection, swelling, bleeding, tooth fractures, and allergic reactions.

2. Oral jewelry needs to be removed prior to taking radiographs. Members of the dental team should be at the forefront of informing patients of the possible deleterious effects of oral jewelry.

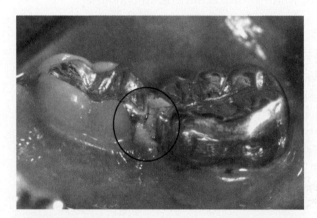

Figure 17-22. Food Impaction. Note the food impaction between the two molar teeth. As this patient chews food, the food is forced between these teeth and produces direct damage to the periodontium. (Courtesy of Dr. Don Rolfs, Wenatchee, WA.)

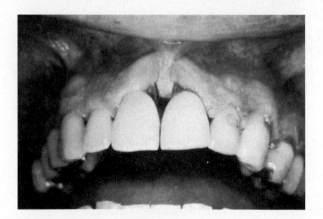

Figure 17-23. Misuse of Toothpick. The interdental papilla between the two central incisors has been destroyed by the patient's habit of repeatedly forcing a toothpick between the teeth. This damage to the papillae is an example of direct damage to the periodontium.

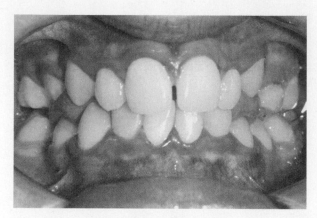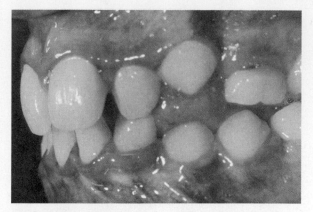

Figure 17-24. Tongue Thrust. Pictured on the left, the facial view of a patient with a tongue thrust. As this patient swallows, the patient applies lateral pressure with her tongue against the teeth. The right-hand photo shows a side view of the tongue thrust. The tongue is visible in the canine region of the mouth as the patient presses her tongue forward when swallowing. (Courtesy of Dr. Don Rolfs, Periodontal Foundations, Wenatchee, WA.)

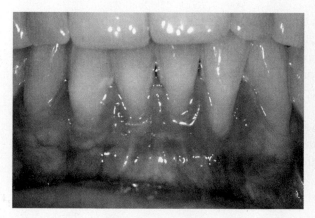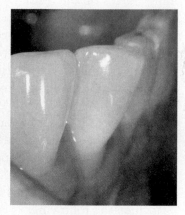

Figure 17-25. Direct Damage to the Periodontium Caused by Traumatic Toothbrushing. This patient overzealously brushes her teeth with a hard-bristle toothbrush. Although overzealous toothbrushing has resulted in minimal gingival inflammation and plaque accumulation seen in this mouth, it has also traumatized the periodontal tissues and caused gingival recession. Note how thin the gingival tissue appears from the facial and the lateral views. (Courtesy of Dr. Hawra Al-Qallaf, Indianapolis, IN.)

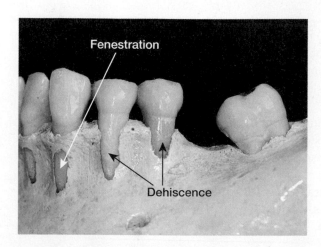

Figure 17-26. Fenestration and Dehiscences.
A fenestration—"window" of bone loss—on the facial aspect of the mandible. Note that the marginal bone is intact in the fenestrated area. Dehiscences, pictured here, are "V-shaped" defects apical to the cementoenamel junctions extending through the marginal bone.

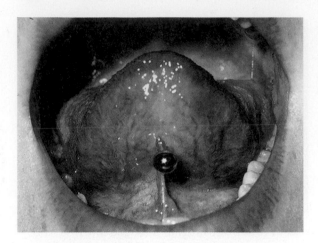

Figure 17-27. Oral Piercing. The metal tongue barbell, pictured here, is a popular object placed in a pierced tongue. (Courtesy of Langlais RP. *Color Atlas of Common Oral Diseases*. 5th ed. Philadelphia, PA: Wolters Kluwer.)

3. **Direct Damage From Occlusal Forces**
   A. **Trauma From Occlusion**
      1. Direct damage to the periodontium can result from *excessive* occlusal (or biting) forces on the teeth.
      2. When excessive occlusal forces cause damage to the periodontium, this is referred to as **trauma from occlusion**. Table 17-2 summarizes definitions of some terms used to describe trauma from occlusion.
         a. When trauma from occlusion occurs, some alveolar bone resorption can result simply because of increased pressure placed on the surrounding alveolar bone.
         b. When there is loss of some alveolar bone due to trauma from occlusion, there can be a more rapid destruction by any existing periodontitis.
      3. A thorough clinical and radiographic exam can frequently reveal signs of trauma from occlusion.
         a. Some of the clinical signs of trauma from occlusion that have been reported include the following:
            1) Tooth mobility
            2) Sensitivity to pressure
            3) Migration of teeth
         b. Some of the radiographic signs of trauma from occlusion that have been reported include the following:
            1) Enlarged, funnel-shaped PDL space
            2) Angular alveolar bone resorption
      4. Trauma from occlusion has been classified in the dental literature for many years as either primary trauma from occlusion or secondary trauma from occlusion.
         a. **Primary trauma from occlusion** is defined as excessive occlusal forces on a sound periodontium with no previous history of periodontal breakdown (Fig. 17-28).
            1) Examples of causes of primary trauma from occlusion include inadvertent placement of a high restoration or insertion of a fixed bridge or partial denture that places excessive force on periodontally healthy supporting teeth.
            2) The changes seen in primary occlusal trauma include a wider PDL space, tooth mobility, and even tooth and jaw pain. These changes are reversible if the trauma is removed.

b. Secondary trauma from occlusion occurs when normal or excessive occlusal forces are placed on teeth with an unhealthy periodontium previously weakened by periodontitis, thus contributing harm to an already damaged periodontium.

1) Secondary trauma from occlusion occurs to a tooth in which the surrounding periodontium has experienced apical migration of the junctional epithelium, loss of connective tissue attachment, and loss of alveolar bone. In this type of trauma, the periodontium was unhealthy prior to experiencing excessive occlusal forces.

2) A tooth with an unhealthy, inflamed periodontium that is subjected to excessive occlusal forces is thought to be more susceptible to more rapid bone loss and pocket formation.

3) Teeth can be tipped laterally easily when subjected to lateral occlusal forces. These tipping forces frequently accompany trauma from occlusion and can create areas of pressure and tension within the PDL that are transmitted to the bone. Figure 17-29 illustrates how this tipping can occur. As alveolar bone loss progresses, this lateral tipping becomes even more likely because of the longer lever arm created by the part of the tooth out of the bone compared to the part of the tooth encased in bone.

4) Teeth with reduced alveolar bone support can have additional damage to the periodontium because of the tipping action of lateral forces placed on the teeth. Figure 17-29 shows a series of drawings that illustrate this concept. Figures 17-30 and 17-31 show radiographs of teeth that have been subjected to secondary occlusal trauma.

TABLE 17-2	TERMS ASSOCIATED WITH TRAUMA FROM OCCLUSION
Term	**Definition**
Trauma from occlusion	Injury to the periodontium resulting from excessive occlusal forces
Primary trauma from occlusion	Injury to a healthy periodontium resulting from excessive occlusal forces
Secondary trauma from occlusion	Injury from normal or excessive occlusal forces applied to a periodontium previously damaged by periodontitis

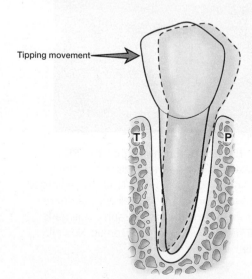

Tipping movement

Figure 17-28. Primary Trauma From Occlusion. Tipping of a tooth within the socket due to lateral occlusal forces often accompanies trauma from occlusion. This tipping can result in areas of pressure and tension within the PDL. In the illustration, "P" indicates an area of pressure in the PDL and alveolar bone. The letter "T" indicates an area of tension. Bone under pressure tends to undergo resorption.

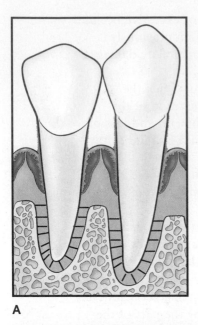
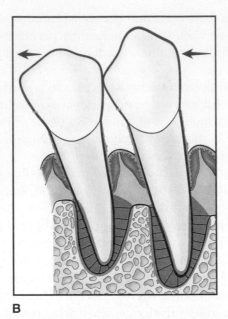
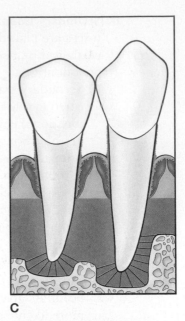

A   **B**   **C**

Figure 17-29. Secondary Trauma From Occlusion: Damage to Teeth With Existing Periodontitis. A.
Teeth with reduced bone height from existing periodontitis. **B.** Teeth being subjected to lateral forces and being moved laterally by those forces. **C.** Additional bone loss to the periodontium as a result of pressure on bone from the lateral tooth movement. The additional bone loss that occurs from secondary trauma from occlusion can further compound the periodontal destruction that occurs due to periodontitis.

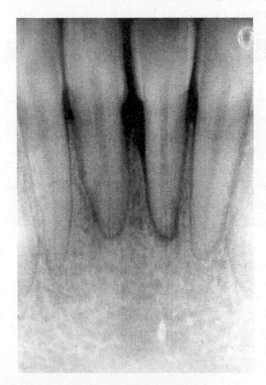

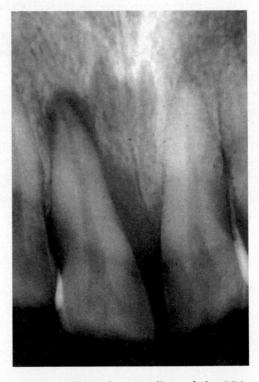

Figure 17-30. Radiographic Evidence of Trauma From Occlusion. Note the dramatic widening of the periodontal ligament space along the lateral root surfaces on the mandibular left central incisor (center tooth on radiograph). The alveolar bone has been destroyed because of the pressure resulting from trauma from occlusion.

Figure 17-31. Enlarged, Funneling of the PDL Space. The maxillary right central incisor has been subjected to trauma from occlusion. Note the enlarged, funnel-shaped widening of the PDL along the entire length of the root. This is the radiographic hallmark of occlusal trauma. (Courtesy of Dr. Donald Newell, Indianapolis, IN.)

B. **Parafunctional Occlusal Forces**

1. A series of other terms has been used to describe occlusal forces. Two of these terms are functional and parafunctional occlusal forces.

   a. **Functional occlusal forces** are the normal forces produced during the act of chewing food (also known as mastication).

   b. **Parafunctional occlusal forces** result from tooth-to-tooth contact made when not in the act of eating.

      1) Examples of these parafunctional habits are clenching of the teeth together as a release of nervous tension or grinding the teeth together for the same release.

         a) **Clenching** is the continuous or intermittent forceful closure of the maxillary teeth against the mandibular teeth.

         b) **Bruxism** is forceful grinding of the teeth.

         c) These parafunctional habits can occur without the person having conscious knowledge of the habit. Some individuals exhibit these habits while asleep.

      2) Parafunctional habits can exert excessive force on the teeth and to the periodontium.

2. There are several clinical therapies that can be used by a dentist to help control the damage from trauma from occlusion.

   a. When the trauma is a result of a faulty bite (referred to as a faulty occlusion), the dentist can make minor adjustments in the bite by selectively reshaping (also known as selective grinding) the occlusal surfaces of the teeth to minimize the damaging forces and eliminate occlusal interferences. This procedure is called an occlusal adjustment.

   b. When the trauma is a result of bruxism, the dentist can fabricate an acrylic appliance known as an occlusal appliance (also referred to as an occlusal splint or a night guard) that can protect the teeth during part of each day. It should be emphasized that an occlusal appliance does not cure bruxism, but rather intervenes by protecting the teeth and implants (if present) from further wear.

4. **Direct Damage Caused by Normal Anatomic Factors.** Typically, normal anatomic factors are not injurious to the periodontium. One exception, however, is a high frenal attachment.

   A. A frenum is a thin fold of mucous membrane with enclosed muscle fibers that attaches the lips to the alveolar mucosa and underlying periosteum (Fig. 17-32). A frenum's primary function is to provide stability to the lips, cheeks, and tongue.

      1. Intraorally, there are four major oral frena: (1) the maxillary labial frenum (connects the upper lip to the gingiva); (2) the mandibular labial frenum (connects the lower lip to the gingiva); (3) the buccal frenum (connects the cheek to the gingiva); and (4) the mandibular lingual frenum (connects the tongue to the gingiva).

      2. Depending on the location, the frenum provides stability to the upper lip, lower lip, cheek, or tongue.

   B. The frenum can be clinically examined by applying light tension to the upper lip, lower lip, or cheek.

   C. A frenum can become a significant problem if tension from lip movement pulls the gingival margin away from the tooth (Figs. 17-33 and 17-34). An abnormal frenal attachment located in close proximity to the gingival margin will distend the gingival sulcus (as the muscular fibers in the frenum repeatedly pull on the gingival margin). This is known as a **frenal pull**. Frenal problems occur most often on the facial surface between the maxillary and mandibular central incisors and in the canine and premolar areas.

D. The presence of any abnormal frenal attachments can be corrected through a procedure known as a frenectomy. However, if the abnormal frenal attachment is not surgically eliminated, the frenum will continually pull down the marginal gingiva and make the exposed root surface more susceptible to plaque biofilm accumulation. This may lead to root caries and/or periodontal disease. If not removed, the health of the tooth and the periodontium may be jeopardized.

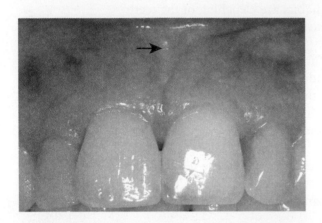

Figure 17-32. Normal Frenal Attachment. Note the healthy band of keratinized tissue separating the maxillary labial frenum from the gingival margin of the maxillary central incisors. Also note the lack of tissue blanching or "pulling" of the gingival margin as tension is applied to the upper lip.

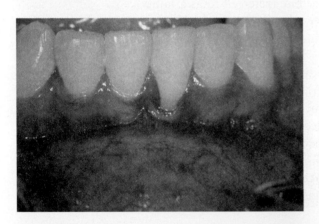

Figure 17-33. Direct Periodontal Damage Caused by a High Frenal Attachment. Note the high frenal attachment between the central incisor teeth. Tension of the lower lip pulls down the gingival margin and contributes to the gingival recession seen on the mandibular left central incisor. Continued tension by the frenum, if not removed, will lead to further progression of tissue breakdown.

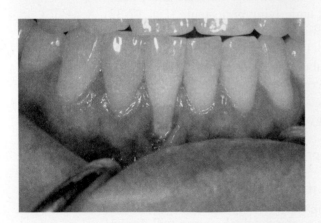

Figure 17-34. Abnormal Frenal Attachment. Note the close proximity of the frenal attachment to the gingival margin of the right central incisor. This patient complains of tooth sensitivity whenever he brushes the exposed root surface, so he does not brush the area very well. Consequently, plaque biofilm has accumulated over the root surface and the marginal gingiva has become severely inflamed.

Chapter Summary Statement

Local contributing factors can increase the risk of developing gingivitis or periodontitis or increase the risk of developing more severe disease when gingivitis or periodontitis are already established. Local factors can increase the risk of periodontal disease by increasing plaque biofilm retention and causing direct damage to the periodontium. As will be discussed in Chapter 20, the dental team must identify these local contributing factors during a clinical assessment so that any local contributing factors can be eliminated or minimized before the disease progresses to a stage that results in permanent damage to the teeth and surrounding periodontium.

Section 5
Focus on Patients

Clinical Patient Care

CASE 1

Examination of a patient reveals gingivitis. In addition, the patient has generalized calculus deposits and numerous restorations with overhangs. What steps might be necessary to bring the gingivitis under control in this patient?

CASE 2

Examination of a patient reveals periodontitis. The patient also has a severe tooth clenching habit. Explain how the tooth clenching habit could be related to the progress of the periodontitis.

Evidence in Action

CASE 1

In a dental hygiene journal, you find an article that refers to mature dental plaque biofilm. Explain what the author means by this term mature dental plaque biofilm.

References

1. Genco RJ. Current view of risk factors for periodontal diseases. *J Periodontol*. 1996;67(10 Suppl):1041–1049.
2. Leknes KN. The influence of anatomic and iatrogenic root surface characteristics on bacterial colonization and periodontal destruction: a review. *J Periodontol*. 1997;68(6):507–516.
3. Pihlstrom B. Treatment of periodontitis: key principles include removing subgingival bacterial deposits; providing a local environment and education to support good home care; providing regular professional maintenance. *J Periodontol*. 2014;85(5):655–656.

 STUDENT ANCILLARY RESOURCES

A wide variety of resources to enhance your learning is available online:

- Audio Glossary
- Book Pages
- Chapter Review Questions and Answers

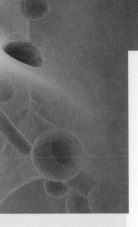

18 Nutrition, Inflammation, and Periodontal Disease

Clinical Application. Though the precise relationship between nutrition and periodontal disease is not fully understood, all members of the dental team must be aware of what is known about this relationship and understand how to apply this information to guide patients with nutritional issues that may have an impact upon periodontal health. This chapter reviews the emerging evidence on the association between nutrition and periodontal disease and provides some valuable recommendations for applying this information to a clinical setting.

Learning Objectives

- Discuss the link between obesity and periodontal disease.
- Discuss the role of polymorphonuclear leukocytes in the production of reactive oxygen species in response to plaque biofilm.
- Discuss how antioxidants may influence periodontal disease onset and progression.
- Describe the proposed roles of micronutrients and macronutrients in periodontal disease.
- List some oral symptoms associated with ascorbic acid deficiency gingivitis.
- Explain the role of dental health care providers in addressing obesity and nutrition in the management of periodontal disease.

Key Terms

Obesity
Body mass index (BMI)
Reactive oxygen species (ROS)
Antioxidants

Micronutrients
Macronutrients
Ascorbic acid deficiency gingivitis

Historically, periodontal disease was seen as an inflammatory disease with limited associations to nutrition. Unlike the link between sugar and dental caries, many early studies into the relationship between nutrition and periodontal disease failed to show associations between nutritional status and periodontal disease. These studies, however, used poor methodologies, tended to study nutrients in isolation, and failed to control for confounding variables (such as smoking). Improved understanding of periodontal disease at the cellular level and more stringent nutritional methodologies have created a renewed interest in the relationship between nutrition and periodontal disease. *Recent research is focused on (1) the association between obesity and periodontal inflammation and (2) the role of antioxidants in the prevention and treatment of periodontal disease.*

Section 1
Association Between Obesity and Periodontal Disease

1. **Obesity Overview**
   A. Obesity is an excess amount of body fat in proportion to lean body mass, to the extent that health is impaired.[1]
      1. The most commonly used measure of body fat is the **body mass index (BMI)**, which is defined as a person's weight in kilograms divided by the square of his/her height in meters. The World Health Organization and the National Heart, Lung, and Blood Institute define overweight as a BMI of 25 to 29.9 and obesity as a BMI of equal to or greater than 30. Over 1.9 billion adults worldwide were overweight in 2014.[2]
      2. More than 65% of the US adult population, 15.8% of children aged 6 to 11 years, and 16.1% of adolescents aged 12 to 19 years, are overweight.[3,4]
      3. More than a third of adults (38%) and 17% of youth (ages 2 to 19) were obese in 2011 to 2014. However, more women over 60 became obese with the prevalence rising to 40% from 31.5% in that group during that time. The CDC data comes from an analysis of the National Health and Nutrition Examination Survey (NHANES) 2011 to 2014 in the United States.[3,4] NHANES is a research study started in the 1960s to assess the health and nutritional status of children and adults in the United States. International trends are similar to those in the USA. The International Obesity Task Force estimates that over 1 billion adults are overweight.[5]
   B. Adipose tissue is a complex and metabolically active endocrine organ that secretes numerous immunomodulatory factors and plays a major role in regulating metabolic and vascular biology.[6] Obese individuals are reported to have elevated levels of circulating tumor necrosis factor-alpha (TNF-α) and interleukin-6 (IL-6) compared to normal weight controls.[7]
2. **The Obesity–Periodontal Disease Link**
   A. Recent research has uncovered a possible a link between obesity and periodontal disease.[8–13]
      1. An analysis of data from the NHANES III involving over 13,000 individuals having one or more sites with clinical attachment loss found a positive correlation between BMI and the severity of periodontal attachment loss.[14]

2. Al-Zahrani and colleagues conducted a study of a representative sample of participants in the NHANES III survey who were 18 years or younger and had undergone a periodontal examination.

   a. The purpose of the study was to examine the relation between body weight and periodontal disease in a representative United States sample. BMI and waist circumference were used as measures of overall and abdominal fat content, respectively.

   b. Study results indicate that even in a younger population, both overall and abdominal obesity are associated with increased prevalence of periodontal disease, while underweight (BMI <18.5) is associated with decreased prevalence.[15]

3. Recent systemic reviews indicate that individuals who are overweight/obese are more likely to suffer from periodontitis compared to individuals of a normal weight.[13,16]

4. In the USA, a case study by the Forsyth Institute reports that obesity is related to a marked increase in plaque biofilm accumulation, attachment loss, deep pockets, bleeding on probing, and an increase in the proportion of *Tannerella forsythia* (*Bacteroides forsythus*).[17]

B. Among lifestyle-related risk factors, smoking has the greatest impact on periodontitis.[18] Both smoking and obesity are independent risk indicators for periodontitis. Nishida and colleagues suggest that obesity is second only to smoking as the strongest lifestyle-related factor for inflammatory periodontal disease destruction.[19]

3. **Biological Mechanisms Linking Obesity With Periodontal Disease.** The mechanism of how obesity modifies the pathogenesis of periodontal disease at the molecular level currently is poorly understood, but what is known is that obesity has several harmful biological effects that might be related to the pathogenesis of periodontitis.[20]

A. **Release of Proinflammatory Cytokines From Adipose Tissue.** Further studies are needed to determine if obesity is a true risk factor for periodontal disease. Several researchers have suggested that the association most likely lies in the commonality of their inflammatory pathways. According to Genco and colleagues, the continuous release of proinflammatory cytokines into the systemic circulation from adipose tissue in obese individuals provides a "systemic inflammatory overload."[14] This relentless release of cytokines provides a possible explanation of how obesity intensifies infections, including periodontal disease.

1. Adipose tissue secretes several cytokines and hormones that are involved in inflammatory processes, suggesting that these pathways are involved in the pathogenesis of obesity and periodontitis. The adverse effect of obesity on the periodontium may be mediated through proinflammatory cytokines like interleukins (IL-1, IL-6, and TNF-α), adipokines (cell-signaling molecules, i.e leptin and adiponectin), and reactive oxygen species (ROS) which may affect the periodontal tissues directly.[21]

   a. Prior to the 1990s, adipose tissue was generally thought of as being inactive and functioning primarily as a tissue containing fat stores, which were available as a reserve source of energy. Research starting in the 1990s, however, made us reevaluate our thoughts on adipose tissue. Adipose tissue is now viewed as a complex, dynamic, metabolically active endocrine organ composed of a variety of cell types. In addition to energy storage, it is now recognized as being involved with metabolic regulation and in immune function.[6,22]

    b. Adipose tissue is a complex of adipocytes with stromal and vascular elements infiltrated with resident lymphocytes and macrophages. It has an extensive distribution throughout the body and may be considered the largest endocrine tissue in the body. In obesity, there is an increase in both fat cell numbers and fat cell size.[6]

    c. Adipose tissue secretes hormones, growth factors, cytokines, and enzymes. These products can affect the overall systemic inflammation and the body's sensitivity to insulin, in turn affecting the whole-body metabolism. Adipose tissue also differs in its ability to produce cytokines based upon its location in the body.

    d. Both harmful and beneficial cytokines can be released from adipose tissue. The adipocytes can provide both the beneficial adiponectin and the proinflammatory cytokines, TNF-α and plasminogen activator inhibitor-1 (PAI-1). In addition, the resident macrophages also secrete TNF-α and IL-6 into the systemic circulation.

2. Adiponectin is a circulating hormone secreted only by adipose tissue and is involved in glucose and lipid metabolism.

    a. Adiponectin production is decreased in obese individuals. It aids in increasing whole-body insulin sensitivity. It has a negative correlation with a person's fat mass.

    b. Low levels of adiponectin are associated with increased systemic inflammation.[23]

3. Leptin is a proinflammatory mediator, whose concentration is dependent upon the energy stored in the body fat.

    a. Leptin has been shown to increase with eating and is elevated in obese individuals, but is found at reduced levels in lean individuals and on fasting. It tends to decrease appetite, but obese individuals may show resistance to its effects leading to no suppression of appetite.[6]

    b. Many researchers consider leptin resistance to be one of the features contributing to obesity's pathology.[23] It has been demonstrated that human leptin is present within healthy gingival tissue and decreases in concentration with increased probing depths.[24]

4. Obesity-associated TNF-α is secreted from both the adipocytes and the macrophages present within the adipose tissue. As people gain weight, there is an increased infiltration of macrophages within their adipose tissue.

    a. This secretion from the adipose tissue is thought to be the greatest contributor of TNF-α to the systemic circulation. It is thought that increased circulating TNF-α from adipose tissue contributes to general systemic inflammation.[8]

    b. TNF-α has been highly implicated in insulin resistance. It is also seen at elevated levels in periodontitis.[8]

5. About 30% of circulating IL-6 is thought to be derived from adipose tissue. Increasing levels of obesity stimulates IL-6 secretion.[25]

    a. An increased risk of developing coronary artery disease is seen with elevated levels of IL-6.[25]

    b. Inflamed periodontal tissues also demonstrate higher levels of IL-6.[26] IL-6 has been shown to stimulate osteoclasts and thus contribute to the alveolar bone loss seen in periodontitis.

6. PAI-1 has been shown to increase in the systemic circulation as adipose tissue increases. It is a protein involved in fibrinolysis and contributes to atherosclerosis. It has been shown to be elevated in periodontal disease.[6]

B. **Increased Levels of Reactive Oxygen Species**

1. Reactive oxygen species (ROS) are chemically active oxygen-containing molecules. ROS can have either physiologic or pathologic properties dependent upon their concentration. ROS have an important role in normal cellular processes and are produced during normal mitochondrial metabolism. At low concentrations, ROS function in cell signaling and allow for proper tissue homeostasis helping to direct normal cellular proliferation, differentiation, and metabolism. At lower levels, ROS can stimulate the growth of epithelial cells and fibroblasts present in the periodontal tissues.[27]

2. Higher concentrations of ROS, however, can lead to tissue damage. Higher levels of ROS can be generated by various cells through exposure to cytokines, bacteria or bacterial products, and tobacco products resulting in elevated levels of ROS with resultant tissue destruction. ROS are also released with platelet activation and from phagocytic cells such as neutrophils and macrophages. This elevation of ROS can lead to periodontal tissue damage.[27]

3. Damage to the periodontal tissues can be prevented or reduced by having adequate stores of antioxidant molecules within the tissues. These antioxidants can include vitamin C and E, β-carotene, selenium, uric acid, and glutathione. These antioxidants can help to prevent the formation of ROS or can help convert them to less reactive forms.[28]

4. An imbalance between ROS production and the antioxidant capacity of the periodontal tissue can lead to the development of periodontal disease. It is likely that the presence of periodontal inflammation results in the body's stores of antioxidants being depleted. The levels of antioxidants in gingival crevicular fluid were determined to be statistically lower in patients with periodontal disease compared to age- and sex-matched controls with periodontal health.[29] While in a survey of over 1,200 Western European men aged 60 to 70, lower serum levels of β-carotene were linked to an increased prevalence of periodontal disease.[30]

5. Emerging scientific evidence indicates that obesity appears to play a role in the multifactorial etiology of periodontitis through the increased production of ROS and an increase in inflammatory cytokines. Figure 18-1 shows a suggested model for the link between obesity and periodontal disease.

4. **The Role of the Dental Team in Managing Obesity and Periodontal Disease**

A. All members of the dental team should be aware of the increasing numbers of obese persons and the significance of obesity as a risk factor for oral health. Addressing obesity in the management of periodontal disease is clearly important in patients who have both conditions. This necessitates the cooperation and collaboration of all health care professionals to educate patients regarding the implications of obesity and periodontitis and to encourage counseling, weight reduction, and treatment.

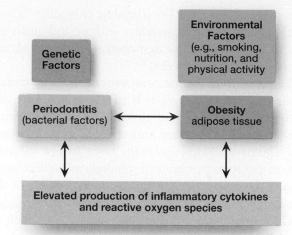

Figure 18-1. Hypothesis Linking Obesity and Periodontal Disease. One hypothesis linking obesity and periodontal disease is that both conditions are associated with an elevated production of both inflammatory cytokines and reactive oxygen species. Of course, both conditions also are affected by other background factors such as genetic factors and environmental factors, which makes identifying a precise link between them difficult.

Section 2
Micronutrients, Antioxidants, and Periodontal Disease

Nutrients are divided into six categories: vitamins, minerals, proteins, lipids, carbohydrates, and water. Micronutrients are nutrients that are needed in microgram to milligram quantities. Vitamins and calcium are two examples of micronutrients. Proteins, lipids, and carbohydrates are macronutrients, which provide energy or calories and are ingested in gram quantities.

1. **Micronutrients and Oxidation**
   A. **Oxidation.** As oxygen interacts with cells of any type—a ripening banana or a cell in the body—oxidation occurs. Oxidation produces some type of change in the cell. The banana may rot or in time, dead body cells are replaced with new cells.
   1. Oxidative stress occurs with the production of harmful molecules called free radicals.
   2. Free radicals containing oxygen, known as reactive oxygen species (ROS), are the most biologically significant free radicals.[28]
   3. It is impossible for the cells of the body to avoid damage by free radicals. Free radicals arise from sources both inside and outside the body. Oxidants develop from processes within the body as the result of normal metabolism and inflammation. Outside the body, free radicals form from environmental factors such as pollution, sunlight, smoking, and radiation.
   4. In response to plaque biofilm, polymorphonuclear leukocytes (PMNs) produce ROS during phagocytosis as part of the host response to infection.[31] These ROS can cause damage to proteins causing fragmentation, peroxidation of lipids, and strand breakage of DNA.
      a. Individuals with periodontal disease have increased numbers of hyperactive PMNs.
      b. It has been suggested that this proliferation results in a high degree of ROS release, culminating in heightened damage to gingival tissue, periodontal ligaments, and alveolar bone.[32]

    c. Studies also have suggested the ROS stimulate osteoclast activation.[33] Compared with healthy controls, patients with periodontitis generate higher levels of ROS. Several studies have demonstrated a correlation between ROS and periodontal disease activity.[28,34–36]

  5. *The damage mediated by ROS can be counteracted by antioxidants.*[37]

B. Antioxidants. Antioxidants are substances that can counteract the damaging effects of the physiological process of oxidation in a living organism.

  1. Nature provides thousands of different antioxidants in fruits, vegetables, nuts, whole grains, and legumes to help protect the body from oxidation.

  2. Dietary antioxidants include vitamins and minerals as well as enzymes (proteins in the body that assist in chemical reactions). Some of the common antioxidants include β-carotene, vitamin C, vitamin E, and selenium.

  3. Data from research suggests that there are mechanisms in which nutrition, particularly antioxidants, can influence periodontal disease onset, progression, and wound healing.[38] Antioxidants are thought to be important in the downregulation of proinflammatory responses. While additional information is needed, it is theorized that nutrients can act as antioxidants that may modulate gingival inflammation.[37,38]

2. Vitamins and Minerals

A. Vitamins. Vitamins are organic compounds that are not synthesized by the body and are necessary for normal metabolism. Vitamin C is the most common water-soluble antioxidant while vitamin E is one of the most common fat-soluble antioxidants.

  1. Vitamin C

    a. Vitamin C is a water-soluble vitamin that cannot be stored by the body.

      1) All plants and most animals can synthesize vitamin C from glucose. On the other hand, humans, nonhuman primates, and a few other animals do not have the appropriate enzymes to synthesize vitamin C. Since the human body lacks the ability to synthesize and store vitamin C, we depend on dietary sources to meet our vitamin C needs.

      2) Vitamin C is found in fresh fruits and vegetables such as oranges, berries, tomatoes, leafy greens, and kiwifruit. Consumption of fruits and vegetables or fortifying diets with vitamin C supplements is essential to avoid ascorbic acid deficiency.

    b. Vitamin C is also known as ascorbic acid. It was named for its ability to cure scurvy. Scurvy is a vitamin C deficiency disease that can lead to muscle weakness, painful and swollen joints, an increased risk of bone fractures, poor wound healing, gingival inflammation, and a weakened periodontal ligament.

    c. The recommended dietary allowance (RDA) for vitamin C is 90 mg for men and 75 mg for women. Smokers are advised to take an additional 35 mg of vitamin C to reduce the oxidative damage caused by smoking.

    d. Dr. James Lind, a British Royal Navy surgeon, discovered in 1753 that through the addition of citrus fruits to the normal shipboard diet, he could prevent the development of scurvy in the sailors. Due to the presence of citrus fruits carried by British ships, British sailors received the name of "limey."[39]

    e. Vitamin C has effective antioxidant properties that are important for maintaining the integrity of cell membranes and protection against the ROS generated during inflammatory responses.[40]

    f. In addition, vitamin C can enhance neutrophil, monocyte, and natural-killer cell functions.[41]

g. Data from NHANES III showed that a lower level of intake of vitamin C lead to an increased risk of having periodontal disease in both current and former smokers.[42] Further analysis demonstrated that by having an increased serum concentration of vitamin C, there was a reduced risk of developing periodontitis.[43]

h. In scurvy, mature collagen fibers do not develop resulting in the presence of immature collagen in the bodily tissues. Vitamin C is needed to modify the amino acids, proline and lysine, for collagen maturation to occur. Collagen is a major component of the periodontium. In ascorbic acid deficiency gingivitis, patients present with tooth mobility (due to the presence of a weakened, immature periodontal ligament).

i. **Ascorbic acid deficiency gingivitis** is an inflammatory response of the gingiva caused by plaque biofilm that is aggravated by chronically low vitamin C (ascorbic acid) levels.

1) Ascorbic acid deficiency gingivitis manifests clinically as bright red, swollen, ulcerated gingival tissue that bleeds with the slightest provocation.[44]

2) An example of infantile vitamin C deficiency is shown in Figures 18-2 and 18-3.

j. In a different case, a 39-year-old woman, presented with severe signs of oral scurvy. Her typical diet consisted of macaroni and cheese, peanut butter, and soda. She could not recall when she had consumed a fruit or vegetable. Her serum vitamin C level was about 10 times below average.[45]

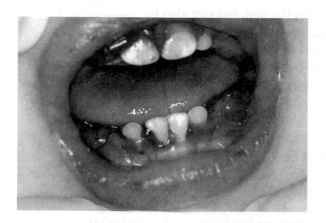

Figure 18-2. Ascorbic Acid Deficiency Gingivitis. This 15-month-old boy had a history of unexplained gingival bleeding for several weeks and fever for 2 days. He had been fed only cow's milk and oatmeal since age 4 months. Laboratory blood tests revealed that his vitamin C levels were low. (Used with permission from Riepe FG, Eichmann D, Oppermann HC, et al. Special feature: picture of the month. Infantile scurvy. *Arch Pediatr Adolesc Med.* 2001;155(5):607–608. All rights reserved.)

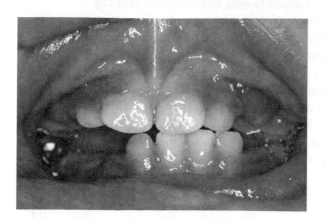

Figure 18-3. After Treatment With Vitamin C. The same boy shown in Figure 18-2 after 3 days' treatment with vitamin C. (Courtesy of Dr. Felix G. Riepe, MD, Christian Albrechts University, Kiel, Germany.)

Section 3
Macronutrients and Periodontal Disease

Proteins, lipids, and carbohydrates are macronutrients, which provide energy or calories. These are eaten in gram quantities versus the micronutrients, which are eaten in milligram to microgram quantities. Many of the pathways to inflammation are related to high caloric intake from refined carbohydrates and oxidative stress, which is stimulated by changes in the metabolism of adipose tissue.[61]

1. **Proteins**
   A. Protein deficiency can have an effect on the host defenses that may modulate the progress of periodontitis. Proteins are needed to provide defensive barriers, such as the junctional and crevicular epithelium. They also contribute to other host immune responses, such as cell-meditated immunity, humoral or antibody mediated immunity, cytokines, and complement molecules. These defenses are impaired with a protein deficiency.
   B. The effect of protein-energy malnutrition on periodontal disease risk was extensively reviewed by Enwonwu and colleagues, who observed that periodontal disease was more prevalent and severe in undernourished individuals than in well-nourished ones.[62] The immune depression that occurs in protein-energy malnutrition promotes vulnerability of the periodontium to inflammatory stimuli from the plaque biofilm.

2. **Refined Carbohydrates and Lipids.** Diets rich in refined carbohydrates and saturated fats may play a role in increasing the risk for periodontal disease. Excessive energy intake causes obesity, which has been shown to be associated with increased risk of periodontitis.
   A. Excess consumption of refined carbohydrates can affect the immune response and may lead to continued destruction of the periodontium in patients with existing periodontitis through mechanisms such as the action of enzymes (i.e., collagenase) and proinflammatory mediators (i.e., IL-1 and IL-6).[61] These destructive mechanisms have been discussed in other chapters of this book.
   B. Diets high in refined carbohydrates and saturated fats cause rapid release of glucose into the bloodstream (Table 18-1). High blood glucose levels increase triglyceride levels and stimulate the release of insulin, which decreases the ability of the body to break down fat stored in adipose depots.[61]
   C. As discussed earlier in this chapter, obesity increases the circulation of ROS, which in turn causes oxidative damage, and progression of periodontal disease.[20]
   D. Omega-3 fatty acids are polyunsaturated lipids, which exhibit anti-inflammatory properties. They are found at high levels in fish oils and in flaxseed oil. The two main omega-3 fatty acids in fish oil are docosahexaenoic acid (DHA) and eicosapentaenoic acid (EPA).
      1. Rats were infected with *Porphyromonas gingivalis* and received a diet containing either fish oil having omega-3 fatty acids or corn oil. Rats receiving the omega-3 fatty acid diet showed less alveolar bone loss and reduced expression of IL-1 and TNF-α. Thus, in the rat model, omega-3 fatty acids reduced the inflammation associated with infection with *P. gingivalis*.[63,64]
      2. NHANES data was evaluated to see if there was a relationship between periodontal disease and the intake of omega-3 fatty acids in 9,182 adults. The data showed that having a higher level of dietary omega-3 fatty acids was associated with a lower level of periodontitis.[65]
      3. Fifty-five adults with moderate periodontitis were enrolled in a study and received capsules containing the omega-3 fatty acid, DHA, or a capsule with a

mixture of soybean and corn oil. Both groups also took 81 mg of aspirin daily and received oral hygiene instruction at the start of the study. No periodontal treatment was provided. At the end of 3 months, the group receiving the omega-3 fatty acid capsules had lower pockets depths and a lower gingival index.[66]

3. **The Role of the Dental Team in Promoting Good Nutrition.**
   A. Making an appropriate connection between diet, nutrients, and periodontal disease can allow clinicians to make specific suggestions to improve a patient's diet. When indicated clinically, nutritional counseling, with an emphasis on periodontal health and root caries prevention, should be offered to periodontal patients. Educating patients about good dietary habits can be accomplished using standard diet forms, counseling techniques, and analysis procedures.
   B. Table 18-1 contains a summary of potential ways that diet and nutrition may modify periodontal disease.

TABLE 18-1	SUMMARY OF THE ASSOCIATION BETWEEN NUTRITION AND PERIODONTAL DISEASE
Dietary Component	**Association With Periodontal Disease**
Dietary antioxidants	Antioxidant status is compromised in periodontal disease.[28,29]
Vitamin C	An epidemiologic study demonstrated a direct association between low vitamin C intake and periodontal disease, especially among smokers.[42]
Vitamin D	An epidemiologic study demonstrated a positive association between low vitamin D intake and gingival inflammation. The anti-inflammatory effects of vitamin D may contribute to a reduction in gingival inflammation.[51,52]
Vitamin E	In vitro studies show that vitamin E can dampen gingival inflammation.[32,55]
Folic acid	Supplementation with folic acid reduces gingival inflammation.[56]
Calcium	Lower intake of calcium has been shown to be independently associated with increased risk of periodontitis.[53,58,59]
Magnesium	Subjects taking magnesium-containing medications have shallower pocket depths and less gingival inflammation.[60]
Protein	Protein malnutrition increases risk and enhances progression of periodontal disease.[62]
Refined carbohydrates and lipids	Excessive energy intake causes obesity, which has been shown to be associated with increased risk of periodontitis. Obesity increases the circulation of ROS which in turn causes oxidative damage and progression of periodontal disease.[20,21,27]
Omega-3 fatty acids	Epidemiologic data shows that a higher intake of omega-3 fatty acids results in a reduced risk of having periodontitis. Subjects taking omega-3 fatty acid in a research study had lower pocket depths and less inflammation after 3 months.[65,66]

Chapter Summary Statement

Although periodontal disease cannot be caused by nutritional deficiencies, some nutritional deficiencies do indeed appear to modify the severity and extent of the periodontal disease.

- Research links specific nutrient deficiencies and foods high in refined carbohydrates to increased inflammation—the very kind that triggers the host-mediated inflammatory response seen in periodontal disease.
- Reports of the relationship between obesity and periodontal disease are increasing. At this time, it is not possible to determine whether obesity predisposes an individual to periodontal disease or periodontal disease affects lipid metabolism, or both. Future longitudinal studies with more precise measures of adiposity on large populations are needed to clarify whether obesity is one of the risk factors for periodontal disease or simply a risk indicator.
- Data from research suggests that there are mechanisms in which nutrition, particularly antioxidants, can influence periodontal disease onset, progression, and wound healing.
- It is wise to counsel patients with periodontal disease to be thoughtful food shoppers and to prepare meals and snacks that are rich in specific nutrients. A nutritionally adequate diet will help to maintain host resistance and to maintain the integrity of the periodontal tissues. At the present time, there is insufficient evidence available to justify treatment with vitamin and mineral supplementation in the adequately nourished individual.

Section 4
Focus on Patients

Clinical Patient Care

Directions for Clinical Patient Cases: Analyze the information and 24-hour diet recall (Tables 18-2 and 18-3) for the two fictitious periodontal patients, to answer the following questions:

1. Can you identify any eating patterns (healthy or unhealthy)? If so, what are they?
2. List diet practices that have the potential to be most detrimental to the individual's periodontal health.
3. List two diet behaviors that the individual could modify to benefit his/her periodontal health.

CASE 1

Fictitious Periodontal Patient—Mr. Phillip Burgess

Mr. Phillip Burgess is a 39-year-old male. Mr. Burgess is 5′8″ in height and weighs 280 pounds (173 cm and 127 kg). His periodontal diagnosis is generalized Stage I, Grade A periodontitis.

TABLE 18-2	MR. BURGESS: 24-HOUR DIET RECALL		
Time	**Food/Beverage**	**Amount**	**Reason**
6:00 AM	2 cups of coffee with nondairy creamer and 2 packets of sugar	2 medium cups	Breakfast
	Honey Nut Cheerios cereal and milk	Medium-sized bowl	
10:00 AM	Apple Danish pastry with icing		Snack
12:00 PM	Double hamburger with cheese, lettuce, tomato, and onion	Supersize	Lunch
	French fries	Large	
	Regular Coke	Large	
2:00 PM	Regular Coke	1 can	Snack
	Bag of potato chips	Small bag	
7:00 PM	Steak	Large	Dinner
	French fries	Large serving	
	Tossed salad with Italian dressing	Small bowl	
	Garlic toast	2 pieces	
	Water		
9:00 PM	Ice cream	Medium bowl	Snack while watching TV

CASE 2

Fictitious Periodontal Patient—Mrs. Glenda Bissada

Mrs. Glenda Bissada is a 70-year-old female. Mrs. Bissada is 5'1" in height and weighs 160 pounds (155 cm and 73 kg). Her periodontal diagnosis is generalized Stage III, Grade B periodontitis.

TABLE 18-3 | MRS. BISSADA: 24-HOUR DIET RECALL

Time	Food/Beverage	Amount	Reason
7:00 AM	Coffee with organic nondairy cream	1 large mug	Breakfast
	Whole-grain English muffin	One	
	Peanut butter and jelly		
10:30 AM	Green grapes	25	Hungry
11:00 AM	M&Ms	3 handfuls	Stressed (arguing with daughter on the phone)
12:30 PM	Philly cheese steak (fried shaved beef, onions, & green peppers, covered with cheese sauce in a large white "hoagie" bun)		Lunch
	Potato chips	One bag	
	Iced tea sweetened with sugar	One glass	
2:00 PM	Caramel-coated popcorn mix	2 handfuls	Stressed/hungry
6:00 PM	Fried hamburger patty with brown gravy		Dinner
	Baked potato with sour cream and real bacon bits		
	Peas		
	Coffee with sugar		
7:00 PM	Glass of water		Thirsty
8:00 PM	Popcorn with butter	Medium bowl	Watching a movie

Ethical Dilemma

Stuart Fisher, your next patient, is new to the practice. He is a 48-year-old male, who is married with three young children. He owns a successful restaurant, where he works as the head chef. As he is self-employed, he doesn't carry dental insurance.

You review Stuart's medical history, and he states that he is scheduled for lap-band surgery next month. Stuart admits that he has neglected his general and oral health for many years, due to his busy lifestyle. He also notes that although he knows better, his diet is poor. After cooking in the restaurant all day and night, the last thing he wants to do is prepare food for himself. So, both before and after work, he stops for "fast food."

Your radiographs and examination reveal that Stuart presents with generalized chronic periodontitis with moderate bone loss throughout his mouth, as well as localized furcation involvement.

You review the treatment plan with Stuart, which includes periodontal instrumentation with anesthesia, nutritional counseling, and referral to a periodontist. Stuart refuses to agree with your suggestions, as he states that he doesn't carry dental insurance. He only scheduled this appointment, as his surgeon required it prior to his surgery. He wants to receive the minimal dental treatment and will not "go for" anything more.

1. What is the best way for you to handle this ethical dilemma?
2. What is the best way to address/discuss Stuart's treatment plan with him?
3. What ethical principles are in conflict in this dilemma?

References

1. Aronne LJ, Segal KR. Adiposity and fat distribution outcome measures: assessment and clinical implications. *Obes Res.* 2002;10 Suppl 1:14S–21S.
2. Obesity and overweight. 2016. Available from: http://www.who.int/mediacentre/factsheets/fs311/en/.
3. Ogden CL, Carroll MD, Lawman HG, et al. Trends in obesity prevalence among children and adolescents in the United States, 1988–1994 through 2013–2014. *JAMA.* 2016;315(21):2292–2299.
4. Flegal KM, Kruszon-Moran D, Carroll MD, Fryar CD, Ogden CL. Trends in obesity among adults in the United States, 2005 to 2014. *JAMA.* 2016;315(21):2284–2291.
5. James PT, Rigby N, Leach R; International Obesity Task Force. The obesity epidemic, metabolic syndrome and future prevention strategies. *Eur J Cardiovasc Prev Rehabil.* 2004;11(1):3–8.
6. Coelho M, Oliveira T, Fernandes R. Biochemistry of adipose tissue: an endocrine organ. *Arch Med Sci.* 2013;9(2):191–200.
7. Dandona P, Aljada A, Bandyopadhyay A. Inflammation: the link between insulin resistance, obesity and diabetes. *Trends Immunol.* 2004;25(1):4–7.
8. Akram Z, Abduljabbar T, Hassan A, Ibrahim M, Javed F, Vohra F. Cytokine profile in chronic periodontitis patients with and without obesity: a systematic review and meta-analysis. *Dis Markers.* 2016;2016:4801418.
9. Akram Z, Safii SH, Vaithilingam RD, Baharuddin NA, Javed F, Vohra F. Efficacy of non-surgical periodontal therapy in the management of chronic periodontitis among obese and non-obese patients: a systematic review and meta-analysis. *Clin Oral Investig.* 2016;20(5):903–914.
10. Duzagac E, Cifcibasi E, Erdem MG, et al. Is obesity associated with healing after non-surgical periodontal therapy? A local vs. systemic evaluation. *J Periodontal Res.* 2016;51(5):604–612.
11. Dalla Vecchia CF, Susin C, Rösing CK, Oppermann RV, Albandar JM. Overweight and obesity as risk indicators for periodontitis in adults. *J Periodontol.* 2005;76(10):1721–1728.
12. Gorman A, Kaye EK, Apovian C, Fung TT, Nunn M, Garcia RI. Overweight and obesity predict time to periodontal disease progression in men. *J Clin Periodontol.* 2012;39(2):107–114.
13. Suvan JE, Petrie A, Nibali L, et al. Association between overweight/obesity and increased risk of periodontitis. *J Clin Periodontol.* 2015;42(8):733–739.
14. Genco RJ, Grossi SG, Ho A, Nishimura F, Murayama Y. A proposed model linking inflammation to obesity, diabetes, and periodontal infections. *J Periodontol.* 2005;76(11 Suppl):2075–2084.
15. Al-Zahrani MS, Bissada NF, Borawskit EA. Obesity and periodontal disease in young, middle-aged, and older adults. *J Periodontol.* 2003;74(5):610–615.
16. Chaffee BW, Weston SJ. Association between chronic periodontal disease and obesity: a systematic review and meta-analysis. *J Periodontol.* 2010;81(12):1708–1724.
17. Socransky SS, Haffajee AD. Periodontal microbial ecology. *Periodontol 2000.* 2005;38:135–187.
18. Eke PI, Wei L, Thornton-Evans GO, et al. Risk Indicators for Periodontitis in US Adults: NHANES 2009 to 2012. *J Periodontol.* 2016;87(10):1174–1185.

19. Nishida N, Tanaka M, Hayashi N, et al. Determination of smoking and obesity as periodontitis risks using the classification and regression tree method. *J Periodontol.* 2005;76(6):923–928.

20. Boesing F, Patiño JS, da Silva VR, Moreira EA. The interface between obesity and periodontitis with emphasis on oxidative stress and inflammatory response. *Obes Rev.* 2009;10(3):290–297.

21. Ylostalo P, Suominen-Taipale L, Reunanen A, Knuuttila M. Association between body weight and periodontal infection. *J Clin Periodontol.* 2008;35(4):297–304.

22. Saely CH, Geiger K, Drexel H. Brown versus white adipose tissue: a mini-review. *Gerontology.* 2012;58(1):15–23.

23. Thanakun S, Pornprasertsuk-Damrongsri S, Izumi Y. Increased oral inflammation, leukocytes, and leptin, and lower adiponectin in overweight or obesity. *Oral Dis.* 2017;23(7):956–965.

24. Dahiya P, Kamal R, Gupta R. Obesity, periodontal and general health: relationship and management. *Indian J Endocrinol Metab.* 2012;16(1):88–93.

25. Makki K, Froguel P, Wolowczuk I. Adipose tissue in obesity-related inflammation and insulin resistance: cells, cytokines, and chemokines. *ISRN Inflamm.* 2013;2013:139239.

26. Khosravi R, Ka K, Huang T, et al. Tumor necrosis factor-alpha and interleukin-6: potential interorgan inflammatory mediators contributing to destructive periodontal disease in obesity or metabolic syndrome. *Mediators Inflamm.* 2013;2013:728987.

27. Ray PD, Huang BW, Tsuji Y. Reactive oxygen species (ROS) homeostasis and redox regulation in cellular signaling. *Cell Signal.* 2012;24(5):981–990.

28. Dahiya P, Kamal R, Gupta R, Bhardwaj R, Chaudhary K, Kaur S. Reactive oxygen species in periodontitis. *J Indian Soc Periodontol.* 2013;17(4):411–416.

29. Brock GR, Butterworth CJ, Matthews JB, Chapple IL. Local and systemic total antioxidant capacity in periodontitis and health. *J Clin Periodontol.* 2004;31(7):515–521.

30. Linden GJ, McClean KM, Woodside JV, et al. Antioxidants and periodontitis in 60-70-year-old men. *J Clin Periodontol.* 2009;36(10):843–849.

31. Roos D, van Bruggen R, Meischl C. Oxidative killing of microbes by neutrophils. *Microbes Infect.* 2003;5(14):1307–1315.

32. Offenbacher S, Odle BM, Green MD, et al. Inhibition of human periodontal prostaglandin E2 synthesis with selected agents. *Agents Actions.* 1990;29(3–4):232–238.

33. Lee NK, Choi YG, Baik JY, et al. A crucial role for reactive oxygen species in RANKL-induced osteoclast differentiation. *Blood.* 2005;106(3):852–859.

34. Waddington RJ, Moseley R, Embery G. Reactive oxygen species: a potential role in the pathogenesis of periodontal diseases. *Oral Dis.* 2000;6(3):138–151.

35. Cao CF, Smith QT. Crevicular fluid myeloperoxidase at healthy, gingivitis and periodontitis sites. *J Clin Periodontol.* 1989;16(1):17–20.

36. Marton IJ, Balla G, Hegedus C, et al. The role of reactive oxygen intermediates in the pathogenesis of chronic apical periodontitis. *Oral Microbiol Immunol.* 1993;8(4):254–257.

37. Ritchie CS, Kinane DF. Nutrition, inflammation, and periodontal disease. *Nutrition.* 2003;19(5):475–476.

38. Chapple IL. Role of free radicals and antioxidants in the pathogenesis of the inflammatory periodontal diseases. *Clin Mol Pathol.* 1996;49(5):M247–M255.

39. Sutton G. Putrid gums and 'dead men's cloaths': James Lind aboard the Salisbury. *J R Soc Med.* 2003;96(12):605–608.

40. Padayatty SJ, Katz A, Wang Y, et al. Vitamin C as an antioxidant: evaluation of its role in disease prevention. *J Am Coll Nutr.* 2003;22(1):18–35.

41. Tauler P, Aguiló A, Gimeno I, et al. Differential response of lymphocytes and neutrophils to high intensity physical activity and to vitamin C diet supplementation. *Free Radic Res.* 2003;37(9):931–938.

42. Nishida M, Grossi SG, Dunford RG, Ho AW, Trevisan M, Genco RJ. Dietary vitamin C and the risk for periodontal disease. *J Periodontol.* 2000;71(8):1215–1223.

43. Chapple IL, Milward MR, Dietrich T. The prevalence of inflammatory periodontitis is negatively associated with serum antioxidant concentrations. *J Nutr.* 2007;137(3):657–664.

44. Riepe FG, Eichmann D, Oppermann HC, Schmitt HJ, Tunnessen WW, Jr. Special feature: picture of the month. Infantile scurvy. *Arch Pediatr Adolesc Med.* 2001;155(5):607–608.

45. Halligan TJ, Russell NG, Dunn WJ, Caldroney SJ, Skelton TB. Identification and treatment of scurvy: a case report. *Oral Surg Oral Med Oral Pathol Oral Radiol Endod.* 2005;100(6):688–692.

46. Siegel C, Barker B, Kunstadter M. Conditioned oral scurvy due to megavitamin C withdrawal. *J Periodontol.* 1982;53(7):453–455.

47. Alhadeff L, Gualtieri CT, Lipton M. Toxic effects of water-soluble vitamins. *Nutr Rev.* 1984;42(2):33–40.

48. Mora JR, Iwata M, von Andrian UH. Vitamin effects on the immune system: vitamins A and D take centre stage. *Nat Rev Immunol.* 2008;8(9):685–698.

49. Bloem MW, Hye A, Wijnroks M, Ralte A, West KP, Jr, Sommer A. The role of universal distribution of vitamin A capsules in combatting vitamin A deficiency in Bangladesh. *Am J Epidemiol.* 1995;142(8):843–855.

50. Anand N, Chandrasekaran SC, Rajput NS. Vitamin D and periodontal health: current concepts. *J Indian Soc Periodontol.* 2013;17(3):302–308.

51. Dietrich T, Joshipura KJ, Dawson-Hughes B, Bischoff-Ferrari HA. Association between serum concentrations of 25-hydroxyvitamin D3 and periodontal disease in the US population. *Am J Clin Nutr.* 2004;80(1):108–113.

52. Dietrich T, Nunn M, Dawson-Hughes B, Bischoff-Ferrari HA. Association between serum concentrations of 25-hydroxyvitamin D and gingival inflammation. *Am J Clin Nutr.* 2005;82(3):575–580.

53. Krall EA, Wehler C, Garcia RI, Harris SS, Dawson-Hughes B. Calcium and vitamin D supplements reduce tooth loss in the elderly. *Am J Med.* 2001;111(6):452–456.

54. Meydani SN, Beharka AA. Vitamin E and immune response in the aged. *Bibl Nutr Dieta.* 2001;(55):148–158.

55. Han SN, Meydani SN. Impact of vitamin E on immune function and its clinical implications. *Expert Rev Clin Immunol.* 2006;2(4):561–567.

56. Yu YH, Kuo HK, Lai YL. The association between serum folate levels and periodontal disease in older adults: data from the National Health and Nutrition Examination Survey 2001/02. *J Am Geriatr Soc.* 2007;55(1):108–113.

57. Green NS. Folic acid supplementation and prevention of birth defects. *J Nutr.* 2002;132(8 Suppl):2356S–2360S.

58. Nishida M, Grossi SG, Dunford RG, Ho AW, Trevisan M, Genco RJ. Calcium and the risk for periodontal disease. *J Periodontol.* 2000;71(7):1057–1066.

59. Al-Zahrani MS. Increased intake of dairy products is related to lower periodontitis prevalence. *J Periodontol.* 2006;77(2):289–294.

60. Meisel P, Schwahn C, Luedemann J, John U, Kroemer HK, Kocher T. Magnesium deficiency is associated with periodontal disease. *J Dent Res.* 2005;84(10):937–941.

61. Chapple IL. Potential mechanisms underpinning the nutritional modulation of periodontal inflammation. *J Am Dent Assoc.* 2009;140(2):178–184.

62. Enwonwu CO, Phillips RS, Falkler WA, Jr. Nutrition and oral infectious diseases: state of the science. *Compend Contin Educ Dent.* 2002;23(5):431–434, 436, 438 passim; quiz 448.

63. Kesavalu L, Bakthavatchalu V, Rahman MM, et al. Omega-3 fatty acid regulates inflammatory cytokine/mediator messenger RNA expression in Porphyromonas gingivalis-induced experimental periodontal disease. *Oral Microbiol Immunol.* 2007;22(4):232–239.

64. Kesavalu L, Vasudevan B, Raghu B, et al. Omega-3 fatty acid effect on alveolar bone loss in rats. *J Dent Res.* 2006;85(7):648–652.

65. Naqvi AZ, Buettner C, Phillips RS, Davis RB, Mukamal KJ. n-3 fatty acids and periodontitis in US adults. *J Am Diet Assoc.* 2010;110(11):1669–1675.

66. Naqvi AZ, Hasturk H, Mu L, et al. Docosahexaenoic Acid and periodontitis in adults: a randomized controlled trial. *J Dent Res.* 2014;93(8):767–773.

 STUDENT ANCILLARY RESOURCES

A wide variety of resources to enhance your learning is available online:

- Audio Glossary
- Book Pages
- Chapter Review Questions and Answers

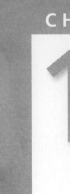

CHAPTER

19 Tobacco, Smoking, and Periodontal Disease

Clinical Application. Smoking may be one of the most significant risk factors in the development and progression of periodontal disease. Dental hygienists have a professional responsibility to provide tobacco cessation services as a routine component of dental hygiene practice. Smoking cessation guidelines recommend that dental team members should check the smoking status of their patients at least once a year and should advise all smokers to stop smoking. This chapter summarizes what is known about tobacco as a risk factor for periodontal disease and provides suggestions for brief, effective tobacco cessation counseling in the dental setting.

Learning Objectives

- Discuss the implications of smoking/the use of tobacco products on periodontal health status.
- Discuss the implications of smoking on the host response to periodontal disease.
- Discuss the effects of smoking on periodontal treatment outcomes.
- Discuss current theories as to why smokers have more periodontal disease than nonsmokers.
- Explain why tobacco cessation counseling is a valuable part of patient care in the dental setting.
- Value the importance of providing tobacco cessation counseling as a routine part of periodontal treatment.

Key Terms

Dental implant
Peri-implant mucositis

Peri-implantitis
Environmental tobacco smoke

Tobacco cessation
counseling

Section 1
Tobacco as a Risk Factor for Periodontal Disease

Inflammation is a critical component of normal tissue repair, as well as being fundamental to the body's defense against infection. Environmental factors, such as smoking, have been reported to modify the host response and hence modify the progression, severity, and outcome of the inflammatory response. Therefore, a comprehensive understanding of how smoking affects inflammation is vital for preventive and therapeutic strategies on a clinical level.

EPIDEMIOLOGY OF TOBACCO IN PERIODONTAL PATIENTS

- Evidence accumulated over the past three decades indicates that cigarette smoking is a very strong risk factor for periodontal disease.[1-4] Cigarette smoking increases the risk for periodontal disease by at least two to three times.[1]
- Tooth loss is the ultimate outcome of untreated periodontitis. Smokers are at higher risk for tooth loss due to periodontal disease.[3,5-7]
- Cigar and pipe smoking are also significant risk factors for attachment loss.[7-9]
- Smokeless tobacco use is associated with severe recession and loss of attachment to buccal surfaces of teeth where the smokeless tobacco was placed.[10]

SMOKING AND PERIODONTITIS

- There is a wealth of literature outlining the role that cigarette smoking has on periodontal disease and treatment, and several reviews cover this topic in detail.[4,11,12]
- Results from the first National Health and Nutrition Examination Survey (NHANES) demonstrated that smokers have greater periodontal destruction than former and never smokers.[8]
- More recently, the NHANES III study concluded that approximately half of periodontitis cases could be attributed to either current (42.9%) smoking or former smoking (10.9%).[8,13] Current estimates indicate smoking also increases the prevalence of periodontitis in excess of 20% in younger segments of the adult population.[7]
- The effect of smoking and periodontal destruction is said to be dose-dependent with total exposure to cigarette smoking being a widely used measure of dose.[7] Heavy smokers (more than 10 cigarettes/day) have greater odds for more severe attachment loss compared to nonsmokers.[14]
- In longitudinal maintenance studies, smoking is strongly correlated to higher rates of tooth loss due to periodontal disease even in patients who were consistently receiving regular periodontal maintenance over a 5-year period.[15-17]
- The Task Force of the 2017 AAP/EFP World Workshop on the Classification of Periodontal and Peri-Implant Diseases and Conditions recognizes that cigarette smoking is a major risk factor for periodontal diseases and peri-implant diseases: (1) smoking increases the rate of progression of periodontitis, (2) it alters the patient's responsiveness to standard therapeutic principles, (3) it influences general health or systemic disease, and (4) it could cause the disease to progress from one stage to the next. Therefore, a clinician should make every effort to assess a patient's smoking status and integrate this pertinent information, along with other risk factors, to formulate the grade of periodontitis. For reference, the reader is referred to Chapter 7 to review the proposed framework for staging and grading periodontitis, according to the 2017 Classification System.

Section 2
Mechanisms of Smoking-Mediated Periodontal Disease

More than 4,000 toxins are present in cigarette smoke including such poisons as carbon monoxide, oxidizing radicals, carcinogens (e.g., nitrosamines), and addictive psychoactive substances such as nicotine.[3,7] Oral problems associated with smoking include halitosis, dry mouth, dental staining (Figs. 19-1 and 19-2), periodontal disease, and cancer.[3,7,12,13] Smoking affects the periodontium in several ways. Some of the possible mechanisms are highlighted in Figure 19-3.

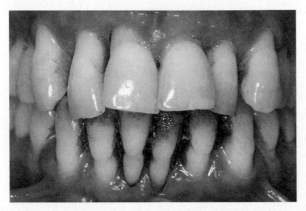
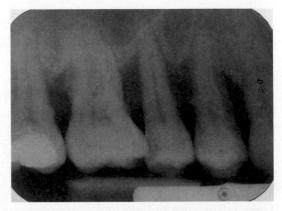

Figure 19-1. Attachment Loss Associated With Smoking. Clinical and radiographic findings show severe horizontal and vertical bone loss that effects the masticatory function of a 37-year old male with a 20 pack-year smoking history. These findings are consistent with the diagnosis of generalized Stage IV, Grade C periodontitis.

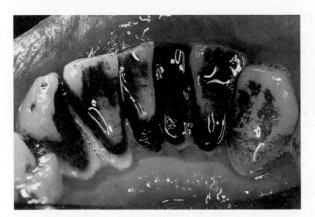
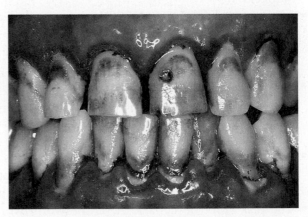

Figure 19-2. Oral Problems Associated With Smoking. Heavy tobacco staining and plaque biofilm accumulation are evident in a smoker along with accompanying signs of periodontitis.

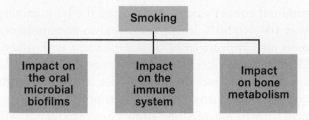

Figure 19-3. Mechanisms of Smoking-Mediated Destruction. Possible impacts of smoking on the periodontium include effects on oral biofilms, the immune system, and alveolar bone.

EFFECTS OF SMOKING ON THE PERIODONTIUM

1. **Impact of Smoking on the Oral Microbial Biofilms**
   A. There are conflicting reports on how smoking affects the oral microflora. A few studies indicate there are no differences in the subgingival bacteria between smokers and nonsmokers.[18–20]
      1. Other investigations, however, show that the subgingival microbial profile associated with periodontitis in smokers is diverse and distinct from that of nonsmokers.[19,21–23]
      2. Multiple studies have shown that plaque biofilm in smokers is more likely to be colonized by *Porphyromonas gingivalis* and other potential periodontal pathogens.[24–28]
      3. More recent studies indicate that smoking is also responsible for depletion of beneficial bacteria along with an increase in pathogenic bacteria such as *Treponema* spp.[29]
   B. Cigarette smoking is associated with a lower oxygen tension in the periodontal pocket and thus is favorable for the growth of anaerobic bacteria.[13]
   C. A recent study by Kumar and colleagues examined the impact of smoking on composition and proinflammatory characteristics of the biofilm during formation. The authors reported that smoking favors early acquisition and colonization of periodontal pathogens in oral biofilms.[21]
2. **Impact of Smoking on the Immune System**
   A. From both a biologic and epidemiologic viewpoint, numerous studies suggest that smoking enhances the risk of periodontal disease.[3,12,30] Smoking affects both the human immune system and cellular and humoral inflammatory response systems.[3,31,32]
   B. Smokers have decreased signs of inflammation and a decreased gingival crevicular blood flow that is indicative of impaired gingival blood flow in smokers. This is due to the vasoconstrictor properties of nicotine.
   C. Although smokers have a higher number of neutrophils, neutrophil function in the peripheral circulation is impaired. Neutrophils have shown decreased adherence, chemotaxis, and phagocytosis in smokers.[33]
   D. Antibody production is another protective mechanism impacted by smoking.[33] Smoking generally decreased IgG$_2$ antibody production that, in turn, leads to decreased serum immunoglobulin G (IgG) concentrations. IgG$_2$ antibody production is also reported to occur in patients with severe forms of periodontitis.[26,33,34]
3. **Smoking and Bone Metabolism**
   A. Bone is one of the tissues most affected by smoking.[35] Smoking is associated with a greater amount of alveolar bone destruction in comparison to nonsmokers.[33,35–37] In a 10-year longitudinal study, reduction in bone height was 2.7 times greater in adult smokers compared to nonsmokers.[35]

1. At least one longitudinal cohort study has reported the bone mineral content among smokers was 10% to 30% lower compared to nonsmokers.[2]

2. Bone loss in smokers also appears to be dose dependent with odds ratios ranging from 3.25 for light smokers to 7.28 for heavy smokers.[38]

B. Although the mechanisms of how nicotine contributes to alveolar bone damage are not fully understood, several pathways have been proposed.

   1. In vitro studies have shown that nicotine suppresses osteoblasts while stimulating alkaline phosphatase activity.[39,40]

   2. Nicotine also increases the secretion of Interleukin-6 (IL-6) and tumor necrosis factor-alpha (TNF-α) in osteoblasts.[41]

   3. Finally, nicotine is also known to alter normal bone remodeling by increasing the release of matrix metalloproteinases.[37]

4. **Impact of Environmental Tobacco Smoke**

   A. Nonsmokers exposed to environmental tobacco smoke (ETS)—"secondhand smoke" or "passive smoking"—are at increased risk for periodontitis. An analysis of NHANES III data concluded that the odds of having periodontitis are 1.6 times higher for nonsmoking adults who are exposed to environmental tobacco smoke than adults who are not exposed to passive smoke.[42]

      1. Sanders and colleagues conclude that exposure to environmental tobacco smoke and presence of severe periodontitis among nonsmokers had a dose-dependent relationship.[43] Their research findings show that individuals exposed to environmental tobacco smoke for 1 to 25 hours per week have a 29% increased risk of severe periodontitis. For those exposed to environmental tobacco smoke for 26 hours or more per week, the odds were twice as high for severe periodontitis as individuals not exposed.

      2. An investigation of 3,137 subjects evaluated the association between environmental tobacco smoke and periodontitis in nonsmokers. This study concluded that adults with high environmental tobacco smoke exposure had two times the odds of periodontitis in comparison with subjects with negligible exposure.[44]

      3. A recent cross-sectional study utilizing NHANES data from 2009 to 2012 concludes that there is a 28% increase in the odds for moderate periodontitis for those with any ETS exposure.[45]

   B. Nishida and colleagues determined that passive smoke exposure was correlated to an elevation of interleukin-1β, albumin, and aspartate aminotransferase (AST) levels in the saliva.[30]

5. **Electronic Cigarettes (ECIGs)**

   A. **The ECIG was introduced to the US market in 2007.** "E-cigarettes" do not contain tobacco. Instead, there is a mechanism that heats up liquid nicotine, which turns into a vapor that smokers inhale and exhale. National youth tobacco surveys demonstrate a threefold increase in the use of ECIGs from 2011 to 2013 in grades 6 to 12. The popularity of ECIGs among youth and its unknown effects long-term is worrisome.[46]

      1. Laboratory analysis of ECIG conducted by the U.S. Food and Drug Administration shows quite clearly that the fluid and aerosol in e-cigarettes contain known toxins, including propylene glycol, heavy metals, volatile organic compounds, and tobacco-specific nitrosamines (http://www.fda.gov/NewsEvents/PublicHealthFocus/ucm173146.htm, Accessed September 29, 2017).

      2. At this time, the possible side effects of inhaling nicotine vapor, as well as other health risks e-cigarettes may pose—both to users and to the public—is unknown.

   B. Some cigarette smokers are utilizing ECIGs as a smoking cessation aid. However, the extent to which ECIGs can help with smoking cessation is unclear.[46]

6. **Waterpipe Smoking (WTS) ("hookah," "Shisha")**
   A. In recent years, along with the use of ECIGs, waterpipes are gaining popularity. The use of a waterpipe is associated with respiratory and cardiovascular problems and also has a significant impact on the oral cavity.
   B. WTS has been found to have significant amounts of nicotine and 27 known or suspected carcinogens.[47]
   C. Higher amounts of nicotine are delivered utilizing WTS compared to cigarettes.[48] During a single WTS episode, waterpipe smokers can inhale over 40 L of smoke compared to 1 L or less for a single cigarette.[47,49]
   D. WTS has been consistently associated with an increase in periodontal pocket depths, loss of clinical attachment, and bone loss compared to nonsmokers.[50-52] Most studies conclude that the impact of WTS is the same as tobacco smoking.[46]
   E. The prevalence of noncigarette tobacco use is on the rise across the globe. Most patients do not associate these habits with smoking. As a result, *practitioners should modify their health history questionnaire to include questions to elicit information about other sources of nicotine.* While cigarette smoking has been steadily but slowly declining in the United States and Canada, the use of alternate tobacco products and their impact on the periodontium cannot be ignored.

EFFECTS OF SMOKING ON PERIODONTAL THERAPY

1. **Impact of Chemical Products and Toxins in Cigarette Smoke on Periodontal Therapy**
   A. Chemical products and toxins in tobacco smoke may delay wound healing by impairing the biologic progression of healing and by inhibiting the basic cellular functions necessary for the initiation of wound healing.[33]
   B. Volatile components of cigarette smoke—namely acrolein and acetaldehyde—may inhibit gingival fibroblast attachment and proliferation. Fibroblasts exposed to nicotine produce less extracellular matrix, less collagen, and more collagenase. These negative effects on fibroblast functions influence wound healing and progression of periodontitis.[3,12]

2. **Smoking and Response to Periodontal Treatment.** Smoking not only increases the risk for developing periodontal disease but also impacts the response to periodontal treatment. Smokers show a poorer response to periodontal therapy compared to nonsmokers.[53-55]
   A. Smokers exhibit less reduction in probing depth and less gain in clinical attachment after treatment compared to ex-smokers or nonsmokers.[56]
   B. In 6-year longitudinal study, nonsmokers had approximately a 50% higher rate of improvement in probing depth and clinical attachment levels after periodontal therapy than did active smokers.[38]
   C. Periodontal treatment in smokers, both surgical and nonsurgical therapies, has been associated with improvements in periodontal outcomes. Comparison of the outcomes, however, showed significantly less improvement in the smokers compared with nonsmokers.[55-63]

Section 3
Smoking and Peri-Implant Disease

A dental implant is a nonbiologic (artificial) device surgically inserted into the jawbone to (1) replace a missing tooth or (2) provide support for a prosthetic denture. The peri-implant tissues are the tissues that surround the dental implant. In many ways, the peri-implant tissues are like the periodontium of a natural tooth. Dental implants are discussed in detail in Chapter 9, Peri-Implant Health and Diseases.

- Peri-implant mucositis (also called peri-implant gingivitis) is plaque-induced gingivitis (with no loss of supporting bone) that is localized in the gingival tissues surrounding a dental implant and is characterized by edema, change in color (red or red-blue), bleeding and/or purulence on probing, with probing depths of equal to or greater than 4 mm, and no evidence of radiographic peri-implant bone loss.[64]
- Peri-implantitis is a more advanced inflammatory disease—essentially periodontitis— that exhibits deep probing depths (5 mm or greater), bleeding on probing (BOP) and/ or purulence, and radiographic evidence of loss of alveolar bone.[65]

THE IMPACT OF SMOKING ON DENTAL IMPLANTS

- Heat produced by smoking, as well as, the toxic by-products of cigarette smoking, such as nicotine, carbon monoxide, and hydrogen cyanide, have been implicated as risk factors for impaired healing after implant surgery.[66]
- Smokers experience almost twice as many implant failures compared with nonsmokers and are more prone to show peri-implant bone loss in the maxilla.[67–74]
- Risk indicators associated with increased peri-implant mucositis and peri-implantitis include poor plaque biofilm control, a history of periodontitis, diabetes, and smoking.[66,70,72–74]
- The combination of smoking and a history of periodontitis (treated or untreated) increase the risk of peri-implant bone loss (Figs. 19-4 and 19-5).[67,73]

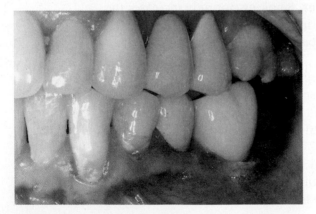

Figure 19-4. Peri-Implant Mucositis. Clinical signs of peri-implant mucositis of the mandibular first molar.

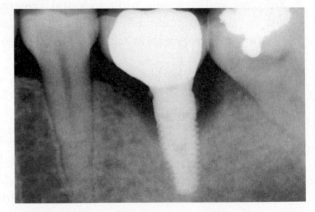

Figure 19-5. Peri-Implantitis. Radiographic evidence of peri-implantitis featuring circumferential angular bone loss.

Section 4
Tobacco Cessation for the Periodontal Patient

EFFECTS OF TOBACCO CESSATION ON THE PERIODONTIUM

There have been few publications in the periodontal literature to specifically address the impact of smoking cessation on the periodontium, most probably because of the common challenges in motivating patients to quit smoking. Fiorini and colleagues conducted a systematic review of the literature to evaluate the effect of smoking cessation on periodontitis progression and response to periodontal therapy. Based on the limited available evidence, Fiorini and colleagues concluded that smoking cessation seems to have a positive influence on periodontitis occurrence and periodontal healing.[1]

1. **The Effect of Smoking Cessation on Periodontal Status**
   A. Current smokers usually have significantly worse periodontal conditions (greater probing depths, more attachment loss, and alveolar bone loss) than either never smokers or former smokers. The NHANES III study concluded that approximately half of periodontitis cases could be attributed to either current smoking (42.9%) or former smoking (10.9%).[8,13]
   B. In general, the periodontal health status of former smokers is not as good as that of never smokers, but is better than that of current smokers.[75] These findings suggest that while the past effects of smoking on the periodontium cannot be reversed, smoking cessation is beneficial to periodontal health.[76]
   C. The American Academy of Periodontology strongly recommends inclusion of tobacco cessation counseling as an integral part of periodontal therapy.[77]
2. **The Effect of Smoking Cessation on Periodontal Treatment Outcomes**
   A. Studies have confirmed that treatment outcomes in former smokers are generally like those that can be expected in never smokers, but are usually better than those that can be expected in current smokers.[76]
   B. The benefits of smoking cessation on the periodontium likely result from (1) a reduction in pathogenic bacteria in the subgingival plaque biofilm, (2) improved circulation in the gingiva, and (3) improvements in the host immune-inflammatory response.

TOBACCO CESSATION COUNSELING IN PERIODONTAL THERAPY

1. **Smoking Cessation and the Prevention of Periodontal Disease**
   A. The knowledge that smoking is a significant risk factor suggests that in smokers, smoking cessation might prevent more periodontal disease than daily plaque control self-care. All patients should be assessed for smoking status and smokers should be given smoking cessation counseling.[78]
   B. Tobacco cessation counseling includes information on smoking cessation and prevention of tobacco use, as well as referrals to other health professionals for tobacco cessation programs.

2. The Role of the Dental Team in Tobacco Cessation Counseling
   A. The World Health Organization (WHO) advocates that all health providers must be involved in tobacco cessation efforts, including oral health professionals who reach a large proportion of the healthy population.[79]
   B. Dental team members have regular contact with patients, are the first to see the effects of tobacco in the mouth and are the only health professionals who frequently see "medically healthy" patients. Dental hygienists, thus, are in an ideal position to reinforce the anti-tobacco message, as well as being able to motivate and support smokers willing to quit.
   C. Dental hygienists have a professional responsibility to provide tobacco cessation services as a routine component of dental hygiene practice. Smoking cessation guidelines recommend that all health professionals, including dental team members, should check the smoking status of their patients at least once a year, and should advise all smokers to stop smoking.[1,79,80]

A USER-FRIENDLY MODEL FOR COUNSELING THE PERIODONTAL PATIENT

1. Counseling Time Commitment. *In the clear majority of cases, dental teams will only be involved in delivering brief advice to smokers. This should take less than 5 minutes of their time.*
2. Key Elements in Providing Brief Advice
   A. All patients should have their smoking/tobacco use status (current, ex-, never smoked) established and checked at regular intervals. This information should be recorded in the patient's chart.
   B. Smokers should then be asked some simple questions, to assess their degree of interest in stopping smoking/tobacco use.
   C. **All smokers and chewers of tobacco should be advised of the value of stopping, and of the health risks of continuing.** The advice should be clear, firm, and personalized.
   D. Although most people know of the risks of tobacco use in relation to cancers and heart disease, fewer are aware of the detrimental effects on the mouth. Dental teams thus have a unique opportunity to highlight the dangers of tobacco use. The early signs of tobacco use—such as tooth staining, changes to the soft tissues and halitosis—are easily identified and are reversible, and this provides a useful means of motivating smokers to stop.
   E. All smokers and chewers of tobacco should be advised of the value of the support offered by quitlines. Quitlines are toll-free telephone centers staffed by trained tobacco cessation experts. It takes as little as 30 seconds to refer a patient to a quitline. Smokers who are interested and motivated to stop should be referred to these services. The U.S. Department of Health and Human Services has a national quitline number: 1-800-QUIT-NOW (1-800-784-8669).
3. **A Pathway and Sample Dialogs for Cessation Counseling.** A tobacco cessation care pathway for dental practice is summarized in Figure 19-6.[81] Boxes 19-1 to 19-3 provide sample dialogs for cessation counseling.

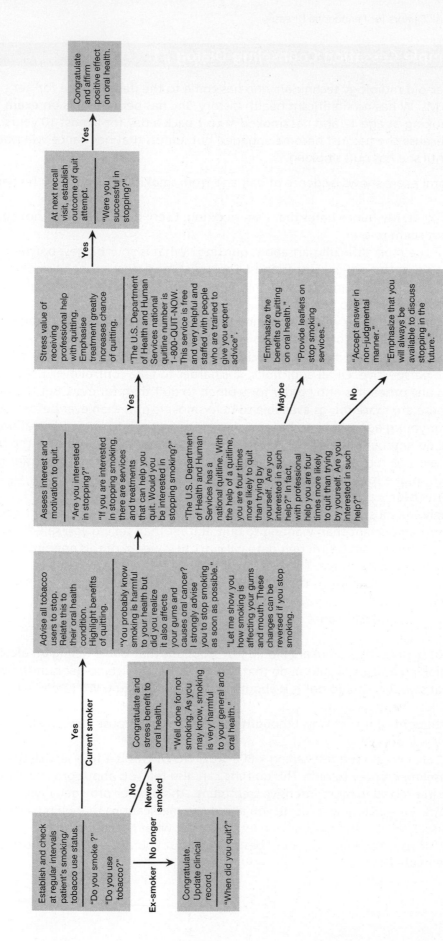

Figure 19-6. A Flowchart for Tobacco Cessation Counseling.

Box 19-1. Sample Cessation Counseling Dialog #1

Ms. W is a 22-year-old radiology technician who has come to the dental office for her bi-annual exam. Ms. W has no significant health history. She has periodontitis on exam. Ms. W began smoking at age 12 and has smoked ¾ to 1 pack a day for almost 10 years. She is very excited because she has just become engaged but admits that her fiancé will not set a wedding date until she has quit smoking.

Clinician: Your oral exam shows evidence of damage from smoking. How do you feel about quitting?

Ms. W: I want to quit. My fiancé hates that I am smoking. Every day I tell myself not to smoke but I just cannot seem to quit.

Clinician: What is the most difficult part about quitting? What is your biggest barrier?

Ms. W: I feel like cigarettes are my best friends! The only time I relax is when I smoke—or when I am out drinking and smoking with my friends. Almost all my friends smoke.

Clinician: Have you ever tried to quit?

Ms. W: Every day!! But nothing works! And then my fiancé yells at me so I feel worse and end up smoking more. I feel so guilty and so embarrassed!

Clinician: It sounds like you are in a vicious circle that is probably making it harder to quit. Let's put this in perspective. Of all addictions, it is harder to take control over the nicotine addiction than any other. It is also harder for women to quit than for men. But the good news is that there are more things available to help smokers quit than ever before. And quitting at your young age will be so beneficial in every way—including your oral health! The longer we do anything, the harder it is to stop. So, stopping now would be the best thing you will ever do for yourself and while it will be very difficult, it will be easier than if you continue to smoke for another 20 years.

Ms. W: What is the best way to quit?

Clinician: Probably the most important thing is for you to do is make the decision to quit. That is even more important than wanting to quit. Rather than telling yourself, "today I am not going to smoke," set a firm quit date within 1 to 2 weeks of this appointment and make plans on how not to smoke. Think of quitting as taking on a new job. With all the other responsibilities you have, quitting should be your priority for about 3 months. And get help—the more support you have the better.

Ms. W: What kind of help? My fiancé tells me to just stop—that if I really wanted to quit I could.

Clinician: A lot of people think smokers should just stop. But that is like telling an alcoholic to just stop drinking and we wouldn't do that. We tell other addicts to get quit therapy and that's what smokers should do! It is about learning how to quit. We rarely get what we want in life unless we work at it.

Ms. W: I never thought of it that way. I thought I couldn't stop because I am weak or just don't have any will power.

Clinician: Not at all. I would suggest calling 1-800-QUIT-NOW. This is a free service that provides counseling on how to quit. This quitline can also tell you about programs near you if you are interested in more intensive treatment. And as your provider, I will assist you in any way I can—including educate you about the medications that help people quit.

Ms. W: Thank you. I will call the quitline and let you know what I decide to do.

Clinician: Good for you. You will miss your "best friend" but your life will be so much better once you have made the break!

Box 19-2. Sample Cessation Counseling Dialog #2

Ms. G is a 50-year-old grant writer who has come to the dental office for follow-up care. Ms. G has type-2 diabetes, COPD (chronic bronchitis), and severe enough periodontal disease that most of her teeth have been extracted in the past few years. Ms. G began smoking at age 13 and has smoked a pack a day for most of her life. About a year ago she decreased her daily consumption to half a pack.

Clinician: Congratulations on being able to cut down on your smoking! Have you thought about quitting completely? We might be able to save your remaining teeth if you are able to quit.

Ms. G: I know I should quit but I really love my cigarettes.

Clinician: Has it been hard for you to cut down?

Ms. G: Actually, it's been horrible.

Clinician: What has been the most difficult part for you?

Ms. G: I can't stop thinking about my next cigarette. I find myself thinking about when I can get the next cigarette in as soon as I put one out!

Clinician: It almost sounds like the cigarettes have become even more important to you since you cut down! While quitting is the most difficult thing you might ever do, it might in fact make your life easier to not have to worry about when you can get in your next cigarette.

Ms. G: That's true—it would be so nice to not to have to think about them anymore.

Clinician: So, you still love your cigarettes but don't love that you are smoking!

Ms. G: Yes that is exactly it. I hate that I am still smoking. I know it is so bad for my health. I feel that I must quit but I have tried to quit before and the longest I have ever gone without a cigarette has only been 4 hours! Cigarettes are the only things that calm me down.

Clinician: How soon do you smoke when you first get up in the morning and do you ever smoke if you wake during the night?

Ms. G: I smoke before my feet hit the ground every morning and I often take a couple of drags if I wake up during the night.

Clinician: It sounds like you have a strong physical addiction as well as a significant psychological addiction. Have you considered using medication to help you quit? You would be a good candidate for pharmacotherapy.

Ms. G: No. I take insulin for my diabetes and I don't want to take anything that would interfere with that.

Clinician: Actually, smoking interferes with controlling your diabetes much more than a quit-smoking medication. And were you aware that with every cigarette your blood sugar goes up? So, your diabetes would be much easier to control if you quit.

Ms. G: I had no idea that was the case.

Clinician: One suggestion would be to look at quitting the same way you look at having diabetes. A nicotine addiction is a chronic condition just as diabetes is. You do whatever you can to control your blood sugar with diet, exercise, and medication to enhance your quality of life and decrease risks—even though you may not want to do all those things. Try to look at quitting that way. Even though you love cigarettes, you will benefit by taking control! Look at quitting as something you are doing for yourself rather than to yourself. That approach may make it easier to let go of smoking.

Ms. G: I like that. It puts me in control of the situation—rather than letting the cigarettes control me! Maybe I will consider trying a medication to help me.

Box 19-3. Sample Smoking Cessation Counseling Dialog #3

Mr. R is a 48-year-old attorney who has come to the dental office for his care. Mr. R has hypertension and high cholesterol. He has periodontal disease on exam. Mr. R began smoking at age 17 and has smoked 2 packs a day for 30 years.

Clinician: As you know, your oral exam shows significant damage from smoking and your blood pressure is elevated today. Have you tried to quit since our last visit?

Mr. R: Not really. And I don't want to talk about it. Everyone is on me. My doctors, my wife, my kids, and now I suppose you are going to give me a hard time too.

Clinician: I don't want to give you a hard time. But I do want you to encourage you to at least try and quit. The more times you try, the more chance you have of success. I am not going to tell you how dangerous it is to smoke. But I am going to remind you that by quitting you can reverse so much of the damage cigarettes have caused in you.

Mr. R: Look I really don't want to quit. I exercise and I watch what I eat. I'll keep coming to you for my teeth and take medicine for my heart problems and hope for the best.

Clinician: You are such a "take charge" person in every other aspect of your life. How about taking control over this addiction rather than hoping for the best?

Mr. R: I will quit when I am ready. I know myself. When I decide to do something, it gets done.

Clinician: Take advantage of that! Consider what is available to help you quit now. It is possible to quit even if you don't want to quit or don't feel ready.

Mr. R: It would get people off my back anyway. My kids nag me every day.

Clinician: People in your life are concerned about you. But you cannot quit for them. You can use the fact that you will have a longer, better quality life with your kids as a motivation though the decision to quit is yours. No one, nothing, can make you quit but there are plenty of us who can help you quit.

Mr. R: If I do this, I am doing it on my own.

Clinician: I understand your wanting to take that approach. However, it would be so much easier if you use a medication. You have been smoking for a long time and a medication would increase your chance of permanent success.

Mr. R: Is it ok to take something with all my heart problems?

Clinician: Absolutely. In fact, the medication, Chantix, has the highest success rates. It should be started 1 to 2 weeks prior to quitting and once there is a therapeutic dose in your system, you should notice a significant decrease in your desire to smoke. I can provide you with more information and arrange for a prescription.

Mr. R: I have heard that makes you feel depressed.

Clinician: That is been reported but only in a tiny minority. Feeling depressed is very common with quitting! I will show you a list of the most common withdrawal symptoms so you will be aware of what to expect. And give you information on the other six FDA-approved medications so you will have all the options. Think about setting a quit date within a couple of weeks and let me know how I can best assist you through the process. I will keep working with you until you are able to quit.

Mr. R: OK I will try but this is just between you and me.

Clinician: I understand and will respect that. At some point people in your life will be aware that you are trying to quit and it might help you to let them know what they can do to help you—including NOT nag you! I am very proud of you for making the attempt. You will not regret it!

Chapter Summary Statement

Tobacco use is a major risk factor for the onset and progression of periodontal disease. Smoking affects the periodontium in several ways by impacting oral biofilms, host immune response, and bone metabolism. There is sufficient evidence for the benefits of tobacco cessation on a wide variety of oral health outcomes, including periodontal treatment. Advice and assistance on tobacco cessation is therefore an integral part in the management of all patients seeking periodontal care.

Section 5
Focus on Patients

Clinical Patient Care

CASE 1

A new patient with severe periodontitis has a history of smoking 1 to 2 packs of cigarettes each day. The patient informs you that he will do "anything" to save his teeth, but that he cannot quit smoking. What counsel would you provide this patient about the effect of the smoking habit on the likelihood of long-term control of his periodontitis?

Clinical Evidence in Action: Clinical Relevance

The current smoking prevalence in the United States is under 15%—why is the focus on helping smokers quit so important?

Fifty years after a momentous report on its hazards, smoking remains the most significant public health predicament. Cigarette smoking is responsible for an estimated 443,000 deaths annually in the United States. Almost 45 million American adults smoke (1). The most vulnerable of our population are most likely to be affected—the less educated, the youth, LGBTQ persons, and minorities. In addition, people who live below the poverty line are 30% more likely to smoke than those who live above it. The prevalence is even higher for those with psychiatric comorbidities.

In its 2014 report, "The Health Consequences of Smoking—50 Years of Progress,"[2] the US Surgeon General concluded that, while significant improvements have been made since the publication of its landmark 1964 report, cigarette smoking remains a major public health problem. It is the leading cause of preventable death, increasing risks of such common causes of mortality as cardiovascular disease, pulmonary disease, and malignancy. Half of those who continue to smoke will die prematurely from a tobacco-related cause.

1. Jamal A, King BA, Neff LJ, Whitmill J, Babb SD, Graffunder CM. Current Cigarette Smoking Among Adults—United States, 2005–2015. *MMWR Morb Mortal Wkly Rep*. 2016;65:1205–1211. DOI: http://dx.doi.org/10.15585/mmwr.mm6544a2.
2. National Center for Chronic Disease Prevention and Health Promotion Office on Smoking and Health. The Health Consequences of Smoking—50 Years of Progress: A Report of the Surgeon General. 2014. Available at: http://www.ncbi.nlm.nih.gov/pubmed/24455788, Accessed February 22, 2017.

Bottom line on Smoking cessation: What should you recommend?

The most recent comprehensive smoking cessation guideline, sponsored by the U.S. Public Health Service, was published in 2008.[1] The U.S. Preventive Services Task Force (USPSTF) recommendation that "clinicians ask all adults about tobacco use and provide tobacco cessation interventions" for those who smoke was issued 1 year later.[2] Since then, countless investigations have assessed the merits of the various cessation medications and counseling designed to help smokers achieve and maintain tobacco abstinence. The most successful practice recommendations are to prescribe varenicline, bupropion, or nicotine replacement as first-line pharmacotherapy for smoking cessation (advising a first-line medication—bupropion, varenicline, nicotine gum, nicotine inhaler, nicotine lozenge, nicotine nasal spray, or nicotine patch—for every patient who smokes is a key component of the 2008 guideline) and provide counseling along with the medication—the combination of medication and counseling has proven to be more effective than either option alone. Despite this evidence, most smokers are still trying to stop on their own and more than 95% of smokers who try to quit without treatment assistance will fail, the majority relapsing within 1 week. Members of the dental team should counsel all tobacco users, even those reluctant to quit, about the benefits of stopping smoking and educate about how to best achieve permanent cessation. As one of the largest cadre of health care professionals, dental hygienists can have an enormous impact. All hygienists have multiple clinical opportunities to encourage smoking cessation and are therefore in a unique position to reduce cigarette consumption and consequently the burden of illness, death, and economic costs resulting from tobacco use.

1. U.S. Public Health Service. A clinical practice guideline for treating tobacco use and dependence: 2008 update. A US Public Health Service Report. *Am J Prev Med*. 2008;35:158–176.
2. U.S. Preventive Series Task Force. Tobacco use in adults and pregnant women: Counseling and interventions. April 2009. Available at: http://www.uspreventiveservicestaskforce.org/PageTopic/recommendation-summary/tobacco-use-in-adults-and-pregnant-women-counseling-and-interventions, Accessed February 22, 2017.

What about the mental health side effects of Chantix (varenicline) and Zyban (bupropion)?

Based on an FDA review of a large clinical trial that the FDA required the drug companies Pfizer and GlaxoSmithKline to conduct, the FDA determined the risk of serious side effects on mood behavior or cognitive abilities with Chantix (varenicline) and Zyban (bupropion) is lower than previously suspected. In fact, because of this trial review, the FDA removed the Black Box Warning (the FDA's most prominent warning for serious mental health side effects) from the Chantix drug label. The language describing the serious mental health side effects seen in patients quitting smoking will also be removed from the Boxed Warning in the Zyban label. The FDA review of the clinical trial results also confirmed that Chantix, Zyban, and nicotine replacement patches were all significantly more effective for helping people quit smoking than placebo. These medications were found to better help people quit smoking regardless of whether they had a history of mental illness. The results of the trial confirm that the benefits of smoking cessation significantly outweigh the risks of these medications and it is incumbent that members of the dental team inform all tobacco users about this new and very important information.[1]

1. https://www.fda.gov/Drugs/DrugSafety/ucm532221.htm.

References

1. Fiorini T, Musskopf ML, Oppermann RV, Susin C. Is there a positive effect of smoking cessation on periodontal health? A systematic review. *J Periodontol.* 2014;85(1):83–91.
2. Gelskey SC. Cigarette smoking and periodontitis: methodology to assess the strength of evidence in support of a causal association. *Community Dent Oral Epidemiol.* 1999;27(1):16–24.
3. Johannsen A, Susin C, Gustafsson A. Smoking and inflammation: evidence for a synergistic role in chronic disease. *Periodontol 2000.* 2014;64(1):111–126.
4. Johnson GK, Guthmiller JM. The impact of cigarette smoking on periodontal disease and treatment. *Periodontol 2000.* 2007;44:178–194.
5. Ahlqwist M, Bengtsson C, Hollender L, Lapidus L, Osterberg T. Smoking habits and tooth loss in Swedish women. *Community Dent Oral Epidemiol.* 1989;17(3):144–147.
6. Holm G. Smoking as an additional risk for tooth loss. *J Periodontol.* 1994;65(11):996–1001.
7. Tonetti MS. Cigarette smoking and periodontal diseases: etiology and management of disease. *Ann Periodontol.* 1998;3(1):88–101.
8. Albandar JM, Streckfus CF, Adesanya MR, Winn DM. Cigar, pipe, and cigarette smoking as risk factors for periodontal disease and tooth loss. *J Periodontol.* 2000;71(12):1874–1881.
9. Tomar SL, Asma S. Smoking-attributable periodontitis in the United States: findings from NHANES III. National Health and Nutrition Examination Survey. *J Periodontol.* 2000;71(5):743–751.
10. Anand PS, Kamath KP, Bansal A, Dwivedi S, Anil S. Comparison of periodontal destruction patterns among patients with and without the habit of smokeless tobacco use—a retrospective study. *J Periodontal Res.* 2013;48(5):623–631.
11. Heasman L, Stacey F, Preshaw PM, McCracken GI, Hepburn S, Heasman PA. The effect of smoking on periodontal treatment response: a review of clinical evidence. *J Clin Periodontol.* 2006;33(4):241–253.
12. Johnson GK, Hill M. Cigarette smoking and the periodontal patient. *J Periodontol.* 2004;75(2):196–209.
13. Johnson GK, Slach NA. Impact of tobacco use on periodontal status. *J Dent Educ.* 2001;65(4):313–321.
14. Grossi SG, Genco RJ, Machtei EE, et al. Assessment of risk for periodontal disease. II. Risk indicators for alveolar bone loss. *J Periodontol.* 1995;66(1):23–29.
15. Chambrone LA, Chambrone L. Tooth loss in well-maintained patients with chronic periodontitis during long-term supportive therapy in Brazil. *J Clin Periodontol.* 2006;33(10):759–764.
16. Martinez-Canut P, Llobell A, Romero A. Predictors of long-term outcomes in patients undergoing periodontal maintenance. *J Clin Periodontol.* 2017;44(6):620–631.
17. McGuire MK, Nunn ME. Prognosis versus actual outcome. IV. The effectiveness of clinical parameters and IL-1 genotype in accurately predicting prognoses and tooth survival. *J Periodontol.* 1999;70(1):49–56.
18. Bostrom L, Bergstrom J, Dahlen G, Linder LE. Smoking and subgingival microflora in periodontal disease. *J Clin Periodontol.* 2001;28(3):212–219.
19. Preber H, Bergstrom J. Occurrence of gingival bleeding in smoker and non-smoker patients. *Acta Odontol Scand.* 1985;43(5):315–320.
20. Stoltenberg JL, Osborn JB, Pihlstrom BL, et al. Association between cigarette smoking, bacterial pathogens, and periodontal status. *J Periodontol.* 1993;64(12):1225–1230.
21. Kumar PS, Matthews CR, Joshi V, de Jager M, Aspiras M. Tobacco smoking affects bacterial acquisition and colonization in oral biofilms. *Infect Immun.* 2011;79(11):4730–4738.
22. Shchipkova AY, Nagaraja HN, Kumar PS. Subgingival microbial profiles of smokers with periodontitis. *J Dent Res.* 2010;89(11):1247–1253.
23. van Winkelhoff AJ, Bosch-Tijhof CJ, Winkel EG, van der Reijden WA. Smoking affects the subgingival microflora in periodontitis. *J Periodontol.* 2001;72(5):666–671.
24. Bagaitkar J, Daep CA, Patel CK, Renaud DE, Demuth DR, Scott DA. Tobacco smoke augments Porphyromonas gingivalis—Streptococcus gordonii biofilm formation. *PLoS One.* 2011;6(11):e27386.
25. Eggert FM, McLeod MH, Flowerdew G. Effects of smoking and treatment status on periodontal bacteria: evidence that smoking influences control of periodontal bacteria at the mucosal surface of the gingival crevice. *J Periodontol.* 2001;72(9):1210–1220.
26. Haffajee AD, Socransky SS. Relationship of cigarette smoking to attachment level profiles. *J Clin Periodontol.* 2001;28(4):283–295.
27. Kamma JJ, Nakou M, Baehni PC. Clinical and microbiological characteristics of smokers with early onset periodontitis. *J Periodontal Res.* 1999;34(1):25–33.
28. Zambon JJ, Grossi SG, Machtei EE, Ho AW, Dunford R, Genco RJ. Cigarette smoking increases the risk for subgingival infection with periodontal pathogens. *J Periodontol.* 1996;67(10 Suppl):1050–1054.
29. Karasneh JA, Al Habashneh RA, Marzouka NA, Thornhill MH. Effect of cigarette smoking on subgingival bacteria in healthy subjects and patients with chronic periodontitis. *BMC Oral Health.* 2017;17(1):64.
30. Nishida N, Yamamoto Y, Tanaka M, et al. Association between passive smoking and salivary markers related to periodontitis. *J Clin Periodontol.* 2006;33(10):717–723.
31. Kinane DF, Chestnutt IG. Smoking and periodontal disease. *Crit Rev Oral Biol Med.* 2000;11(3):356–365.
32. Palmer RM, Wilson RF, Hasan AS, Scott DA. Mechanisms of action of environmental factors—tobacco smoking. *J Clin Periodontol.* 2005;32 Suppl 6:180–195.
33. Jacob V, Vellappally S, Smejkalova J. The influence of cigarette smoking on various aspects of periodontal health. *Acta Medica.* 2007;50(1):3–5.
34. Mooney J, Hodge PJ, Kinane DF. Humoral immune response in early-onset periodontitis: influence of smoking. *J Periodontal Res.* 2001;36(4):227–232.
35. Bergstrom J, Eliasson S. Cigarette smoking and alveolar bone height in subjects with a high standard of oral hygiene. *J Clin Periodontol.* 1987;14(8):466–469.
36. Kerdvongbundit V, Wikesjo UM. Effect of smoking on periodontal health in molar teeth. *J Periodontol.* 2000;71(3):433–437.
37. Razali M, Palmer RM, Coward P, Wilson RF. A retrospective study of periodontal disease severity in smokers and non-smokers. *Br Dent J.* 2005;198(8):495–498; discussion 485.

38. Grossi SG, Zambon JJ, Ho AW, et al. Assessment of risk for periodontal disease. I. Risk indicators for attachment loss. *J Periodontol.* 1994;65(3):260–267.

39. Fang MA, Frost PJ, Iida-Klein A, Hahn TJ. Effects of nicotine on cellular function in UMR 106-01 osteoblast-like cells. *Bone.* 1991;12(4):283–286.

40. Rosa GM, Lucas GQ, Lucas ON. Cigarette smoking and alveolar bone in young adults: a study using digitized radiographs. *J Periodontol.* 2008;79(2):232–244.

41. Kamer AR, El-Ghorab N, Marzec N, Margarone JE, 3rd, Dziak R. Nicotine induced proliferation and cytokine release in osteoblastic cells. *Int J Mol Med.* 2006;17(1):121–127.

42. Yamamoto Y, Nishida N, Tanaka M, et al. Association between passive and active smoking evaluated by salivary cotinine and periodontitis. *J Clin Periodontol.* 2005;32(10):1041–1046.

43. Sanders AE, Slade GD, Beck JD, Agustsdottir H. Secondhand smoke and periodontal disease: atherosclerosis risk in communities study. *Am J Public Health.* 2011;101 Suppl 1:S339–S346.

44. Sutton JD, Ranney LM, Wilder RS, Sanders AE. Environmental tobacco smoke and periodontitis in U.S. non-smokers. *J Dent Hyg.* 2012;86(3):185–194.

45. Sutton JD, Salas Martinez ML, Gerkovich MM. Environmental Tobacco Smoke and Periodontitis in United States Non-Smokers, 2009 to 2012. *J Periodontol.* 2017;88(6):565–574.

46. Ramoa CP, Eissenberg T, Sahingur SE. Increasing popularity of waterpipe tobacco smoking and electronic cigarette use: Implications for oral healthcare. *J Periodontal Res.* 2017;52(5):813–823.

47. Shihadeh A, Schubert J, Klaiany J, El Sabban M, Luch A, Saliba NA. Toxicant content, physical properties and biological activity of waterpipe tobacco smoke and its tobacco-free alternatives. *Tob Control.* 2015;24 Suppl 1:i22–i30.

48. Eissenberg T, Shihadeh A. Waterpipe tobacco and cigarette smoking: direct comparison of toxicant exposure. *Am J Prev Med.* 2009;37(6):518–523.

49. St Helen G, Benowitz NL, Dains KM, Havel C, Peng M, Jacob P, 3rd. Nicotine and carcinogen exposure after water pipe smoking in hookah bars. *Cancer Epidemiol Biomarkers Prev.* 2014;23(6):1055–1066.

50. Natto S, Baljoon M, Abanmy A, Bergstrom J. Tobacco smoking and gingival health in a Saudi Arabian population. *Oral Health Prev Dent.* 2004;2(4):351–357.

51. Natto S, Baljoon M, Bergstrom J. Tobacco smoking and periodontal bone height in a Saudi Arabian population. *J Clin Periodontol.* 2005;32(9):1000–1006.

52. Natto S, Baljoon M, Bergstrom J. Tobacco smoking and periodontal health in a Saudi Arabian population. *J Periodontol.* 2005;76(11):1919–1926.

53. James JA, Sayers NM, Drucker DB, Hull PS. Effects of tobacco products on the attachment and growth of periodontal ligament fibroblasts. *J Periodontol.* 1999;70(5):518–525.

54. Machuca G, Rosales I, Lacalle JR, Machuca C, Bullon P. Effect of cigarette smoking on periodontal status of healthy young adults. *J Periodontol.* 2000;71(1):73–78.

55. Preber H, Bergstrom J. The effect of non-surgical treatment on periodontal pockets in smokers and non-smokers. *J Clin Periodontol.* 1986;13(4):319–323.

56. Kaldahl WB, Johnson GK, Patil KD, Kalkwarf KL. Levels of cigarette consumption and response to periodontal therapy. *J Periodontol.* 1996;67(7):675–681.

57. Ah MK, Johnson GK, Kaldahl WB, Patil KD, Kalkwarf KL. The effect of smoking on the response to periodontal therapy. *J Clin Periodontol.* 1994;21(2):91–97.

58. Grossi SG, Skrepcinski FB, DeCaro T, Zambon JJ, Cummins D, Genco RJ. Response to periodontal therapy in diabetics and smokers. *J Periodontol.* 1996;67(10 Suppl):1094–1102.

59. Kinane DF, Radvar M. The effect of smoking on mechanical and antimicrobial periodontal therapy. *J Periodontol.* 1997;68(5):467–472.

60. Miller PD, Jr. Root coverage with the free gingival graft. Factors associated with incomplete coverage. *J Periodontol.* 1987;58(10):674–681.

61. Preber H, Bergstrom J. Effect of cigarette smoking on periodontal healing following surgical therapy. *J Clin Periodontol.* 1990;17(5):324–328.

62. Rosen PS, Marks MH, Reynolds MA. Influence of smoking on long-term clinical results of intrabony defects treated with regenerative therapy. *J Periodontol.* 1996;67(11):1159–1163.

63. Tonetti MS, Pini-Prato G, Cortellini P. Effect of cigarette smoking on periodontal healing following GTR in infrabony defects. A preliminary retrospective study. *J Clin Periodontol.* 1995;22(3):229–234.

64. Sanz M, Chapple IL, Working Group 4 of the VIII European Workshop on Periodontology. Clinical research on peri-implant diseases: consensus report of Working Group 4. *J Clin Periodontol.* 2012;39 Suppl 12:202–206.

65. Tomasi C, Derks J. Clinical research of peri-implant diseases—quality of reporting, case definitions and methods to study incidence, prevalence and risk factors of peri-implant diseases. *J Clin Periodontol.* 2012;39 Suppl 12:207–223.

66. Levin L, Schwartz-Arad D. The effect of cigarette smoking on dental implants and related surgery. *Implant Dent.* 2005;14(4):357–361.

67. Anner R, Grossmann Y, Anner Y, Levin L. Smoking, diabetes mellitus, periodontitis, and supportive periodontal treatment as factors associated with dental implant survival: a long-term retrospective evaluation of patients followed for up to 10 years. *Implant Dent.* 2010;19(1):57–64.

68. Cavalcanti R, Oreglia F, Manfredonia MF, Gianserra R, Esposito M. The influence of smoking on the survival of dental implants: a 5-year pragmatic multicentre retrospective cohort study of 1727 patients. *Eur J Oral Implantol.* 2011;4(1):39–45.

69. Charalampakis G, Rabe P, Leonhardt A, Dahlen G. A follow-up study of peri-implantitis cases after treatment. *J Clin Periodontol.* 2011;38(9):864–871.

70. Heitz-Mayfield LJ. Peri-implant diseases: diagnosis and risk indicators. *J Clin Periodontol.* 2008;35(8 Suppl):292–304.

71. Heitz-Mayfield LJ, Huynh-Ba G. History of treated periodontitis and smoking as risks for implant therapy. *Int J Oral Maxillofac Implants.* 2009;24 Suppl:39–68.

72. Klokkevold PR, Han TJ. How do smoking, diabetes, and periodontitis affect outcomes of implant treatment? *Int J Oral Maxillofac Implants.* 2007;22 Suppl:173–202.

73. Koldsland OC, Scheie AA, Aass AM. Prevalence of implant loss and the influence of associated factors. *J Periodontol.* 2009;80(7):1069–1075.

74. Rodriguez-Argueta OF, Figueiredo R, Valmaseda-Castellon E, Gay-Escoda C. Postoperative complications in smoking patients treated with implants: a retrospective study. *J Oral Maxillofac Surg.* 2011;69(8):2152–2157.

75. Bolin A, Eklund G, Frithiof L, Lavstedt S. The effect of changed smoking habits on marginal alveolar bone loss. A longitudinal study. *Swed Dent J.* 1993;17(5):211–216.

76. Preshaw PM, Heasman L, Stacey F, Steen N, McCracken GI, Heasman PA. The effect of quitting smoking on chronic periodontitis. *J Clin Periodontol.* 2005;32(8):869–879.

77. Position paper: tobacco use and the periodontal patient. Research, Science and Therapy Committee of the American Academy of Periodontology. *J Periodontol.* 1999;70(11):1419–1427.

78. Binnie VI. Addressing the topic of smoking cessation in a dental setting. *Periodontol 2000.* 2008;48:170–178.

79. Walt G. WHO's World Health Report 2003. *BMJ.* 2004;328(7430):6. doi: 10.1136/bmj.328.7430.6.

80. West R, McNeill A, Raw M. Smoking cessation guidelines for health professionals: an update. Health Education Authority. *Thorax.* 2000;55(12):987–999.

81. Needleman I, Warnakulasuriya S, Sutherland G, Bornstein MM, Casals E, Dietrich T, et al. Evaluation of tobacco use cessation (TUC) counselling in the dental office. *Oral Health Prev Dent.* 2006;4(1):27–47.

 ## STUDENT ANCILLARY RESOURCES

A wide variety of resources to enhance your learning is available online:

- Audio Glossary
- Book Pages
- Chapter Review Questions and Answers

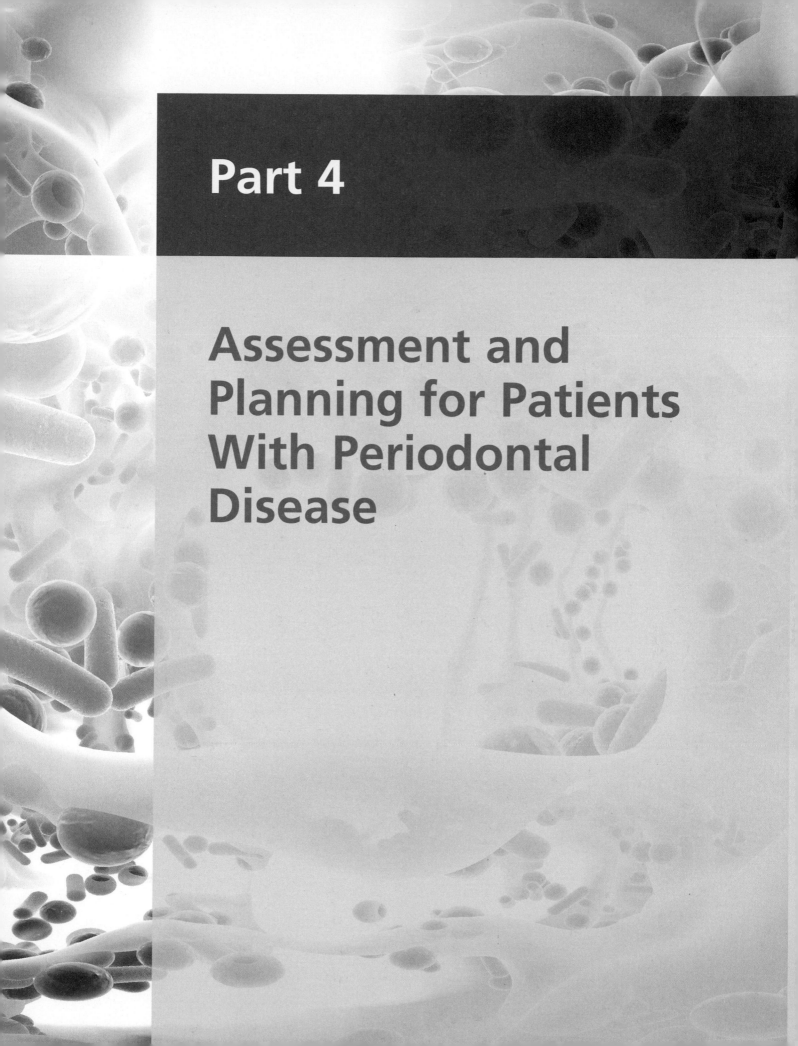

Part 4

Assessment and Planning for Patients With Periodontal Disease

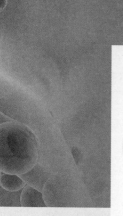

Clinical Application.
Clinical periodontal assessment is a critical step in the care all patients with periodontal diseases. A careful and meticulous clinical periodontal assessment serves as the foundation for assigning a periodontal diagnosis, developing plans for treating patients, and monitoring the success or failure of periodontal treatment performed. The rigorous standards of care in effect today require every clinician participating in patient care to be familiar with the details of performing and documenting a clinical periodontal assessment. This chapter describes how to perform a clinical periodontal assessment, how to document the findings of the assessment, and how to perform calculations needed during the assessment.

Learning Objectives

* List the components of a comprehensive periodontal assessment.

* Describe how to evaluate each component of a comprehensive periodontal assessment.

* Explain how to calculate the width of attached gingiva.

* Explain how to calculate clinical attachment level given several different clinical scenarios.

* Compare and contrast a periodontal screening examination and a comprehensive periodontal assessment.

* Given a clinical scenario, calculate and document the clinical attachment levels for a patient with periodontitis.

Key Terms

Clinical periodontal
  assessment
Baseline data
Comprehensive periodontal
  assessment
Exudate
Horizontal tooth mobility

Vertical tooth mobility
Fremitus
Furcation probes
Attached gingiva
Mucogingival defects
Clinical attachment level

Periodontal screening
  examination
Periodontal Screening and
  Recording
World Health Organization
  probe
Gingival crevicular fluid

Section 1
Overview of the Periodontal Assessment Process

1. Clinical periodontal assessment is a fact-gathering process designed to provide a comprehensive picture of the patient's periodontal health status.
   A. **Importance of Periodontal Assessment**
      1. This assessment is one of the most important duties performed by any dental team.
         a. The dental team is obligated to perform and document findings of a periodontal assessment for every patient when he/she first enters the dental practice and periodically thereafter.[1-5]
         b. Periodontal assessment requires meticulous attention to detail since successful patient care is dependent on a thorough and accurate periodontal evaluation.
      2. The information gathered during the clinical periodontal assessment forms the basis of both a periodontal diagnosis and an individualized treatment plan for the patient.
   B. **Objectives of Periodontal Assessment.** The objectives of the clinical periodontal assessment process include the following:
      1. Detect clinical signs of inflammation in the periodontium.
      2. Identify damage to the periodontium already caused by disease or trauma.
      3. Provide the dental team with data used to assign a periodontal diagnosis and a tooth-by-tooth prognosis.
      4. Document features of the periodontium to serve as baseline data for long-term patient monitoring.
   C. **Two Types of Periodontal Assessment.** Two commonly used periodontal assessments are the periodontal screening examination and the comprehensive periodontal assessment.
      1. **Periodontal Screening Examination.** Periodontal screening examination is a quick information-gathering process that may be used to determine if a more thorough comprehensive periodontal assessment (see below) is needed to formulate a diagnosis.
      2. **Comprehensive Periodontal Assessment.** Comprehensive periodontal assessment is an in-depth information-gathering process used to gather the detailed data needed to document the complete periodontal health status of a patient.
2. Standard of Care
   A. *The standard of care for dentists and dental hygienists is to complete an accurate and thorough periodontal assessment on every patient.*
   B. Without a thorough clinical periodontal assessment, periodontal diseases are often not diagnosed or are misdiagnosed, inevitably leading to either undertreatment or overtreatment of the patient.
3. Documentation of Assessment Findings
   A. The clinical periodontal assessment is not complete until all of the information gathered during the assessment has been accurately recorded in the patient's dental chart.
   B. The importance of the accuracy of the documentation cannot be overstated.
      1. Findings documented during the clinical periodontal assessment serve as baseline data used to evaluate the success or failure of an episode of periodontal therapy. Baseline data refers to clinical information gathered at the initial appointment that can be used for comparison to clinical information gathered at a subsequent appointment.
      2. Documented findings also provide the baseline data used in the long-term monitoring of the patient's periodontal health status. An example of when patient monitoring may occur is at periodontal maintenance visits following successful treatment.

Section 2
The Comprehensive Periodontal Assessment

A comprehensive periodontal assessment is an intensive clinical periodontal evaluation used to gather information about the periodontium. This section of the chapter outlines the clinical features that should be noted and documented during a comprehensive periodontal assessment. It is important to note that special precautions are necessary when examining dental implants. These examination techniques are presented in Chapter 9.

The comprehensive periodontal assessment normally involves the evaluation of (1) clinical features such as probing depth measurements, bleeding on probing, presence of exudate, level of the free gingival margin, level of the mucogingival junction, tooth mobility, furcation involvement, presence of calculus, presence of plaque biofilms, gingival inflammation, and presence of local contributing factors and (2) radiographic features such as the level of the alveolar crest, pattern of the trabecular bone, width of the PDL space, and presence or absence of the lamina dura. A more in-depth description of radiographic assessment is discussed in Chapter 21. Findings obtained from a comprehensive periodontal assessment will provide vital information of the overall health of the periodontium and enable proper periodontal diagnosis.

It should be noted that there are a number of excellent electronic tools that can be used while performing a comprehensive periodontal assessment; for example, periodontal probes are available that can record probing depths directly in computer software. The discussion in this chapter focuses only on the basic concepts underlying each of the clinical factors being assessed with the knowledge that a clinician who understands the basic concepts can easily apply any of the available electronic tools appropriately.

COMPONENTS OF THE COMPREHENSIVE PERIODONTAL ASSESSMENT

1. **The Gingiva.** The comprehensive periodontal assessment includes evaluation of the health of the gingival tissues including assessment of tissue color, contour, consistency, and texture. These clinical features are discussed in Chapter 5, Clinical Features of the Gingiva. The landmarks of the gingival tissues are pictured in Figure 20-1.

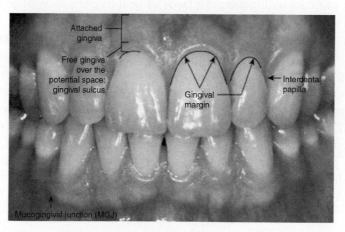

Figure 20-1. Landmarks of the Gingival Tissues. Important gingival landmarks include the gingival margin, the interdental papilla, free gingiva, attached gingiva, and mucogingival junction. (Used with permission from Wilkins EM. *Clinical Practice of the Dental Hygienist.* 12th ed. Philadelphia, PA: Wolters Kluwer; 2017.)

A. Gingival Inflammation

1. A thorough periodontal assessment includes recording the overt clinical signs of inflammation. The overt clinical signs of inflammation of the gingiva include erythema (redness) and edema (swelling) of the gingiva resulting in readily identifiable changes in gingival color and contour.

2. It is always important to be aware that inflammation can be present in the deeper structures of the periodontium without necessarily involving any obvious visual signs of inflammation of the gingival margin.

   a. When assessing the presence of inflammation, it is important to remember that bleeding on probing also can be a sign of inflammation.

   b. Thus, when a clinician is identifying gingival inflammation for purposes of planning treatment, the visible signs such as color, contour, and consistency changes in the gingiva must be correlated with the other signs such as bleeding on probing or the presence of exudate.

B. Level of the Free Gingival Margin. The level of the free gingival margin in relationship to the cementoenamel junction (CEJ) should be recorded on the dental chart. This level can simply be drawn on the facial and lingual surfaces of the dental chart. The photographs in Figure 20-2 show examples of the three possible relationships that may exist between the free gingival margin and the CEJ.

1. **Free gingival margin can be slightly coronal to (above) the CEJ.** This is the natural level of the gingival margin and represents the expected position of the gingival margin in the absence of disease or trauma.

2. **Free gingival margin can be significantly coronal to the CEJ.** The gingival margin can be significantly coronal to the CEJ due to (1) swelling (edema), (2) overgrowth (as seen in patients taking certain medications), or (3) increase in fibrous connective tissue (as seen in long-standing inflammation of tissue).

3. **Free gingival margin can be apical to the CEJ.** This relationship, known as gingival recession, results in exposure of a portion of the root surface.

C. Recession of the Gingival Margin

1. Gingival recession is the displacement of the gingival soft tissue margin apical to the CEJ which results in exposure of the root surface.[6] This is a common clinical condition, and research indicates it presents in at least one or more tooth surfaces in 23% of US adults between 30 and 90 years of age.[6–8]

2. The prevalence of gingival recession has been shown to increase with age and can occur in patients with good standards of oral hygiene as well as those with poor oral hygiene and periodontal disease.[8]

3. The etiology of gingival recession is often multifactorial. Chan and colleagues[9] categorize the etiological factors of gingival recession under predisposing factors and precipitating factors. Predisposing factors include anatomical factors, inflammation, high frenal attachments, and a lack of adequate keratinized gingiva. Precipitating factors include traumatic forces (i.e., excessive brushing), habits (i.e., oral piercings), plaque-induced inflammation, and certain dental procedures (such as subgingival restorations).

4. The severity of gingival recession can be classified using the Miller classification system for gingival recession.[10] This classification system is outlined in Figure 20-3A–D.

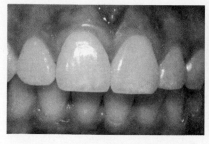
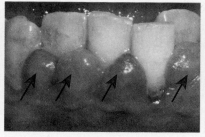
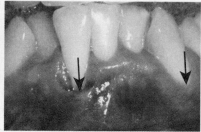

Figure 20-2. Level of the Free Gingival Margin. The photo on the left is an example of the gingival margin in health—slightly coronal to the CEJ. The center photo shows swollen gingiva where the gingival margin is coronal to the CEJ. In the photograph on the right, the gingival margin on the canine teeth is apical to the CEJ (recession of the gingival margin).

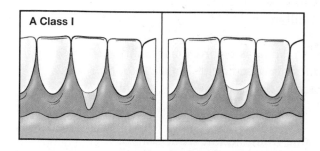

Figure 20-3A. Miller Class I Defect. In a Miller Class I gingival defect, the recession is isolated to the facial surface and the interdental papillae fill the adjacent interdental spaces. Class I recession does not extend to the mucogingival line.

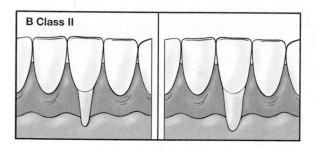

Figure 20-3B. Miller Class II Defect. In a Miller Class II gingival defect, the recession is isolated to the facial surface and the papillae remain intact and fill the interdental spaces. Class II recession does extend to or beyond the mucogingival line into the mucosa.

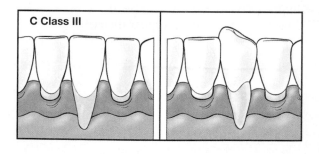

Figure 20-3C. Miller Class III Defect. In a Miller Class III gingival defect, the recession is quite broad with the interdental papillae missing due to damage from disease. The Class III defect extends to or beyond the mucogingival line into the mucosa.

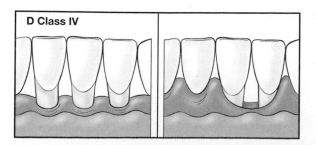

Figure 20-3D. Miller Class IV Defect. In a Miller Class IV gingival defect, the recession extends to or beyond the mucogingival junction with severe loss of interproximal alveolar bone resulting in open interdental areas.

Figures 20-3A–D. The Miller Classification System for Gingival Recession.

D. **Level of Mucogingival Junction**
1. The level of the mucogingival junction represents the junction between the keratinized gingiva and the nonkeratinized mucosa. The level of the mucogingival junction is used in calculation of the width of the attached gingiva as will be described later in this section.
2. The mucogingival junction is usually readily visible since the keratinized gingiva is normally pale pink and opaque while the surface of the mucosa consists of thin, translucent tissue (Fig. 20-4).
3. Occasionally, the mucogingival junction can be difficult to detect visually. In this case, the tissue can be manipulated by pulling on the patient's lip or pushing on the tissue with a blunt instrument to distinguish the moveable mucosa from the more firmly attached gingiva.

E. **Probing Depth Measurements.** Probing depth measurements are made from the free gingival margin to the base of the pocket (or base of the sulcus).
1. Probing depths are recorded to the nearest full millimeter. Measurements are normally rounded up to the next higher whole number (e.g., a reading of 3.5 mm is recorded as 4 mm, and a 5.5 mm reading is recorded as 6 mm).
2. Probing depth measurements are recorded for six specific sites on each tooth: (i) distofacial, (ii) middle facial, (iii) mesiofacial, (iv) distolingual, (v) middle lingual, and (vi) mesiolingual.

F. **Bleeding on Probing**
1. Bleeding on gentle probing represents bleeding from the soft tissue wall of a periodontal pocket where the wall of the pocket is ulcerated (i.e., where portions of the epithelium have been destroyed) (Fig. 20-5).
2. Bleeding can occur immediately after the site is probed or can be slightly delayed after probing. An alert clinician will observe each site for a few seconds before moving on to the next site.

G. **Presence of Exudate**
1. Exudate (sometimes referred to as suppuration) is pus that can be expressed from a periodontal pocket. Pus is composed mainly of dead white blood cells and can occur in response to any infection, including periodontal disease.
2. Exudate can be recognized as a pale yellow material oozing from the orifice of a pocket. It is usually easiest to detect when the gingiva is manipulated in some manner. Figure 20-6 depicts the use of light finger pressure on the gingiva to reveal the presence of exudate. Figure 20-7 illustrates the clinical appearance of exudate in a patient with periodontitis.

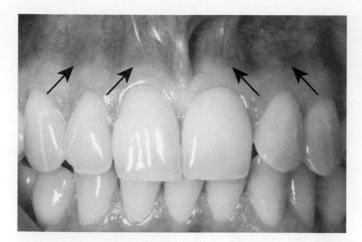

Figure 20-4. Mucogingival Junction. The mucogingival junction represents the junction between the keratinized gingiva and the nonkeratinized mucosa and is usually readily visible.

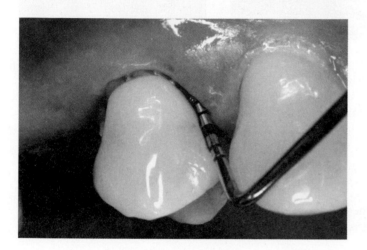

Figure 20-5. Bleeding Site. Bleeding from the soft tissue wall is a sign of disease. This bleeding was evident upon gentle probing. (Courtesy of Dr. Richard Foster, Guilford Technical Community College, Jamestown, NC.)

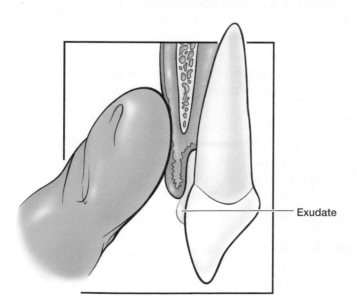

Exudate

Figure 20-6. Using Finger Pressure to Detect Exudate. Exudate can be detected in a periodontal pocket by placing an index finger on the soft tissue in the area of the pocket and exerting light pressure. This light pressure can force the exudate out of the pocket, making it readily visible to the clinician.

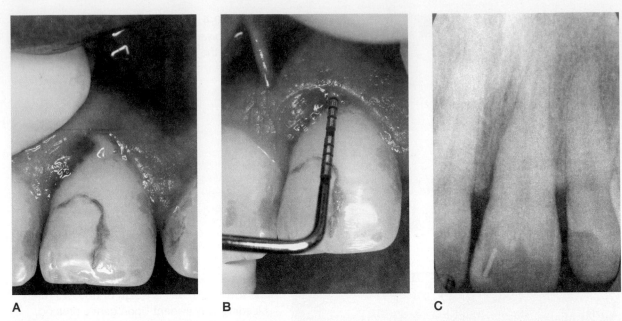

Figure 20-7. Exudate. A. Pressure with the clinician's finger on the gingiva reveals exudate from the gingival tissue adjacent to the central incisor. **B.** Exudate also is visible during probing. **C.** Radiograph of the same incisor shown in Figure 20-3A and 20-3B. (Courtesy of Dr. Richard Foster, Guilford Technical Community College, Jamestown, NC.)

2. The Teeth

  A. Tooth Mobility and Fremitus

    1. Horizontal tooth mobility, movement of a tooth in a facial-to-lingual direction, is assessed using the blunt ends of two dental instrument handles on either side of the tooth (Fig. 20-8).

      a. Alternating moderate pressure is applied in the facial-lingual direction against the tooth first with one, then the other instrument handle.

      b. Mobility can be observed by using an adjacent tooth as a stationary point of visual reference during attempts to move the tooth being examined.

    2. Vertical tooth mobility, the ability to depress the tooth in its socket, can be assessed using the end of an instrument handle to exert pressure against the occlusal or incisal surface of the tooth (Fig. 20-9).

    3. Even though the periodontal ligament allows some slight movement of the tooth in its socket, the amount of this natural tooth movement is so slight that it cannot normally be seen with the naked eye. Thus, when visually assessing mobility, the clinician should expect to find no visible movement in a periodontally healthy tooth.

    4. There are many rating scales for recording clinically visible tooth mobility. One useful scale is indicated in Table 20-1.

    5. In some dental offices, the dentist may also wish to assess fremitus.

      a. Fremitus is a palpable or visible movement of a tooth when in function.

      b. Fremitus can be assessed by gently placing a gloved index finger against the facial aspect of the tooth as the patient either taps the teeth together or simulates chewing movements. Fremitus is easy to detect if the finger pressure is gentle.

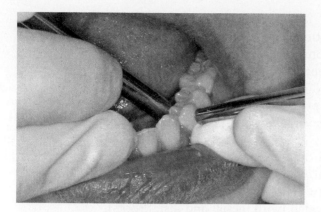

Figure 20-8. Determining Horizontal Tooth Mobility. To determine buccolingual mobility, the blunt ends of two instrument handles are applied to the tooth to see if it can be displaced buccolingually. Light, alternating force is applied with the instrument handles to detect movement relative to the adjacent teeth. (Used by permission from Scheid RC, Woelfel JB. *Woelfel's Dental Anatomy: Its Relevance to Dentistry*. 7th ed. Philadelphia, PA: Lippincott Williams & Wilkins; 2007.)

TABLE 20-1	SCALE FOR RATING VISIBLE TOOTH MOBILITY
Classification	**Description**
Class 1	Slight mobility, up to 1 mm of horizontal displacement in a facial-lingual direction
Class 2	Moderate mobility, greater than 1 mm but less than 2 mm of horizontal displacement in a facial-lingual direction
Class 3	Severe mobility, greater than 2 mm of displacement in a facial-lingual direction or vertical displacement (tooth depressible in the socket)

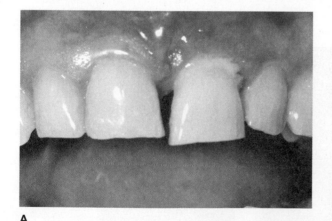

A

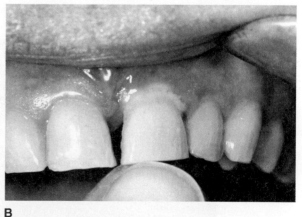

B

Figure 20-9. Vertical Tooth Mobility. A. The patient came to the dental office complaining of a loose tooth. Note the supraeruption of the maxillary left central incisor. **B.** The patient then demonstrated how he could push this tooth upward by applying pressure with his index finger against the incisal edge. This central incisor has vertical mobility. (Courtesy of Dr. Don Rolfs, Wenatchee, WA.)

B. Furcation Involvement

1. A furcation probe is used to assess furcation involvement on multirooted teeth. Most molar teeth are multirooted, but some maxillary premolar teeth also develop with two roots creating the potential for a furcation involvement.

2. Furcation probes are curved, blunt-tipped instruments that allow easy access to the furcation areas; straight periodontal probes cannot be relied upon to detect furcation involvements accurately. The most common type of furcation probe is known as the Nabers Probe.

3. Furcation involvement occurs on a multirooted tooth when periodontal infection invades the area between and around the roots, resulting in a loss of attachment and loss of alveolar bone between the roots of the tooth.

   a. Mandibular molars are usually bifurcated (with mesial and distal roots), with potential furcation involvement on both the facial and lingual aspects of the tooth (Fig. 20-10).

   b. Maxillary molar teeth are usually trifurcated (with mesiobuccal, distobuccal, and palatal roots) with potential furcation involvement on the facial, mesial, and distal aspects of the tooth.

   c. Maxillary first premolars that have bifurcated roots (buccal and palatal roots) have the potential for furcation involvement on the mesial and distal aspects of the tooth.

4. Furcation involvement frequently signals a need for periodontal surgery after completion of nonsurgical therapy, so detection and documentation of furcation involvement is a critical component of the comprehensive periodontal assessment.

5. Furcation involvement should be recorded using a scale that quantifies the severity (or extent) of the furcation invasion. Table 20-2 shows a commonly used scale for rating furcation invasions of multirooted teeth. This scale is known as the Glickman Furcation Classification system.

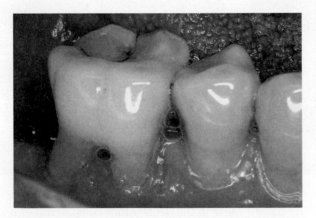 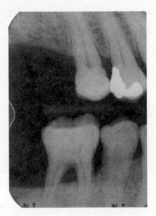

Figure 20-10. Furcation Involvement. The photograph on the left shows a furcation involvement as viewed from the facial aspect of a mandibular first molar. On the right, a radiograph of the same molar tooth shows bone loss between the roots of this molar.

TABLE 20-2	SCALE FOR RATING FURCATION INVOLVEMENT
Classification	**Description**
Class I	Incipient (early) furcation involvement; the tip of the Nabers probe tip can detect the curvature of the furcation concavity, but cannot enter inside the furcation.
Class II	A Nabers probe penetrates the furcation greater than 1 mm, but does not pass completely through the furcation.
Class III	The probe passes completely through the furcation, but the furcation entrance is not clinically visible because the soft tissue remains coronal to the furcation. In mandibular molars, the probe passes completely through the furcation between the mesial and distal roots. In maxillary molars, the probe passes between the mesiobuccal and distobuccal roots and will touch the palatal root.
Class IV	Same as Class III furcation, except that the entrance to the furca is clinically visible because of advanced gingival recession.

C. **Presence of Calculus Deposits on the Teeth**
   1. The presence of dental calculus on the teeth should be noted since these deposits must later be identified and removed as part of the nonsurgical therapy.
   2. Calculus is a local contributing factor in both gingivitis and periodontitis; thus, the identification and removal of these deposits is a critical component of successful patient treatment.
   3. Calculus deposits can be located through several techniques that include the following:
      a. Direct visual examination using a mouth mirror to locate supragingival deposits.
      b. Visual examination while using compressed air to dry the teeth to aid in locating supragingival deposits.
      c. Tactile examination using an explorer to locate subgingival calculus deposits.

D. **Presence of Plaque Biofilm on the Teeth**
1. The presence of plaque biofilm on the teeth should be noted during a comprehensive periodontal assessment since these deposits contain living periodontal pathogens that can lead to both gingivitis and periodontitis.
2. Plaque biofilms can be identified using disclosing dyes or by moving the tip of an explorer or a periodontal probe along the tooth surface adjacent to the gingival margin.
3. There are many ways to record the presence of plaque biofilms, but most dental offices record the results of the plaque assessment in terms of the percentage of tooth surfaces with plaque biofilm evident at the gingival margin. A useful formula for recording plaque percentages is shown in Box 20-1.
   a. Note that in using the calculation shown in Box 20-1, a plaque score of 90% indicates that 90% of the total available tooth surfaces have plaque biofilm at the gingival margin.
   b. One goal of therapy would be for the patient to learn and perform biofilm control measures that would bring the plaque score as close to 0% as possible (or at least to bring the percentage of tooth surfaces with plaque biofilm as low as possible).
4. As discussed previously in this book, plaque biofilm is the primary etiologic factor for both gingivitis and periodontitis. Identification of the presence and distribution of plaque biofilm on the teeth is a critical piece of information needed when planning appropriate therapy and patient education.

Box 20-1. Formula for Calculating Plaque Percentages

$$\frac{\text{Number of tooth surfaces with plaque}}{\text{Total number of tooth surfaces}} \times 100 = \text{percentage score}$$

---

3. **Local Factors and Radiographic Evidence**
   A. **Presence of Local Contributing Factors**
   1. A thorough periodontal assessment will always include identification of local contributing factors.
   2. These factors are discussed in Chapter 17. The plan for treatment for any periodontal patient will always include measures to eliminate or to minimize the impact of these local factors.
   B. **Radiographic Evidence of Alveolar Bone Loss.** Radiographic interpretation is discussed in Chapter 21.
   1. It is important for the clinician to remember, however, that radiographs play an important role in arriving at the periodontal diagnosis and in developing an appropriate plan for nonsurgical periodontal therapy.
   2. Radiographic evidence of alveolar bone loss is always an important part of a clinical periodontal assessment.

COMPONENTS OF THE COMPREHENSIVE PERIODONTAL ASSESSMENT THAT REQUIRE CALCULATIONS

Some judgments that are made as part of a comprehensive periodontal assessment require some calculations. The most common features that may require some calculations are the width of the attached gingiva and clinical attachment level.

1. **Width of Attached Gingiva**
   A. **Description.** The attached gingiva is the part of the gingiva that is firm, dense, and tightly connected to the cementum on the cervical-third of the root or to the periosteum (connective tissue cover) of the alveolar bone. The attached gingiva lies between the free gingiva and the alveolar mucosa, extending from the base of the sulcus (or pocket) to the mucogingival junction (Fig. 20-11).
   1. The functions of the attached gingiva are to keep the free gingiva from being pulled away from the tooth and to protect the gingiva from trauma.
   2. The width of the attached gingiva is not measured on the palate since it is not possible to determine where the attached gingiva ends and the palatal mucosa begins.
   3. *The attached gingiva does not include any portion of the gingiva that is separated from the tooth by a crevice, sulcus, or periodontal pocket.*
   4. Although the attached gingiva is keratinized tissue, the width of the attached gingiva is not synonymous with the width of keratinized tissue. To calculate the width of keratinized tissue, the width of the attached gingiva and the width of the free gingiva are added together.

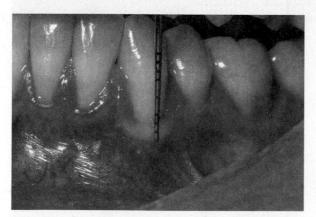
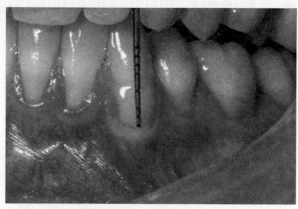

A

B

Figure 20-11. Width of Attached Gingiva. A. The total width of the gingiva from the gingival margin to the mucogingival junction is 2 mm. **B.** The probing depth—from the gingival margin to the base of the pocket—is 1 mm. Thus, this site has 1 mm of attached gingiva. (Used by permission from Scheid RC, Woelfel JB. *Woelfel's Dental Anatomy Its Relevance to Dentistry.* 7th ed. Philadelphia, PA: Lippincott Williams & Wilkins; 2007.)

B. Significance of Inadequate Attached Gingiva and Keratinized Gingiva

1. The width of the attached gingiva and the width of the keratinized gingiva are important clinical features for the dentist to keep in mind when planning restorative procedures. An adequate band of keratinized gingiva may be a prerequisite to maintain periodontal health and unaltered attachment levels on restored teeth. However, if a submarginal restoration is placed on a tooth with a narrow band of keratinized gingiva, the submarginal restoration may result in gingival inflammation and periodontal breakdown. It is conceivable that on a tooth with a narrow band of keratinized tissue, the submarginal restoration could act as a plaque retentive area that is difficult to keep clean. Therefore, it is important to use the information collected during the comprehensive periodontal assessment to calculate this clinical feature.

2. Mucogingival defects are deviations from the normal anatomic relationship between the gingival margin and the mucogingival junction.

   a. Common mucogingival conditions are recession and reduction or absence of keratinized tissue.

   b. With increased attachment loss, the base of a pocket may eventually extend beyond the mucogingival junction (thus, this site has no attached gingiva). When the periodontal probe extends apical to the mucogingival junction, a mucogingival defect is present.

   c. Areas with a lack of keratinized gingiva can be difficult to clean, leading to biofilm accumulation.

Box 20-2. Calculating the Width of Attached Gingiva

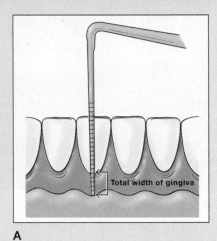

A

Figure 20-12A

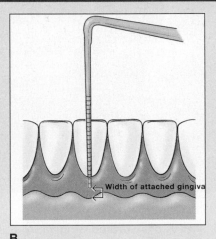

B

Figure 20-12B

Formula: To calculate the width of attached gingiva (WAG) at a specific site, measure the width of the keratinized gingiva (WKG) and subtract the probing depth (PD) from the total width using the steps below (WKG – PD = WAG).

Step 1: Place a periodontal probe on the outside of the tissue and measure from the gingival margin to the mucogingival junction. This measurement provides the total width of keratinized tissue.

Step 2: Measure the sulcus or pocket depth (from the gingival margin to the base of the sulcus or pocket).

Step 3: The width of the attached gingiva is calculated by subtracting the probing depth from the total width of the keratinized gingiva.

C. **Calculating the Width of Attached Gingiva.** The method for calculation of the width of attached gingiva is shown in Box 20-2 (Fig. 20-12). Note that the information needed to calculate the width of the attached gingiva already would have been recorded during the periodontal assessment.

2. **Clinical Attachment Level (CAL)**

   A. **Definition.** The clinical attachment level (CAL) is a clinical measurement of the true periodontal support around the tooth as measured with a periodontal probe. Box 20-3 outlines a comparison of probing depths and CALs.

   B. **Significance of Clinical Attachment Levels**

   1. An attachment level measurement is a more accurate indicator of the periodontal support around a tooth than is a probing depth measurement.

      a. Probing depths are measured from the free gingival margin to the base of the sulcus or pocket. The position of the gingival margin may change with tissue swelling, overgrowth of tissue, or recession of tissue. Since the position of the gingival margin can change (move coronally or apically), probing depths do not provide an accurate means to monitor changes in periodontal support over time in a patient.

      b. On the other hand, CAL provides an accurate means to monitor changes in periodontal support over time. The CAL is calculated from measurements made from a fixed point on the tooth that does not change (i.e., the CEJ of the tooth).

   2. The presence of loss of attachment is a critical factor in distinguishing between gingivitis and periodontitis.

      a. Inflammation with no attachment loss is characteristic of gingivitis.

      b. Inflammation with attachment loss is characteristic of periodontitis.

Box 20-3. Comparison of Probing Depths and Clinical Attachment Levels

Monitoring the periodontal support of teeth over time is a vital component of long-term care of patients with periodontal disease. There are two measurements used to describe the amount of periodontal support for teeth: (1) probing depths and (2) clinical attachment levels (CALs). Probing depths are frequently used, whereas CALs are less commonly used. Clinicians should be aware that the use of probing depths alone may not be in some patients' best interests.

- **Probing depths** alone are not the most reliable indicators of the amount of periodontal support for a tooth. Probing depths are measured from the gingival margin; the position of the gingival margin often changes over time. Changes in the level of the gingival margin occur with gingival swelling, overgrowth of gingiva, or gingival recession. So, a change in probing depth over time may indicate a change in the amount of periodontal support for a tooth, but it may also only indicate that there has been some change in the level of the gingival margin (which may well be unrelated to the actual periodontal support of the tooth).

- **Clinical attachment levels (CALs)** are the preferred and more accurate indicators of the actual amount of periodontal support for a tooth. CAL measurements are made from a fixed point that does not change (i.e., the CEJ of the tooth). Therefore, when there is a change in the CAL over time, this change reflects an accurate measurement of a true change in the periodontal support of a tooth.

C. **Calculating the Clinical Attachment Level**
   1. **When the gingival margin is near the CEJ.** When the gingival margin is at its natural location (i.e., *slightly* coronal to the CEJ of the tooth),[11] the probing depth and the CAL readings are the same for all practical purposes (Fig. 20-13A).
   2. **When the gingival margin is significantly coronal to the CEJ (i.e., there is gingival enlargement).** When gingival enlargement is present, a straight calibrated periodontal probe is used to measure the distance that the gingival margin is coronal to the CEJ (Fig. 20-13B). Remember that the natural position for the gingival margin is either at or slightly coronal to the CEJ, but there are many instances when the gingival margin will be found to be significantly (several millimeters) coronal to the CEJ. If the gingival margin is significantly coronal to the CEJ, the distance between the margin and the CEJ is estimated using the following technique:
      a. Position the tip of the straight calibrated probe at a 45-degree angle to the tooth surface.
      b. With light force, slowly move the probe beneath the gingival margin until the junction between the enamel and cementum is detected.
      c. Measure the distance between the gingival margin and the CEJ, and measure the probing depth at this site.
      d. Subtract the distance from the gingival margin to the CEJ from the probing depth to determine the CAL at the site.
   3. **When the gingival margin is apical to the CEJ (i.e., the gingival margin is recessed with root exposure).** When gingival recession is present, a straight calibrated periodontal probe is used to measure the distance the gingival margin is apical to the CEJ (Fig. 20-13C), and the same probe is used to measure the probing depth at the site. Both of these measurements will have been made and recorded as part of the comprehensive periodontal assessment. To calculate the CAL, simply add these two measurements (i.e., the amount of gingival recession plus the amount of the probing depth at the site).
D. **Recording the Gingival Margin on a Periodontal Chart.** Customarily, the notations 0, –, or + are used to indicate the position of the gingival margin with respect to the CEJ on a periodontal chart (Box 20-4).

Box 20-4. Notations That Indicate the Position of the Free Gingival Margin

- A zero **(0)** indicates the free gingival margin is *slightly* coronal to the CEJ. In health, the free gingival margin should be at this level.
- A negative number **(–)** indicates the free gingival margin significantly covers the CEJ. This is also known as negative recession.
- A positive number **(+)** indicates the free gingival margin is apical to the CEJ. This is also known as positive recession.

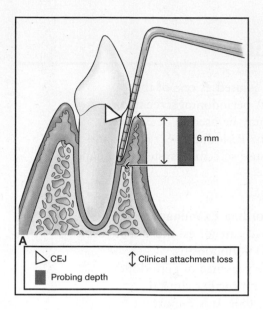

Figure 20-13A. Calculating Clinical Attachment Level when the Gingival Margin is slightly coronal to the Cementoenamel Junction. When the gingival margin is slightly coronal to the CEJ, no calculations are needed since the probing depth and the clinical attachment level are equal.

For example:
Probing depth measurement: 6 mm
Gingival margin level: 0 mm
Clinical attachment loss: 6 mm

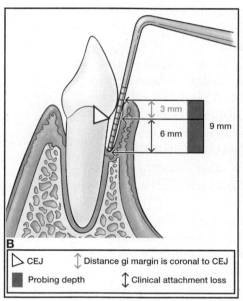

Figure 20-13B. Calculating Clinical Attachment Level when the Gingival Margin is significantly coronal to the Cementoenamel Junction. When the gingival margin is significantly coronal to the CEJ, the CAL is calculated by SUBTRACTING the gingival margin level from the probing depth.

For example:
Probing depth measurement: 9 mm
Gingival margin level: −3 mm
Clinical attachment loss: 6 mm

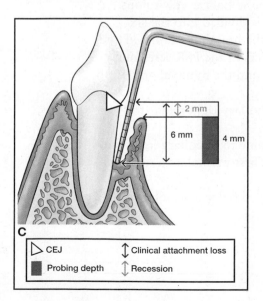

Figure 20-13C. Calculating Clinical Attachment Level in the Presence of Gingival Recession. When recession is present, the CAL is calculated by ADDING the probing depth to the gingival margin level.

For example:
Probing depth measurement: 4 mm
Gingival margin level: +2 mm
Clinical attachment loss: 6 mm

Section 3
Periodontal Screening Examination

In some dental offices, a periodontal screening examination is used as one of the first steps in evaluating the periodontal status of a patient. A periodontal screening examination is a rapid, inexpensive screening process that may be used to determine if a more comprehensive periodontal assessment is necessary. The Periodontal Screening and Recording (PSR) examination is one example of an easy-to-use screening system that can aid in the detection of periodontal disease.

1. Periodontal Screening and Recording (PSR) Examination
   A. Characteristics of the Periodontal Screening and Recording Examination
      1. The PSR can help separate patients into three broad categories: those that seem to have (1) periodontal health, (2) gingivitis, or (3) periodontitis.
      2. When the PSR screening examination indicates the presence of periodontal health or gingivitis, except in a very few instances no further clinical periodontal assessment may be needed beyond the PSR. It is important to note that individual states have different rules related to the use of this type of screening examination.
   B. Techniques for Performing the PSR Screening Examination
      1. Special Probe. A World Health Organization (WHO) probe is used for this examination. The WHO probe has a colored band (called the reference mark) located 3.5 to 5.5 mm from the probe tip (Fig. 20-14). This color-coded reference mark is used when performing the PSR screening examination.
         a. Instead of reading and recording six precise measurements per tooth, the clinician only needs to observe the position of the color-coded reference mark in relation to the gingival margin and a few other clinical features such as the presence of bleeding on probing, the presence of calculus, or the presence of an overhang on a restoration.
         b. Each of the sextants is examined as a separate unit during the PSR screening (i.e., only one PSR code number will be assigned to the entire sextant).
         c. *Only one PSR code is recorded for each sextant in the mouth.* Each sextant is assigned a single PSR code; the highest code obtained for the sextant is recorded.
         d. An "X" is recorded instead of a PSR code if the sextant is edentulous.
      2. One Code Per Sextant. Using the PSR, the mouth is divided into the six sextants (segments) listed below. Each sextant of the mouth is examined and assigned an individual PSR code. The unique aspects of the PSR screening system are the manner in which the probe is read and the minimal amount of information that needs to be recorded.
         a. Maxillary right posterior sextant: terminal maxillary right molar to maxillary right first premolar
         b. Maxillary anterior sextant: maxillary right canine to maxillary left canine
         c. Maxillary left posterior sextant: maxillary left first premolar to terminal maxillary left molar
         d. Mandibular left posterior sextant: terminal mandibular left molar to mandibular left first premolar

    e. Mandibular anterior sextant: mandibular left canine to mandibular right canine

    f. Mandibular right posterior sextant: mandibular right first premolar to terminal mandibular right molar

3. Probing Technique

    a. The probe is "walked" circumferentially around each tooth in the sextant being examined. Walking a periodontal probe refers to moving the probe in small increments circumferentially around a tooth.

    b. The color-coded reference mark is monitored continuously as the probe is walked around each tooth. At each site probed, the color-coded reference mark will be (a) completely visible, (b) partially visible, or (c) not visible at all.

2. The PSR Codes

A. Use of PSR Codes

    1. A PSR code is assigned to each sextant according to the criteria shown in Figure 20-14. *The code assigned to a sextant should represent the most advanced periodontal finding on any tooth in that sextant.*

    2. The PSR codes are used to guide further clinical documentation.

        a. For some patients with low PSR codes in all sextants (codes 0, 1, or 2), the PSR screening may be adequate documentation of the patient's periodontal health status. *Note, however, that the dentist may request a comprehensive periodontal assessment even when low PSR codes are found, since many periodontal conditions must be monitored in more detail than that included in the PSR.* In other words, the benefits of the PSR system does not supplant the wealth of additional information garnered from a thorough comprehensive periodontal assessment.

        b. For patients with higher PSR codes in one or more sextants (codes 3 or 4), a comprehensive periodontal examination should be performed as outlined previously in Section 2 of this chapter.

B. Cautions for Interpreting PSR Codes. The PSR codes can mislead a clinician in certain patients.

    1. As already pointed out, lower codes usually mean periodontal health or gingivitis, and higher codes usually mean periodontitis. *When interpreting the results of the PSR, the clinician must be alert for teeth with gingival enlargement or gingival recession. In the presence of either of these conditions, the PSR can give misleading results.*

    2. Another shortcoming is that the partial recording approach of the PSR index may grossly underestimate the severity of periodontal destruction because it only relies on probing depth measurements, but fails to quantify the amount of clinical attachment loss.

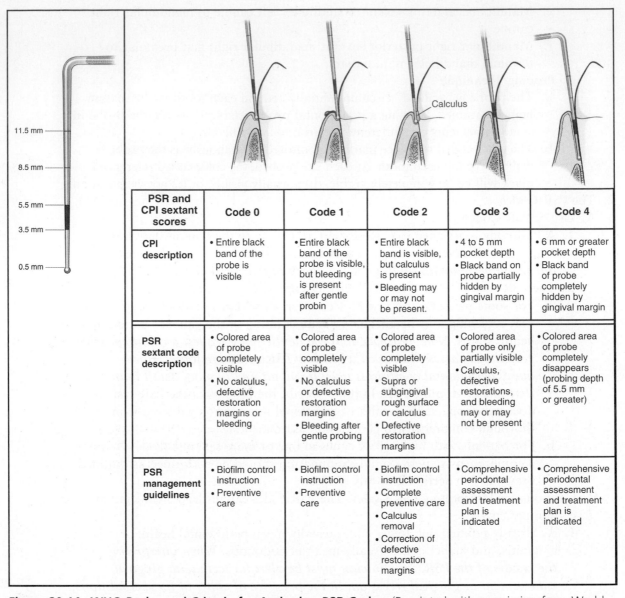

PSR and CPI sextant scores	Code 0	Code 1	Code 2	Code 3	Code 4
CPI description	• Entire black band of the probe is visible	• Entire black band of the probe is visible, but bleeding is present after gentle probin	• Entire black band is visible, but calculus is present • Bleeding may or may not be present.	• 4 to 5 mm pocket depth • Black band on probe partially hidden by gingival margin	• 6 mm or greater pocket depth • Black band of probe completely hidden by gingival margin
PSR sextant code description	• Colored area of probe completely visible • No calculus, defective restoration margins or bleeding	• Colored area of probe completely visible • No calculus or defective restoration margins • Bleeding after gentle probing	• Colored area of probe completely visible • Supra or subgingival rough surface or calculus • Defective restoration margins	• Colored area of probe only partially visible • Calculus, defective restorations, and bleeding may or may not be present	• Colored area of probe completely disappears (probing depth of 5.5 mm or greater)
PSR management guidelines	• Biofilm control instruction • Preventive care	• Biofilm control instruction • Preventive care	• Biofilm control instruction • Complete preventive care • Calculus removal • Correction of defective restoration margins	• Comprehensive periodontal assessment and treatment plan is indicated	• Comprehensive periodontal assessment and treatment plan is indicated

Figure 20-14. WHO Probe and Criteria for Assigning PSR Codes. (Reprinted with permission from World Health Organization. *Oral Health Surveys: Basic Methods*. 5th ed. Section 1: Basic Principles of Clinical Oral Health Surveys. Geneva: WHO; 2013:pp. 48, 51.)

Section 4
Supplemental Diagnostic Tests

1. Overview of Supplemental Diagnostic Tests
   A. Clinical periodontal assessment using the parameters discussed in Section 2 will result in an accurate periodontal diagnosis and can serve as a sound basis for designing an appropriate plan for therapy for the patient with periodontal disease. There are, however, a number of supplemental diagnostic tests that can be used for certain patients.
   B. Clinicians might consider using some of these supplemental tests for patients that have refractory forms of periodontitis.
   C. There are a number of supplemental tests that have been suggested for use, and much research is continuing related to these types of tests. Most of these tests fall into three general types:
      1. Tests related to bacteria
      2. Tests that analyze gingival crevicular fluid content
      3. Tests for genetic susceptibility to periodontal disease
   D. It is critical for the clinician to realize that based upon current research, there is currently no supplemental diagnostic test that stands out as the gold standard. Thus, supplemental diagnostic tests should not be routinely ordered for all patients with periodontal disease unless the disease is refractory or the disease is considered to be too complex to diagnose with conventional methods alone.
2. Tests Related to Bacteria
   A. Table 20-3 presents an overview of the tests related to bacteria. It is important to keep in mind that conventional periodontal therapy brings periodontal pathogens to low enough levels that disease progression can be halted without the need for identifying specific periodontal pathogens in most patients.

TABLE 20-3	TESTS RELATED TO BACTERIA	
Test Name	**Purpose of Test**	**Special Considerations**
Phase contrast microscopic study of plaque sample	Used for patient education and motivation	Test cannot identify specific bacterial species
Culture and sensitivity	Used to determine the sensitivity of bacteria to specific antibiotics	Sampling techniques for this test and the transport of bacterial samples to the laboratory are difficult
Deoxyribonucleic acid (DNA) probe analysis	Used to identify specific periodontal pathogens in a patient's mouth	Only a few bacterial species can be identified by this test

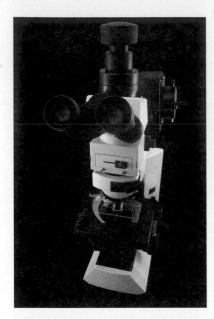
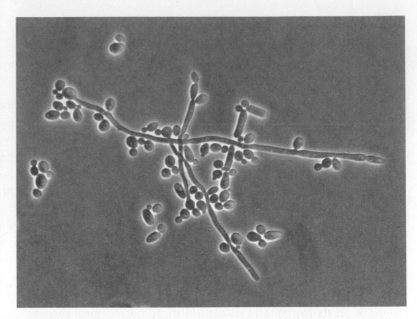

Figure 20-15. Microscope and Microorganisms. On the left, an example of a phase contrast microscope. The photograph on the right shows the opportunistic fungus, *Candida albicans*. Oral candidiasis is a fungal infection caused by the overgrowth of *C. albicans*, which causes creamy white lesions on the tongue and lining of mucous membranes of the oral cavity.

    B. Patient Education Tool: Phase Contrast Microscope
        1. The advantage of the phase contrast microscope is that it enables patients to view live microorganisms and to actually see the live motion of the spirochetal microorganisms (Fig. 20-15).
        2. Effective communication is essential skill for the dental hygienist. Viewing live microorganisms is an effective tool to educate patients by allowing them to view the live microorganisms which are contributing to their periodontal disease breakdown.
        3. Phase contrast microscopy is an effective means of microscopically monitoring motile (movable) bacteria, such as *Treponema*. However, the utility of phase contrast microscope is limited since it cannot be used to identify nonmotile, nonspirochetal periodontopathic species such as *Porphyromonas gingivalis* or *Aggregatibacter actinomycetemcomitans*. Thus, the diagnostic capabilities of phase contrast microscope is limited and is not recommended for routine use in clinical settings.
   3. Tests That Analyze Gingival Crevicular Fluid Content
    A. Gingival Crevicular Fluid
        1. Gingival crevicular fluid is the fluid that flows into the sulcus from the adjacent gingival connective tissue; the flow is slight in health and increases in the presence of inflammatory disease. The advantage of analyzing gingival crevicular fluid is that it provides site-specific information about the inflammatory status of a specific periodontal site.
        2. Gingival crevicular fluid originates in connective tissue and flows into periodontal pockets. It has long been believed that this gingival crevicular fluid can contain markers for periodontal disease progression, and quite a bit of research time has been devoted to the study of this fluid.
        3. In a clinical setting, obtaining gingival crevicular fluid from all sites in an individual's mouth may be prohibitive (too time-consuming and too costly).

B. **Examples of Gingival Crevicular Contents That Have Been Studied**
  1. Collagenase (an enzyme that breaks down collagen) is an example of one of the gingival crevicular fluid contents that has been studied, though no test for this is currently in widespread use.
  2. Prostaglandin E2 is another such gingival crevicular fluid constituent that has been studied. Prostaglandin E2 is a cyclooxygenase product which is a major mediator that contributes to inflammatory reactions such as those seen in periodontal disease.

C. **Tests for Genetic Susceptibility to Periodontal Disease**
  1. Genetic Susceptibility
     a. It is obvious that a patient's genetic makeup affects susceptibility to many diseases including periodontal disease.
     b. This genetic makeup is inherited and cannot normally be altered.
  2. Tests for Interleukin-1
     a. One test for genetic susceptibility to periodontal disease has been studied extensively and has resulted in a test that has been marketed to clinicians. The first version of this test was the PST Genetic Susceptibility Test from Interleukin Genetics Incorporated, Waltham, MA. In 2013, the company released a new version of this genetic susceptibility test, called Interleukin's PerioPredict Genetic Risk Test.
     b. Both of these tests identify patients who are genetically predisposed to produce high levels of interleukin-1 (an inflammatory mediator produced in response to the presence of periodontal pathogens).
        1. Higher levels of interleukin-1 in patients tend to predispose the patients to more inflammation in the periodontium and has been associated with increased risk for severe and progressive periodontal disease.[12]
        2. It has been reported that 30% of the people in the United States have the genetic makeup to produce high levels of interleukin-1 in response to periodontal pathogens.

4. **The Future.** It would be extremely helpful if clinicians had access to a diagnostic test that could reliably predict which individuals are susceptible for future periodontal breakdown. It would also be helpful to have a diagnostic test which could accurately indicate the current status of disease activity. It is safe to assume that as more research is completed, additional useful clinical tests will be developed in this area.

Chapter Summary Statement

The information gathered by the members of the dental team during the clinical periodontal assessment forms the basis for an individualized treatment plan for the patient. This chapter discusses two types of clinical periodontal assessment: a periodontal screening examination and the comprehensive periodontal assessment. The Periodontal Screening and Recording (PSR) is an example of a quick periodontal screening system for the detection of periodontal disease.

The comprehensive periodontal assessment is a complete, more thorough clinical periodontal assessment used to gather information about the periodontium. The information collected in a comprehensive periodontal assessment includes probing depth measurements, bleeding on probing, presence of exudate, level of the free gingival margin, level of the mucogingival junction, tooth mobility, furcation involvement, presence of calculus, presence of plaque biofilm, gingival inflammation, radiographic evidence of alveolar bone loss, and presence of local contributing factors. In addition, as part of the comprehensive periodontal assessment, several measurements—namely, the width of the attached gingiva and the clinical attachment levels—must also be calculated. Measuring clinical attachment level is the gold standard in determining whether gingivitis or periodontitis is present at a site of inflammation.

Supplemental diagnostic tests are indicated for certain patients and may provide critical information that will aid in formulating a diagnosis. However, at this time, there is no established, standardized protocol to justify the routine use of supplemental diagnostic test for all individuals.

To summarize, performing a careful and thorough periodontal assessment is necessary to identify the type of periodontal disease and monitor disease activity. All members of the dental team must be capable of performing a meticulous periodontal assessment. Furthermore, as new supplemental diagnostic assessments emerge, clinicians must be able to think critically about these tests, understand the strength and limitations of each test, and analyze the outcomes of these tests based on sound scientific evidence.

Section 5
Focus on Patients

Clinical Patient Care

CASE 1

While visiting a dental office, you observe a member of the dental team performing a periodontal assessment. You note that while searching for furcation invasion, the clinician is using a straight calibrated periodontal probe. What critical information might be lost because of instrument selection for this step in a periodontal assessment?

CASE 2

During a comprehensive periodontal assessment, you note severe inflammation of the gingiva over the facial surface of a lower right molar tooth. On the dental chart you are using, there is no obvious mechanism to record this important piece of periodontal information. How should you proceed?

CASE 3

During a periodontal assessment of a periodontitis patient, you are trying to determine the clinical attachment level on the facial surface of a canine tooth. On the facial surface of the canine tooth, you have measured 3 mm of gingival recession and a probing depth of 6 mm. How much attachment has been lost on the facial surface of this canine tooth?

Ethical Dilemma

Your next patient is Marlene Perkins, who is a new patient to your practice. She is a 37-year-old married mother of two small daughters, who works part-time as a lawyer. Her chief complaint is "bleeding gums." She left her last dental practice because she questioned if she was receiving quality dental services.

The radiographs, you have taken today, show that there is very slight horizontal bone loss on her anterior teeth. Marlene's pocket readings range from 1 to 4 mm throughout her mouth, and there is generalized bleeding on probing. She presents with heavy plaque biofilm and moderate supragingival and subgingival calculus, although states that she had her teeth cleaned 4 months ago. She states that she "isn't a very good flosser, and was always reprimanded by the hygienist at her former dental practice, to do a better job."

She notes that she has a history of periodontal disease in her family, as both her mother and father have had "extensive gum surgeries." She asked the dentist and hygienist in her last practice if periodontal disease was hereditary and if there was a way to predict if she also would have periodontal disease. She was told that each person is an individual, and that if she "took care of her teeth and gums," she would be just fine.

1. What is the best way for you to handle this ethical dilemma?
2. What is the best way to address/discuss Marlene's treatment plan?
3. What ethical principles are in conflict in this dilemma?

References

1. American Academy of Periodontology. Comprehensive periodontal therapy: a statement by the American Academy of Periodontology*. *J Periodontol.* 2011;82(7):943–949.

2. Armitage GC. Diagnosis of periodontal diseases. *J Periodontol.* 2003;74(8):1237–1247.

3. Leisnert L, Hallstrom H, Knutsson K. What findings do clinicians use to diagnose chronic periodontitis? *Swed Dent J.* 2008;32(3):115–123.

4. Van Aelst L, Cosyn J, De Bruyn H. [Guidelines for periodontal diagnosis in Belgium]. *Rev Belge Med Dent.* 2008;63(2):59–63.

5. Ziada H, Irwin C, Mullally B, Allen E, Byrne PJ. Periodontics: 1. Identification and diagnosis of periodontal diseases in general dental practice. *Dent Update.* 2007;34(4):208–210, 213–14, 217.

6. Kassab MM, Cohen RE. The etiology and prevalence of gingival recession. *J Am Dent Assoc.* 2003;134(2):220–225.

7. Albandar JM, Kingman A. Gingival recession, gingival bleeding, and dental calculus in adults 30 years of age and older in the United States, 1988–1994. *J Periodontol.* 1999;70(1):30–43.

8. Baker P, Spedding C. The aetiology of gingival recession. *Dent Update.* 2002;29(2):59–62.

9. Chan HL, Chun YH, MacEachern M, Oates TW. Does gingival recession require surgical treatment? *Dent Clin North Am.* 2015;59(4):981–996.

10. Miller PD, Jr. A classification of marginal tissue recession. *Int J Periodontics Restorative Dent.* 1985;5(2):8–13.

11. Gargiulo AW, Wentz FM, Orban B. Dimensions and relations of the dentogingival junction in humans. *J Periodontol.* 1961;32(3):261–267.

12. Giannobile WV, Braun TM, Caplis AK, Doucette-Stamm L, Duff GW, Kornman KS. Patient stratification for preventive care in dentistry. *J Dent Res.* 2013;92(8):694–701.

 STUDENT ANCILLARY RESOURCES

A wide variety of resources to enhance your learning is available online:

- Audio Glossary
- Book Pages
- Chapter Review Questions and Answers

21 Radiographic Analysis of the Periodontium

Clinical Application. Interpretation of dental radiographic images is an integral part of the diagnosis and treatment planning for patients with most types of periodontal diseases. Though interpretation of dental radiographs can be far from straightforward, all the members of the dental team will need to rely on their skills in radiographic interpretation on a daily basis. This chapter outlines basic information related to the analysis of dental radiographic images that members of the dental team can use as a springboard for further study of this topic.

Learning Objectives

- Describe dental radiographic characteristics of the healthy periodontium.
- Describe early dental radiographic evidence of periodontal disease.
- Name some techniques that can be employed with periodontal patients to obtain good quality dental radiographs.
- Explain the basic principles of the vertical bitewing technique.
- Describe the limitations of dental radiographs that all clinicians should keep in mind when viewing radiographs.
- Explain the difference between vertical and horizontal alveolar bone loss as seen in dental radiographs.
- Given a selection of sample dental radiographs, apply the information from this chapter when analyzing those radiographs.

Key Terms

Radiolucent
Radiopaque
Cortical bone
Lamina dura

Crestal irregularities
Triangulation
Horizontal bone loss
Vertical bone loss

Cone beam computed
  tomography

Section 1
Radiographic Appearance of the Periodontium

No comprehensive periodontal evaluation is complete without supplementing the information obtained during the clinical evaluation with information obtained from high-quality dental radiographs.[1,2] All dental clinicians must be able to recognize certain radiographic signs associated with periodontal diseases. The level of the alveolar bone is usually considered among the most important of the features revealed by dental radiographs, but there are many other, sometimes subtle, features that can be important for the clinician to note when viewing dental radiographs. Not all structures of the periodontium are even visible on dental radiographic images; some periodontal structures, such as the gingiva, cannot normally be seen on a dental radiograph. Examples of other features that may provide important information include features, such as the appearance of the interdental alveolar bone crests, the size and shape of the tooth roots, the relationship between adjacent tooth roots, the condition of the alveolar bone in furcation areas, and the presence of certain local contributing factors.

1. **Radiolucent Versus Radiopaque Structures.** Structures (or materials) that can be viewed on a dental radiograph are described as either *radiolucent* or *radiopaque* depending upon the degree of penetration of these structures by x-rays used in dental radiography.
   A. **Radiolucent** structures are those that are easily penetrated by x-rays.
      1. Most of the x-ray beams will be able to pass through these structures to expose the radiographic film. Thus, on the completed radiograph, radiolucent areas appear as dark gray to black.
      2. Examples of radiolucent structures that can be seen on dental radiographs are the tooth pulp, the periodontal ligament space, bone loss due to a periapical abscess, marrow spaces in the bone, and alveolar bone loss defects due to periodontitis.
   B. **Radiopaque** structures are those that absorb or resist penetration by x-rays.
      1. Most of the x-ray beams will not be able to pass through these structures to expose the radiographic film. Thus, radiopaque areas appear light gray to white on the completed radiograph.
      2. Examples of radiopaque structures are tooth enamel, dentin, metallic tooth restorations (such as amalgam restorations or gold restorations), some composite restorations, pulp stones, and alveolar bone supporting the tooth roots.
   C. It should be noted that many periodontal and tooth-associated structures allow only limited (but not total) penetration of the x-rays. These structures will appear as various subtle shades of gray on the completed radiograph. At times, these subtle differences can be confusing to clinicians.
2. **Radiographic Features of Parts of the Periodontium.** One of the components of the periodontium that can be identified on radiographic images includes the alveolar bone itself, and it is important for clinicians to become very familiar with the radiographic appearance of this tooth-supporting bone (Fig. 21-1).
   A. **Cortical Bone**
      1. **Cortical bone** is the outer surface of a bone and is composed of layers of bone closely packed together.

a. In the maxilla, the cortical bone is usually a thin shell covering the outer surface of the maxilla.

b. In the mandible, the cortical bone is usually a dense layer of bone covering the outer surface of the mandible.

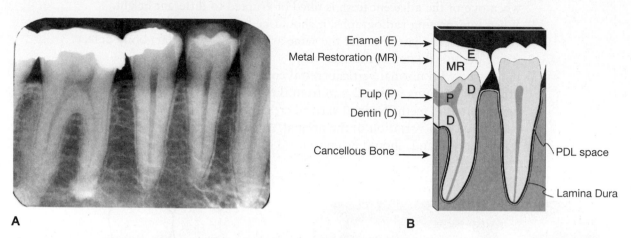

A   **B**

Figure 21-1. Radiographic Structures of the Periodontium. The dental radiograph (A) and drawing (B) provide points of reference for many of the features discussed in this chapter.

2. Radiographic Appearance of cortical and cancellous bone
   a. Both cortical bone and cancellous bone can be identified on dental radiographs.
   b. One example of cortical bone is the inferior border of the mandible which often appears on the radiograph as a thick white border. Another example of cortical bone is the interdental crestal bone.
   c. One example of cortical bone that needs to be evaluated on dental radiographs is the interdental alveolar crest. In health, interdental alveolar crests between the teeth of both jaws appear on the dental radiographs as thin white lines on the outside of crestal bone.
   d. The lattice-like pattern of the cancellous bone that fills the interior portion of the alveolar process also appears on the dental radiograph. This cancellous bone appears as a pattern of delicate white tracings within the bone.

B. **Level of the Alveolar Crest in Health**
   1. The normal level of the alveolar bone crest (as it appears on a radiograph) is located approximately 2 mm apical to (or below) the cementoenamel junction (CEJ).
   2. *The level of the alveolar bone crest in relationship to the CEJ is one indicator of periodontal health that should always be noted when analyzing a dental radiograph.*

C. **Contour of the Alveolar Crest in Health**
   1. The contour of the interproximal alveolar crest in health is parallel to an imaginary line drawn between the CEJs of adjacent teeth. *The contour of the crest of the interproximal bone is another indicator of periodontal health that should always be noted when analyzing a dental radiograph.*
   2. In posterior sextants, the normal contour of the interproximal crest can vary depending upon the actual levels of the CEJs of the adjacent teeth.
      a. Horizontal crest contour. The crest of the interproximal bone will have a horizontal contour when the CEJs of the adjacent teeth are at the same level. Figure 21-2 shows an example of posterior teeth with horizontal crest contours.

    b. Vertical (or angular) crest contour.

        1) The crest of the interproximal bone will have a vertical or angular contour when one of the adjacent teeth is tilted or erupted to different height. Figure 21-3 shows an example of posterior teeth with an angular contour when one of the adjacent teeth is tilted or erupted to different height.

        2) When interpreting radiographs, it should be kept in mind that normal vertical crestal contour is not the same as a vertical (angular) bony defect (to be discussed later in this chapter.)

        3) In an area with normal vertical crestal contour, the interproximal bone level remains within 2 mm from the level of the CEJ of the approximating teeth. Normal vertical crestal contour should be considered as a variation of the normal. A vertical (angular) bony defect, on the other hand, should be considered as pathology.

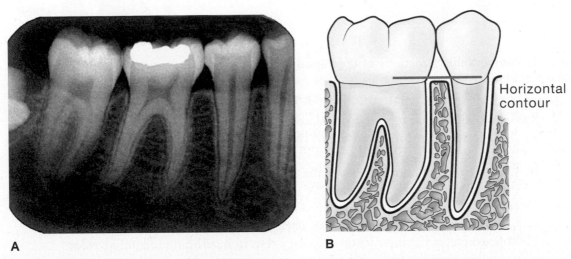

A   **B**

Figure 21-2. A. Normal Alveolar Bone Height. This radiograph shows a normal alveolar bone height that is 1.5 to 2 mm below and parallel to the cementoenamel junction. In this example, alveolar crest is a dense radiopaque line as it would normally appear in health. **B. Horizontal Crest Contour.** The crest of the interproximal bone will have a horizontal contour when the CEJs of the adjacent teeth are at the same level. Note that the crest parallels an imaginary line drawn between adjacent CEJs.

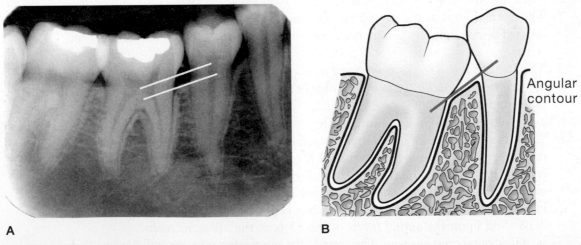

A   **B**

Figure 21-3. Vertical (or Angular) Crest Contour. A. The crest of the interproximal bone will have a vertical or angular contour when one of the adjacent teeth is tilted or erupted to a different height. **B.** Note that this crest also parallels an imaginary line drawn between adjacent CEJs, though the adjacent CEJs are at different levels. Also note that the interproximal bone level is still within 2 mm of the CEJ level of the approximating teeth.

D. **Shape and Character of the Alveolar Crestal Bone Crest in Health**
1. The surfaces of the interdental bone crests are smooth and covered with a thin layer of cortical (dense, hard) bone that may appear as a thin, white line on a radiograph.
2. One of the most important radiographic features of the alveolar crest is that it forms a smooth intact surface between adjacent teeth with only the width of the periodontal ligament space separating it from the adjacent root surface.
   a. The crest of the interdental bone between incisor teeth is usually thin and somewhat pointed in appearance because of the relative close proximity of the adjacent tooth roots of anterior teeth.
   b. The crest of the interdental bone between the posterior teeth is usually flat or slightly rounded because of the relatively greater distance between adjacent tooth roots (Fig. 21-4).
3. *The shape and character of the alveolar bone crest are other indicators of periodontal health that should always be noted when analyzing a dental radiograph.*
E. **Lamina Dura**
1. The alveolar bone proper is the thin layer of dense bone that lines a normal tooth socket. In radiographic images, the alveolar bone proper is referred to as the lamina dura.
2. *The presence of the lamina dura is another indicator of periodontal health that should always be noted when analyzing a dental radiograph.*
3. On a dental radiograph, the lamina dura appears as a continuous white (radiopaque) line around the tooth root (Fig. 21-5).
4. Note that on a radiograph, the lamina dura is continuous with the cortical bone layer of the crest of the interdental septa.

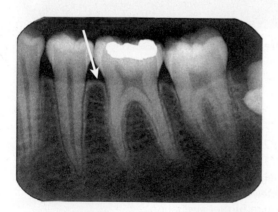

Figure 21-4. Alveolar Crest. The alveolar crest (indicated by an *arrow*) forms a smooth intact surface between adjacent teeth and displays a relatively flat contour.

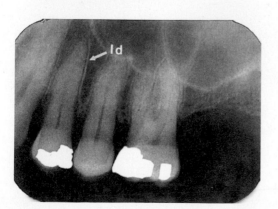

Figure 21-5. Lamina Dura and Periodontal Ligament Space. The lamina dura (*ld*) appears as a continuous white line around the tooth root. The periodontal ligament space will usually appear as a thin black line around the tooth root, but is actually filled with soft tissue (the periodontal ligament and associated soft tissue structures).

F. **Periodontal Ligament Space**

1. The space between the tooth root and the lamina dura of the socket is filled with the periodontal ligament tissue. The periodontal ligament tissue functions as the actual attachment of the tooth to the lamina dura of the socket.

2. *The appearance of the periodontal ligament space is another indicator of periodontal health that should always be noted when analyzing a dental radiograph.*

3. As already noted, the periodontal ligament tissue does not resist penetration of x-rays and, therefore, appears on the radiograph as a thin radiolucent black line surrounding the tooth root. The precise appearance of the lamina dura on a dental radiograph can be affected by the complex contours of individual tooth roots or by changing the angulation of the x-ray tube (Fig. 21-6).

4. Extremely widened periodontal ligament spaces always need to be evaluated further (Fig. 21-7).

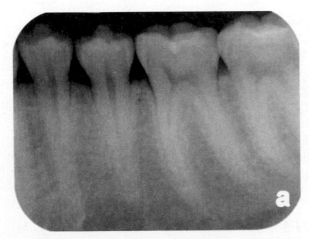 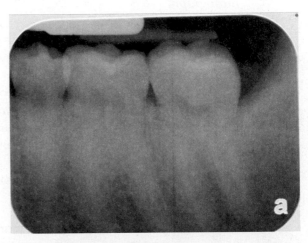

Figure 21-6. Appearance of the Lamina Dura on Two Different Radiographs. These two radiographs were taken at the same appointment from a single patient. In the left radiograph, the lamina dura is distinct and well-defined. However, in the right periapical radiograph, the lamina dura appears fuzzy and is difficult to detect in some areas due to differences in x-ray tube angulation.

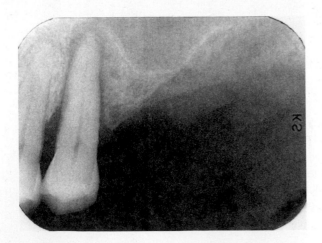

Figure 21-7. Extreme Widening of the PDL Space. This maxillary second premolar has an extremely widened periodontal ligament space. This completely abnormal appearance of the PDL space will require further evaluation.

Section 2
Use of Radiographic Images During Periodontal Evaluation

1. **Review of Some Basic Techniques for Obtaining Good Quality Radiographs.** There are many outstanding textbooks available that explain dental radiology in detail. Such detail is not appropriate for this textbook, but the following are a few straightforward suggestions to consider when dental radiographs are intended for use as adjuncts to clinical periodontal evaluations.

   A. **Long-cone Paralleling Technique for Periapical Radiographs.** The long-cone paralleling technique can provide radiographs that are more anatomically accurate when compared with other intraoral radiographic techniques (such as the bisecting angle technique).

   B. **Long-cone Paralleling Technique for Bitewing Radiographs.** Combining the long-cone paralleling technique with the use of bitewing radiographs can provide excellent information about periodontal structures.[3–5]

   1. Note that a dental radiograph taken with poor technique can result in excessive vertical angulation and can obscure alveolar bone loss associated with periodontitis.

   2. If poor techniques in positioning the radiographic film or x-ray beam are employed, periapical radiographs may overestimate or underestimate the actual outline of the alveolar bone (Fig. 21-8).

      a. For this reason, many clinicians utilize bitewing radiographs as the primary radiographs used to evaluate crestal bone height (rather than periapical radiographs).

      b. It should be noted again that proper long-cone paralleling technique can minimize distortion of crestal bone height on periapical radiographic images and improve their usefulness.

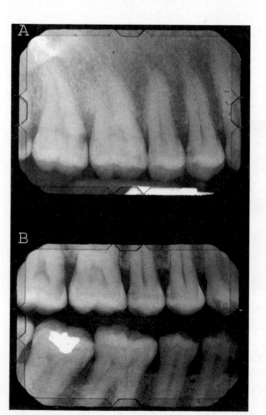

Figure 21-8A. Excessive Vertical Angulation. Note how the crestal bone height is distorted in the periapical radiograph shown here as opposed to the bitewing radiograph shown below.

Figure 21-8B. Bitewing Radiograph. This bitewing radiograph shows the same maxillary teeth as the one with excessive vertical angulation above. Note the striking difference between the apparent bone height on these radiographs.

C. **Vertical Bitewing Technique for Periodontal Patients.** Extensive alveolar bone loss can be obscured unless vertical bitewing radiographs are used.

1. Alveolar bone loss of 5 mm or greater may cause the coronal bone to be poorly visualized or not seen at all on normal bitewing radiographic images.
2. Vertically oriented bitewings may be used in these situations to increase visualization of the alveolar bone.
3. An adaptor is available for most film holders to accomplish this vertical orientation.
4. Using the vertical bitewing technique, the long axis of the film is rotated 90 degrees to be perpendicular to the occlusal plane (Fig. 21-9).
5. Vertical bitewing radiographic images show more of the coronal bone than regular bitewings especially when the teeth are widely separated by the film holder (Fig. 21-10).

D. **Long-Grayscale/Low Contrast Images in Periodontal Patients.** Long-grayscale/low contrast radiographic images have many visible shades of gray that make it easier to see some of the subtle changes such as alveolar bone loss in periodontal disease. These images can be obtained using high kVp exposures (70 to 100 kVp) or using digital imaging software adjustments to maximize the gray scale of normally exposed images. In addition, many software programs now provide presets to optimize for detection of periodontal disease.

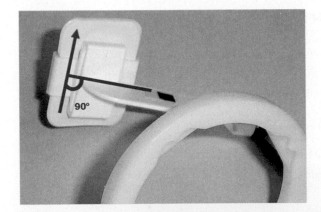

Figure 21-9. Film Placement for Vertical Bitewing. A #2 periapical film positioned for taking a vertical bitewing radiograph. Note how the film is rotated 90 degrees from the usual orientation.

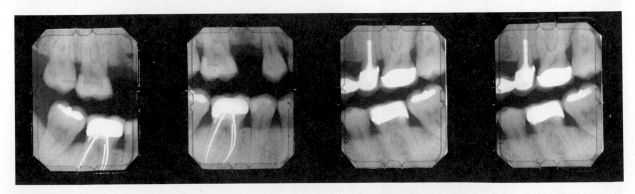

Figure 21-10. Four-Film Vertical Bitewing Series. Note how much coronal bone is visible on these vertical bitewings despite the separation of the teeth by the positioning device.

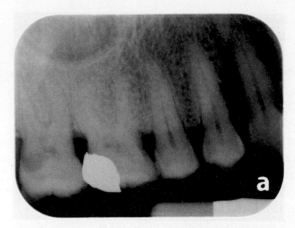
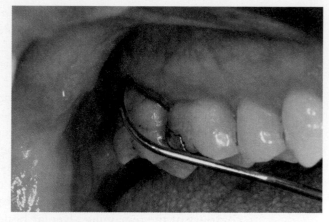

Figure 21-11. Limitations of Two-Dimensional Conventional Radiographs. As seen in the radiograph on the left, the overlying buccal cortical plate and the underlying palatal root obscure any radiographic sign of a mid-buccal furcation on the maxillary molars. As seen in the photograph, however, clinical evaluation of the area with a Nabers probe reveals the presence of a furcation invasion on the maxillary second molar. (Courtesy of Dr. Jennifer Chang, University of Texas Dental School at Houston, TX.)

2. **Limitations of Dental Radiographs During Periodontal Evaluation.** Despite the high value of the information obtained from dental radiographs, there are several limitations in the use of these dental radiographs that should always be kept in mind by the wise clinician. Some of these limitations are outlined below.

   A. **Radiographs are two-dimensional images of three-dimensional structures.** A radiograph provides a two-dimensional image of a very complex three-dimensional structure (i.e., a tooth and the surrounding supporting structures). The fact that the radiograph is a two-dimensional image can often be misleading to the viewer. Two examples that frequently cause confusion during radiographic interpretation are (1) that the buccal alveolar bone can hide bone loss on the lingual aspect of a tooth and (2) that the palatal root makes it difficult to visualize furcation alveolar bone loss on a maxillary molar tooth (Fig. 21-11).

   B. **Information obtained from a dental radiograph is primarily limited to information about calcified structures.** This fact has already been discussed, but is important enough to state again. Radiographic images do not normally provide information about the noncalcified components of the periodontium which, of course, play a leading role in the development and progress of periodontitis.

   C. **Radiographs provide only limited information about certain critical aspects of the periodontium.** Dental radiographic images *do not reveal* the following: the presence or absence of periodontal pockets, the presence of early stages of alveolar bone loss, the precise morphology of any existing alveolar bone destruction, the presence of tooth mobility, early furcation alveolar bone loss, the level of the epithelial attachment on the tooth, or information about periodontal disease activity. These limitations are discussed below.

      1. Dental radiographs do not reveal the presence or absence of periodontal pockets.
         a. Since the periodontal pocket is composed of soft tissue, it will not be visible on the radiograph.
         b. The only reliable method of locating a periodontal pocket and evaluating its extent is by careful periodontal probing.

      2. Dental radiographs do not reveal the presence of early stages of alveolar bone loss.
         a. The very earliest signs of periodontitis must be detected clinically, not radiographically.

    b. *It should be noted that by the time bone loss due to periodontitis becomes detectable on the dental radiograph, the disease usually has progressed well beyond the earliest stages.*

3. Dental radiographs do not reveal the precise morphology of any existing alveolar bone destruction.

    a. Conventional dental radiographs cannot accurately display the precise shape of alveolar bone deformities because these are not three-dimensional images. For instance, any bony changes that occur in the buccal or lingual cortical bony plate cannot be identified on a conventional radiograph because it is obscured by the dense root structure. As such, it is very difficult to detect a bony fenestration or dehiscence from a conventional radiograph (Fig. 21-12).

    b. Alveolar bone loss from periodontitis can result in complex and convoluted contours of the remaining alveolar bone that may not be detectable on a conventional radiograph.

4. Dental radiographs do not always reveal the presence of alveolar bone loss in furcation areas.

    a. Radiographic images frequently appear to show more interradicular bone (alveolar bone between the roots of the teeth) than is actually present. The facial and lingual aspects of the alveolar bone will often be superimposed over the furcation and hide bone loss from view, thereby obscuring the presence and the extent of the furcation invasion (Fig. 21-13).

    b. Also, slight variations in alignment of the x-ray beam may conceal the presence or extent of furcation alveolar bone loss.

    c. Furcation involvement (attachment and bone loss between the roots) must be evaluated by clinical examination with a curved furcation probe, as discussed in Chapter 20.

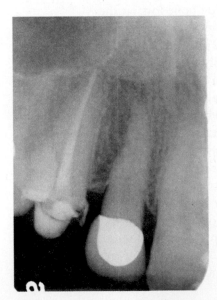 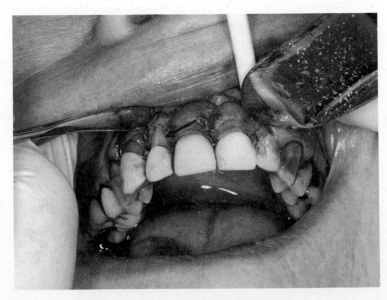

Figure 21-12. Bony Dehiscence. The radiograph fails to reveal the presence of a bony dehiscence. A periodontal flap is a surgical procedure in which incisions are made in the gingiva or mucosa to allow for separation of the soft tissues from the underlying tooth roots and underlying alveolar bone. In the case depicted above, the radiograph fails to reveal the presence of a bony dehiscence. However, the flap elevation reveals that the root of the maxillary lateral incisor is denuded of its facial bony plate. This complete loss of overlying cortical bone is known as a bony dehiscence. (Note: crowns were placed on the maxillary canine and central incisor soon after the radiograph was taken, but prior to flap surgery.) (Courtesy of Dr. Jennifer Chang, University of Texas Dental School at Houston, TX.)

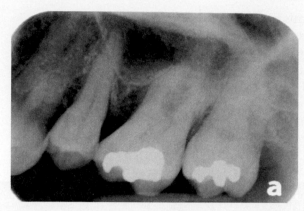
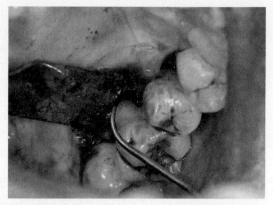

Figure 21-13. Limitation of Radiographs in Detecting Furcation Bone Loss. An angular defect on the mesial of the maxillary first molar is clearly visible on the periapical radiograph. However, following flap reflection, a mesiobuccal furcation invasion that was not radiographically apparent is present. (Case Courtesy of Dr. Takkaki Kishimoto, Fukuoka, Japan.)

5. Dental radiographs do not reveal the presence of tooth mobility. While it is indeed possible to visualize the width of some periodontal ligament spaces on dental radiographs, the only accurate way to determine the presence of tooth mobility is during the clinical evaluation.
6. Dental radiographs do not reveal the level of the epithelial attachment on the tooth.
   a. Since the epithelial attachment to the tooth is soft tissue, this structure will not be shown on a dental radiograph.
   b. The only way to identify the level of epithelial attachment is through careful periodontal probing.
7. Dental radiographs do not reveal any information about periodontal disease activity.
   a. Radiographic images do not reveal that periodontal disease activity is taking place at the time the radiographs were taken. They only show what destruction has happened at some time in the past (i.e., before the radiograph was taken—in some cases even years before).
   b. It is important to remember that the radiographic examination itself is never a satisfactory substitute for a clinical periodontal assessment.
3. **Benefits of Dental Radiographs During Periodontal Evaluation.** Despite the limitations of dental radiographs, the periodontal evaluation is *never* complete without supplementing clinical information with accurate radiographic images. Examples of what dental radiographs may reveal are bony changes associated with periodontitis, important aspects of the tooth root morphology, the relationship of the maxillary sinus to the periodontal deformity, widening of periodontal ligament space, advanced furcation bone loss, alveolar bone loss due to periodontal abscesses, and the presence of some local factors such as overhanging restorations, marginal ridge height discrepancies, open contacts and calculus (Table 21-1).
   A. **Assessment of Alveolar Bone Changes.** As already discussed, by the time alveolar bone loss is detectable on the dental radiograph, the disease usually has progressed well beyond the earliest stages. Nevertheless, it is important to examine each radiograph for the earliest radiographic signs of periodontal disease.

Two early radiographic signs of periodontitis are (1) crestal irregularities and (2) triangulation of the periodontal ligament space.

1. Crestal Irregularities. Crestal irregularities are the appearance of breaks or fuzziness associated with the interdental crest instead of a nice clean line at the crest of the interdental alveolar bone (Fig. 21-14).

2. Triangulation (Funneling). Triangulation is the widening of the periodontal ligament space caused by the resorption of bone along either the mesial or distal aspect of the interdental (interseptal) crestal bone (Fig. 21-15).

TABLE 21-1	RADIOGRAPHIC SIGNS ASSOCIATED WITH PERIODONTAL DISEASE
Condition	**Radiographic Sign(s)**
Early bony changes	Break or fuzziness at the crest of the interdental alveolar bone Widening of the periodontal ligament space at crestal margin
Horizontal bone loss	Can be measured from a plane that is parallel to a tooth-to-tooth line drawn from the CEJs of adjacent teeth
Vertical bone loss	Seen as more bone loss on the interproximal aspect of one tooth than on the adjacent tooth; bone level is at an angle to a line joining the CEJs
Bone defects	Are radiolucent due to bone loss and therefore visible on radiographic images, although three-dimensional structure may be hard to determine
Furcation alveolar bone loss	Loss of alveolar bone in furcation area may be detectable as a triangular radiolucency especially on mandibular molars
Unfavorable crown-to-root ratio	Seen as a greater portion of the tooth coronal to the alveolar crest compared to the portion of tooth structure apical to the alveolar crest
Peri-implant bone loss	Bone loss around a dental implant

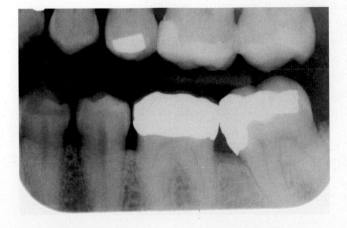

Figure 21-14. Crestal Irregularities. The interproximal crestal bone level between the mandibular first molar and the mandibular second molar appears indistinct and irregular. Additionally, note the overhanging restorative margin on the mesial of the mandibular second molar that is contributing to the localized crestal irregularity.

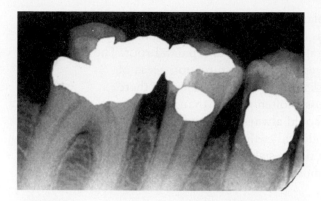

Figure 21-15. Triangulation. The crestal bone between these mandibular teeth demonstrates triangulation, a pointed, triangular appearance.

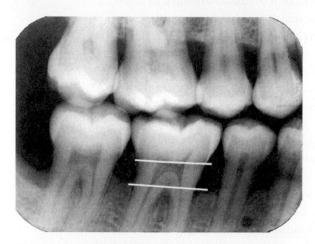

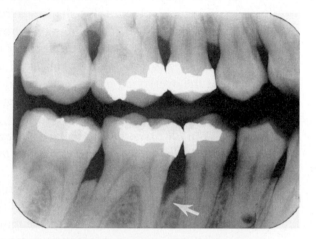

Figure 21-16. Horizontal Bone Loss. Horizontal bone loss is parallel to an imaginary line drawn between the CEJs of adjacent teeth.

Figure 21-17. Vertical Bone Loss. The arrow points to vertical bone loss on the mesial surface of the mandibular first molar.

B. **Horizontal Versus Vertical Alveolar Bone Loss due to Periodontitis.** Alveolar bone loss from periodontitis is described as either horizontal bone loss or vertical bone loss.
   1. The extent and direction of bone loss is determined using the CEJ of adjacent teeth as the points of reference.
   2. Horizontal bone loss is alveolar bone loss that is parallel to an imaginary line drawn between the CEJs of adjacent teeth (Fig. 21-16). In health, the normal horizontal bone levels are within 2 mm from the CEJ. On the other hand, a crestal bone level greater than 2 mm from the CEJ is defined as exhibiting horizontal bone loss.
   3. Vertical (or angular) bone loss occurs when there is greater bone destruction on the interproximal aspect of one tooth than on the adjacent tooth so that the bone meets the tooth at an acute angle (Fig. 21-17). The presence of vertical bone loss is often a radiographic diagnostic sign of severe periodontitis.[2]
C. **Assessment of Alveolar Bone Loss in a Furcation**
   1. As mentioned previously, furcation alveolar bone loss will not usually be seen on the dental radiograph until the bone destruction extends past the furcation area.
      a. Furcation bone loss on mandibular molar teeth is easier to detect on a dental radiograph than furcation bone loss on maxillary molar teeth. Furcation bone loss is easier to detect on mandibular molar teeth because mandibular molars have only two roots, a mesial root and a distal root (Fig. 21-18). On the radiograph, the clinician can usually visualize a diminished radiodensity between these two roots.

    b. Furcation bone loss on maxillary molar teeth is more difficult to detect on a radiograph than furcation bone loss on mandibular molars. Maxillary molars have three roots, a mesiobuccal, distobuccal, and palatal root. The palatal root is often superimposed over some of the furcation areas of the tooth on the radiograph and masks (hides) any radiolucency there.

  2. It is a general rule that furcation bone loss is often *greater* than what the radiograph reveals. All furcation areas should always be probed with a curved periodontal probe during a clinical periodontal evaluation.

  3. If severe alveolar bone loss is evident on the mesial or distal surface of any multirooted tooth (especially maxillary molars), furcation involvement should be suspected.

    a. On a radiograph, an interproximal furcation invasion appears as a small, triangular radiographic shadow across the mesial or distal root of a maxillary molar. This finding is known as a furcation arrow (Fig. 21-19).

    b. However, as previously discussed, the furcation arrow may be difficult to visualize from a radiograph due to the complex root anatomy or thickness of the overlaying buccal cortical bone. In addition, it is important to keep in mind that the absence of a furcation arrow is not indicative of an absence of a bony furcation involvement.

    c. *As in all cases, the presence of furcation bone loss must be confirmed clinically with a curved furcation probe.*

D. Assessment of Peri-Implant Bone Loss

  1. Two-dimensional radiographs are useful in detecting peri-implant bone loss (bone loss around a dental implant) (Fig. 21-20).

  2. Peri-implant bone loss is one of the major signs of peri-implantitis. In its simplistic terms, peri-implantitis is defined as an oral inflammatory process that affects the soft tissue and the hard tissue around an osseointegrated implant.

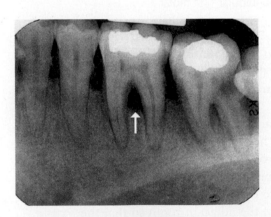

Figure 21-18. Furcation Involvement. The furcation alveolar bone loss is easily visible on the mandibular first molar in this radiograph. Bone loss in a furcation area to this degree is usually accompanied by a finding of furcation involvement during the clinical evaluation.

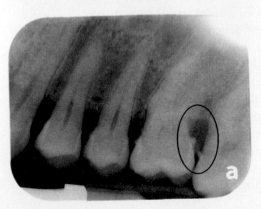

Figure 21-19. Furcation Arrow. Note the small, triangular radiolucent shadow (*circled*) that falls across the distobuccal root of the maxillary first molar. This shadow indicates an interproximal furcation invasion.

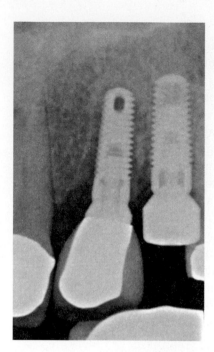

Figure 21-20. Radiographic Sign of Peri-Implantitis. Note the loss of radiodensity around this osseointegrated implant. This is indicative of peri-implant bone loss.

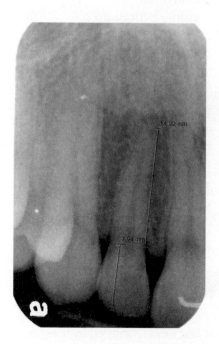

Figure 21-21. Favorable Crown-to-Root Ratio. An example of a favorable crown-to-root ratio. Note that the crown-to-root ratio on the maxillary lateral incisor is approximately 1:2.

E. **Special Considerations in the Assessment of Alveolar Bone Loss**
1. The clinician should keep in mind that the radiograph reveals the bone *remaining* rather than the amount of bone lost. The amount of bone loss needs to be *estimated* as the difference between the level of the remaining bone and the expected bone height.
2. Alveolar bone loss can occur on any or all surfaces of a tooth; however, tooth roots tend to mask (or hide) bone loss on the facial and lingual surfaces of the teeth.

F. Assessment of Crown-to-Root Ratio

1. The crown-to-root ratio is a measure of the length of the tooth coronal to the alveolar crest of bone compared with the length of the root embedded in the bone, as determined using a periapical radiograph.

   a. The crown-to-root ratio determines the ability of a tooth to be maintained without becoming mobile and eventually lost.

   b. The crown-to-root ratio is determined using a radiograph of the tooth.

   c. The ideal crown-to-root ratio is approximately 1:2 (Fig. 21-21).

2. The crown-to-root ratio plays an important role in determining the periodontal prognosis of an individual tooth. It should also be a key consideration when evaluating if a tooth is suitable to act as an abutment for a fixed or removal denture prosthesis.

G. Recognition of Local Contributing Risk Factors on Dental Radiographs. In some instances, it is possible to identify local contributing risk factors for periodontitis on dental radiographs. Examples of local contributing risk factors that may be revealed by the dental radiograph are calculus deposits and faulty restorations.

1. Calculus Deposits. The only accurate way to detect calculus deposits is with an explorer, however, large calculus deposits may indeed be visible on a dental radiograph.

2. Faulty Restorations. Faulty dental restorations are common contributing factors in patients with periodontal disease. In many cases, faulty restorations can be detected on a radiograph (Fig. 21-22).

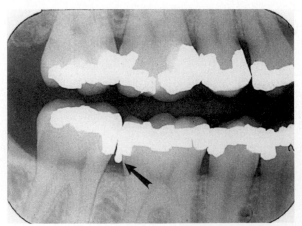
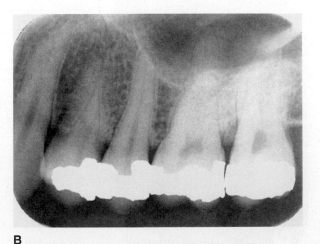

A   **B**

Figure 21-22. Faulty Restorations. A. The distal surface of the mandibular first molar, indicated by the arrow, has a faulty restoration that can harbor plaque biofilm and prevents thorough daily self-care. **B.** The distal proximal tooth surface of the maxillary first molar and the mesial tooth surface of the second molar have been restored but the restorations do not reproduce their original shape and contour. These faulty contours can allow food impaction at the site which, in turn, may cause direct damage to the periodontium at the site.

4. **Beyond Conventional Dental Radiography.** Modern radiology offers an interesting array of imaging methods that have been suggested for possible use in place of conventional dental radiography. One of these imaging methods is the use of cone beam computed tomography (CBCT) (Fig. 21-23). Dental cone beam computed tomography is a radiographic imaging method that generates detailed three-dimensional images of the periodontium as well as of other structures of the head and neck (Fig. 21-24).

A. Accurate three-dimensional images are indispensable for treatment planning for the surgical placement of dental implants. CBCT imaging is in common use for implant procedures, as well as, for complex surgeries involving the head and neck structures, such as orthognathic surgery.

B. Most dental clinicians rely on conventional intraoral radiographs, *not CBCT* scans, to detect and diagnose interproximal bone loss. This is because CBCT performance has not yet been confirmed as superior to that provided by conventional intraoral radiographs in the detection of interproximal bone loss.

C. CBCT imaging does not allow for distinguishing different types of soft tissue, such as discriminating junctional epithelium from connective tissue.

D. Also, unfortunately at this point, CBCT emits higher absorbed radiation doses to patients when compared with conventional dental radiography.

E. From the research available, there does not appear to be sufficient scientific evidence to justify the *routine* use of CBCT for the diagnosis and treatment planning for patients with periodontitis with infrabony/intrabony periodontal defects or furcation defects.[6]

F. Recently, the American Academy of Periodontology convened an expert panel to assess the clinical value of using CBCT to diagnose, treatment plan, and manage periodontal disease. While the expert panel believed that the application of CBCT imaging could have potential value, *the consensus was that there is currently limited evidence to support the routine use of CBCT in routine periodontal treatment planning.* However, the panel suggested that CBCT imaging may be a useful adjunctive diagnostic tool to evaluate selected periodontal cases on a case-by-case basis.[7]

G. Newer technologies, such as CBCT, offer interesting promise when compared with conventional radiography. However additional research is needed to confirm their value in the routine management of periodontitis patients.

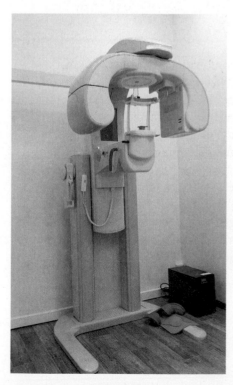 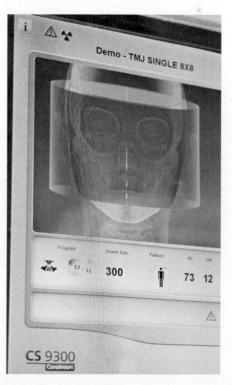

Figure 21-23. Dental Cone Beam Computed Tomography. On the left, an example of a digital dental CBCT machine. The photograph on the right shows an example of the digital image on a computer screen.

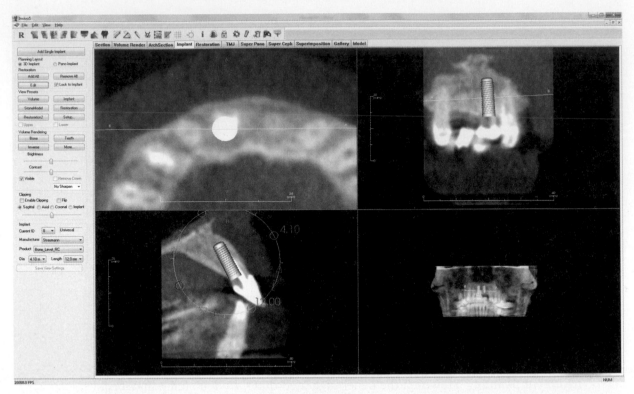

Figure 21-24. CBCT Images. Initial imaging assessment during the implant treatment planning stage is best achieved with CBCT imaging. CBCT imaging allows the clinician to visualize the dentition, maxillofacial skeleton, and the anatomic vital structures in three-dimensions during the presurgical diagnostic phase. Pre-implant surgical CBCT significantly reduces the risk of incorrect implant placement which can compromise the outcome of implant therapy.

Chapter Summary Statement

The use of dental radiographs to supplement information obtained during a clinical periodontal assessment is a critical step in patient care. While there are limitations in the information obtained from conventional dental radiographs, these radiographic images are still an important diagnostic aid in the examination and diagnosis of patients with periodontitis. Radiographic images can be extremely useful tools in the detection of alveolar bone changes due to periodontitis such as crestal irregularities, triangulation, interseptal bone loss, in addition to the detailed assessment of alveolar bone defects and furcation alveolar bone loss.

According to the current best available evidence, CBCT imaging plays a vital role in providing important information for treatment planning of implant or advanced oral reconstructive surgery. However, for the management and treatment planning of periodontitis cases, the routine use of CBCT may provide little information that is not otherwise revealed by conventional intraoral radiographs.

Section 3
Focus on Patients

Clinical Patient Care

CASE 1

Mr. Jones is a new patient in your dental office. He brings with him some recent full-mouth radiographs that reveal no evidence of alveolar bone loss. While studying a copy of the patient's dental chart, you note that there is a diagnosis of Stage II, Grade A periodontitis. How might you explain the apparent discrepancy between the lack of radiographic evidence of bone loss and the diagnosis of periodontitis?

CASE 2

During a periodontal assessment for a new patient, you detect clinical attachment loss. When you suggest that the patient needs dental radiographs, the patient objects because she does not want to be exposed to "unnecessary x-rays." How might you address the patient's concerns?

CASE 3

While reviewing a new set of dental radiographs for a patient, you note numerous sites of obvious alveolar bone loss. How can you determine if the radiographs display horizontal or vertical bone loss?

Ethical Dilemma

Philomena C. is your first patient of the morning. She was born in Italy, and moved to the United States with her family when she was 10. She is a 60-year-old homemaker, who appears slightly overweight, and admits to high blood pressure and high cholesterol, both controlled by medication. She has been a patient in the practice of your dentist's sister, Dr. Lynne, who has an office across town, for the last 30 years. She recently decided to change dental practices as our office is near her residence.

Philomena has been faithful with her recall visits, and has followed all the treatments that Dr. Lynne and the various hygienists have suggested during her years as a patient in that practice, including routine radiographs.

You begin probing, and Philomena questions what you are doing. She states that "no one has ever done that to her teeth and gums," and quite frankly finds it very uncomfortable. Philomena says that she thought her oral health could be evaluated by the "full set of x-rays" that she received every few years.

Your clinical exam reveals that Philomena presents with generalized tooth mobility and early furcation involvement, especially on the maxillary molars. Her probe readings are generalized 4 to 6 mm in the posterior sextants. She assumed that her mouth was in good health, and is shocked to find out otherwise.

1. What ethical principles are in conflict in this dilemma?
2. What is the best way for you to handle this ethical dilemma?
3. What is the best way to address/discuss Philomena's treatment plan?

References

1. Armitage GC; Research, Science and Therapy Committee of the American Academy of Periodontology. Diagnosis of periodontal diseases. *J Periodontol.* 2003;74(8):1237–1247.
2. Bragger U. Radiographic parameters: biological significance and clinical use. *Periodontol 2000.* 2005;39:73–90.
3. Mol A. Imaging methods in periodontology. *Periodontol 2000.* 2004;34:34–48.
4. Tugnait A, Clerehugh V, Hirschmann PN. The usefulness of radiographs in diagnosis and management of periodontal diseases: a review. *J Dent.* 2000;28(4):219–226.
5. Tugnait A, Clerehugh V, Hirschmann PN. Radiographic equipment and techniques used in general dental practice: a survey of general dental practitioners in England and Wales. *J Dent.* 2003;31(3):197–203.
6. Nikolic-Jakoba N, Spin-Neto R, Wenzel A. Cone-Beam Computed Tomography for Detection of Intrabony and Furcation Defects: A Systematic Review Based on a Hierarchical Model for Diagnostic Efficacy. *J Periodontol.* 2016;87(6):630–644.
7. Mandelaris GA, Scheyer ET, Evans M, Kim D, McAllister B, Nevins ML, et al. American Academy of Periodontology Best Evidence Consensus Statement on Selected Oral Applications for Cone-Beam Computed Tomography. *J Periodontol.* 2017;88(10):939–945.

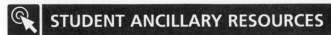

STUDENT ANCILLARY RESOURCES

A wide variety of resources to enhance your learning
is available online:

- Audio Glossary
- Book Pages
- Chapter Review Questions and Answers

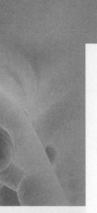

22 Best Practices for Periodontal Care

Clinical Application.

All clinicians face the daunting task of ensuring that they are providing the best possible care for their patients. Dental hygienists must commit to staying updated in their knowledge about periodontal diseases and the care patients with these diseases require. Faced with the fact that there is continuous publication of scientific information about these topics, sifting through information to find the most appropriate and applicable is both time-consuming and challenging. This chapter outlines strategies that any dental hygienist (or any member of the dental team) can employ to ensure that he or she is indeed able to provide patient care that is based upon the best scientific evidence available.

Learning Objectives

- Summarize how the explosion of knowledge is impacting practitioners and patients.
- Identify the three components of evidence-based decision-making.
- Discuss the benefits and limitations of experience.
- Describe the role of the patient in the evidence-based model.
- List locations for accessing systematic reviews.
- Explain the difference between a peer-reviewed journal and trade magazine.
- State three desired outcomes from attending continuing education courses.
- Formulate a question using the PICO process.

Key Terms

Best practice
Association
Causal factor
Evidence-based practice
Confirmation bias

Best evidence
Levels of evidence
Systematic review
PICO process
Databases

Cochrane oral health database
MEDLINE
PubMed
Peer-reviewed journals

Section 1
What Is Best Practice?

Providing the best possible care to patients is the foremost goal of all dental health care providers. Yet, it is generally acknowledged that periodontal care may vary from office to office and even by regions of the country. *As new procedures and techniques become available, hygienists committed to excellence must regularly update and adapt their strategies for providing patient care.* The approach known as "best practice" is an important tool in helping hygienists provide high quality care to their patients.

1. **Overview of the Concept of Best Practice**
   A. **Definition.** Best practice refers to practices/treatments/therapies that are based on the best available evidence.[1]
   B. **Goals and Considerations**
      1. The goal of best practice is the use of concepts, interventions, and treatments that are known to promote a higher quality of care.
         a. The outcomes should be measurable such as a reduction in probing depths.
         b. The outcome should be reproducible. For example, if a technique produces a certain result on one patient, it is reasonable to expect a similar outcome when the technique is used with other patients.
      2. Best practice is derived from evidence-based care. It is the process of using the best available evidence in patient interventions.[1]
2. **Circumstances That Prompted the Best Practice Approach to Patient Care**
   A. **Direct Access to Rapidly Emerging Clinical Research Information**
      1. Volume of Information
         a. Studies on new techniques, tests, procedures, and products for periodontal care is emerging at an astonishing rate. Hundreds of articles are published in dental journals each year.
         b. In addition to the information in dental journals, relevant articles are published each year in medical and specialty journals. An example of articles in other disciplines that are relevant to periodontal health are those on the topic of the oral/systemic link, important research on this topic can be found in journals such the *New England Journal of Medicine* or *Diabetes Care*.
      2. Direct Access to Information
         a. In the past, dental health care providers relied on what they learned in school and the advice of recognized experts to determine how to provide care. Patients had little or no input into this process. Knowledge of new or cutting-edge research was limited to a few practitioners with access to an educational or health care institution.
         b. With the digital media, clinicians and patients have instant access to the results of federally funded clinical trials on treatment methods, equipment, and materials. PubMed, a gateway to more than 23 million research citations, can be accessed by anyone for free.
         c. There are now more than 10,000 open access scholarly journals. Open access means that the scientific studies and papers are open to any reader—health care provider or patient without any financial, legal, or technical barriers.

  d. *Practicing dental hygienists are expected to remain current with new techniques, devices, and materials and make judgments about whether something newer will result in improvements in periodontal care.* Research has shown that there is an inverse relationship between the number of years in practice and the quality of care provided. This means the longer you are in practice, the more at-risk you are for providing a lower quality of care.[2]

B. **Active Patient Role in Decision-Making**
  1. Before the widespread use of information technology, patients depended on the expertise of a health care provider for advice, and in most cases accepted that advice without question.
  2. Many of today's patients expect to be a partner in the decision-making process about their own periodontal care. Patients may arrive at the dental office with information downloaded from the Internet. Patients who are more engaged in their health care experience report a better experience and three to five times greater satisfaction with their providers.[3]

3. **Ability to Interpret the Literature**
  A. **Not All Studies Are Significant to Clinical Care.** Even though hundreds of studies are published yearly, not all are valid and even fewer are significant enough on their own to merit a change in clinical care.
    1. The merit or weight of study is influenced by its design. For example, a randomized clinical trial is considered a higher level of evidence than a case series.
    2. No study is completely free of bias. Reputable journals require investigators to declare a conflict of interest and disclose corporate financial support for studies.
    3. Many studies either are not designed to provide an answer to the needs of the clinician or provide results that are too weak to merit implementation.
  B. **New Does Not Necessarily Mean Better**
    1. New treatments and products need to demonstrate consistent superiority to established methods.
    2. Some new products and therapies are also significantly costlier to implement, and these costs are ultimately passed down to patients.
  C. **Associations Are Not the Same as Cause and Effect**
    1. An association is a relationship between an exposure and a disease that implies the exposure *might* cause the disease.[4]
    2. A causal factor (causality) is an event or condition that plays a role in producing an occurrence of a disease.[4] An example of a causal factor is exposure to the bacterium called *Mycobacterium tuberculosis*. Exposure to this bacterium may cause an individual to develop the infectious disease tuberculosis (TB).
    3. Finding an association between an event and a disease does not make it causal.
      a. Over the past several years, many studies have looked at the relationship between periodontal disease and a host of systemic conditions.
      b. For instance, while many studies do show that periodontal disease is *associated* with cardiovascular disease, at the time of this writing, periodontal disease cannot be said to be a causal factor for cardiovascular disease.[4]

Section 2
Role of Evidence-Based Decision-Making in Best Practice

1. **Introduction to Evidence-Based Decision-Making.** Knowledge of the most recent and relevant evidence is the foundation for best practice. The ADHA advocates evidence-based, patient/client-centered *dental hygiene* practice.
   A. **Definition.** The ADHA defines **evidence-based practice** as the conscientious, explicit, and judicious use of current best evidence in making decisions about the care of individual patients. The practice of evidence-based dental hygiene requires the integration of individual clinical expertise and patient preferences with the best available external clinical evidence from systematic research.[5]
   B. **Why is there a need for evidence-based decision-making?**
      1. Evidence-based dentistry is "an approach to caring for patients that is intended to increase the likelihood that a patient will receive optimal care."
      2. There is often a wide variation in treatment recommendation among practitioners. Evidence-based care seeks to reduce this disparity to ensure that all patients have access to the highest quality treatments.[6]
      3. The translation of research findings into sustainable improvements in treatment outcomes is challenging. The Agency for Healthcare Research and Quality notes it can take up to 20 years for original research to become part of routine clinical practice.[7]
      4. There are barriers to the implementation of evidence-based care. Staying current requires a time commitment. Having access to the best evidence may require a journal subscription or professional association membership to access peer-reviewed journals and/or clinical standards.[8]
      5. New evidence that conflicts with the practitioner's views, beliefs, attitudes, and experiences can also be a barrier to implementing evidence-based care.[8] Dental hygienists may encounter challenges with this when trying to implement new evidence-based interventions or protocols that are not aligned with the doctor or practice's personal philosophy.
   C. **About Evidence-Based Decision-Making**
      1. Evidence-based decision-making emerged from the work of Dr. David Sackett and others at McMaster University in Ontario, Canada. Dr. Sackett is credited with crafting the term. Another driver of evidence-based decision-making is Archie Cochrane, a Scottish physician. Dr. Cochrane championed the use of randomized clinical trials to evaluate medical treatments. The Cochrane Collaboration is named after him.[6,9]
      2. Evidence-based decision-making includes three foundational elements: (1) incorporation of the best scientific evidence with (2) the health care provider's clinical expertise and judgment, and (3) patient's preferences and values. Figure 22-1 illustrates these three foundational elements of evidence-based health care. Box 22-1 provides an example of evidence-based practice.
      3. Evidence is not meant to replace experience or clinical skills. The addition of evidence to decision-making brings balance to the process. It helps close the gap between "what we do" and science.[8] It can enhance patient care and outcomes.[8]

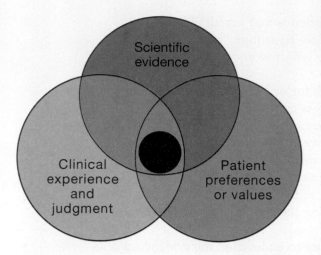

Figure 22-1. The Three Foundational Elements of Evidence-Based Health Care. Evidence-based care has three equal components: scientific evidence, clinical experience, and patient preferences or values.

Box 22-1. Evidence-Based Practice: An Example

Evidence-based practice is built on information obtained from research.

For example, perhaps a dental hygienist was taught in school that ultrasonic instrumentation should be used sparingly and only for the removal of large supragingival calculus deposits. In addition, the hygienist learned in school that hand instruments produce the best results for periodontal instrumentation.

After reading current research on ultrasonic instrumentation, the hygienist learns that modern slim-tipped ultrasonic instruments can be used subgingivally and that a combination of ultrasonic and hand instrumentation leads to excellent results.

This evidence motivates the dental hygienist to attend a continuing education course on ultrasonic instrumentation and to incorporate ultrasonic instrumentation in treating patients with periodontitis.

D. **Foundational Elements of Evidence-Based Decision-Making**
   1. Evidence-based care recognizes that essential skills are needed to engage in evidence-based decision-making and obtain the best health outcomes.[9,10]
      a. Over time, health care providers gain clinical expertise by engaging in clinical experiences (i.e., treating patients and observing the results).
      b. Patients' preferences may be the result of many factors including past dental experiences, current medical and dental status, perceived needs, health values, and economic considerations.
      c. The most challenging essential skill for a health care professional to develop is the ability to assess "evidence."
   2. Clinical experience is both valuable and limiting. It signifies the ability of a clinician to grow in skill and knowledge through experience.
      a. Experience helps the practitioner make thoughtful clinical judgments about the applicability of research findings to individual patient situations. Yet, all patients are different; they may present with complicated or complex medical and dental histories.
      b. Experience is valuable when it is used as a learning rather than reinforcement tool. Ideally, a clinician uses his or her clinical experiences in making better treatment decisions.

   c. Experience can be limiting. The limitation is that not all individuals are able to learn and grow from experience. To acquire "practical wisdom", the clinician needs to learn how to be reflective and analyze his or her own performance.

      1) There is a human tendency to look for or interpret information that confirms our beliefs. This tendency is called **confirmation bias**.

      2) Confirmation bias can lead practitioners to misinterpret information based on beliefs, positive or negative, about a treatment or device.

3. Patient preference or values is an important consideration in treatment selection. If due consideration is not given to the individual patient's preferences, values, and concerns as well as their unique clinical circumstances, the likelihood of the patient fully accepting the clinician's recommendation is diminished.

   a. It is the dental hygienist's responsibility to understand the evidence and its implications for periodontal treatment and communicate it effectively to a patient. Ultimately, it will be the patient who chooses which therapy he or she prefers.

   b. While patients have choices, practitioners have the responsibility to recommend treatment that is safe, evidence-based, clinically sound, high quality, and equitable.[5] In helping a patient decide which periodontal treatment is right for him or her, there are several elements that should be discussed, including:

      1) The evidence about a particular treatment option.

      2) The treatment of choice based on sound evidence.

      3) All possible evidence-based treatment alternatives.

      4) The risks of no treatment at all.

   c. In addition to the efficacy of a proposed treatment, a patient may place equal weight on other aspects of treatment such as:

      1) Cost. Patients usually are concerned about what a treatment will cost. In addition, patients decide if the treatment has benefits that they perceive as being worth the cost.

      2) Pain. Assurances about pain control and management help lessen these concerns.

      3) Time lost from work. Different jobs and work environments have varying levels of flexibility in allowing employees time off for health-related matters.

      4) Impact on family. Caregivers of young children or elderly family members may feel that they do not have the time to devote to periodontal treatment. Individuals with chronic health problems may believe that periodontal care is no longer a priority.

      5) Insurance benefits. A practice reality is that patients will sometimes choose care based on what insurance will pay for versus the full treatment recommendation. However, it should be communicated to the patient that insurance coverage is not the same as the standard of care.

2. **Evaluation of Scientific Evidence. All scientific evidence is not created equal.**

  A. **Levels of Evidence.** Best evidence is the highest level of evidence available for a specific clinical question.

    1. Levels of evidence is a ranking system used in evidence-based care to describe the strength of the results measured in a clinical trial or research study. In simple terms, one way of looking at levels of evidence is as follows (the higher the level, the better the quality; the lower, the greater the bias). Figure 22-2 illustrates the levels of evidence.

2. Based on a hierarchy of levels of evidence, systematic reviews constitute the highest level of current best evidence, and expert opinion is lower-level evidence.

3. The highest level of evidence available represents the current best evidence for a specific clinical question.

B. **Systematic Reviews: The gold standard in evidence-based care**

1. A systematic review attempts to identify, appraise, and synthesize all the empirical evidence that meets pre-specified eligibility criteria to answer the given research questions.[11]

   a. The systematic review process was developed to minimize bias and ensure transparency.[12]

   b. Methods used in conducting a systematic review need to be adequately documented so they can be replicated.[12]

   c. When conducted well, a systematic review should provide the best possible estimate of any true effect.[12]

2. Systematic reviews are, by their very nature, efficient. As an information management tool, they provide a way of coping with large volumes of data in a concise and manageable form.

   a. With more than two million articles published in medical and dental journals annually, it is impossible for one health care provider to read and utilize all the new information.

   b. Systematic reviews of randomized clinical trials represent one of the highest levels of evidence.[11,12]

   c. Systematic reviews also facilitate the development of clinical practice guidelines by bringing together all that is known about a given topic in a nonbiased manner. This provides useful mechanisms for bringing research to practice.[8]

3. Because of the emphasis on evidence-based care, there are more systematic reviews conducted in dentistry than ever before.

4. The systematic review makes incorporating evidence-based care easier. In the past, practitioners were encouraged to do their own searching for research. Since most busy practitioners do not have the time or expertise to do this, the systematic review fills this gap.

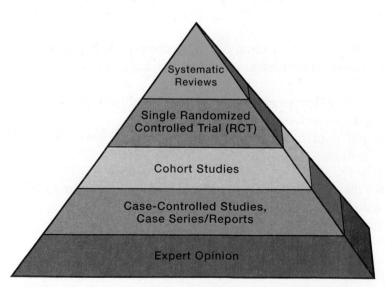

Figure 22-2. Levels of Evidence. The importance or merit of a research study usually is evaluated through its design. Systematic reviews and randomized controlled trials represent the best levels of evidence. Case reports and expert opinion are the lowest levels of evidence.

Section 3
Finding Clinically Relevant Information

Today, all that is required to have access to research information is a computer with Internet access. Determining which studies are of the highest evidence and the most clinically relevant for a particular need is much more challenging. The most comprehensive process for finding and critically evaluating clinical evidence involves a five-step process. This five-step process is summarized in Box 22-2. Steps 1 to 3 of this five-step process are discussed below.

Box 22-2. Five-Step Process for Finding and Evaluating Clinical Evidence[a]

1. Develop an answerable clinical question from a patient problem or need.
2. Conduct a computerized search to locate the best available evidence.
3. Critically appraise the evidence for clinical applicability.
4. Apply the results to your particular clinical situation.
5. Evaluate the process and the results.

[a]Adapted from Forrest JL, Overman P. Keeping current: a commitment to patient care excellence through evidence-based practice. *J Dent Hyg.* 2013;87 Suppl 1:33–40.

---

1. **Developing an Answerable Question.** A clinical question may develop from questions that arise relative to patient care or from an area in which the hygienist wants updated knowledge. In order to find the best information to help patients, it is fundamental to learn how to ask the "right questions." This is more challenging than it seems. It involves converting problems into answerable questions.
   A. **Use Four Components to Structure the Question.** The structure for asking a clear and focused question entails four critical components, known as the PICO process.[9] The PICO process involves the combination of four separate components to form an answerable question: "Patient, Intervention, Comparison, and Outcome."
      1. P (Patient or Problem). An example of the P component might be "*A periodontal maintenance patient with bleeding and gingivitis.*"
      2. I (Intervention)
         a. An intervention is a specific diagnostic test, treatment, adjunctive therapy, medication, product, or clinical procedure.
         b. An example of an intervention being questioned is "*brushing and daily home irrigation.*"
      3. C (Comparison)
         a. Identifies the specific alternative therapy or device that you wish to compare to the main intervention.
         b. An example of the "C" segment of the question is "*compared to brushing and flossing.*"
      4. O (Outcome)
         a. Identifies the measurable outcome you plan to accomplish, improve, or influence.
         b. An example of the "O" segment of the question is "*reduce gingivitis and bleeding within 4 weeks.*"

B. Formulate the Question. Once each of the PICO components has been determined, the clinician combines them into an answerable question. Using the above examples, the question would read: *"For a periodontal maintenance patient with bleeding and gingivitis, will brushing and daily home irrigation OR brushing and flossing provide a better reduction in bleeding and gingivitis within 4 weeks?"*

2. **Conduct a computerized search to find the best evidence.**
   A. **Databases**
      1. The most efficient way to go about finding relevant research is to use an online index of published articles, such as PubMed, MEDLINE, or Cumulative Index of Nursing and Allied Health Literature (CINAHL).
      2. These indexes—known as **databases**—list all articles published in each period of time by journals in a particular profession or group of professions.
      3. **MEDLINE** is the U.S. National Library of Medicine's (NLM) premier database that contains over 26 million references to journal articles in life sciences with a concentration on biomedicine. MEDLINE enables quick access to locate relevant clinical evidence in the published dental/periodontal literature (Fig. 22-3).
         a. A distinctive feature of MEDLINE is that the records are indexed with NLM Medical Subject Headings (MeSH).
         b. Anyone can access MEDLINE for free using **PubMed**—a gateway hosted by the National Library of Medicine.

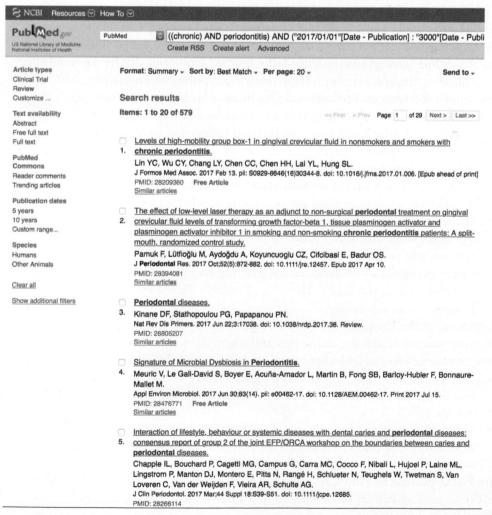

Figure 22-3. PubMed Website. PubMed search results for the topic "chronic periodontitis." (Courtesy of the U.S. National Library of Medicine, Bethesda, MD.)

B. **Systematic Reviews.** Many health care providers do not have the time or expertise needed to do their own systematic reviews of a question. Fortunately, there are numerous trustworthy resources for busy practitioners who want to implement high-quality science into patient care.

1. **The Cochrane Oral Health Database of Systematic Reviews**
   a. The Cochrane Oral Health database was established in 1993 by a British epidemiologist, who recognized that ready access to systematic reviews of available evidence would facilitate better-informed decisions by health care providers.
   b. The Cochrane Database of Systematic Reviews includes systematic reviews of health care interventions that are produced and disseminated by Cochrane Oral Health; a global not-for-profit organization.
      1) The Cochrane Library is published online. Abstracts of reviews are free.
      2) Also, many health science libraries subscribe to the Cochrane databases so that faculty and students have online access.
   c. The Cochrane Review group relevant to periodontics is the "Oral Health Review Group." An example of a systematic review conducted by the Oral Health Group is on the topic of psychological interventions to improve adherence to oral hygiene instructions in adults with periodontal diseases.
   d. A complete listing of topics and abstracts can be accessed at http://oralhealth.cochrane.org/

2. **The PubMed Clinical Query: The National Library of Medicine**
   a. One feature of the MEDLINE database is the PubMed Clinical Query, which provides specialized searches using an evidence-based filter.
   b. An online tutorial for the PubMed Clinical Query tool can be accessed online at http://www.nlm.nih.gov/bsd/disted/pubmedtutorial/020_570.html

3. **Systematic Reviews by Professional Organizations.** Many professional organizations are developing systematic reviews. The American Dental Association recently developed a web-based Center for Evidence-Based Dentistry (http://ebd.ada.org).

4. **Systematic Reviews in Evidence-Based Journals**
   a. Evidence-based journals publish summaries of valid research studies to simplify the evidence-based process for dental health care providers.
   b. For example, *The Journal of Evidence-Based Dental Practice* scans the top dental journals and a panel reviews the selected articles for clinical relevance to practice.
   c. Other examples of evidence-based journals include *Evidence-Based Dentistry, Evidence-Based Medicine, Evidence-Based Healthcare*, and *Evidence-Based Nursing*.

5. **Appraisal of the Evidence for Clinical Applicability.** In medicine, the use of point-of-care electronic databases and algorithms are emerging to help practitioners evaluate and implement evidence-based decision-making.[10]
   a. The use of electronic records is integral to this process as it allows individual patient characteristics to be automatically linked to the best evidence.[10]
   b. Table 22-1 outlines pre-appraised evidence resources including interactive drug databases that are a key part of clinical care decision support systems.[10]

3. **Using the PICO Process to Find Clinically Relevant Information.** Figure 22-4 shows how the PICO process can be incorporated in a three-step approach to finding clinically relevant information.

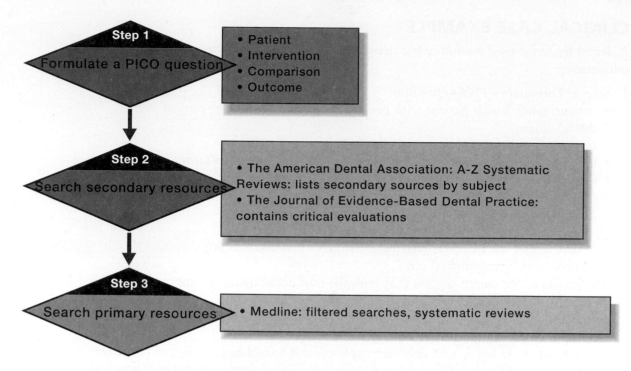

Figure 22-4. Strategy for Finding Clinically Relevant Evidence. The Centre for Evidence-Based Medicine recommends a straightforward approach based on (1) formulating a PICO question, (2) searching evaluated (secondary) resources, and (3) then examining primary text documents.

CLINICAL CASE EXAMPLE

A dental hygienist used the following steps to find evidence-based clinically relevant information.

1. Step 1: Formulate a PICO Question.
   * Patient: *adult female patient with generalized periodontitis; new patient in the dental office*
   * Intervention: *periodontal instrumentation*
   * Comparison: *full-mouth disinfection versus quadrant instrumentation*
   * Outcome: *resolution of inflammation*
   * Question: *For a patient with chronic periodontitis, will full-mouth disinfection OR quadrant instrumentation provide a better reduction in inflammation?*
2. Step 2: Search online evidence-based sources:
   a. ADA Center for Evidence-Based Dentistry at http://ebd.ada.org
   b. PubMed at http://pubmed.gov
3. The results of the search suggest that both the traditional quadrant approach and the newer full-mouth debridement could be equally effective (Box 22-3).
4. In this instance, the dental hygienist presented both options to the patient, explaining that both treatment options are equally effective.
5. The patient chose full-mouth debridement because it would be less disruptive for her to be away from work for 1 day rather than four shorter appointments over a period of several weeks.

Box 22-3. Search Results

Main Results

The search identified 216 abstracts. Review of these abstracts resulted in 12 publications for detailed review. Finally, seven randomized controlled trials (RCTs) which met the criteria for eligibility were independently selected by two review authors. None of the studies included reported on tooth loss. All treatment modalities led to significant improvements in clinical parameters after a follow-up of at least 3 months. For the secondary outcome, reduction in probing depth, the mean difference between full-mouth disinfection and control was 0.53 mm (95% confidence interval (CI) 0.28 to 0.77) in moderately deep pockets of single-rooted teeth and for gain in probing attachment 0.33 mm (95% CI 0.04 to 0.63) in moderately deep single- and multirooted teeth. Comparing FMD and FMS, the mean difference in one study for gain in probing attachment amounted to 0.74 mm in favor of FMS (95% CI 0.17 to 1.31) for deep pockets in multirooted teeth, while another study reported a mean difference for reduction in bleeding on probing of 18% in favor of FMD (95% CI −34.30 to −1.70) for deep pockets of single-rooted teeth. No significant differences were observed for any of the outcome measures, when comparing full-mouth disinfection and control.

Authors' Conclusions

In patients with chronic periodontitis in moderately deep pockets slightly more favorable outcomes for pocket reduction and gain in probing attachment were found following full-mouth disinfection compared to control. However, these additional improvements were only modest and there was only a very limited number of studies available for comparison, thus limiting general conclusions about the clinical benefit of full-mouth disinfection.

TABLE 22-1 | PRE-APPRAISED EVIDENCE RESOURCES[a]

Level 6 Clinical Decision Support Systems: Interactive Drug Databases

Clinical Key	http://www.clinicalkey.com
Comprehensive Drug Database; Interactions	http://www.lexi.com
Integrative Medicine with Evidence-Based Grading System	http://www.naturalstandard.com
Up-to-date	http://www.uptodate.com

Level 5 Summaries: Clinical Practice Guidelines

American Academy of Pediatric Dentistry	http://www.aapd.org/media/policies.asp
American Academy of Periodontology	http://www.perio.org/resources-products/posppr2.html
ADA Clinical Recommendations	http://ebd.ada.org/ClinicalRecommendations.aspx
ADHA Position Papers and Consensus Statements	http://www.adha.org/profissues/index.html
American Heart Association	http://my.americanheart.org/professional/Statements-Guidelines/Statements-Guidelines_UCM_316885_Sub-HomePage.jsp
Centers for Disease Control and Prevention	http://www.cdc.gov/OralHealth/guidelines.htm
PubMed (article type limited to "Practice Guideline")	http://pubmed.gov
Scottish Intercollegiate Guidelines Network	http://www.sign.ac.uk/guidelines/index.html
The Evidence-Based Dental Library	http://www.ebdlibrary.com

Level 4 Synopses of Systemic Reviews: Critically Appraised Systemic Reviews

ADA Center for Evidence-Based Dentistry (Critical Summary)	http://ebd.ada.org/SystemicReviews.aspx
Database of Abstracts of Reviews of Effects (DARE)	http://www.crd.york.ac.uk/crdweb/SearchPage.asp
PubMed (look for comments on systemic reviews)	http://pubmed.gov
Evidence-Based Dentistry	http://www.nature.com/ebd/index.html
Journal of Evidence-Based Dental Practice	http://www.jebdp.com

Level 3 Systemic Reviews

ADA Center for Evidence-Based Dentistry	http://ebd.ada.org/SystemicReviews.aspx
Cochrane Database of Systemic Reviews	http://www.thecochranelibrary.com
PubMed (article filter limit to "systemic review")	http://pubmed.gov
Evidence-Based Dentistry	http://www.nature.com/ebd/index.html
Journal of Evidence-Based Dental Practice	http://www.jebdp.com

Level 2 Synopses of Individual Studies: Critically Appraised Randomized Controlled Trials (RCTs)

Database of Abstracts of Reviews of Effects (DARE)	http://www.crd.york.ac.uk/crdweb/SearchPage.asp
PubMed (limit to "RCT" or "clinical trial"; look for comments)	http://pubmed.gov
Evidence-Based Dentistry	http://www.nature.com/ebd/index.html
Journal of Evidence-Based Dental Practice	http://www.jebdp.com

Level 3 Original Studies: Individual Research Studies (Original studies & not pre-appraised)

PubMed (limit to "RCT" or "clinical trial")	http://pubmed.gov
Journal publications, that is, Journal of Dental Hygiene, International Journal of Dental Hygiene, dental specialty groups, etc.	http://www.adha.org/publications/index.html jada.ada.org http://www.ifdh.org/publications.html

[a]Courtesy of Miller SA and Forrest JL, National Center for Dental Hygiene Practice & Research, 2012 (Forrest JL, Overman P. Keeping current: a commitment to patient care excellence through evidence-based practice. *J Dent Hyg.* 2013;87(Suppl 1):33–40.).

Section 4
Lifelong Learning Skills for Best Practice

One of the most challenging aspects of best practice involves self evaluation. Practitioners continually need to think about whether the care they are providing is still the best level care. There are several questions a dental hygienist should think about on a regular basis.

1. **How sure am I that what I do is right?**
   A. **Do I know where to access systematic reviews? Do I keep up with journal reading?**
      1. Peer-Reviewed Journals. **Peer-reviewed journals** (also called refereed journals) use a panel of experts to review research articles for study design, statistics, and conclusions. Peer-reviewed journals:
         a. Are good sources for randomized clinical trials and learning about new research findings; sometimes will publish systematic reviews.
         b. May be expensive to purchase a subscription; some highly ranked peer-reviewed journals from professional associations have begun allowing free access to full studies 6 months after publication.
         c. Are a good source of higher levels of evidence—systematic reviews and randomized clinical trials.
      2. Practice or Trade Magazines
         a. Can be commercial in nature
         b. May or may not be peer-reviewed; generally provide more of the "expert" opinion
         c. May or may not be supported with references
         d. Vary widely in quality
         e. Provide the lowest quality of evidence
      3. Textbooks
         a. Provide a broad overview of a subject
         b. May not provide specifics on the research
         c. May be dated because of the amount of time involved in writing and publishing a textbook; always check the publication date
   B. **Do I attend continuing education courses? How do I decide which courses to attend?**
      1. Content: Is the subject matter something you like or something that you need? It is important to take the time to evaluate learning/practice needs. Conferring with co-workers or your employer can facilitate more objective choices.
      2. Speaker: Is he or she an expert, a facilitator, or both? A well-rounded speaker will provide information on the latest research findings along with providing some practical advice based on experience.
      3. Outcomes: A well-rounded continuing education course will do three things[13]:
         a. Re-affirm: The course information provides support for your current ways of providing treatment.
         b. Re-energize: The course supports changes in areas that you have previously identified, and provides the motivation and impetus to begin making those changes.
         c. Re-examine: The course addresses new research findings that merit further study and investigation as to the appropriateness of incorporation into practice.

C. **Am I active in my professional association?**
1. Networking with colleagues exposes dental hygienists to other practicing professionals who can provide guidance and mentoring to younger members.
2. Membership in a professional organization can provide free access to peer-reviewed journals.
3. Active membership provides the opportunity to help shape evidence-based policies and guidelines for the organization.
4. Provides immediate access to any Clinical Practice Guidelines the association may develop.

D. **How well developed is my clinical judgment?** Am I able to combine evidence and clinical experience to make a good decision?

E. **Do I take into consideration what my patient wants?**
1. Do I listen to my patients?
2. Do I provide them with enough information and direction to make a good decision?
3. Do I respect their autonomy and choices?

F. **Are there things that I should stop doing?** Am I holding on to what I do because "that's what I learned in school" even though it was several years ago?

G. **Are there things I need to change?**
1. Are there better, more efficient, or cost-effective tools available such as specific diagnostic tests, treatments, adjunctive therapies, medications, products, or procedures than what I am currently using?
2. Do I have the appropriate amount of time scheduled or equipment provided for the highest level of patient care?

H. **Professional Responsibilities and Considerations**
1. Per the ADHA Standards for Clinical Dental Hygiene Practice, dental hygienists are responsible and accountable for their dental hygiene practice, conduct, and decision-making.[5]
2. Dental hygienists need to be able to access and utilize current, valid, reliable evidence in clinical decision-making through analyzing and interpreting the literature and other resources.[5]
3. Dental hygienists need to maintain awareness of changing trends in dental hygiene, health, and society that impact dental hygiene care.[5]
4. Dental hygienists need to participate in activities to enhance and maintain continuing competence and address professional issues as determined by appropriate self-assessment.[5]
5. Dental hygienists need to commit to lifelong learning to maintain competence in an evolving health care system.[5]

Chapter Summary Statement

Best practice is a process of care with the goal of achieving consistent, superior patient outcomes. Best practice is founded on evidence-based data. The highest ranked level of evidence today is the systematic review; an evaluation of a body of research on a treatment or device through rigorous scientific methods to determine the overall validity and clinical applicability of that treatment or device. In addition to scientific data, best practice incorporates sound clinical judgment and patient values into the process. Achieving best practice requires that dental hygienists question and think about what they are doing and be open to learning new techniques. By using this approach to periodontal care, hygienists can meet the challenges of continuing to provide quality care in a rapidly changing field of dental health care.

Section 5
Focus on Patients

Clinical Patient Care

CASE 1

You have just started working in a new office and find that the other dental hygienist in the practice, Debbie, "doesn't believe" in using the ultrasonic equipment. Debbie states she has been practicing for 20 years, that is what she learned in school and she knows what she sees; good results with hand scaling. It is a little intimidating since you have less experience (only 5 years) but have routinely used ultrasonic instruments and mention to her "that is what you learned in school." For a while you pass it off as no big deal, a difference of opinions, but because Debbie didn't use the ultrasonic equipment, the equipment in the office is old and doesn't function at the level it should. You speak to your employer about getting a new machine, but he said, "Debbie doesn't use it, why do you?"

1. How would you answer your employer?
2. What types of evidence would you try to locate to justify your position?
3. Where would you search?
4. What types of key words would you use?
5. How would you manage your conflict with Debbie?

CASE 2

Your patient, Ms. Karen Jones, is a healthy, nonsmoking 30-year-old. Her only medication is birth control pills of 5 years' duration, and a daily multivitamin. She has been coming in for regular maintenance every 6 months. She brushes two times per day and flosses when she remembers, perhaps once a week and she states she finds the procedure difficult. The exam shows some 4 mm probing depths and significant bleeding. As you have done several times in the past, you show the patient how to use the manual brush and floss and really "lay it on the line" about improving oral health and warn her she will need to come in more frequently if her habits do not improve. The patient states that "she tries" and is visibly upset when she leaves office. While you hate to see her upset, you hope she finally got the message.

About a month after her visit, you get a message that Karen Jones would like you to call her. When you reach Karen, she tells you that she just heard on a national newscast that "flossing has no proven medical benefits." Karen reports she read more about it on the internet, and talked to a relative who is also a dental hygienist. She has learned about automatic toothbrushes, interdental brushes, and oral irrigators, and how they could help her. In fact, she has purchased one of everything, and feels her mouth is improving. Not only that, the oral irrigating device makes the task so much easier. And she loves the convenience of those tiny brushes after lunch when she is at work. "Why didn't you tell me about this!" she demands. "I am unhappy, and going to have my records transferred elsewhere!"

1. What are some of the reasons the dental hygienist may have for not telling Karen about these products?
2. Ethically, is not telling a patient about all self-care products that have evidence to support their use the same as not telling a patient about all available professional treatment options? Why or why not?
3. What steps could the dental hygienist take to improve her knowledge on self-care products?

Evidence in Action

USING THE EVIDENCE TO COMMUNICATE WITH PATIENTS

Dental hygienists have an ethical obligation to recommend treatments based on the best available evidence. It is essential that clinicians learn how to effectively communicate these recommendations to patients. Patients will often have questions that reflect their own values, expectations, and perceived oral health needs. Acknowledging and respecting patient concerns are a key part of responding to questions and counseling them about preferred treatments and any evidence-based alternatives.

It is common for patients to question why nonsurgical periodontal therapy is recommended. When practitioners are up-to-date and aware of current evidence, locating that evidence and providing an answer that knowledgably addresses the patients concerns and needs is much easier.

For example, a clinical practice guideline from the American Dental Association on nonsurgical treatment of periodontitis provides practitioners with a third-party, evidence-based recommendation on the treatment of choice for nonsurgical periodontal therapy.[14] Knowledge of documents that support everyday practice also helps align all members of the dental team to support a best practice treatment and provides strong documentation to the patient.

Ethical Dilemma

You have been working as a hygienist in the same periodontal practice for the last 10 years and are quite happy there. There are four dentists in the group, so you have a very full schedule, which allows you to work 4 10-hour days. The practice is very flexible and generous with their resources and benefits. They pay for continuing education courses for all staff members. Unfortunately, you haven't taken any courses since you have worked there, even though you know you are in violation of your state practice act. You have been very busy in your personal life over the last number years, as you got engaged, married, had two children within the span of 2 years, and are now caring for your aging parents. You just can't squeeze anything else into your life.

Your next patient, Richie G., is a 63-year-old real estate agent, who was referred to your practice for a periodontal evaluation 3 months ago. Richie comes armed with questions, articles, and information that he has downloaded from the internet. Although Dr. Willis, the periodontist, suggested periodontal surgery for Richie's treatment, Richie is inquiring about laser procedures as well as bone and tissue regeneration. He asks for your opinion on the articles and studies he has in hand, and if you think there are superior options to "gum surgery."

While you want Richie to be a partner in the decision about his periodontal care, you feel very uncomfortable discussing this with him. You know you are not current in your dental knowledge, and do not know how to accurately interpret the literature Richie presents to you. Unfortunately, you have not updated or adapted your own treatment strategies, and still rely on what you learned in school over 10 years ago.

1. What ethical principles are in conflict in this dilemma?
2. What is the best way for you to handle this ethical dilemma?

References

1. The University of Iowa College of Nursing. Csomay Center—Best practices for healthcare professionals. Available from: https://nursing.uiowa.edu/hartford/best-practices-for-healthcare-professionals, Accessed October 10, 2017.

2. Choudhry NK, Fletcher RH, Soumerai SB. Systematic review: the relationship between clinical experience and quality of health care. *Ann Intern Med.* 2005;142(4):260–273.

3. Alston C, Paget L, Halvorson G, et al. *Communicating with Patients on Health Care Evidence.* Washington, DC: Institute of Medicine of the National Academies; 2012. Available at: www.iom.edu/evidence

4. Brunette DM. Causation, association and oral health—systemic disease connections. In: Glick M, ed. *The Oral-Systemic Health Connection: A Guide to Patient Care.* Chicago, IL: Quintessence Publishing Co.; 2014:24–47.

5. American Dental Hygienists' Association. Standards for Clinical Dental Hygiene Practice. Revised 2016. Access Supplement 2016. Available at: https://www.adha.org/resources-docs/2016-Revised-Standards-for-Clinical-Dental-Hygiene-Practice.pdf, Accessed October 10, 2017.

6. Bader JD. Introduction to evidence-based dentistry. *Int J Evid Based Pract Dent Hygienist.* 2015;1(1):9–16.

7. Fact Sheet: Translating Research into Practice (TRIP) - II. Agency for Healthcare Research and Quality. Available at: https://archive.ahrq.gov/research/findings/factsheets/translating/tripfac/trip2fac.pdf, Accessed October 10, 2017.

8. Kishore M, Panat SR, Aggarwal A, Agarwal N, Upadhyay N, Alok A. Evidence based dental care: integrating clinical expertise with systematic research. *J Clin Diagn Res.* 2014;8(2):259–262.

9. Frantsve-Hawley J, Clarkson JE, Slot DE. Using the best evidence to enhance dental hygiene decision-making. *J Dent Hyg.* 2015;89(Suppl 1):39–42.

10. Forrest JL, Overman P. Keeping current: a commitment to patient care excellence through evidence-based practice. *J Dent Hyg.* 2013;87 Suppl 1:33–40.

11. The Cochrane Library. About the Cochrane Review. What is a systematic review? Available at: http://www.cochranelibrary.com/about/about-cochrane-systematic-reviews.html, Accessed October 10, 2017.

12. McCool R, Glanville J. What is a systematic review? *Int J Evid Based Pract Dent Hygienist.* 2015;1:19–27.

13. Jahn CA. Product focus: continuing education. *Access.* 2008;22:30–32.

14. Smiley CJ, Tracy SL, Abt E, et al. Systematic review and meta-analysis on the nonsurgical treatment of chronic periodontitis by means of scaling and root planing with or without adjuncts. *J Am Dent Assoc.* 2015;146(7):508–524 e5.

Recommended Readings

Abrahamyan L, Pechlivanoglou P, Krahn M, et al. A practical approach to evidence-based dentistry: IX: how to appraise and use an article about economic analysis. *J Am Dent Assoc.* 2015;146(9):679–689.e1.

Brignardello-Petersen R, Carrasco-Labra A, Booth HA, et al. A practical approach to evidence-based dentistry: how to search for evidence to inform clinical decisions. *J Am Dent Assoc.* 2014;145(12):1262–1267.

Brignardello-Petersen R, Carrasco-Labra A, Glick M, Guyatt GH, Azarpazhooh A. A practical approach to evidence-based dentistry: understanding and applying the principles of EBD. *J Am Dent Assoc.* 2014;145(11):1105–1107.

Brignardello-Petersen R, Carrasco-Labra A, Glick M, Guyatt GH, Azarpazhooh A. A practical approach to evidence-based dentistry: III: how to appraise and use an article about therapy. *J Am Dent Assoc.* 2015;146(1):42–49.e1.

Brignardello-Petersen R, Carrasco-Labra A, Glick M, Guyatt GH, Azarpazhooh A. A practical approach to evidence-based dentistry: IV: how to use an article about harm. *J Am Dent Assoc.* 2015;146(2):94–101.e1.

Brignardello-Petersen R, Carrasco-Labra A, Glick M, Guyatt GH, Azarpazhooh A. A practical approach to evidence-based dentistry: V: how to appraise and use an article about diagnosis. *J Am Dent Assoc.* 2015;146(3):184–191.e1.

Carrasco-Labra A, Brignardello-Petersen R, Azarpazhooh A, Glick M, Guyatt GH. A practical approach to evidence-based dentistry: X: how to avoid being misled by clinical studies' results in dentistry. *J Am Dent Assoc.* 2015;146(12):919–924.

Carrasco-Labra A, Brignardello-Petersen R, Glick M, Guyatt GH, Azarpazhooh A. A practical approach to evidence-based dentistry: VI: how to use a systematic review. *J Am Dent Assoc.* 2015;146(4):255–265.e1.

Carrasco-Labra A, Brignardello-Petersen R, Glick M, Guyatt GH, Neumann I, Azarpazhooh A. A practical approach to evidence-based dentistry: VII: how to use patient management recommendations from clinical practice guidelines. *J Am Dent Assoc.* 2015;146(5):327–336.e1.

STUDENT ANCILLARY RESOURCES

A wide variety of resources to enhance your learning is available online:

- Audio Glossary
- Book Pages
- Chapter Review Questions and Answers

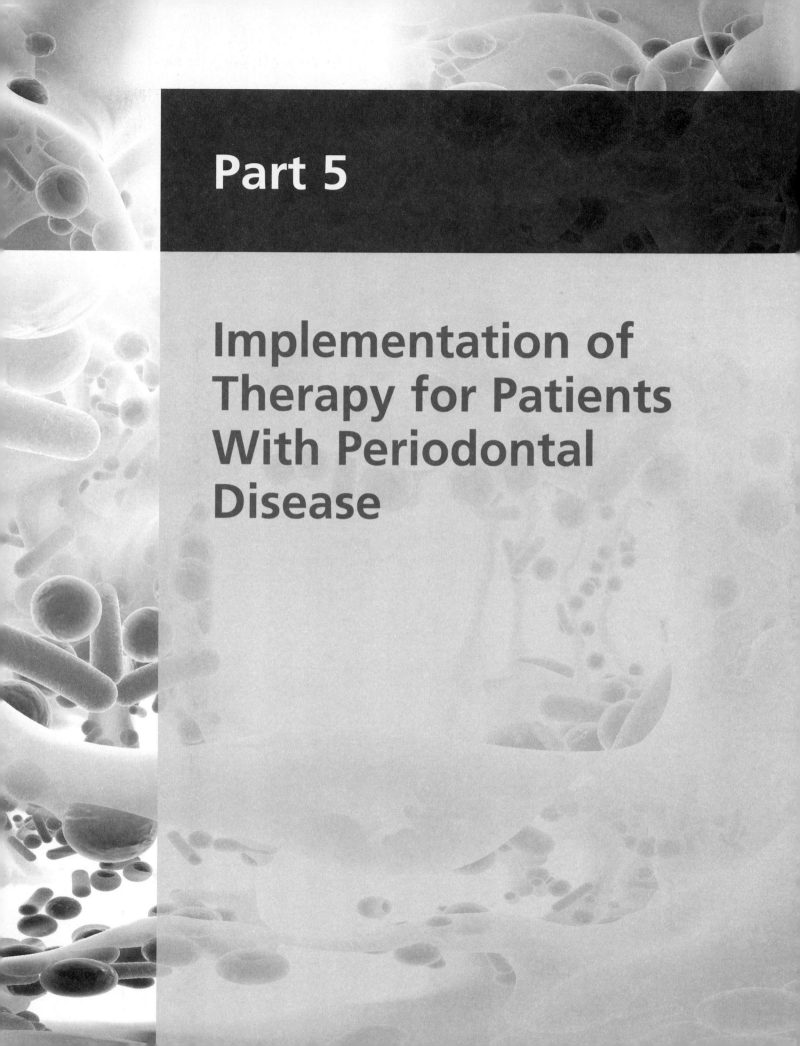

Part 5

Implementation of Therapy for Patients With Periodontal Disease

23 Iatrosedation: Easing and Managing Pediatric Patient Fears

Clinical Application.
"No man stands so tall as when he stoops to help a child." This James Dobson quote helps to frame the special relationship that exists between adults who serve children. Likewise, this quote is appropriate for adults who serve children in a pediatric dental setting. It has been demonstrated in the literature that early oral health experiences serve as an influential and foundational role for patients' decisions and motivations to seek, access, and utilize dental care as adults.[1–3] As a dental team member, the hygienist is in a key position to promote a positive and productive environment for pediatric dental patients. This chapter introduces several topics relevant to a concept of fear/anxiety management known as iatrosedation and behavioral guidance. This chapter will provide an outline of practical iatrosedation strategies based on evidence-based guidelines from behavioral psychology, child developmental, and behavioral dentistry principles.

Learning Objectives

- Define pharmacosedation and iatrosedation.
- Discuss the importance of iatrosedation and behavioral guidance for the pediatric dental patient.
- Describe the role and effect of growth and development in patient behavior and outcomes.
- Discuss the variables that may impact the behavior of pediatric dental patients.
- During role plays or in the clinical setting, demonstrate effective communication with pediatric dental patients and their parents or caregivers.
- Discuss the behavioral guidance strategies for a range of pediatric dental patients representing all stages of growth and development.
- Review techniques for safe and effective application of distraction techniques with pediatric patients.
- Demonstrate how to perform a knee-to-knee oral screening exam for infants and toddlers, gain access to a child's mouth, and restrain a child's body movements during an oral screening exam.

Key Terms

Objective fear
Subjective fear
Pharmacosedation
Iatrosedation
Engagement behaviors

Disengagement behaviors
Nonpharmacological therapy
Frankl Behavioral Rating Scale
Tell-Show-Do
Positive reinforcement

Distraction
Modeling
Systematic desensitization
Pediatric dentistry triad
Knee-to-knee position

Section 1
Dental Anxiety and the Pediatric Dental Patient

Dental fear and anxiety are major contributors to the reluctance of people in North America and across the world to obtain dental services. Most patients are afraid of three things at the dental office—fear of loss of control, fear of embarrassment, or fear of pain. The overall effect of dental anxiety appears to be multifaceted, such that the individual not only avoids his/her dental appointments but also tends to have worse oral health. The incidence of dental fear and anxiety appears to be relatively consistent throughout the world, with some subgroups reporting higher levels than others. This chapter addresses the general concept of iatrosedation or how the dental clinician utilizes his or her behaviors to help alleviate pediatric dental patient fears.

1. **Dental Anxiety in Relation to Dental Treatment.** According to various studies, the prevalence of dental fear and anxiety among *pediatric patients* ranges between 5% and 20%.[4-7] In a recent study assessing the prevalence of dental fear and anxiety among 308 *adult patients* in various private practice settings, White et al. identified several sources of dental fear and anxiety in adults: (1) fear of dental experience, (2) previous negative dental experience, (3) cost of treatment, (4) gag reflex, and (5) fear of bad news.[8] While this study examined dental fear and anxiety among an adult cohort, it is possible that these same factors may also play a role in evoking similar responses from a fearful and anxious pediatric patient.

   A. **Causes of Dental Fear in Children.** Children experience dental anxiety just as adults do, and this fear is intensified by a sense of the unknown. They just do not know what to expect during the dental appointment, and that is scary.

      1. It is important for the practitioner to understand where dental anxiety originates in children. There are essentially two types of dental fear: objective and subjective fear.

         a. **Objective fear** is one that results from a direct experience. Objective fear is created when a child has a negative experience in the dental office, such as feeling pain or not understanding precisely what is happening. The next time the child is scheduled for a dental visit, he or she would be fearful due to this prior painful or frightening experience. The only way to overcome objective fear is to return to the dentist and replace these negative experiences with positive ones. Over time, as a child becomes more comfortable with the dental setting and more familiar with the dental practitioner, his/her anxiety will subside.

         b. **Subjective fear** is one that does not spring from a prior experience. This fear may result from images of terrifying dentists on television, playground horror stories from classmates, or by sensing mom's anxiety before her own dental appointment.

      2. McElroy was responsible for the earliest reference to behavior management in the dental literature in 1895.[9] He wrote *"Although the operative dentistry may be perfect, the appointment is a failure if the child departs in tears."* This was the first time the success of a dental visit for a child was not measured by simply completing the dental treatment at hand.

   B. **Managing Dental Fear.** When helping fearful dental patients cope with anxiety, the two primary techniques used in contemporary dentistry are (1) pharmacosedation and (2) iatrosedation.

1. **Pharmacosedation** is defined as the act of making calm with the administration of anxiety reduction medications, such as a barbiturate or benzodiazepine.
    a. Managing pediatric dental patients with medication can be quite challenging, even for the most experienced dental clinician. It requires a strong understanding of human anatomy and physiology, a deep familiarity with the pharmacologic mechanisms of action of a large number of anxiolytic/sedative agents, and a thorough grasp of current pharmacosedative techniques and technology.
    b. In some pharmacosedative cases, even a skilled dental practitioner may require the help of an individual who has undergone advanced specialized training in anesthesiology (i.e., a dental anesthesiologist, nurse anesthetist).
2. Iatrosedation was developed and defined by Dr. Nathan Friedman as the act of making calm by the doctor's behavior ("*iatro*" means pertaining to a doctor or treatment; "*-sedation*" means the act of calming).[2] Behavior in this sense includes a broad spectrum of verbal and nonverbal communication (behavior). The Mosby's Dental Dictionary defines **iatrosedation** as a relaxed state induced by actions rather than drugs; a method of anxiety reduction that is psychologically based.
    a. Iatrosedation encompasses a range of nonpharmacological techniques in reducing the dental patient's anxiety. **Nonpharmacological therapy** means any therapy that does not include sedative or anxiolytic drugs or medications.
    b. Iatrosedation is a technique for helping anxious patients of any age; however, this technique is particularly useful when treating pediatric and special needs individuals.

2. **Factors That Influence Appointment Outcomes in Pediatric Patients.** The pediatric patient is shaped by their environmental influences. These influences include family and external influences, patient influences, and the influence of the clinician and office setting.[1,3,10–15]

A. **Family and External Influences**
    1. Parental anxiety: Parents or caregivers who exhibit high anxiety in their daily life or the dental office setting typically can affect the child's behavior negatively. This is especially true of the effect of maternal anxiety (Fig. 23-1).
    2. Parental/caregiver factors such as parental age, health, or education.
    3. Stability of the child's day-to-day life including emotional stability of parents/caregivers or such factors as the stability of the marital relationship.
    4. Family culture and beliefs. Is health a priority in the family value system?
    5. Parental/caregiver attitudes: Parental or caregiver attitudes have the potential to impact the child's demeanor. This influence is based on parenting styles such as overprotective, overindulgence, under affectionate, rejecting, and authoritarian.

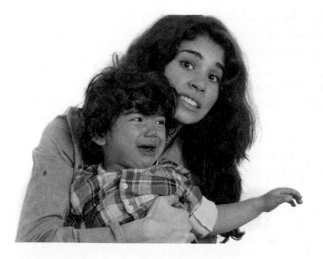

Figure 23-1. Parental Anxiety. A child's behavior may be adversely influenced by a parent or caregiver who exhibits high anxiety in the dental setting.

B. **Patient Factors**

1. **Developmental Factors.** In 1959, Dr. Erik Erikson articulated a comprehensive theory that identifies a series of eight stages which a healthy developing individual should pass through from infancy to late adulthood—infant, toddler, preschooler, grade-schooler, teenager, young adult, middle-age adult, older adult.[16] The following is an outline description of Erickson's stages of development from infant to adolescent and the impact in the dental setting.

   a. Infants—Babies: Birth to age 2
      1) Children learn to sit, stand, walk, and run.
      2) Vocally infants progress from babbling to using simple sentences.
      3) They can identify familiar faces and progress through periods of being friendly and then fearful of strangers.
      4) At this age, a child is too young to cooperate with dental procedures.

   b. Toddlers—Preschoolers: Ages 3 to 5 years
      1) Children develop autonomy (self-confidence and independence) and initiative.
      2) Toddlers thrive in a controlled and structured environment.
      3) They are able to follow simple instructions.
      4) At this age, children welcome an active role in the dental treatment experience.

   c. School Age Children: Ages 6 to 12 years
      1) School-aged children have smooth and strong motor skills with variable physical abilities.
      2) Children develop a sense of body image around age 6.
      3) This is the period of socialization; children are learning to get along with others.
      4) They are learning the rules and regulations of society.
      5) At this stage, children begin to overcome fears of new objects and situations.

   d. Adolescent—Teenagers: Ages 13 to 18 years
      1) At this stage in development, the individual should respect the dental team member as a person.
      2) The hygienist should treat adolescents respectfully according to their advanced level of maturity.
      3) If an adolescent is acting out in a negative way, it is likely the result of his/her own self-esteem or self-image issues.
      4) During this period of development, the individual is responsive to direct focus and empathy.

2. **Patient Temperament.** The temperament of the pediatric patient plays a major role in determining or gauging their appointment outcomes.

   a. Easy: These children have a positive attitude, are pleasant, adaptable, and willing to try new things.

   b. Slow to warm-up: Typically, this describes the shy patient. This child is slow to adapt to new things, but will become comfortable once he or she gets acquainted with the environment.

   c. Difficult: This group of children are challenging dental patients. They have difficulty with routines, sleeping, are disengaging, and are neither accepting nor adaptable to change. They may be awkward in social settings.

    d. Patient's Medical History. Patients who have had positive medical experiences in the past are more likely to cooperate during a dental visit. Those who have had medical challenges or negative medical experiences may have a difficult time at the dental office.

    e. Patient's Awareness of Dental Concern. A child with an existing dental concern (such as pain, inflammation or trauma) may have a tendency toward negative behavior because the child is aware there is a problem that needs to be treated.

3. **Dental Team Factors.** Behavioral guidance and management of the child and adolescent patient are necessary to establish a relationship between the patient, parent/caregiver, and the hygienist. Oftentimes, there are aspects of the relationship that are beyond the control of the dental hygienist. Aspects of the relationship that are within the control of the clinician include:

    a. Being mindful of personal and office appearance

    b. Acknowledging the parent while not allowing a parent/caregiver to interfere with direct communication with the child

    c. Maintaining interest, concern, humor, and confidence when interacting with the patient and parent/caregiver

    d. Using subtle commands, rather than making suggestions or asking questions

    e. Maintaining a readiness and willingness to be firm

    f. Avoiding fear-promoting words and always explaining before doing

    g. Keeping appointments short and at an optimum time for the patient

4. **Additional Factors.** Other factors that may influence appointment outcomes are summarized in Box 23-1.

Box 23-1. Examples of Additional Patient Factors

Variables that can influence the outcomes for the pediatric dental patient:

- Readiness for learning
- Motivation
- Language development
- Dental anxiety of parents/caregivers and siblings
- Behavioral diagnosis or problems (ADHD, Autism)
- Physical handicaps
- Emotional development
- Academically gifted

Section 2
Behavioral Assessment of the Pediatric Patient

Dental fear has been related to personality, increased general fears, previous painful dental experiences, parental dental fear, age, and gender. When treating a pediatric patient, the first issue of concern is the child's behavior. One of the most challenging issues for the clinician is to anticipate what type of behavior can be expected from a child or adolescent patient. A child who arrives at the dental office crying or screaming is obviously fearful. On the other hand, a child who is quiet or withdrawn is exhibiting behavior that is difficult to read. In order to prevent disruptive behavior, it is imperative to identify the dentally anxious child at the earliest possible age. For this purpose, different types of behavioral measuring scales have been used to assess dental fear. Behavioral assessment tools are helpful tools to classify behavior and more effectively care for children and adolescents.

1. **Behavioral Management**
   A. **Impact of Clinician Behaviors.** The success or failure of iatrosedation can hinge on the behavior and demeanor of the dental practitioner. For example, a dental practitioner who has a soothing demeanor and a good bedside manner will be able to allay and calm an anxious pediatric patient much better than a jittery and nervous practitioner. These same behaviors can also be used by the dental practitioner to manage the anxiety of an adult patient or a patient with special needs.
      1. As a vital member of the dental team, the dental hygienist plays a critical role in the success of the dental team by establishing and shaping the pediatric dental patient's perceptions, beliefs, and experiences around dentistry.
      2. It is imperative for the clinician to be able to recognize and address the dental fears and anxieties that the pediatric patient population may experience, and utilize effective behavioral management strategies to promote a positive dental experience (i.e., helping the child patient cope and find success in the dental setting).
   B. **Body Language Assessment.** Behavior management begins the moment the child enters the dental environment. Engagement and *disengagement* are important signals to monitor in the patient's body language.
      1. Engagement behaviors indicate interest, receptivity, or agreement. Good eye contact, smiling, and open body posture are all signs of engagement.
      2. Disengagement behaviors signal that a person is bored, angry, or defensive. If someone is disengaged, the amount of eye contact decreases; people tend to look away from things that distress them. Disagreement also shows up in compressed lips, clenched jaw muscles, or a head turned slightly away. If the child in the waiting room sits with his feet wrapped around the legs of the chair, he may be anxious and disengaged.
   C. **Pre-appointment Evaluations.** Pre-appointment evaluations can help with predicting behavior outcomes.[17] The medical history taking aspect of the first visit provides an excellent opportunity for the dental team to assess the potential behavior of the child. The objectives of a behavioral assessment tool are twofold: (1) to learn about patient and parental concerns, and (2) to gather information that would allow the clinician to estimate the cooperative ability of the child. Figure 23-2 provides examples of questions used to predict a child's behavior in a dental setting.

Child Survey

DIRECTIONS: Place a checkmark in the column that best describes your child's behavior.

How afraid is your child of...	Not at all	A bit afraid	Fairly afraid	Very afraid
1. new situations or unfamiliar people?				
2. getting a shot at the doctor's office?				
3. having a medical examination?				
4. having a dental problem (something wrong with his/her mouth)?				
5. people wearing uniforms?				
6. coming to the dental office today?				

Figure 23-2. Behavioral Assessment Tool. Shown here is an example of a short questionnaire to assess the potential behavior of a child before his first dental visit. While taking the medical history, the parent or caregiver can be asked to complete a brief behavioral questionnaire. Several negative responses on the behavior assessment tool can indicate a potentially challenging outcome for the patient's visit and alert the clinician to a potential behavioral problem that may complicate the dental appointment.

2. **Behavioral Assessment Tools.** Behavioral assessment scales are helpful tools to classify and document behavior of children and adolescents. Documentation of a child's behavior during a series of appointments, or over a period of years, can assist in behavior management.
   A. **Frankl Behavioral Rating Scale**
      1. One of the most widely used systems was introduced by Frankl et al. in 1962. It is referred to as the Frankl Behavioral Rating Scale.[1,18] The scale divides observed behavior into four categories: definitely negative, negative, positive, and definitely positive. A detailed description of the scale is provided in Table 23-1.
      2. The Frankl scale lends itself to a shorthand form of documentation in the chart or computerized record. A child displaying positive cooperative behavior can be identified by jotting down (+) or (+/+). Conversely, uncooperative behavior can be noted by (–) or (–/–).
      3. When documenting the behavioral assessment at the conclusion of the visit in the patient record, it is important to be very descriptive on key aspects of the responses. Sample observations could be "*(–) the patient cried, was withdrawn and required lots of reminders to stay open for most of the visit*" or "*(+/+) the patient was pleasant and talkative. She hopped up into the big girl chair and was very interested in having her favorite bubble gum tooth sparkles.*"
      4. If behavior ranges from negative to positive during a visit, a simple notation could be (– > +). The management technique can also be recorded: "*patient responded well to the T (Tell), S (Show), D (Do) technique.*"

TABLE 23-1 | FRANKL BEHAVIORAL SCALE

Patient Record Notation		Patient Behavior
(–/–)	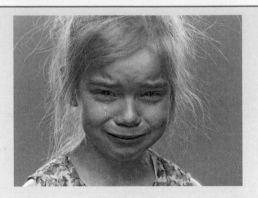	**Rating –/–** Refusal of treatment; forceful crying, fearfulness, or any overt evidence of extreme negativism
(–)	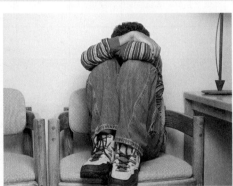	**Rating –** Reluctance to accept treatment; uncooperativeness, some evidence of negative attitude, sullen and withdrawn
(+)	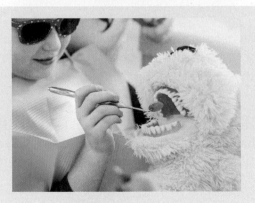	**Rating +** Acceptance of treatment; cautious at times; willingness to cooperate with the dentist, at times with reservation, but the patient follows directions cooperatively
(+/+)	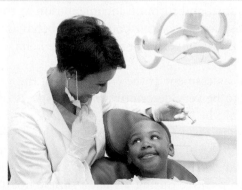	**Rating +/+** Good rapport with the clinician, interest in dental procedures, laughter and enjoyment

Section 3
Iatrosedation Techniques With Pediatric Patients

The dental hygienist plays a critical role in shaping the pediatric dental patient's perceptions and beliefs about dental care. Often, the hygienist is the first member on the dental team to have a significant interaction with the child patient during his or her initial office visits. Iatrosedation is an effective behavioral management approach to overcome dental fear and anxiety in adults and children. The end-result of effective iatrosedation is to make the dental visit more pleasant for both the patient and members of the dental team, facilitate the delivery of high quality dental care, and improve outcomes of treatment.

There are several methods of timely and appropriate behavioral interventions with pediatric and special needs patients.[1,19–23] This section presents seven common behavioral guidance practices effective when working with pediatric patients in the dental setting. *Many of the behavioral guidance techniques prescribed for the pediatric patient population would serve to ease the fears in adult patients.* It is imperative to realize that behavioral guidance starts with clinician! See Table 23-2 for a summary of key points.

TABLE 23-2	BEHAVIORAL GUIDANCE TO REDUCE ANXIETY[1,20]
Tell-Show-Do	Informing the patient of what will happen, demonstrating it, and then performing that part of the procedure
Nonverbal Communication	The clinician reinforces desired behavior and guides behavior through body language, contact, posture, and facial expression
Voice Control	A controlled modulation of the clinician's voice volume, tone, or pace to influence and direct the patient's behavior
Positive Reinforcement	Offering a tangible or social reward in response to the patient having a desired behavior
Distraction	Directing the patient's attention from a behavior, thought, or feeling to something else
Modeling	Providing the patient an example or demonstration about how to behave constructively
Systematic Desensitization	Reducing the patient's anxiety by initially presenting a situation or object that evokes a little fear, and then progressively presenting stimuli that are more fear-provoking

1. **Effective Techniques for Easing Patient Fears**
    A. **Tell-Show-Do**
        1. The Tell-Show-Do approach is a cornerstone method of behavioral shaping used to help children. Tell-Show-Do is one of the most effective approaches when working with pediatric patients. See this approach illustrated in Table 23-3.
        2. The objective of the Tell-Show-Do approach is to familiarize the patient with the dental setting, and expose the child to the dental procedure and instruments. This reinforces desired behavior by gaining the patient's trust and empowers him/her regarding the experience.

TABLE 23-3 | TELL-DO-SHOW APPROACH

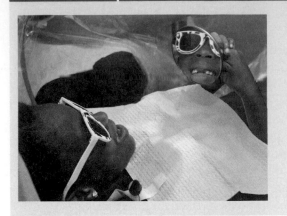

TELL.

- A verbal explanation of a procedure using words that are appropriate to the stage and level of development of the patient.
- Explain to the patient what you are going to do and orient them in the patient mirror.

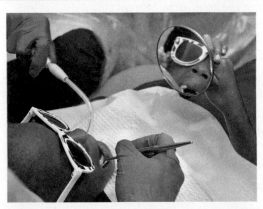

TELL.

- Use visual, auditory, olfactory, and tactile aspects of the procedure to help the child to understand.
- Explain to the patient what you are going to do and introduce the procedure using the mouth mirror and saliva ejector or "straw."

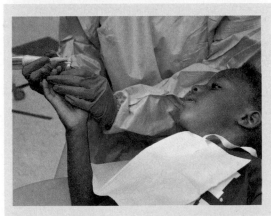

SHOW.

- A demonstration of the procedure for the patient.
- For example, lightly applying a rubber prophy cup on the child's fingernail allows the patient to see, hear (whirring sound of the handpiece), and feel this procedure.

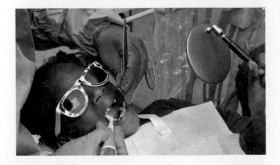

DO. Begin the rubber cup polishing procedure.

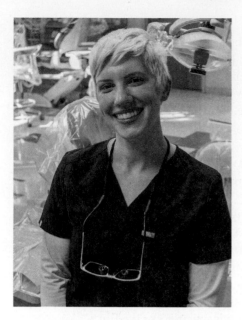

Figure 23-3. Behavioral Guidance Starts With You. A positive experience for a child patient starts with the clinician's body language, posture, facial expression, and tone of voice.

B. Nonverbal Communication

1. The clinician models and guides the desired behavior through his or her own body language, contact, posture, and facial expression (Fig. 23-3).
2. The objective of nonverbal behavioral modeling is to establish positive rapport with the patient to gain desirable behavior.

C. Voice Control

1. The clinician employs a controlled volume, tone, and pace when speaking to influence and direct the patient's behavior.
2. The objective is to gain the patient's attention and compliance.

D. Positive Reinforcement

1. Positive reinforcement is the addition of a tangible or social reward following a desired behavior that makes it more likely that the behavior will occur again in the future.
   a. The clinician rewards appropriate behaviors in order to strengthen the recurrence of those behaviors. For example, the clinician rewards a child with a colorful sticker for sitting still while the clinician exposed a digital radiograph.
   b. Social rewards include positive voice modulation, facial expression, verbal praise, and appropriate physical demonstrations of affection by members of the dental team.
   c. Nonsocial rewards include tokens, toys, and stickers.
2. The objective of positive reinforcement is to reinforce desired behaviors.

E. Distraction

1. Distraction is the technique of diverting the patient's attention away from a procedure that the child may perceive as unpleasant. Giving patients something else to focus on is especially effective. Examples of distraction techniques are listening to music through ear buds, watching videos on a ceiling-mounted monitor, squeezing a stress ball, or cuddling a stuffed toy.
2. The objective is to build trust between the clinician and patient and avert patient avoidance behavior.

F. Modeling

  1. **Modeling** is the technique of learning new skills by observing and then imitating another person, such as a parent or another patient, who performs the *behavior* to be acquired. This approach works well in a dental office with an open bay concept where the child is able to watch another patient demonstrating positive behavior during the procedure. For example, a child observes the dental clinician using dental instruments in another patient's mouth.

  2. The objective of modeling is to reinforce desired behavior by allowing a child to observe a patient who is tolerating the treatment well.

G. Systematic Desensitization

  1. **Systematic desensitization** is the technique for reducing a patient's anxiety by initially presenting a situation or object that evokes a little fear, and then progressively presenting stimuli that are more fear-provoking.

     a. Oftentimes, having the patient do a "getting acquainted" visit to the office is helpful if a child has a history of anxiety in new situations or with the pediatrician. For example, the first visit might consist of visiting a treatment room, riding up and down in a dental chair, and having water sprayed in the mouth from a dental "water squirter" (with no actual treatment being performed at this visit).

     b. It is also helpful to educate the parents on the language used in the office as well as establish expectations for the future visit. Box 23-2 provides some examples of word substitutions for dental terminology.

     c. "Mapping out" the experience of a dental appointment with visual aids as brochures or "My First Dental Visit" books can help desensitize the patient and ensure a successful visit.

  2. The objective of systematic desensitization is to create a positive experience by slowly introducing a child to the dental setting.

Box 23-2. Examples of Word Substitutions of Dental Terminology for the Pediatric Patient

Dental Terminology	Word Substitute
• Dental light	• *Flashlight*
• Saliva ejector	• *Straw*
• High evacuation suction	• *Mouth vacuum*
• Air syringe	• *Air dryer*
• Water syringe	• *Water squirter*
• Explorer	• *Tooth counter*
• Scaler	• *Tooth scrubber*
• Prophy angle	• *Tooth tickler*
• Prophy paste	• *Tooth sparkler*
• Sealant	• *Tooth paint*
• Etchant	• *Tooth soap*
• Radiographs	• *Tooth picture*
• Fluoride	• *Tooth vitamin*

H. **The Pediatric Dentistry Triad: Clinician—Patient—Parent/Caregiver**
   1. With the majority of adult patients, the clinician–patient interaction should be a one-to-one relationship.
   2. For pediatric or special needs patients, the clinician interacts not only with the patient, but also with parents and caregivers. This three-way relationship is known as the **pediatric dentistry triad**.[1,22,25] It is important for the hygienist to establish a positive rapport with parents and caregivers as Figure 23-4 illustrates. Parents and caregivers need to know that all members of the dental team are competent and care about the best outcomes for the child.
      a. Partnering with the child and the parent/caregiver facilitates achieving a positive outcome to the dental visit for the child.
      b. Educating the parent/caregiver about the planned treatment and anticipated treatment outcomes is helpful in setting expectations and avoiding "over-involvement" of the parent/caregiver during the appointment.
      c. Involving the parent/caregiver as a "silent observer" is a means to support a one-on-one relationship between the child and the dental clinician.

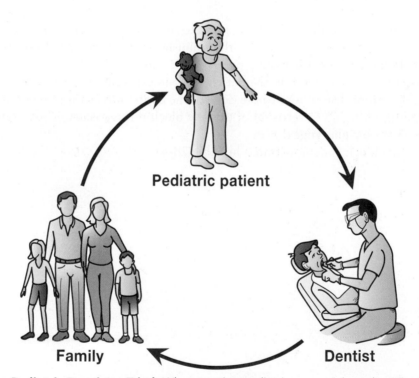

Figure 23-4. The Pediatric Dentistry Triad. When treating pediatric or special needs patients, the clinician establishes a relationship with the patient and his or her parents or caregivers.

3. The most important goal of the dental visit is for the child to have a positive experience. In order to accomplish this all members of the dental team should:
   a. Establish positive communication with the patient and parent/caregiver.
   b. Build a trusting relationship with the patient and parent/caregiver.
   c. Strive to alleviate fear and anxiety for the child patient.
   d. Promote a positive attitude towards oral health in general with the entire family.
   e. Deliver quality and competent dental oral health care.

2. **Adaptive Support.** On some occasions, it becomes necessary to utilize an adaptive support tool such as a bite block when working with pediatric dental patients.
   A. A bite block is a wedge-shaped device with the rubber-like texture that is placed between a patient's teeth and used to assist the patient to keep the mouth open wide during a procedure. The bite block also serves a "resting place" that allows the patient to relax his jaws when holding the mouth open for prolonged procedures such as application of pit and fissure sealants.
   B. Bite blocks come in different sizes; therefore, it is important to select the proper fit. To achieve maximum mouth opening, the bite block should be placed more posteriorly.
      1. Informed consent should be obtained prior to using a bite block. For patients under the age of consent or adults with diminished mental capacity, informed consent should be obtained from a parent or caregiver.[28-30]
      2. Prior to placing a bite block in the patient's mouth, it is imperative to securely attach a length of dental floss to the device. The dental floss should be of an adequate length to aid in retrieval of the bite block if it is dislodged and falls into the posterior pharyngeal area.
      3. Use of a bite block is demonstrated in Table 23-4.

TABLE 23-4	APPLICATION OF A DENTAL BITE BLOCK

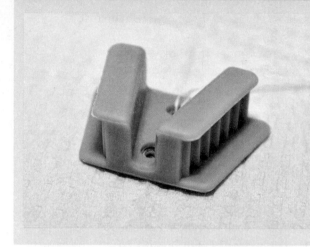

1. Select a bite block of appropriate size for the patient's mouth. Attach approximately a 12-inch length of dental floss to the bite block.

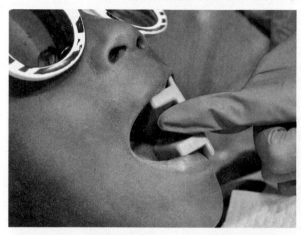

2. Gently guide the bite block along the occlusal surfaces of the teeth.

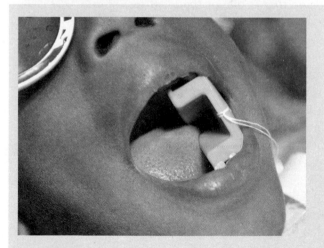

3. Ensure a comfortable fit of the bite block in the patient's mouth. Note that the dental floss is positioned to aid in retrieval of the bite block.

3. **The Infant Oral Exam**
   A. **Guidelines for Infant Oral Health Care.** The American Academy of Pediatric Dentistry[31,32] makes recommendations that relate to the role of the dental hygienist in infant oral health care:
      1. Every infant should receive an oral health risk assessment from his or her primary medical care provider or dental health care provider by 6 months of age.
      2. Parents or caregivers should establish a dental home for infants by 12 months of age.
      3. Health care professionals and all stakeholders in children's health should support the identification of a dental home for all infants at 12 months of age.
   B. **Role of the Hygienist in Guidance and Counseling**
      1. The guideline that the infant should have the "first dental visit by the child's first birthday" places the dental hygienist in a prime position to engage in infant oral health care. A benefit of this philosophy is that it exposes pediatric patients to the dental setting at an early age. The hygienist will be able to educate parents and caregivers on setting the pediatric patient on an early path to oral health.
      2. The 2017 American Academy of Pediatric Dentistry guidelines on anticipatory guidance/counseling is defined as the process of providing practical, developmentally appropriate information about children's health to prepare parents and caregivers for significant physical, emotional, and psychological milestones. The recommended topics for parent and caregiver counseling that relate to the role of the dental hygienist include oral hygiene and dietary habits.
   C. **The Knee-to-Knee Technique for the Initial Infant Dental Visit**
      1. Proper positioning of the child is critical to conducting an effective and efficient clinical exam in a young child. In general, the knee-to-knee position should be used with children ages 6 months to 3 years, or up to age 5 with children who have special health care needs. Children older than 3 may be able to sit alone in the dental chair. *The knee-to-knee positioning is one of the most secure and effective approaches for the infant dental visit.*
      2. In order to perform the infant oral exam, the child needs to be in a safe and secure position, usually held by his or her parent or caregiver.
         a. The dental hygienist and the parent/caregiver sit on two chairs facing one another and take a seat with knees touching to make a table. They can use a patient pillow; however, this is not necessary.
         b. Knee-to-knee positioning may be accomplished with the child on the dental chair and the parent and clinician on dental stools. Alternatively, the child sits on the parent's lap with the parent and clinician seated on dental stools or office chairs.
         c. It is important that there is adequate light available or an assistant could hold a flashlight to help visualize the patient's mouth.
         d. Refer to Figures 23-5 to 23-10 for detailed illustration of this approach.

D. *CELEBRATE* the end of the visit. Accentuate the positives and do not focus on the negatives.

1. Keep in mind the patient's level of growth and development. Crying at this stage and age is to be expected and within normal limits.

2. Take this opportunity to also celebrate with the parent/caregiver who helped the child have a successful visit. Reassure the parent/caregiver that an uncooperative or tearful child is to be expected and that behavior should improve over time with increased maturity of the patient.

3. Reinforce the need for good oral hygiene, fluoride applications, and healthy nutrition habits.

E. **Practical Considerations for Providing Care for Pediatric Patients.** The primary aim is to provide quality care for the pediatric patient that will minimize disruptive behavior, promote a positive psychological response to treatment, and promote patient safety and welfare. To achieve this end, a consideration should be made in three practical areas: the practice environment, patient scheduling, and parental presence or absence in the exam room.

1. Office environment and design: The overall office environment should be comfortable and inviting for families. To achieve this effect, some offices have themes, bright colors, designated areas for play with toys and/or video games, as well as adult areas with beverage centers.

2. Scheduling: When scheduling it is helpful to consider the patient's age and development. Children ages 5 and under as well as those with special health care needs typically benefit from appointment times in the morning. Avoiding nap time or other disruptive times of the day helps the dental team support positive behavioral outcomes.

3. Parental Involvement:

   a. The literature has demonstrated that children's behavior is unaffected by parental presence or absence. However, the exception to this effect has been found in young children under the age of 4 years old. Typically, this demographic of children demonstrates better behavior with their parent or caregiver present.[24-27]

   b. It is normal for a child under the age of 4 to experience separation anxiety at this stage in development. It has been shown that this is a strong indicator of dental anxiety. Therefore, it appears that parental presence is helpful with the younger dental patient, but has no positive impact on older children. It is helpful for all members of the dental team to discuss these expectations with parents and caregivers.

   c. If the decision is made to allow parents into the dental treatment room, the clinician needs to establish positive communication with the adult and set expectations. In doing so, the clinician should avoid allowing the parent or caregiver to become a distraction during treatment by:

      1) Disrupting direct clinician communication with the child by controlling the conversation or providing incorrect instructions.

      2) Repeating (echoing) the clinician's instructions to the child.

      3) Attempting to "coach" or "cheer the patient on" during the appointment in a disruptive manner.

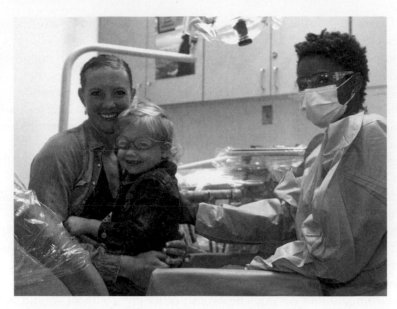

Figure 23-5. Step 1. Knee-to-Knee Technique: Make Positioning Fun.

- Have the child sit on the parent's lap in a straddle position with the child facing the parent/caregiver.
- The clinician faces the parent and approaches the parent until their knees touch, forming a bridge. A pillow may be used to help secure the patient.
- Ask the parent to gently lean the child back onto the clinician's lap.
- The parent may hold the child's hands to avoid having the child interfere with the clinical examination.
- Another important tip: keep child's legs around the caregiver's waist during the exam. This will also aid in restraining the child's body movement.

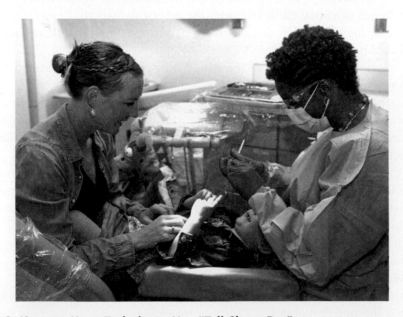

Figure 23-6. Step 2. Knee-to-Knee Technique: Use "Tell-Show-Do."

- Even when approaching the knee-to-knee position with the young child, utilizing Tell-Show-Do is critical. This allows the patient to warm up to the "fun" instruments that will be used during the visit.
- Beginning with introducing the dental mirror also aids in desensitizing the patient.

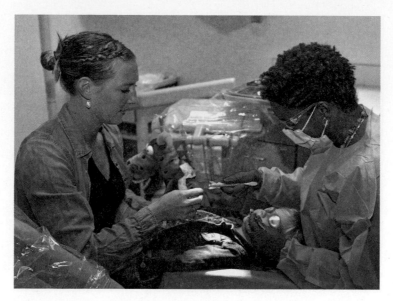

Figure 23-7. Step 3. Knee-to-Knee Technique: Partner With the Parent or Caregiver.

- Invite the parent to partner with you with the Tell-Show-Do approach.
- Allow mom to demonstrate how she brushes the child's teeth at home.
- This allows the patient to become more comfortable with having dental instruments in the mouth.

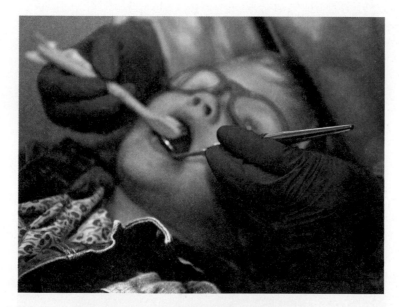

Figure 23-8. Step 4. Knee-to-Knee Technique: Toothbrush Prophylaxis.

- A toothbrush is effective in removing plaque biofilm in most young children. It is also nonthreatening to young children and serves to demonstrate the proper brushing technique to the caregiver.
- Clinical examination of the teeth and soft tissues can be accomplished while counting the child's teeth aloud. Many clinicians make a game of this task, singing songs, engaging the child's attention, and if all else fails, distracting the child with a brightly colored toy.
- Praise the child at each step for cooperation and good behavior.

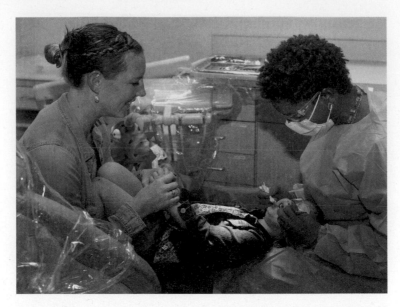

Figure 23-9. Step 5. Knee-to-Knee Technique: Alternate Position for Unhappy Patient.

- Controlling the child's body movement, particularly leg movements, can be achieved by the caregiver gently resting his/her arms on the child's bent legs, enfolding the child's body in a snug "hug."
- Mom holds the patient's hands and secures the patient's legs with her forearms. The patient remains safe even in this position and when the patient is unhappy.

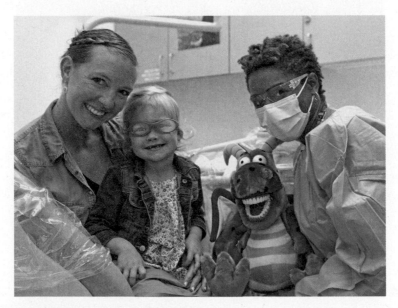

Figure 23-10. Step 6. Knee-to-Knee Technique: Celebrate.

- Celebrate the dental visit by highlighting the positives.
- If the patient is unhappy still try to celebrate the end of the visit.
- Celebrate the positives.
- Provide lots of praise and prizes!

Chapter Summary Statement

Iatrosedation and behavioral guidance are effective strategies to implement for the child and adolescent patient population. Therefore, it is critical that all members of the dental team understand the importance of behavioral guidance and be comfortable with implementing these techniques as part of patient care when indicated. The ability to communicate well with the child and the parent/caregiver, express empathy, and project calmness are necessary skills to promote positive behavior and reduce disruptive behavior. The behavioral guidance assessments and techniques described in this chapter are universal strategies and approaches used in pediatric dentistry. When appropriately used, iatrosedation and behavioral guidance techniques set the tone of the dental appointment as a positive experience, and provide the child patient with a rewarding opportunity to gain faith in their clinician and acquire confidence in their own abilities to overcome previously conceived fears and anxiety associated with dental treatment.

Section 4
Focus on Patients

Evidence in Action

DIRECTIONS: For each patient case answer the following:

1. How would you rate this patient's behavior based on the Frankl Scale of Behavioral Assessment?
2. What behavior guidance techniques would you use to help this patient have a successful visit?

CASE 1: A 4-year-old female patient with past medical history of allergy to penicillin and eczema happily greets you in the lobby. She hops into the dental chair and is eager to have dental treatment. During the procedure, she is very cooperative and talkative.

CASE 2: A healthy 3-year-old male patient walks into the treatment area clenching his mother's hands and offers you little eye contact. He is hesitant to sit in the dental chair and requires a great deal of coaxing to participate with the treatment. He begins to cry out during the prophy and during the entire appointment, but keeps his mouth open.

CASE 3: A healthy 2-year-old male patient and his older sister arrive for their appointments. The older sister is seen first and the younger brother is able to watch the entire visit. After completion of the older sister's appointment, you now ask the 2-year-old to sit in his very own "big boy chair." After modeling with his older sister, the patient sits in the chair by himself. The patient is attentive and cooperative for the visit.

CASE 4: A healthy 6-year-old female patient reluctantly greets you in the lobby. As you approach the treatment area, the patient announces loudly that she doesn't want to have her teeth brushed today. She then refuses to sit in the dental chair, sits on the floor and holds on to the base of an extra chair for parents in the room. Mom is able to convince the patient to sit in the chair with promises to buy a treat at McDonald's following the visit if the treatment is completed. The patient attempts to bite your finger and intentionally spits out the prophy paste in your face.

PATIENT CASE

A 4-year-old new patient presents to your dental team's office and has a past medical history of asthma that is controlled as needed (prn) with Claritin and Albuterol. In the lobby, he screams and kicks when asked to put down a video game and come to the treatment room. Once back in the treatment area he enjoys playing with the toys, but won't let go of mom's arm when it's time to sit in the dental chair.

1. Consider this patient's stage of development both physically and emotionally and assess his current behavior.
2. Explain the approaches to behavioral guidance strategies and alternatives that may be utilized to help this patient have a successful visit.

Clinical Patient Care

PATIENT CASE 1: You plan to take bitewing radiographs on a healthy 3-year-old female patient. She refuses to open her mouth for the radiograph after happily sitting in the chair.

• What behavioral guidance approaches might you use with this 3-year-old patient?
• If the patient decides to cooperate and accomplishes having the radiographs taken, how would you assess her behavior based on the Frankl scale?

PATIENT CASE 2: A patient with Down syndrome is excited about his recall exam today. He gives you a big hug in the lobby, eagerly walks into the treatment area. During the oral exam, you notice there is moderate gingivitis in the anterior sextants of the maxillary and mandibular teeth. When you attempt to instrument these areas, the patient tightly purses his lips and refuses to keep his mouth open.

• How would you proceed with this visit?
• What special considerations should you make with a child diagnosed with Down syndrome?
• Based on the Frankl scale of behavioral assessment, how would you rate this patient's behavior?

Ethical Dilemma

CASE 1

Mom presents with her 17-year-old son, George, with a medical history of Asperger syndrome, developmental delay and dairy allergy. George's caregiver, Nona, usually comes to all medical and dental visits, but is going to be running late for today's appointment. George's mother has multiple appointments scheduled for the day and insists that her son's appointment begin without Nona's assistance.

George is cooperative about walking to the treatment room, but is hesitant to sit in the dental chair. George's mother begins to physically push George into the chair stating he just needs a gentle nudge. George's mother asks the hygienist to help her to "force her son into the chair" and becomes upset when the hygienist declines to do so.

Fortunately, Nona arrives. It takes 10 minutes to coax George into the dental chair. Nona suggests that the appointment be rescheduled because George is "having a bad day." George's mother refuses to reschedule saying that "George only requires a bit of tough love."

George remains uncooperative, squeezing his lips closed, and struggling. The entire time, George's mother is adamant that the dental team help her force the George to complete his treatment today. She states she had put a lot of effort and time into bringing George to the dental office today. She asks the hygienist for his/her opinion about trying to continue with treatment today.

1. What is the best approach for behavioral guidance for a special needs patient?
2. Should a dental clinician continue to "push" a patient to complete treatment? Does this change in the case of an emergency?
3. Are there ethical principles in conflict in this case?

References

1. Avery DR, Dean JA, McDonald RE. *McDonald and Avery's Dentistry for the Child and Adolescent*. 10th ed. St. Louis, MO: Elsevier; 2016:700.
2. Friedman N. Iatrosedation: the treatment of fear in the dental patient. *J Dent Educ*. 1983;47(2):91–95.
3. Krikken JB, Vanwijk AJ, Tencate JM, Veerkamp JS. Child dental anxiety, parental rearing style and dental history reported by parents. *Eur J Paediatr Dent*. 2013;14(4):258–262.
4. Chhabra N, Chhabra A, Walia G. Prevalence of dental anxiety and fear among five to ten year old children: a behaviour based cross sectional study. *Minerva Stomatol*. 2012;61(3):83–89.
5. Klingberg G, Broberg AG. Dental fear/anxiety and dental behaviour management problems in children and adolescents: a review of prevalence and concomitant psychological factors. *Int J Paediatr Dent*. 2007;17(6):391–406.
6. Lee CY, Chang YY, Huang ST. Prevalence of dental anxiety among 5- to 8-year-old Taiwanese children. *J Public Health Dent*. 2007;67(1):36–41.
7. Saatchi M, Abtahi M, Mohammadi G, Mirdamadi M, Binandeh ES. The prevalence of dental anxiety and fear in patients referred to Isfahan Dental School, Iran. *Dent Res J (Isfahan)*. 2015;12(3):248–253.
8. White AM, Giblin L, Boyd LD. The prevalence of dental anxiety in dental practice settings. *J Dent Hyg*. 2017;91(1):30–34.
9. Wright GZ, Kupietzky A, eds. *Behavior management in dentistry for children*. 2nd ed. Ames, IA: John Wiley & Sons Inc.; 2014:248.
10. Dentistry AAOP. Overview: AAPD reference manual. *Pediatr Dent*. 2017;39(6):5–7.
11. Goleman J. Cultural factors affecting behavior guidance and family compliance. *Pediatr Dent*. 2014;36(2):121–127.
12. Havelka C, McTigue D, Wilson S, Odom J. The influence of social status and prior explanation on parental attitudes toward behavior management techniques. *Pediatr Dent*. 1992;14(6):376–381.
13. Klein H. Psychological effects of dental treatment on children of different ages. *J Dent Child*. 1967;34(1):30–36.
14. Shinde SD, Hegde RJ. Evaluation of the influence of parental anxiety on children's behavior and understanding children's dental anxiety after sequential dental visits. *Indian J Dent Res*. 2017;28(1):22–26.
15. Zhou Y, Cameron E, Forbes G, Humphris G. Systematic review of the effect of dental staff behaviour on child dental patient anxiety and behaviour. *Patient Educ Couns*. 2011;85(1):4–13.
16. Erikson EH. *Childhood and Society*. Reissue edition ed. New York: Norton; 1993:445.
17. Wright GZ, Stigers JI. Nonpharmacologic management of children's behaviors. In: Dean JA. *McDonald and Avery's Dentistry for the Child and Adolescent*. 10th ed. St. Louis, MO: Elsevier; 2016:700.

18. Frankl SN, Shiere FR, Fogels HR. Should the parent remain with the child in the dental operatory? *J Dent Child.* 1962;29:150–163.

19. Adair SM, Waller JL, Schafer TE, Rockman RA. A survey of members of the American Academy of Pediatric Dentistry on their use of behavior management techniques. *Pediatr Dent.* 2004;26(2):159–166.

20. Dentistry AAOP. Behavior guidance for the pediatric dental patient. *Pediatr Dent.* 2017;39(6):246–259.

21. Folayan MO, Idehen E. Factors influencing the use of behavioral management techniques during child management by dentists. *J Clin Pediatr Dent.* 2004;28(2):155–161.

22. Peretz B, Kharouba J, Blumer S. Pattern of parental acceptance of management techniques used in pediatric dentistry. *J Clin Pediatr Dent.* 2013;38(1):27–30.

23. Singh H, Rehman R, Kadtane S, Dalai DR, Jain CD. Techniques for the behavior management in pediatric dentistry. *Int J Sci Stud.* 2014;2(7):269–272.

24. Peretz B, Zadik D. Attitudes of parents towards their presence in the operatory during dental treatments to their children. *J Clin Pediatr Dent.* 1998;23(1):27–30.

25. Peretz B, Zadik D. Parents' attitudes toward behavior management techniques during dental treatment. *Pediatr Dent.* 1999;21(3):201–204.

26. Pfefferle JC, Machen JB, Fields HW, Rosnick WR. Child behavior in the dental setting relative to parental presence. *Pediatr Dent.* 1982;4(4):311–316.

27. Ramos ME, Kao JY, Houpt M. Attitudes of pediatric dentists toward parental presence during dental treatment of children. *J N J Dent Assoc.* 2010;81(3):32–37.

28. Dentistry AAOP. Informed consent. *Pediatr Dent.* 2017;39(6):397–399.

29. LeBlang TR, Roso AJ, White C. Informed consent to medical and surgical treatment. In: Sanbar SS. *Legal Medicine.* 6th ed. St. Louis, MO: Mosby; 2004:750.

30. Sfikas PM. A duty to disclose. Issues to consider in securing informed consent. *J Am Dent Assoc.* 2003;134(10):1329–1333.

31. Perinatal and infant oral health care. *Pediatr Dent.* 2017;39(6):208–212.

32. Dentistry AAOP. Guideline on periodicity of examination, preventive dental services, anticipatory guidance/counseling, and oral treatment for infants, children, and adolescents. *Pediatr Dent.* 2017;39(6):188–196.

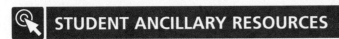

STUDENT ANCILLARY RESOURCES

A wide variety of resources to enhance your learning is available online:

- Audio Glossary
- Book Pages
- Chapter Review Questions and Answers

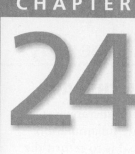

Clinical Application. Treating patients with periodontal diseases is a dynamic process
that requires constant monitoring and continual reassessment of ongoing therapy. Periodontal therapy
is often divided into phases and one of the first phases of therapy following comprehensive periodontal
assessment is the nonsurgical therapy phase. Members of the dental team need to have a clear
understanding of the importance of nonsurgical periodontal therapy and the decisions that are required
following this therapy. This chapter provides an overview of nonsurgical periodontal therapy, discusses
some of the problems that can arise during this therapy, and outlines the decisions needed following
re-evaluation of the nonsurgical therapy.

Learning Objectives

- Explain the term and name four goals for nonsurgical periodontal therapy.
- Explain the role of interdisciplinary collaborative care in nonsurgical periodontal therapy.
- Write a typical treatment plan for nonsurgical therapy for (1) a patient with dental biofilm-induced
  gingivitis and (2) a patient with generalized stage I, grade A periodontitis.
- Describe the type of healing to be expected following instrumentation of root surfaces.
- Explain strategies for managing dental hypersensitivity during nonsurgical therapy.
- Explain why re-evaluation is an important step during nonsurgical therapy.
- List steps in an appointment for re-evaluation of the results of nonsurgical therapy.
- Describe the rationale and list the indications for referring a patient to a periodontist.

Key Terms

Nonsurgical periodontal therapy
Interdisciplinary care
Periodontal instrumentation

Long junctional epithelium
Dentinal hypersensitivity
Re-evaluation

Nonresponsive disease sites
Co-management

Section 1
Overview of Nonsurgical Periodontal Therapy

UNDERSTANDING NONSURGICAL PERIODONTAL THERAPY

1. **Nonsurgical Periodontal Therapy Defined.** Nonsurgical periodontal therapy is a term used to describe the many nonsurgical steps used to eliminate inflammation in the periodontium of a patient with periodontal disease. The goal is to return the periodontium to a healthy state that can then be maintained by a combination of both professional care and patient self-care.
   A. **The "Gold Standard"**
      1. Nonsurgical periodontal therapy is a cornerstone of periodontal therapy and the first recommended approach to control periodontal infections.
      2. Although, nonsurgical periodontal therapy has evolved over the years, it is still the "gold standard" to which other treatment methods are compared.[1-4]
   B. **Alternate Terminology**
      1. Many terms have been used to describe nonsurgical periodontal therapy, and this fact may create some confusion. Some of the other terms that have been used to describe this same phase of treatment include initial periodontal therapy, initial therapy, hygienic phase, anti-infective phase, cause-related therapy, phase I treatment, and soft tissue management.
      2. Nonsurgical periodontal therapy, however, is one of the most frequently used terms for this phase of periodontal care.
2. **What Does Nonsurgical Periodontal Therapy Include?** Nonsurgical periodontal therapy includes self-care education, periodontal instrumentation, and the use of chemical agents to prevent or control periodontal disease. It is convenient to view nonsurgical periodontal procedures as the initial step in the periodontal treatment for a patient, but for many patients, nonsurgical periodontal therapy is all that is needed to bring periodontal disease under control. The use of chemical agents in periodontal care is presented in Chapter 27.
3. **What Are the Broad Objectives of Nonsurgical Periodontal Therapy?** Ideally, nonsurgical periodontal therapy should (1) eliminate both living bacteria in the microbial biofilm and calcified biofilm microorganisms (dental calculus) from the tooth surface and adjacent soft tissues, (2) eliminate inflammation of the periodontium, and (3) return the periodontium to a healthy state that can then be maintained by a combination of patient self-care and professional care.
4. **Philosophy for Nonsurgical Periodontal Therapy**
   A. The basic philosophy for developing a sensible plan for nonsurgical periodontal therapy should be to plan treatment that will provide for the control, elimination, or minimization of (1) primary etiologic factors for periodontal disease, (2) local risk factors for periodontal disease, and (3) systemic risk factors for periodontal disease.
   B. Procedures included in a plan for nonsurgical periodontal therapy should be selected to meet the needs of each individual patient; therefore, nonsurgical therapy plans can vary from patient to patient.
5. **General Principles of Controlling Periodontal Infection**
   A. **Patient Self-Care**
      1. Patients can remove *supragingival* plaque biofilm with daily brushing and use of interdental aids and/or water flossing devices.
      2. Unfortunately, studies show that many patients lack the motivation or skills to sustain a biofilm-free dentition over a substantial period of time.

3. Clinical trials indicate that self-care alone, without the routine professional care, usually does not provide for long-term success in reversing gingivitis.[5-8]

B. **Professional Care**

1. Ramseier and colleagues examined a group of subjects first in 1970 and again in 2010 to assess long-term attachment loss and periodontitis-related tooth loss. The results of this study conclude that calculus removal, biofilm control, and the control of gingivitis *are essential* in preventing disease progression, further loss of attachment, and ultimately tooth loss.[9]

2. Routine periodontal instrumentation is required to keep the *subgingival* microbial biofilm under control.[3]

3. Adequate removal of *subgingival* biofilm is virtually impossible for patients to achieve on their own.[10,11]

4. Studies indicate that periodontal instrumentation is needed approximately every 3 months to disrupt the harmful biofilm and to prevent or reverse any damage to the periodontal attachment apparatus.[2] Another reason for a 3-month recall is the need for continuous self-care coaching and patient motivation.

5. Over time, in patients with good compliance and with demonstrably stable supra- and subgingival environments, maintenance intervals may be extended.

6. **Factors Influencing Nonsurgical Therapy Outcomes.** Not all patients respond well to nonsurgical periodontal therapy.

A. **Patient Compliance Factors.** Poor patient compliance with daily self-care and regular professional maintenance appointments are common factors in unfavorable treatment outcomes.

B. **Lifestyle or Systemic Factors.** Systemic diseases/conditions and local factors may give rise to an increased prevalence, incidence or severity of gingivitis and periodontitis.[12,13]

C. **Disease Factors.** Some cases of periodontitis are refractory and do not respond favorably in spite of well-executed nonsurgical periodontal therapy and patient self-care. In such a scenario, referral to a periodontist is prudent.

GOALS OF NONSURGICAL PERIODONTAL THERAPY

Nonsurgical periodontal therapy constitutes the first step in controlling periodontal infections. The goals of nonsurgical periodontal therapy are discussed below and summarized in Box 24-1.

1. **Goal 1: To minimize the bacterial challenge to the patient**

A. Control of the bacterial challenge usually involves intensive training of the patient in appropriate techniques for self-care in combination with frequent professional care for the removal of calculus deposits and bacterial products from tooth surfaces.[1]

B. Removal of calculus deposits and bacterial products contaminating the tooth surfaces is an important step in achieving control of the bacterial challenge. Calculus deposits are always covered with living microbial biofilms that are associated with continuing inflammation if not removed.[14]

2. **Goal 2: To eliminate or control local contributing factors for periodontal disease**

A. Local contributing factors can increase the risk of developing periodontitis in localized sites. For example, defective restorations with overhangs can lead to plaque biofilm retention in a localized area. Local contributing factors are discussed in Chapter 17.

B. Biofilm retention at a site over time allows periodontal pathogens to live, multiply, and lead to damage of the periodontium.

C. A thorough plan for nonsurgical periodontal therapy will always include minimizing the impact of local environmental contributing factors.

3. **Goal 3: To minimize the impact of systemic factors for periodontal disease**
   A. It is apparent that there are certain systemic diseases or conditions that can increase the risk of developing periodontitis or can increase the risk of developing more severe periodontitis where periodontitis already exists.[13]
      1. Systemic diseases or conditions such as diabetes mellitus may have a significant impact on long-term treatment outcomes.[15–19] Genetic susceptibility to periodontal disease is responsible for at least some disease occurrence.[20,21]
      2. Smoking is a highly significant risk factor for periodontitis.[12,22]
         a. Smokers exhibit compromised healing following nonsurgical and surgical therapy compared with nonsmokers or former smokers.
         b. *Since the majority of patients who do not respond well to therapy are smokers, smoking education and cessation programs should be included as part of a comprehensive nonsurgical periodontal treatment plan when indicated.*
      3. Systemic factors are discussed in Chapter 16 of this book.
   B. A thorough plan for nonsurgical therapy always includes measures to minimize the impact of systemic risk factors. For example, a periodontitis patient with a family history of diabetes mellitus should be evaluated to rule out undiagnosed diabetes as a contributing systemic factor to the periodontitis. This medical evaluation should occur as part of the nonsurgical periodontal therapy. Another example would be that a patient who smokes should receive smoking cessation counseling.

4. **Goal 4: To stabilize the attachment level**
   A. The ultimate goal of nonsurgical periodontal therapy in periodontitis patients is to stabilize the level of attachment by eliminating inflammation in the periodontium.
   B. Stabilization of the attachment level by eliminating inflammation involves control of all of the factors listed in the other goals of nonsurgical periodontal therapy.

Box 24-1. Goals of Nonsurgical Periodontal Therapy

Goal 1: To minimize the bacterial challenge to the patient
Goal 2: To eliminate or control local environmental risk factors for periodontal disease
Goal 3: To minimize the impact of systemic risk factors for periodontal disease
Goal 4: To stabilize the attachment level by eliminating inflammation

---

TYPES OF PROCEDURES INCLUDED IN NONSURGICAL THERAPY

Box 24-2 lists some of the nonsurgical therapy procedures that the dental team may utilize for patients. The list of procedures that may be included in nonsurgical therapy is lengthy, but it should be evident that while some of the procedures are included in the treatment of all patients, other procedures are utilized only rarely. Since each patient presents unique treatment challenges, members of the dental team will need to customize the selection of the nonsurgical procedures included for each individual.

1. **Customized Patient Education and Self-Care Instructions**
   A. Patient education is a vital component of nonsurgical periodontal therapy. The dental team should ensure, from the onset of treatment, that the patient understands the long-term implications of periodontitis, both in terms of treatment effects and the risks of nontreatment. Patients should be made aware that once the active phase of treatment is completed, they will require regular maintenance appointments to keep their periodontal condition stable.
   B. Another important aspect of nonsurgical periodontal therapy is effective daily self-care by the patient. Thus, patients need to be taught self-care skills and also be motivated to use those skills. These important topics are discussed in Chapters 25 to 27.
2. **Instrumentation of Tooth Surfaces.** Periodontal instrumentation is always an important component of nonsurgical periodontal therapy. The thoroughness of periodontal instrumentation determines the overall success of nonsurgical periodontal therapy in most patients.
3. **Use of Antimicrobial Agents.** A variety of antimicrobial agents are available in the form of irrigation solutions and gel applications. Antimicrobial agents are discussed in Chapter 27.
4. **Use of Adjunctive Supragingival and Subgingival Irrigation.** Some patients may benefit in supplementing their routine home oral hygiene regimen with an oral irrigation device. The rationale and the indications for oral irrigation devices are discussed in Chapter 26.
5. **Correction of Local Contributing Factors.** Correction of local contributing factors such as overhanging margins on restorations or control of food impaction is a critical component of nonsurgical periodontal therapy in many patients. In some cases, surgical therapy is necessary to gain better access to the local contributing factor so as to completely eliminate it, as in the case of a large subgingival restorative overhang. Local contributing factors are discussed in Chapter 17.
6. **Interprofessional Collaboration for Correction of Systemic Risk Factors**
   A. The American Dental Hygienists Association defines interdisciplinary care as two or more health care providers working within their respective disciplines who collaborate with the patient and/or caregiver to develop and implement a care plan.[23] Interprofessional collaboration values a team-based approach which emphasizes responsibility, accountability, communication, and cooperation between medical professionals, dental professionals, and allied health professionals to promote patient-centered care and positive outcomes.
   B. Correction of systemic risk factors such as undiagnosed diabetes is a critical component of nonsurgical periodontal therapy in some patients. This component often demands careful coordination of care with other health care providers such as physicians in light of the close interrelationship between oral health and systemic health. Systemic conditions that amplify susceptibility to periodontal diseases are discussed in Chapter 16. Additionally, the influence of periodontal disease on systemic health is discussed in Chapter 34.
7. **Modulation of Host Defenses.** When indicated, modulation of host defenses can also be a component of nonsurgical periodontal therapy. Modulation of host defenses is discussed in Chapter 28.

Box 24-2. Procedures That May Be Included in Nonsurgical Periodontal Therapy

1. Customized self-care instructions including
   a. Mechanical plaque biofilm control
   b. Chemical plaque biofilm control
   c. Adjunctive supragingival and subgingival oral irrigation
2. Periodontal instrumentation of tooth surfaces
3. Use of antimicrobial agents
4. Correction of local contributing factors
5. Interdisciplinary care for correction/control of systemic risk factors
6. Modulation of host defenses

NONSURGICAL THERAPY RELATED TO THE PERIODONTAL DIAGNOSIS

Nonsurgical periodontal therapy is indicated for many patients, if not all patients. It may be helpful to view some common periodontal diagnoses and to see how nonsurgical periodontal therapy normally relates to these diagnoses.

1. **A Diagnosis of Dental Biofilm-Induced Gingivitis**
   A. Nonsurgical periodontal therapy is the primary type of care provided for most patients with dental biofilm-induced gingivitis.
   B. Thorough nonsurgical therapy can normally bring dental biofilm-induced gingivitis under control and bring it to a point that periodontal health can be maintained by a combination of both professional care and patient self-care.
   C. This general relationship between nonsurgical therapy and a diagnosis of dental biofilm-induced gingivitis should not be interpreted to mean that patients with this diagnosis never need periodontal surgery, since periodontal surgery is sometimes needed to correct other existing problems (i.e., gingival recession or gingival overgrowth) in gingivitis patients.

2. **A Diagnosis of Stage I or II With Grade A Periodontitis**
   A. Thorough nonsurgical therapy can also bring many cases of incipient or moderate periodontitis under control and bring it to a point that periodontal health can be maintained by a combination of both professional care and patient self-care.[24–27]
   B. It should be noted that some patients with this type of periodontitis diagnosis may require periodontal surgery if the periodontium does not respond favorably to standard nonsurgical treatment principles.[28]
   C. Periodontal surgery is sometimes used to correct other problems (i.e., gingival recession) and may indeed be indicated in any patient.
   D. A patient with a periodontitis grade of Grade A exhibits few risk factors is more responsive to standard periodontal therapy. Nonetheless, it is important to periodically monitor and continually reassess an individual's periodontitis grade at each recall visit to identify any potential future risk factors (i.e., patient resumes smoking habit) that may alter the estimate of the future course of the disease.

3. **A Diagnosis of Stage III or Stage IV With Grade B or C Periodontitis**
   A. For most patients with Stage III or Stage IV periodontitis, control of the periodontitis requires thorough nonsurgical periodontal therapy, more advanced periodontal procedures, such as periodontal surgery. As explained in Chapter 7, both stage III and stage IV represent a periodontitis that is characterized by

significant periodontal breakdown which severely jeopardizes the support and function of the dentition.

B. Although periodontal surgery is frequently indicated for patients with more advanced periodontitis, it should be understood that *most patients with periodontitis can benefit from undergoing nonsurgical therapy prior to periodontal surgical intervention.*

C. Nonsurgical periodontal therapy is frequently successful in minimizing the extent of any surgery subsequently needed and may be needed to improve the outcomes of that periodontal surgery.

D. A patient with a periodontitis grade of Grade B or C exhibits several known risk factors (i.e., smoking factors, systemic factors, etc.) that increase the likelihood of the disease progressing at a greater rate than is typical for the majority of the population and are less responsive to standard periodontal therapies. Thus, such a patient will require more intensive management of their condition and will need to be continually reassessed to identify any newly emerging future risk factors that may alter the estimate of the future course of the disease.

TYPICAL TREATMENT PLANS FOR NONSURGICAL PERIODONTAL THERAPY

A treatment plan for nonsurgical therapy is a list of nonsurgical procedures or interventions that addresses a patient's periodontal health needs as identified during the periodontal assessment. Although it is critical for a treatment plan for nonsurgical therapy to meet the needs of each individual patient, new clinicians often find it helpful to view examples of typical treatment plans. A properly designed treatment plan for nonsurgical periodontal therapy could include procedures to be carried out *by the dental hygienist, by the dentist, or by the patient. It is important to keep in mind that the examples of the typical treatment plans provided below are intended to augment, not replace, the sound clinical judgement of the dental provider. In turn, the obligation of the practitioner is to design an individualized treatment plan that is tailored to specifically address the needs of an individual patient.*

1. **Examples of Typical Treatment Plans**
   A. **Dental Biofilm-Induced Gingivitis.** A typical plan for nonsurgical therapy for a patient with moderate dental biofilm-induced gingivitis might include the following:
      1. Customized self-care instructions including patient education and motivation.
      2. Periodontal instrumentation (typically a dental prophylaxis in American Dental Association terminology).
      3. Elimination of plaque retentive factors such as overhanging restorations, caries, or ill-fitting dental prostheses.
      4. Re-evaluation of the patient's periodontal status.
         a. Response to nonsurgical therapy is normally delayed, since it takes some time for the body defense mechanisms to respond to individual treatment steps.
         b. Because of this delay time in healing, the dental team is obligated to re-evaluate the results of nonsurgical periodontal therapy after a period of healing to ensure that all appropriate measures have been included and to identify any other measures that might be needed.
         c. It is wise for the dental team to include this re-evaluation step in the plan for nonsurgical therapy so that the patient has a clear understanding from the outset how future treatment decisions will be made.

B. Stage I or Stage II With Grade A Periodontitis. As already discussed, it is always important to customize the nonsurgical therapy for the needs of each patient, but again it may be helpful to look at a typical nonsurgical plan for a patient with incipient or moderate periodontitis. This typical plan might include the following:

1. Customized self-care instructions including patient education and motivation.
2. Periodontal instrumentation (typically scaling and root planing in American Dental Association terminology).
3. Control of local risk factors to include steps such as removal of overhanging restorations, restoration of caries, or minimizing excessive occlusal forces.
4. Correction of systemic risk factors to include steps such as smoking cessation counseling or referral for control of diabetes.
5. Re-evaluation of patient's periodontal status.

C. Stage III or Stage IV With Grade B or C Periodontitis. Most patients with stage III or stage IV periodontitis exhibit complicating factors such as advanced attachment loss, deep probing depths, advanced alveolar bone loss, furcation involvements, or mucogingival problems that require some more advanced treatment procedures later in therapy.

1. A typical treatment plan for nonsurgical therapy for a patient with stage III or stage IV periodontitis may require periodontal surgery as part of the treatment plan.

   a. Members of the dental team should be aware of the possible need for periodontal surgical intervention in patients with more advanced periodontitis.

   b. As the severity of periodontitis increases, it becomes more likely that periodontal surgery will be needed to bring the disease under control.

   c. The need for periodontal surgical therapy should be re-evaluated after the completion of nonsurgical periodontal therapy. Surgical periodontal therapy is discussed in Chapter 29.

Section 2
Mechanical Nonsurgical Therapy

OVERVIEW OF INSTRUMENTATION IN NONSURGICAL THERAPY

1. **Periodontal Instrumentation During Nonsurgical Therapy.** It is generally accepted that removal of pathogenic microorganisms that form plaque biofilms and calculus on cementum is the major goal of periodontal instrumentation.
   A. **Plaque Biofilm**
      1. Because of the structure of biofilms, physical removal of plaque biofilm is the most effective mechanism of control, though chemical agents are sometimes used to improve the patient response to these procedures.
      2. Most subgingival biofilm within pockets *cannot* be reached by brushes, floss, or antibacterial rinses.
         a. For this reason, frequent periodontal instrumentation of subgingival root surfaces to remove or disrupt plaque biofilms mechanically is an essential component of the treatment of most patients with periodontitis.
         b. In fact, periodontal instrumentation is likely to remain an important component of nonsurgical periodontal therapy for the foreseeable future.
   B. **Calculus Deposits**
      1. Removal of calculus deposits from tooth surfaces is a critical component in any plan for nonsurgical periodontal therapy.
      2. Calculus deposits harbor living bacterial biofilms; thus, if the calculus remains, so do the bacteria, making it impossible to re-establish periodontal health. Calculus removal is always a fundamental part of nonsurgical periodontal therapy.
2. **Preservation of Root Cementum During Periodontal Instrumentation**
   A. **Cementum's Role in the Periodontium**
      1. Cementum is a key component of periodontal tissues, and its preservation is of paramount importance for the quality of healing at completion of periodontal both nonsurgical and surgical treatment modalities.
      2. Cementum can influence the activities of periodontal cells and may play an important regulatory role in periodontal treatment. *The ideal outcome for periodontal therapy arises from the removal of supragingival and subgingival biofilm and calculus while preserving root cementum.*
      3. Periodontal reattachment or new attachment as end-result of therapy strongly relies on the presence of cementum after root instrumentation. *Improper or aggressive mechanical instrumentation may reduce the thickness or eventually remove all the cementum over the root surface. This will result in exposure of dentin to the oral environment and make the tooth more susceptible to root caries or dentinal hypersensitivity.*
      4. Cementum provides tooth attachment and maintenance of occlusal relationships between the jaws.
   B. **Historical Perspectives Regarding Cementum Removal**
      1. Previously it was accepted that bacterial endotoxins or bacteria penetrate the cementum of periodontally diseased root surfaces.
      2. This concept resulted in the removal of all or most of the cementum as a primary endpoint of periodontal healing.[29,30]
      3. More specifically, the goal of periodontal therapy was to obtain a treated root surface with smooth and hard surface characteristics that was free of endotoxins.[29,31]

C. **Current Evidence-Based Perspectives Regarding Cementum Removal**

1. In contrast, recent studies report that endotoxins are not located within cementum[20,32] and removal of cementum is not necessary for a successful periodontal treatment.[33]

2. The preservation of cementum on the root surface was further supported by Saygin et al. who reported that cementum was necessary for new attachment and as a source of growth factors.[34,35]

3. Furthermore, Grzesik and Narayanan suggested that cementum plays an important regulatory role in periodontal regeneration.[36]

4. *From these studies, it can be concluded that conservation of cementum is necessary for optimal periodontal health as well as for periodontal regeneration.*

5. During periodontal instrumentation, the extent of instrumentation should be limited to that needed to obtain a favorable tissue response. Root surfaces should be instrumented only to a level that results in resolution of tissue inflammation in the periodontal tissues.

3. **Evolving Instrumentation Terminology.** There has been some evolution in the terminology associated with dental calculus and plaque biofilm removal over the past years. The careful reader will be wise to note the terminology that appears in many dental hygiene journals and textbooks compared to the terminology in dental journals and textbooks. The differences in this terminology are described below.

A. **Traditional Instrumentation Terminology.** Traditional instrumentation terminology uses the terms scaling and root planing. As traditionally defined, *scaling* is instrumentation to remove plaque biofilm and calculus off the root surface while *root planing* is a treatment procedure designed to remove diseased cementum that is contaminated with toxins or microorganisms.

B. **Emerging Instrumentation Terminology**

1. Recently in the dental hygiene literature, increasing numbers of authors are using new terminology that reflects modern therapy better than the traditional terminology. The term "periodontal instrumentation" or "periodontal debridement" is suggested to replace the older terms scaling and root planning.

2. Periodontal instrumentation (periodontal debridement) is defined as the removal or disruption of plaque biofilm, its byproducts, and biofilm retentive calculus deposits from coronal tooth surfaces and tooth root surfaces to the extent needed to re-establish periodontal health and restore a balance between the bacterial flora and the host's immune responses.

C. **Considerations Regarding Emerging Terminology and Insurance Codes**

1. Insurance codes are numeric codes to identify different dental procedures. The most important use of codes is for insurance billing purposes. Insurance codes are entered on insurance forms indicating the dental treatment listed by the appropriate procedure code number. In the United States, insurance codes are published in the *American Dental Association Current Dental Terminology*. These codes are very specific and should be reviewed carefully before specific dental treatment is coded.

2. The *ADA Current Dental Terminology* continues to use the traditional terms "prophylaxis" and "scaling and root planing" to describe periodontal instrumentation. This difference in terminology can be confusing to clinicians.

   a. Although the term periodontal instrumentation/debridement as defined in the dental hygiene literature may describe modern periodontal therapy better than older terms, this terminology has not yet replaced the older terms as recognized by the ADA. For this reason, many dentists have been reluctant to embrace the new terminology without changes in ADA codes.

b. Some authors and clinicians have redefined the term "root planing" so that its meaning is similar to that of periodontal instrumentation/debridement. This approach of redefining the term root planing can be confusing, however, because it is difficult to determine which definition of "root planing" any one person is using.

c. At this time, *dental team members should use the currently accepted insurance codes when filling out insurance forms and in communications with insurance companies or other third-party payers.*

END POINT FOR INSTRUMENTATION DURING NONSURGICAL THERAPY

The end point of periodontal instrumentation is to return the tissues of the periodontium to a state of health. In this context health means periodontal tissues that are free of inflammation.

1. Healing Following Nonsurgical Instrumentation
   A. After thorough periodontal instrumentation, some healing of the periodontal tissues will normally occur.
      1. The primary type of healing in a site of attachment loss after periodontal instrumentation is through the formation of a long junctional epithelium.
         a. As inflammation in the periodontium resolves, epithelial cells can readapt to the root surface as shown in Figure 24-1.
         b. This adaptation of the epithelial cells to the root surface is referred to as a long junctional epithelium.
      2. **It is important to realize that following periodontal instrumentation, there normally is** *no formation of new alveolar bone, new cementum, or new periodontal ligament.* In other words, nonsurgical periodontal instrumentation does *not* stimulate periodontal regeneration.
   B. Clinically, nonsurgical periodontal therapy, including instrumentation, may certainly result in reduced probing depths. Figure 24-2 shows examples of various soft tissue responses to thorough periodontal instrumentation.
      1. The reduced probing depths result from the formation of a long junctional epithelium combined in many instances with resolution of gingival edema that is usually a part of the inflammatory process. Figure 24-3 shows how some of this reduction in probing depth can occur at the base of a periodontal pocket.
      2. Thus, one important clinical feature to monitor following periodontal instrumentation, in addition to clinical attachment loss, is the probing depths.
      3. It should be noted at this point that there are other clinical signs that can correlate with inflammation that can be expected to change following periodontal instrumentation (i.e., bleeding on probing).
2. **Assessing Tissue Healing.** Tissue healing does not occur overnight, and in many patients, it is not possible to assess the true tissue response until at least 1 month after the completion of periodontal instrumentation. Assessing tissue healing during and following nonsurgical therapy is discussed in Section 3 of this chapter.

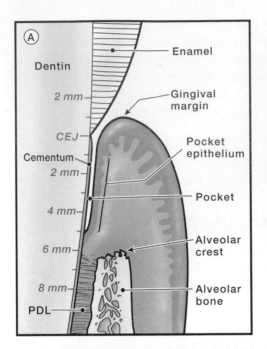
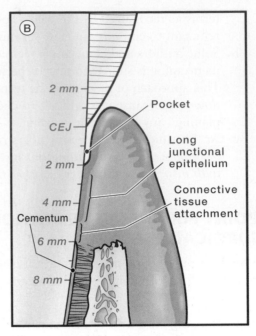

Figure 24-1. Healing After Nonsurgical Periodontal Instrumentation. The drawing on the left depicts the tissue before therapy; the periodontal pocket has a probing depth of 6 mm. The drawing on the right depicts the tissue after periodontal therapy; the tissue healing is through the formation of a long junctional epithelium. This results in a probing depth of 3 mm. Note that there is no formation of new bone, cementum, or periodontal ligament during the healing process that occurs after nonsurgical periodontal instrumentation.

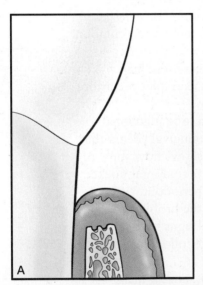
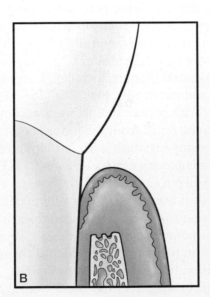
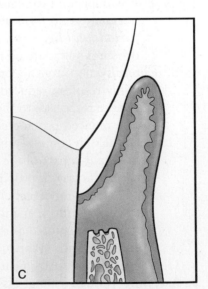

Figure 24-2. Soft Tissue Responses to Thorough Periodontal Instrumentation. This figure shows some of the possible tissue changes that can occur following thorough periodontal instrumentation of a root surface:
A. There can be complete resolution of the inflammation resulting in shrinkage of the tissue and a shallow probing depth.
B. There can be readaptation of the tissues to the root surface with a long junctional epithelium resulting in a shallow probing depth.
C. There can be very little change in the level of the soft tissues resulting in a residual periodontal pocket.

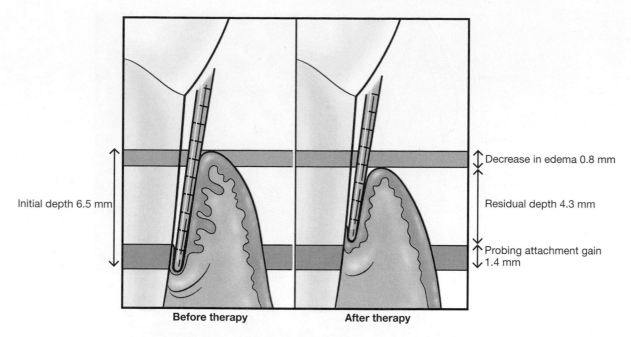

Figure 24-3. Details of Healing at the Base of a Pocket Following Periodontal Instrumentation. Since the tip of a periodontal probe can easily penetrate inflamed soft tissue in the base of periodontal pocket, the probing depth can decrease a small amount following instrumentation because the tissues at the base of the pocket can be much more resistant to deeper penetration by the probe. This figure also depicts a slight decrease in gingival edema resulting from resolution of inflammation in the tissue.

DENTINAL HYPERSENSITIVITY ASSOCIATED WITH NONSURGICAL THERAPY

Dentinal hypersensitivity as described in this section is not really a periodontal disease or a periodontal condition. It is not even considered a pathologic condition since "sensitive" dentin histologically looks the same and physiologically behaves the same as "nonsensitive" dentin. In fact, some clinicians believe that the sharp pain characteristic of dentinal hypersensitivity may be the normal pulpal response when the dentin is exposed to the oral environment. However, dentinal hypersensitivity appears so frequently during successful nonsurgical periodontal therapy that clinicians need to be aware of this condition, understand its origin, and understand therapies for the condition. On the other hand, it should be kept in mind that not all teeth with exposed dentin are sensitive to mechanical, chemical, osmotic, tactile, or thermal stimuli; in such situations, the open dentinal tubule is covered by a protective smear layer protecting it from the external stimuli.

1. **Introduction to Dental Hypersensitivity**
   A. **Dentinal hypersensitivity** (also referred to as dentinal sensitivity) is a short, sharp, painful reaction that occurs when areas of exposed dentin are subjected to mechanical, thermal, or chemical stimuli. For example, an individual might experience sensitivity while brushing, when eating cold foods such as ice cream, or when eating sweet, sour, or acidic foods such as grapefruit. In some patients simply breathing in cold air while walking outside on a cold day can produce this painful reaction.
   B. **Anatomy of the Dento-Pulpal Complex**
      1. Throughout the thickness of the dentin, there are long, miniature branching tunnels known as dentinal tubules. The dentinal tubes are typically oriented perpendicular to the long axis of the tooth (Fig. 24-4).

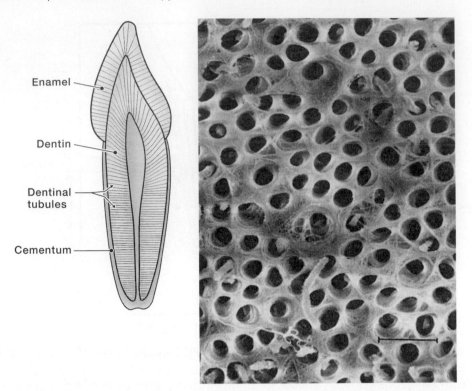

Figure 24-4. Dentinal Tubules. The drawing on the left shows the numerous dentinal tubules that penetrate the dentin. On the right, a scanning electron micrograph of the cross section of dentinal tubules adjacent to the pulp chamber of a human tooth. The black line engraved in the lower right is 10 microns long. (Used by permission from Melfi RC, Alley KE. *Permar's Oral Embryology and Microscopic Anatomy*. 10th ed. Philadelphia, PA: Lippincott Williams & Wilkins; 2000:120, Figure 5-8.)

    2. Within each dentinal tubule is an odontoblastic process which is a direct extension of a cell in the tooth pulp known as an odontoblast (Fig. 24-5) and dentinal fluid which is extracellular fluid that surrounds the odontoblastic process.

    3. One of the functions of cementum is to protect the underlying radicular dentin. As long as the cementum remains intact and covers the radicular dentin, the underlying dentin will be protected from any external stimuli that could potentially trigger the pain associated with dentinal hypersensitivity.

C. Mechanism of Dentinal Hypersensitivity

    1. Dentinal hypersensitivity develops in two phases. First, the dentin loses its protective cementum covering (lesion localization). This leads to exposure of the dentinal tubules to the oral environment (lesion initiation).

    2. There are three theories which have been proposed to explain the mechanism behind dentinal hypersensitivity.

        a. Direct Stimulation Theory

            1) Under this theory, it was previously postulated that the pulpal nerve could extend through the entire extent of the dentinal tubule. As such, any external stimulus that acts upon the exposed dentinal tubules could potentially activate the nerve ending.

            2) However, this theory lost much credence as it was later found that pulpal nerve endings do not traverse through the entire length of the dentinal tubule and innervate the outer dentin which is the most sensitive part of the root.[37]

b. Odontoblastic Transducer Mechanism Theory

    1) It was previously postulated that the odontoblasts themselves act as receptor cells which relay signals to a nerve terminal. This, in turn, would stimulate the pain fibers in the pulp and trigger the sudden sharp pain sensation characteristic of dentinal hypersensitivity.[38]

    2) This theory, however, lost much support when subsequent microscopic studies failed to show synapses between odontoblasts and nerve terminals.[39]

c. Hydrodynamic Theory

    1) This theory proposes that movement of the dentinal fluid in the tubules activates nerve cell endings that initiate the pain response at the dentin-pulpal complex.[40]

    2) Stimuli—such as cold thermal stimulus, hot thermal stimulus, evaporative stimulus—cause the dentinal fluid to shift back-and-forth within the tubule. This movement of the fluid, in turn, excites the nerve cell endings and triggers the sharp pain response characteristic of dentinal hypersensitivity.

    3) The hydrodynamic theory would explain why some patients with dentinal hypersensitivity may experience sharp pain when inhaling cold air through the mouth. *Currently, the Hydrodynamic Theory is the most widely accepted theory to explain dentinal hypersensitivity.*

2. Precipitating Factor for Hypersensitivity

    A. Dentinal hypersensitivity is usually associated with recession of the gingival margin. Factors which can cause apical displacement of the gingival margin include traumatic toothbrushing, dental erosion, and periodontitis. Even nonsurgical periodontal therapy can cause the gingival margin to recede because of the resolution of swelling of the gingiva. In fact, approximately half of patients who undergo scaling and root planing experience post-treatment dentinal hypersensitivity.[41]

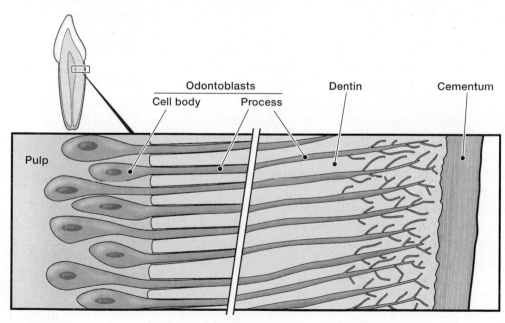

Figure 24-5. Odontoblastic Process. The odontoblastic cell process in the dentinal tubule often fills the part of the dentinal tubule closest to the pulp but can extend farther from the pulp toward the junction of the dentin with the enamel or cementum.

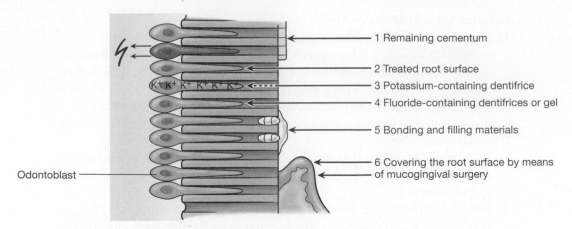

1 Remaining cementum

2 Treated root surface

3 Potassium-containing dentifrice

4 Fluoride-containing dentifrices or gel

5 Bonding and filling materials

6 Covering the root surface by means of mucogingival surgery

Odontoblast

Figure 24-6. The Various Possibilities for Dentinal Tubules Following Therapy. Chemicals can be used to occlude the dentinal tubules and to eliminate or minimize associated dentinal sensitivity. Another treatment modality is mucogingival surgery to cover the exposed root surface, thereby eliminating dentinal hypersensitivity. Soft tissue grafts will also provide a more esthetic outcome as it reestablishes the natural contours and harmony of the gingival margin of the affected tooth with adjacent teeth.

B. **Dentinal Hypersensitivity Following Periodontal Instrumentation**
   1. It should be noted that most dentinal hypersensitivity following periodontal instrumentation is mild and resolves within a few weeks *if the exposed root surfaces are kept biofilm free by thorough self-care.*
   2. In its more severe forms, however, dentinal hypersensitivity can result in so much discomfort that it can prevent a patient from performing thorough self-care. It is fortunate that most instrumentation of root surfaces does not result in the development of dentinal hypersensitivity.
   3. Sensitivity may not occur in some instances because instrumentation of root surfaces can result in a smear layer of dentin that covers the root surfaces and blocks the tubules. This so-called "smear layer" refers to crystalline debris from the tooth surface that covers or plugs the dentinal tubules during the instrumentation; this smear layer blocks the tubules, inhibits fluid flow, and prevents the development of sensitivity.
3. **Strategies for Managing Patients With Dentinal Hypersensitivity.** There are a number of strategies that have been recommended for dealing with dentinal hypersensitivity (Fig. 24-6). These strategies range from simply allowing the open dentinal tubules to seal themselves to performing periodontal surgery. Each of the strategies has proved successful for some patients. Table 24-1 provides an overview of chemical agents that have been investigated for the control of dentinal hypersensitivity by occluding dentinal tubules.
A. **Periodontal Instrumentation in Patients With Existing Dental Hypersensitivity**
   1. For teeth with existing dentinal hypersensitivity, instrumentation of hypersensitive root surfaces can result in eliciting the sharp pain during a clinical procedure such as periodontal instrumentation or drying the tooth with a compressed stream of air.
   2. Since many patients have existing dentinal hypersensitivity, it is critical for dental hygienists to ask patients about hypersensitive teeth prior to attempting a clinical procedure such as periodontal instrumentation.
   3. For patients with existing hypersensitivity, local anesthesia can be used to control any discomfort that might arise during thorough instrumentation.

B. **Patient Education—A Critical Element in Patient Management.** In the patient's eyes, the development of the tooth sensitivity could well appear to be simply a result of the nonsurgical treatment. In reality most often the sensitivity results from areas where clinical attachment loss has previously occurred as a result of existing periodontitis. An appropriate strategy for managing patients undergoing nonsurgical periodontal therapy would include educating patients about the possibility of developing hypersensitivity following the procedure. This warning should be given before beginning any treatment and should be part of the discussion preceding informed consent. It may be helpful to provide the patient with the following facts before initiating instrumentation:
1. Sensitivity to cold can increase following periodontal instrumentation.
2. If sensitivity resulting from periodontal instrumentation occurs, it will usually gradually disappear over a few weeks.
3. *Thorough daily plaque biofilm removal during self-care is one of the most important factors in the prevention and control of sensitivity.* It should be noted that without meticulous self-care, treatments for dentinal hypersensitivity are usually not successful.
4. If dentinal hypersensitivity becomes an ongoing problem, recommendations for in-home therapies can be made that can enhance its resolution, but immediate results should not be expected.

C. **Occluding Patent (Open) Dentinal Tubules With In-Home Therapies**
1. One important strategy for managing patients with dentinal hypersensitivity involves applying chemicals to the exposed root surface that can help occlude (or block) the openings of the dentinal tubules.
2. The chemicals used to occlude the dentinal tubules often eliminate or minimize associated sensitivity. The mechanism of action of these chemicals has been reported to be precipitating minerals or precipitating proteins within open dentinal tubules resulting in sealing the openings of the tubules.
3. Many of these chemical agents are available in special formulations of toothpastes, and there are a variety of toothpastes specifically formulated to aid in desensitizing teeth.[42–45] Many chemical agents have been reported to help in some patients. Examples of some of the more common chemical agents in toothpaste formulations for dentinal hypersensitivity are potassium nitrate, strontium chloride, sodium citrate, and fluorides. Table 24-1 includes an overview of some of the chemical agents that have been investigated for control of hypersensitivity by blocking dentinal tubules.
4. The reported efficacy of the chemical agents in controlling dentinal hypersensitivity varies, but this strategy remains the most commonly utilized treatment for this condition.

D. **Occluding Patent Tubules With In-Office Therapies**
1. There are also professionally applied in-office products that contain chemicals that also have been reported to decrease dentinal hypersensitivity.
2. A variety of chemical agents have been utilized in in-office remedies for dentinal hypersensitivity. Examples of chemicals that have been reported to decrease hypersensitivity following in office applications are potassium oxalate, ferric oxalate, and fluorides solutions, or fluoride varnishes.
3. Note that Table 24-1 includes an overview of some of the chemical agents that have been investigated for control of hypersensitivity by blocking dentinal tubules.

E. **Desensitizing Nerves Associated With the Tubules.** It has also been reported that applying certain chemicals to the root surface can block the nerve receptors in or near the tooth pulp from activating the painful response.
   1. The chemical agents that can be used to block the nerve receptors from activating a painful response include potassium salts (such as potassium nitrate); potassium nitrate is the active ingredient found in some desensitizing toothpastes and has been shown to be effective in decreasing sensitivity in some patients.
   2. It is thought that potassium depolarizes the nerve fibers associated with the odontoblastic processes thus preventing pain signals from traveling to the brain.

F. **Treating Exposed Dentin Surfaces With Lasers**
   1. Lasers have been used to treat exposed hypersensitive dentin surfaces with some success.
   2. The mechanism of action of lasers in decreasing dentinal hypersensitivity is not clear at this point.

G. **Blocking Dentinal Tubules With Restorative Materials**
   1. One strategy for blocking some dentinal tubules is to cover the exposed dentin surface with a bonding agent—the same kinds of materials that can sometimes be used to restore caries.
   2. Since the exposure of dentin at some sites can be associated with missing tooth structure resulting from abrasion or erosion of the root surface, bonding a restorative material over that surface can not only block exposed dentinal tubules, it can also restore any missing tooth structure.
   3. Examples of restorative materials that have been used to block dentinal tubules include oxalic acid and resin, glass ionomer cements, composites, and dentin bonding agents.

H. **Blocking Dentinal Tubules With a Periodontal Surgical Procedure**
   1. Another strategy for blocking the open dentinal tubules is to cover the root surface with a gingival grafting material.
   2. This approach can result in rebuilding the gingiva to a more natural level that covers an exposed tooth root, covering the dentinal tubules.

TABLE 24-1	**OVERVIEW OF AGENTS THAT HAVE BEEN INVESTIGATED FOR THE CONTROL OF HYPERSENSITIVITY BY OCCLUDING DENTINAL TUBULES**

Agents that can precipitate proteins that can occlude dentinal tubules

• Glutaraldehyde	• Zinc chloride
• Silver nitrate	• Strontium chloride

Agents that can precipitate minerals that can occlude dentinal tubules

• Sodium fluoride	• Calcium phosphate
• Stannous fluoride	• Calcium carbonate
• Strontium chloride	• Arginine
• Potassium oxalate	• Bioactive glass

Section 3
Decisions Following Nonsurgical Therapy

THE RE-EVALUATION APPOINTMENT

Re-evaluation refers to a formal step after the completion of nonsurgical therapy. During the re-evaluation appointment, the members of the dental team perform another periodontal assessment to gather information about the patient's periodontal status and determine how well the periodontium has responded to initial therapy. After comparison with the periodontal status at the time of the initial assessment, the team members make several critical clinical decisions regarding management of the patient's periodontal condition. The re-evaluation is described in detail below.

1. The Re-evaluation Appointment
    A. **Timing of a Re-evaluation**
        1. Periodontal tissue healing does not occur immediately, and in most cases it is not possible to determine the true tissue response for at least 1 month after the completion of nonsurgical periodontal therapy.
        2. Members of the dental team should usually schedule an appointment for a re-evaluation of a periodontitis patient 4 to 6 weeks after completion of nonsurgical therapy.
    B. **Understanding the Steps in a Re-evaluation.** The steps in a typical re-evaluation appointment usually include those listed below (Box 24-3):
        1. The first step in the re-evaluation appointment is to do a medical status update for the patient. Of course, this is the first step in any patient appointment.
        2. The second step is to perform a thorough clinical periodontal assessment; the nature of a clinical periodontal assessment has already been described in Chapter 19.
        3. The third step is to do a comparison of the results of the patient's initial periodontal assessment with the results of the patient's re-evaluation assessment.
        4. The fourth step is to make appropriate decisions related to the next steps in therapy.
2. Options for Treatment Following Re-evaluation
    A. **Managing Nonresponsive Disease Sites.** During the re-evaluation, members of the dental team may identify nonresponsive disease sites.
        1. Nonresponsive disease sites are areas in the periodontium that show deeper probing depths, continuing loss of attachment, or continuing clinical signs of inflammation in spite of the nonsurgical therapy provided. As explained in Chapter 7, this would be consistent with the characteristics of a refractory periodontitis.

Box 24-3. Steps in a Typical Re-evaluation Appointment

1. Update the medical status of the patient.
2. Perform a periodontal clinical assessment.
3. Compare the initial periodontal assessment with the re-evaluation assessment.
4. Make decisions related to the next steps in periodontal therapy.

2. Nonresponsive sites should be carefully rechecked for thoroughness of self-care and rechecked for the presence of residual calculus deposits.

3. If plaque biofilm is discovered at a nonresponsive site, the site should be thoroughly deplaqued with an ultrasonic instrument (unless ultrasonic instrumentation is contraindicated for this patient), and the patient should receive additional self-care motivation and training.

4. If calculus is found at a nonresponsive site, additional periodontal instrumentation should be performed.

5. When nonresponsive sites are encountered, the members of the dental team should also consider the possibility that other factors might be contributing to the disease process (such as undiagnosed diabetes or smoking).

6. In some patients, the nonresponsive disease sites may also require the use of antimicrobial agents.

7. Some nonresponsive sites represent areas of more advanced destruction from the disease process that will need more advanced care such as periodontal surgery.

B. **Performing Additional Nonsurgical Therapy.** It is common for the re-evaluation step to indicate the need for additional nonsurgical periodontal therapy by the dental team, and there are several reasons for this.

1. Self-care efforts by the patient, though improved, may not be adequate for control of inflammation in the periodontium.

2. Subgingival calculus deposits are difficult to remove especially in the presence of inflammation resulting in edematous tissue.

3. An unsuspected systemic condition may be contributing to the disease process.

C. **Establishing a Program for Periodontal Maintenance**

1. Following appropriate treatment, all patients with periodontitis should be placed on a program of periodontal maintenance.

2. Periodontal maintenance includes all measures used by the dental team and the patient to keep periodontitis under control; periodontal maintenance is discussed in Chapter 30.

3. The goal of periodontal maintenance is to prevent the recurrence of periodontal diseases.

4. At each periodontal maintenance recall visit, the dental practitioner performs a clinical reassessment of the periodontium to determine if the periodontitis is controlled. If the periodontium appears stable and the periodontitis is controlled, periodontal maintenance should be performed. However, if the periodontium is inflamed and there are signs of disease reoccurrence, then site-specific or full-mouth periodontal instrumentation should be performed. If the disease has severely deteriorated, then referral to a periodontist for surgical therapy is recommended.

D. **Recognizing the Need for Periodontal Surgery**

1. The need for some types of periodontal surgery can often be determined at the time of the initial periodontal assessment.

2. Periodontal surgery to control chronic periodontitis or to regenerate damaged periodontal tissues, however, is frequently best identified at the time of the re-evaluation; periodontal surgery and its indications are discussed in Chapter 29.

THE RELATIONSHIP OF NONSURGICAL RE-EVALUATION TO OTHER STEPS IN TREATMENT

Figure 24-7 illustrates how re-evaluation of nonsurgical periodontal therapy relates to the other steps in the overall management of a periodontal patient.

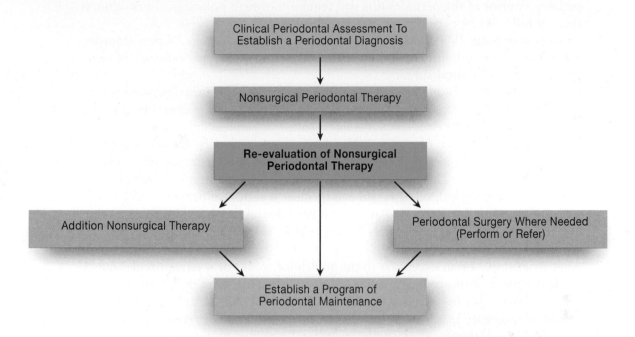

Figure 24-7. Diagram Illustrating How Re-evaluation of Nonsurgical Periodontal Therapy Relates to Other Steps in the Overall Management of a Periodontal Patient. Re-evaluation of nonsurgical therapy would be performed following the therapy. Decisions made at the re-evaluation will primarily involve additional nonsurgical therapy, periodontal surgery, and periodontal maintenance.

THE RELATIONSHIP BETWEEN NONSURGICAL AND SURGICAL THERAPY

Periodontal surgery can play an important role in therapy for certain patients, and this topic will be discussed in Chapter 29 of this textbook. However, at the time of re-evaluation, members of the dental team should be aware of the general relationship between nonsurgical periodontal therapy and periodontal surgery and should be able to discuss the possible need for periodontal surgery with patients.

1. **Indications for Surgical Therapy.** As a general rule, periodontal surgery will be needed by patients with more advanced periodontal conditions. Table 24-2 shows an overview of the general relationship of nonsurgical periodontal therapy to surgical periodontal treatment for patients with various periodontal conditions.
   A. **Patients with dental biofilm-induced gingivitis.** For most patients with plaque-induced gingivitis, the gingivitis can be controlled with nonsurgical therapy alone, and only rarely will periodontal surgery be a part of the treatment recommended.

B. **Patients with Stage I/II Periodontitis.** For most patients with Stage I periodontitis, the periodontitis can be controlled with nonsurgical therapy alone, and only occasionally will periodontal surgery be a part of the treatment recommended.

C. **Patients with Stage III Periodontitis.** For some patients with Stage III periodontitis, the periodontitis can be controlled with nonsurgical therapy alone. For other patients, control of the periodontitis will require thorough nonsurgical periodontal therapy followed by periodontal surgery.

D. **Patients with Stage IV Periodontitis.** For most patients with Stage IV periodontitis, control of the periodontitis will require thorough nonsurgical periodontal therapy followed by periodontal surgery.

2. **Exceptions.** There will always be exceptions to the general guidelines described above.

A. One example of an exception would be a patient with moderate dental biofilm-induced gingivitis where the gingivitis has resulted in gingival enlargement. It is common for some types of gingival enlargement to require periodontal surgery to eliminate the enlargement, improve esthetics, or provide for improved access for effective self-care. This type of surgical therapy is known as a gingivectomy. A patient with drug-induced gingival enlargement would also benefit from undergoing a gingivectomy. However, as all periodontal therapies, long-term benefit can only be sustained with effective patient motivation and continuous reinforcement of patient self-care.

B. Another example of an exception to the guidelines would be a patient with Stage I, grade A periodontitis accompanied by severe gingival recession on a tooth. Though surgery is not normally needed in patients with stage I periodontitis, periodontal surgery may well be needed to correct the gingival recession and/ or address the patient's chief complaints (typically related to gingival esthetics or thermal sensitivity).

TABLE 24-2	INDICATIONS FOR NONSURGICAL AND SURGICAL THERAPY	
Disease Status	**Nonsurgical Therapy**	**Surgical Therapy**
Dental biofilm-associated gingivitis	Always indicated	Usually not indicated
Stage I periodontitis	Always indicated	Usually not indicated
Stage II periodontitis	Always indicated	Usually not indicated
Stage III periodontitis	Always indicated	Sometimes indicated
Stage IV periodontitis	Always indicated	Usually indicated

RECOGNIZING THE NEED FOR REFERRAL TO A PERIODONTIST

Although the general dental team can and should treat most patients with dental biofilm-induced gingivitis and most patients with periodontitis, the need for referral of some patients from a general dental office to a periodontist is always a possibility that should be considered. Making the important decision of where the patient should receive periodontal therapy is not always easy. The members of the team should discuss this issue in detail to determine the comfort level for treating periodontitis patients within the general dental practice. There are occasions when, due to the extent and complexity of a case, a referral to a periodontist is indicated. Box 24-4 lists some of the primary reasons to refer to a periodontist.[46–51]

Certain patients may benefit from co-management by a general dental practice and periodontal office. Co-management is defined as the shared responsibility and accountability for the care of a patient. Referral of patients with periodontal problems to a periodontist depends on several factors, including:

- The severity of disease and complexity of treatment required
- The patient's desire to see a specialist or undergo specialist treatment
- The general practitioner's knowledge, experience, and training to treat patients with a range of periodontal problems
- The presence of other complicating factors such as the patient's medical history

---

Box 24-4. Clinical or Risk Factors Indicating Patients Who Would Likely Benefit From Co-management by a Periodontist

- Unresolved inflammation or continued loss of bone and/or attachment, despite nonsurgical periodontal therapy
- Managing a Stage III or Stage IV periodontitis which exhibits severe periodontal destruction
- Intensive management of a Grade B or Grade C periodontitis
- Non–plaque-induced conditions requiring specialist care, such as treatment gingival recession defects attributed to non-periodontitis reasons
- Patients requiring surgical procedures involving tissue augmentation or regeneration, including management of mucogingival problems, infrabony defects, and furcation invasions
- Patients requiring surgery involving bone removal (e.g., crown lengthening)
- Patients requiring surgery associated with osseointegrated implants
- Patients with medical history that significantly affects medical management (e.g., head/neck radiotherapy, intravenous bisphosphonate therapy, bleeding disorders)
- Patients that the general dental office team does not feel comfortable treating, for any reason

Chapter Summary Statement

Nonsurgical periodontal therapy refers to all the initial steps used by the dental team to bring gingivitis and periodontitis under control. The goals of nonsurgical periodontal therapy are to control the bacterial challenge to the patient, to minimize the impact of systemic risk factors, to eliminate or control local environmental risk factors, and to stabilize the attachment level. The precise steps included in nonsurgical periodontal therapy should depend on the specific needs of each individual patient.

A vital component of a plan for nonsurgical periodontal therapy is periodontal instrumentation. Biofilms are resistant to topical chemical control; therefore, mechanical periodontal instrumentation of subgingival root surfaces is an essential component of successful nonsurgical periodontal therapy. Dentinal hypersensitivity may occur in some areas of exposed dentin. Thorough daily self-care is the most important factor in the prevention and control of hypersensitivity, but some patients with dentinal hypersensitivity will need additional measures.

Re-evaluation is an important step in nonsurgical periodontal therapy. During re-evaluation the dental team determines the patient's need for additional nonsurgical therapy, referral of the patient for periodontal surgery, or enrollment of the patient in a periodontal maintenance program.

Section 4
Focus on Patients

Clinical Patient Care

CASE 1

Mr. H. just returned for a 6-week re-evaluation appointment following nonsurgical periodontal therapy for periodontitis. Clinically, Mr. H. exhibits poor tissue healing and generalized plaque biofilm.

Though the patient denies having diabetes, the patient does report having several close family members with this disease.

Make a list of steps your dental team might include in an appropriate plan for nonsurgical periodontal therapy for this new patient.

CASE 2

At the time of re-evaluation for a patient with a diagnosis of periodontitis, your dental team identifies a few sites of residual subgingival calculus deposits and documents totally ineffective patient self-care. How should the members of your dental team manage the oral health needs of this patient?

CASE 3

Ms. J is a 22-year-old pregnant female who presents to your office with periodontal disease. She reports a chief complaint "My gums are bleeding a lot when I brush." She is currently in her second trimester and is unsure if she should be receiving dental treatment at this time. What steps would you take with her physician to coordinate her care? Also, how would you explain to the patient that dental treatment during the second trimester of pregnancy is safe and beneficial to the fetus and the mother?

CASE 4

Mr. R is a 44-year-old male who presents to your office with painful, bleeding gingiva and a fetid odor. He appears thin and emaciated. During your exam, he states "My gum line just seems to be sloughing off." You suspect that he may be suffering from necrotizing periodontal disease and an undiagnosed immunocompromised disorder. He reports that he has not seen a physician in the last 7 years. As part of your comprehensive periodontal examination, how would you motivate the patient to seek a medical evaluation? Also, if he undergoes a medical evaluation and is diagnosed with an immunocompromised disorder, how would this affect your dental management of this patient?

CASE 5

One of your patients who has been undergoing nonsurgical periodontal therapy seems a bit upset when he comes in another appointment. After being seated in your treatment room, he states that he gets a sharp pain in his teeth when he tries to eat his favorite desert, ice cream. How should you proceed based upon the patient's complaint?

CASE 6

Mr. A is a 76-year-old patient who reports to your office for a routine periodontal maintenance. He is currently undergoing hemodialysis. What steps would you take with his physician to coordinate proper management of his dental care? Also, what affects does hemodialysis have on the planned dental treatment?

CASE 7

Mr. B is a 63-year-old patient who presents to your office for a comprehensive periodontal evaluation. He reports a history of leukemia that he is currently managing with his physician. During your examination, you note that the gingiva generally appears swollen with spontaneous hemorrhaging. What steps would you take with his physician to coordinate proper management of his dental care?

Ethical Dilemma

You are a retired librarian who just recently lost your husband. You grew up, went to college, married and raised a family all in the same town in which you were born. You are fortunate to be surrounded by many family members and long-time friends.

You are currently a patient in Dr. Jay Mack's periodontal practice, and have been for the last 15 or so years. You see Evelyn, the older of the two hygienists in the practice, every 3 months. The only supplemental aids she has suggested that you use, in addition to tooth brushing, are "tufted floss and a tongue scraper."

You are very active in your church and community. At your weekly bridge club gathering, several other participants mention that they also are patients in Dr. Mack's practice. Further discussions revealed that all the patients who saw Evelyn were instructed to use tufted floss and tongue scrapers, for their self-care. However, those patients who saw Anne, the younger hygienist, were instructed to use a variety of self-care aids. It sounds like Anne recommends different aids based on each individual patient's needs. Your bridge partner, Florence who also sees Evelyn, the hygienist, says her teeth are very sensitive to hot, cold, and sweets, yet has only been instructed and educated in the use of tufted floss and a tongue scraper as well.

You wonder why so many patients with differing needs receive the same instructions from the dental hygienist, Evelyn.

1. What ethical principles are in conflict in this dilemma?
2. Should you meet with Dr. Mack to discuss your concerns?
3. How should this ethical dilemma be handled?

References

1. Drisko CH. Nonsurgical periodontal therapy. *Periodontol 2000.* 2001;25:77–88.
2. Lindhe J, Nyman S. Long-term maintenance of patients treated for advanced periodontal disease. *J Clin Periodontol.* 1984;11(8):504–514.
3. Smiley CJ, Tracy SL, Abt E, et al. Evidence-based clinical practice guideline on the nonsurgical treatment of chronic periodontitis by means of scaling and root planing with or without adjuncts. *J Am Dent Assoc.* 2015;146(7):525–535.
4. Tanwar J, Hungund SA, Doddani K. Nonsurgical periodontal therapy: A review. *J Oral Res Rev.* 2016;8:39–44.
5. De la Rosa M, Zacarias Guerra J, Johnston DA, Radike AW. Plaque growth and removal with daily toothbrushing. *J Periodontol.* 1979;50(12):661–664.
6. Listgarten MA, Lindhe J, Hellden L. Effect of tetracycline and/or scaling on human periodontal disease. Clinical, microbiological, and histological observations. *J Clin Periodontol.* 1978;5(4):246–271.
7. Listgarten MA, Schifter CC, Laster L. 3-year longitudinal study of the periodontal status of an adult population with gingivitis. *J Clin Periodontol.* 1985;12(3):225–238.
8. Macgregor ID, Rugg-Gunn AJ, Gordon PH. Plaque levels in relation to the number of toothbrushing strokes in uninstructed English schoolchildren. *J Periodontal Res.* 1986;21(6):577–582.
9. Ramseier CA, Anerud A, Dulac M, et al. Natural history of periodontitis: Disease progression and tooth loss over 40 years. *J Clin Periodontol.* 2017;44(12):1182–1191.
10. Axelsson P, Nystrom B, Lindhe J. The long-term effect of a plaque control program on tooth mortality, caries and periodontal disease in adults. Results after 30 years of maintenance. *J Clin Periodontol.* 2004;31(9):749–757.
11. Page RC, Offenbacher S, Schroeder HE, Seymour GJ, Kornman KS. Advances in the pathogenesis of periodontitis: summary of developments, clinical implications and future directions. *Periodontol 2000.* 1997;14:216–248.
12. Position paper: tobacco use and the periodontal patient. Research, Science and Therapy Committee of the American Academy of Periodontology. *J Periodontol.* 1999;70(11):1419–1427.
13. Kinane DF, Marshall GJ. Periodontal manifestations of systemic disease. *Aust Dent J.* 2001;46(1):2–12.
14. Rabbani GM, Ash MM, Jr., Caffesse RG. The effectiveness of subgingival scaling and root planing in calculus removal. *J Periodontol.* 1981;52(3):119–123.
15. Teng YT, Taylor GW, Scannapieco F, et al. Periodontal health and systemic disorders. *J Can Dent Assoc.* 2002;68(3):188–192.
16. Scannapieco FA. Position paper of The American Academy of Periodontology: periodontal disease as a potential risk factor for systemic diseases. *J Periodontol.* 1998;69(7):841–850.
17. Jindal A, Parihar AS, Sood M, Singh P, Singh N. Relationship between Severity of Periodontal Disease and Control of Diabetes (Glycated Hemoglobin) in Patients with Type 1 Diabetes Mellitus. *J Int Oral Health.* 2015;7(Suppl 2):17–20.
18. Grossi SG, Genco RJ. Periodontal disease and diabetes mellitus: a two-way relationship. *Ann Periodontol.* 1998;3(1):51–61.
19. Casanova L, Hughes FJ, Preshaw PM. Diabetes and periodontal disease: a two-way relationship. *Br Dent J.* 2014;217(8):433–437.

20. Michalowicz BS, Wolff LF, Klump D, et al. Periodontal bacteria in adult twins. *J Periodontol*. 1999;70(3):263–273.

21. Hodge P, Michalowicz B. Genetic predisposition to periodontitis in children and young adults. *Periodontol 2000*. 2001;26:113–134.

22. Tonetti MS. Cigarette smoking and periodontal diseases: etiology and management of disease. *Ann Periodontol*. 1998;3(1):88–101.

23. Association ADH. ADHA Policy Manual. Chicago, IL: ADHA; 2016. Available from https://www.adha.org/resources-docs/7614_Policy_Manual.pdf. Accessed September 7, 2018.

24. Badersten A, Nilveus R, Egelberg J. Effect of nonsurgical periodontal therapy. I. Moderately advanced periodontitis. *J Clin Periodontol*. 1981;8(1):57–72.

25. Cobb CM. Clinical significance of non-surgical periodontal therapy: an evidence-based perspective of scaling and root planing. *J Clin Periodontol*. 2002;29 Suppl 2:6–16.

26. Greenstein G. Nonsurgical periodontal therapy in 2000: a literature review. *J Am Dent Assoc*. 2000;131(11):1580–1592.

27. Lowenguth RA, Greenstein G. Clinical and microbiological response to nonsurgical mechanical periodontal therapy. *Periodontol 2000*. 1995;9:14–22.

28. Stambaugh RV, Dragoo M, Smith DM, Carasali L. The limits of subgingival scaling. *Int J Periodontics Restorative Dent*. 1981;1(5):30–41.

29. Jones WA, O'Leary TJ. The effectiveness of in vivo root planing in removing bacterial endotoxin from the roots of periodontally involved teeth. *J Periodontol*. 1978;49(7):337–342.

30. O'Leary TJ. The impact of research on scaling and root planing. *J Periodontol*. 1986;57(2):69–75.

31. Chace R. Subgingival curettage in periodontal therapy. *J Periodontol*. 1974;45(2):107–109.

32. Moore J, Wilson M, Kieser JB. The distribution of bacterial lipopolysaccharide (endotoxin) in relation to periodontally involved root surfaces. *J Clin Periodontol*. 1986;13(8):748–751.

33. Nyman S, Westfelt E, Sarhed G, Karring T. Role of "diseased" root cementum in healing following treatment of periodontal disease. A clinical study. *J Clin Periodontol*. 1988;15(7):464–468.

34. Narayanan AS, Bartold PM. Biochemistry of periodontal connective tissues and their regeneration: a current perspective. *Connect Tissue Res*. 1996;34(3):191–201.

35. Saygin NE, Giannobile WV, Somerman MJ. Molecular and cell biology of cementum. *Periodontol 2000*. 2000;24:73–98.

36. Grzesik WJ, Narayanan AS. Cementum and periodontal wound healing and regeneration. *Crit Rev Oral Biol Med*. 2002;13(6):474–484.

37. Frank RM, Steuer P. Transmission electron microscopy of the human odontoblast process in peripheral root dentine. *Arch Oral Biol*. 1988;33(2):91–98.

38. Rapp R, Avery JK, Strachan DS. Possible role of the acetylcholinesterase in neural conduction within the dental pulp. In: Finn SB, ed. *Biology of the Dental Pulp Organ, A Symposium*. Tuscaloosa, AL: University of Alabama Press; 1968:309–331.

39. Pashley DH. Dynamics of the pulpo-dentin complex. *Crit Rev Oral Biol Med*. 1996;7(2):104–133.

40. Brännström M. A hydrodynamic mechanism in the transmission of pain-produced stimuli through the dentine. In: Anderson DJ, ed. *Sensory Mechanisms in Dentine*. Oxford, England: Pergamon; 1963:73–79.

41. von Troil B, Needleman I, Sanz M. A systematic review of the prevalence of root sensitivity following periodontal therapy. *J Clin Periodontol*. 2002;29 Suppl 3:173–177; discussion 195–196.

42. Kimura Y, Wilder-Smith P, Yonaga K, Matsumoto K. Treatment of dentine hypersensitivity by lasers: a review. *J Clin Periodontol*. 2000;27(10):715–721.

43. Li Y. Innovations for combating dentin hypersensitivity: current state of the art. *Compend Contin Educ Dent*. 2012;33 Spec No 2:10–16.

44. Schwarz F, Arweiler N, Georg T, Reich E. Desensitizing effects of an Er:YAG laser on hypersensitive dentine. *J Clin Periodontol*. 2002;29(3):211–215.

45. Verma SK, Maheshwari S, Singh RK, Chaudhari PK. Laser in dentistry: An innovative tool in modern dental practice. *Natl J Maxillofac Surg*. 2012;3(2):124–132.

46. Darby I, Barrow SY, Cvetkovic B, et al. Periodontal treatment in private dental practice: a case-based survey. *Aust Dent J*. 2017;62(4):471–477.

47. Dockter KM, Williams KB, Bray KS, Cobb CM. Relationship between prereferral periodontal care and periodontal status at time of referral. *J Periodontol*. 2006;77(10):1708–1716.

48. Dowell P, Chapple IL; British Society of Periodontology. The British Society of Periodontology referral policy and parameters of care. *Dent Update*. 2002;29(7):352–353.

49. Ryder MI, Armitage GC. Minimally invasive periodontal therapy for general practitioners. *Periodontol 2000*. 2016;71(1):7–9.

50. Wadia R. Periodontal disease in general practice—an update on the essentials. *Dent Update*. 2014;41(5):467–469.

51. Williams KB, Burgardt GJ, Rapley JW, Bray KK, Cobb CM. Referring periodontal patients: clinical decision making by dental and dental hygiene students. *J Dent Educ*. 2014;78(3):445–453.

25 Patient's Role in Nonsurgical Periodontal Therapy

Clinical Application. For nearly every patient with periodontal disease, the patient's own efforts at self-care play a role in the outcome of nonsurgical periodontal therapy. Sometimes the self-care techniques required for a patient with periodontitis are far more complicated than the self-care efforts required by a patient with a healthy periodontium. Self-care for a periodontal patient must accommodate changes in the periodontium due to disease—examples of such changes include open embrasure spaces, exposure of root concavities, and attachment loss, as well as, patient ability and interest. This chapter provides guidance for clinicians working together with patients to collaboratively select and use appropriate self-care devices.

Learning Objectives

- In a classroom or laboratory setting, explain the criteria for selection and correctly demonstrate the use of the following to an instructor: power toothbrush and the interdental aids presented in this chapter.

- Explain why interdental care is of special importance for a patient with periodontitis.

- In a clinical setting, recommend, explain, and demonstrate appropriate interdental aids to a patient with type III embrasure spaces. Assist the patient in selecting an appropriate interdental aid that the patient is willing to use on a daily basis.

- Explain how the presence of exposed root concavities in a dentition would influence your selection of effective self-care aids.

- State the rationale for tongue cleaning and in the clinical setting, recommend and teach tongue cleaning to an appropriate patient.

Key Terms

Co-therapist
Volatile sulfur compounds

Gingival embrasure space (Type I, II, III)
Root concavity

Section 1
Patient Self-Care in Nonsurgical Therapy

Nonsurgical periodontal therapy includes all nonsurgical treatment and educational measures used to help control gingivitis and periodontitis, such as patient self-care, periodontal instrumentation, and chemical plaque control.

1. **Patient as Co-Therapist.** Because periodontitis is plaque biofilm-associated disease, a key element of nonsurgical periodontal therapy must be directed toward its daily control by the patient.
   A. Successful nonsurgical periodontal therapy always involves the patient in a collaborative coaching program on self-care techniques.
   B. The patient's efforts at self-care are essential to the disease control and the outcome of therapy. Some dental teams refer to the patient as having the role of co-therapist in the process of nonsurgical periodontal therapy.
      1. This concept of the patient as co-therapist is used to underscore the vital role the patient plays in the daily self-management of biofilm and the stabilization of periodontitis.
      2. The patient should be actively involved in making decisions about his or her own healthcare and be willing to make a long-term commitment to meticulous self-care and regular professional care.
   C. Mechanical biofilm removal includes self-care efforts by the patient on a daily basis and subgingival periodontal instrumentation by the dental hygienist at regular intervals.
2. **Self-Care**
   A. **What is Self-Care?** There is no single accepted definition of self-care. One that has been developed for people with chronic diseases is "the actions individuals take to lead a healthy lifestyle; to meet their social, emotional, and psychological needs; to care for their long-term condition and prevent further illness or accident."[1] A recent systematic review found that periodontitis was associated with having a negative impact on the quality of life. The more severe the disease, the greater the impact.[2]
      1. Self-care education involves instruction on the use and frequency of a product. For example, suggesting the addition of a product such as interdental aid to the daily routine.
      2. The self-care plan should involve collaboration between the dental hygienist and patient.
         a. The dental hygienist needs to provide input and support while at the same time taking into consideration the patient's interest and abilities. Optimally, the final decision on self-care devices is made collaboratively.
         b. Recommending a device that the clinician likes but that the patient dislikes will not contribute to patient motivation and compliance.
         c. Collaboration hinges on good communication so the dental hygienist needs to provide education and instruction using empathy and words that the patient understands.
   B. **Goals of Self-Care.** The goal of self-care is improved oral health via optimal biofilm removal and the elimination of bleeding and inflammation.
   C. **Self-Care Aids Employed in Biofilm Control**
      1. Toothbrushing is the most frequently used aid for biofilm removal. Generally, brushing is the only daily form of self-care performed by most patients. *Interdental aids are necessary for most patients and critical for periodontal maintenance patients as the interdental area is generally not accessible to toothbrushing.*
      2. Tongue cleaning on a daily basis helps control halitosis and may contribute to a healthy periodontal environment.

Section 2
Self-Care Challenges for Patients With Periodontitis

1. **Anatomical Challenges for the Patient With Periodontitis.** Due to attachment loss, the dentition of an individual with periodontitis often presents anatomical challenges to effective biofilm control, such as recession of the gingival margin, type of embrasure spaces, and exposed root concavities.

   A. **Gingival Embrasure Spaces.** The gingival embrasure space is the small triangular open space (apical to the contact area) between the curved proximal surfaces of two teeth. The three types of embrasure spaces are shown in Figures 25-1 to 25-3.

      1. In health, the interdental papilla fills the gingival embrasure space. Dental floss is effective in areas of normal gingival contour.

      2. *The tissue destruction characterized by periodontitis usually results in an interdental papilla that is reduced in height or missing, resulting in an open embrasure space. Dental floss is not effective in areas with open embrasure spaces.*

      3. Analysis of the gingival embrasure spaces is critical in determining which interdental aid is likely to be most effective in control of plaque biofilms. Table 25-1 summarizes aids for interdental biofilm removal.

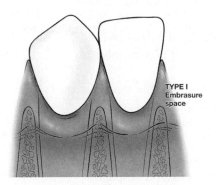

Figure 25-1. Type I Embrasure—space filled by the interdental papilla. For the patient with excellent self-care compliance and good manual dexterity, dental floss is an effective means of biofilm control.

TYPE I
Embrasure
space

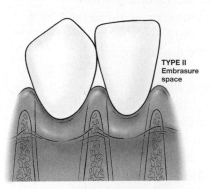

Figure 25-2. Type II Embrasure—height of interdental papilla is reduced. Interdental brushes and wooden toothpicks are effective means of biofilm control.

TYPE II
Embrasure
space

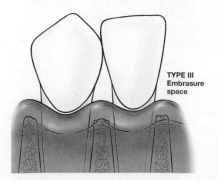

Figure 25-3. Type III Embrasure—the interdental papilla is missing. Interdental brushes and end-tuft brushes are effective means of biofilm control.

TYPE III
Embrasure
space

B. **Exposed Root Concavities.** A root concavity is a trench-like depression in the root surface. Root concavities commonly occur on the proximal surfaces of anterior and posterior teeth and the facial and lingual surfaces of molar teeth.

1. In health, root concavities are covered with alveolar bone and help to secure the tooth in the bone.

2. Periodontitis results in the apical migration of the junctional epithelium, loss of connective tissue, and destruction of alveolar bone. This tissue destruction results in the exposure of root concavities to the oral environment (either in the presence of tissue recession or, frequently, within a periodontal pocket).

3. Figure 25-4 shows the root surface of a mandibular canine covered in a colored powder; the colored powder represents plaque biofilm. Figures 25-5A,B and 25-6 demonstrate the ineffectiveness of dental floss in cleaning the root concavity of a maxillary premolar.

4. Figures 25-5C,D and 25-6 demonstrate the effectiveness of an interdental brush in cleaning the root concavity of a maxillary premolar. Note that only the interdental brush is effective in reaching the concave surface of the root concavity.

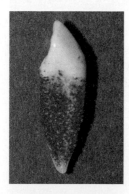

Figure 25-4. Anatomical Challenge: Biofilm Removal From Root Concavity. The proximal surface of this mandibular canine is covered with colored powder representing plaque biofilm. Figure 25-5A,B, below, compares the effectiveness of dental floss and an interdental brush in removing biofilm from an exposed root cavity.

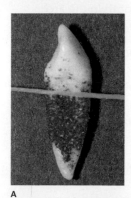
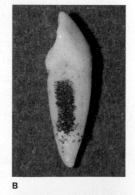

Figure 25-5A,B. Use of Dental Floss for Biofilm Removal. As seen in figures **A** and **B**, dental floss is not effective in removing the powder (simulated biofilm) from the exposed root concavity.

A

B

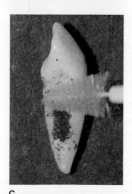
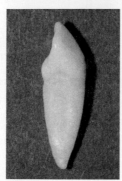

Figure 25-5C,D. Use of an Interdental Brush for Biofilm Removal. As seen in figures **C** and **D**, an interdental brush effectively removes the powder (simulated biofilm) from the root concavity.

C

D

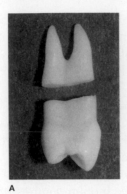
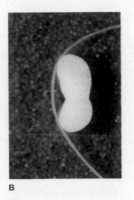
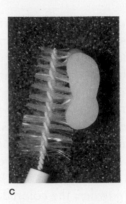

A   B   C

Figure 25-6. Application of Interdental Aids to Root Concavity in Cross Section. A. A maxillary premolar (side view) is cut to expose a cross section of the root. **B.** The root of the same maxillary premolar viewed in cross section; dental floss is unable to clean the root concavity. **C.** The bristles of the interdental brush extend into the root cavity for successful biofilm removal.

TABLE 25-1	AIDS FOR INTERDENTAL PLAQUE BIOFILM REMOVAL	
Interdental Aid	**Description/Example**	**Indications for Use**
Dental floss	Unwaxed or waxed thread made of silk, nylon, or plastic monofilament fibers	A patient with type I embrasure spaces and excellent compliance to self-care regime
Floss holders	Handheld device to hold the floss or single-use device containing a segment of dental floss (Reach Access Flosser, Glide Floss Picks)	A patient with type I embrasure spaces who is motivated but has dexterity issues
Tufted dental floss	Thickened yarn-like dental floss (J & J Superfloss)	Type II embrasure spaces, fixed bridges, distal surface of last tooth in the arch, proximal surfaces of widely spaced teeth
Interdental brush	Tiny nylon brushes on a handle (Butler Gum Proxabrush) Some brands come in varying sizes (TePe Interdental Brushes)	Type II or Type III embrasure spaces. Distal surface of last tooth in the arch, exposed furcation areas that permit easy insertion of the brush Embrasure spaces with exposed proximal root concavities
End-tuft brush	Small bristle tuft on a toothbrush-like handle (Butler End-Tuft Brush)	Type III embrasure spaces, distal surface of the last tooth in arch, lingual surfaces of mandibular teeth, crowded or mis-aligned teeth, exposed furcation areas
Pipe cleaner	Standard pipe cleaner cut into 3-inch lengths	Type III embrasure spaces, exposed furcation areas that permit insertion
Toothpick in holder	A round toothpick in a plastic handle (Marquis Perio-Aid)	Type II or III embrasure spaces, biofilm removal at gingival margin, furcation areas or root concavities
Triangular wooden wedge	A triangular-shaped toothpick generally made of basswood (J & J Stim-U-Dent)	Type II or III embrasure spaces

2. **Selecting Interdental Aids for the Patient With Periodontal Disease**
   A. **Dental Floss**
      1. Description. Dental floss is unwaxed or waxed thread made of silk, nylon, or plastic monofilament fibers used to remove dental plaque biofilm from the proximal surfaces of teeth.
      2. Effectiveness. While floss tends to be the primary recommendation of most dental hygienists, patient compliance is low. *It has also been shown that a significant number of those that do floss are not able to perform the function effectively.*[3]
         a. Evidence indicates that a variety of alternative interdental aids are as effective or more effective than dental floss in removing biofilm and in reducing bleeding and gingivitis.[4]
            1) When added to toothbrushing, a study found that dental floss has been shown to significantly reduce bleeding compared to toothbrushing alone.[5]
            2) Two systematic reviews of dental floss added to manual toothbrushing found in most cases, the addition of dental floss does not increase biofilm removal or reduce gingivitis.[6,7] The authors conclude that practitioners need to determine on an individual basis whether effective flossing is a reasonable and achievable goal.[6]
            3) Two systematic reviews have looked at the ability of dental floss to reduce interproximal caries. Even though conventional wisdom has long advocated for flossing to reduce decay, no scientific studies have been conducted on adults to evaluate the ability of dental floss to reduce or prevent interproximal decay. The absence of this evidence does not mean flossing may not have an effect on interproximal decay; however, it does mean the flossing has not been proven to prevent decay.[7,8]
            4) It may be easier for some individuals to use floss via a floss holder. Flossing via floss holder has been shown to be as effective as handheld floss and a mechanism for increasing the development of a flossing habit.[9] There are many variations of floss holders. Some require manually wrapping the floss onto the holder. Others may be single-use devices with the floss already in place (Fig. 25-7).
         b. *When given a choice, patients often prefer other types of interdental cleaners to dental floss.*[4]
         c. Flossing may not be as effective for periodontal patients; recession, attachment loss, and size of the gingival embrasure space are limiting factors.[4]
         d. A water flosser has also been shown to be an effective alternative to dental floss, appropriate for patients with many types of oral anatomy and conditions.[4] The topic of irrigation is discussed in detail in Chapter 26.
         e. Some mouth rinses have been shown to be an effective alternative to dental floss. Mouth rinses are discussed in detail in Chapter 27.
      3. Indications for Recommendation of Dental Floss
         a. Type I embrasures. Dental floss is effective in removing biofilm from tooth crowns and the convex root surfaces in the region of the cementoenamel junction (CEJ). *Dental floss is not effective in removing biofilm from root concavities and grooves.*
         b. Recommended for patients with excellent compliance with self-care. Patient compliance with dental flossing is low with many patients being unable or unwilling to perform daily flossing.[3]

c. Patients who participate in crafting hobbies such as knitting, crocheting, needlepoint or woodworking may be good candidates for dental floss as they are likely more adept and comfortable at using their hands.

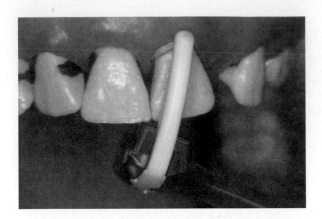

Figure 25-7. Technique for Use of Floss Holder. Flossing via a floss holder is as effective as handheld flossing provided the patient uses proper technique. The dental floss should be wrapped around the proximal tooth surface in a similar manner to the technique employed with handheld floss.

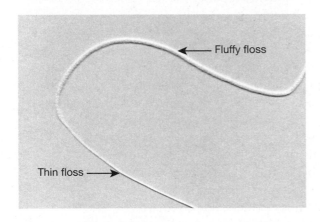

Figure 25-8. Tufted Dental Floss. This aid is a specialized type of floss consisting of a fluffy segment of yarn-like floss attached to a segment of thin floss.

B. Tufted Dental Floss
  1. Description. A specialized type of dental floss that has a segment of ordinary floss attached to a thicker, fluffy, yarn-like segment of floss (Fig. 25-8).
  2. Indications
     a. For type II embrasures.
     b. To clean under the pontic of a fixed bridge.
     c. To clean the distal surface of the last tooth in the arch.
     d. To remove plaque biofilm from the proximal surfaces of widely spaced teeth.
  3. Technique
     a. For interdental proximal surfaces, the fluffy part of the floss is used interdentally in a C-shape against the tooth, applying pressure with a slight sawing motion against first one proximal surface and then the adjacent proximal tooth surface.
     b. For fixed bridges, the tufted floss is threaded under the pontic and used to clean the undersurface of pontic. Next, the distal surface of the mesial abutment tooth and the mesial surface of the distal abutment tooth are cleaned using the tufted floss.

C. Interdental Brush

1. **Description.** Tiny conical or "pine tree" shaped nylon bristle brush attached to a handle (Fig. 25-9). Brushes are available in different diameters so that the best size can be selected. The size of the embrasure space determines the correct diameter of the bristle part of the brush. There should be a slight bit of resistance as the brush is moved back and forth between the teeth. Often it is necessary to use different size brushes within one mouth.

2. **Indications**
   a. A systematic review of interdental brushes found inconclusive evidence to determine whether interdental brushes removed more plaque than flossing.[10]
   b. Interdental brushes are recommended for biofilm removal in type II and III embrasure spaces (Fig. 25-10). Interdental brushes should not be used where the interdental papilla fills the interdental space.
   c. *The bristles of an interdental brush are very effective at cleaning root concavities.*

3. **Technique.** The brush is inserted into the open interdental space and slid in and out of the embrasure space for several strokes. *Always use the interdental brush without toothpaste.* Figure 25-11A–D shows techniques for use of interdental brushes.

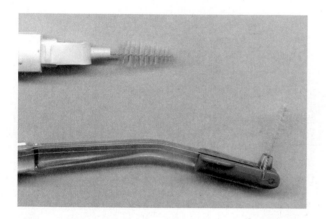

Figure 25-9. Interdental Brushes. Interdental brushes are one of the most useful aids for cleaning root concavities.

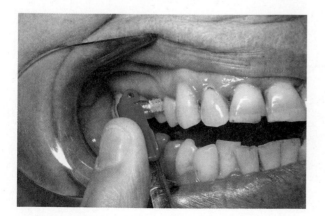

Figure 25-10. Use of Interdental Brush. (Courtesy of Dr. Deborah Milliken, South Florida Community College.)

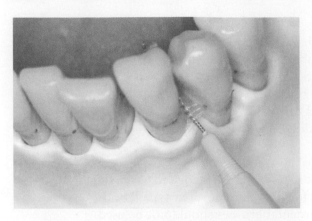

Figure 25-11. Procedure for Use of an Interdental Brush. A. The brush handle is held between the thumb and index finger and the brush gently pushed between the teeth. The brush should be maintained at a 90-degree angle to the long axis of the tooth.

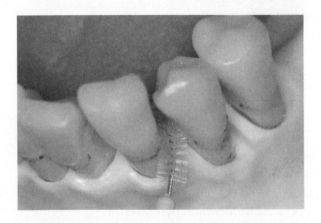

B. The bristles can be adapted to tooth surfaces with slight pressure and varying the angle of insertion. For optimal biofilm removal, the brush is slid in and out of the space using the entire length of the bristle part of the brush.

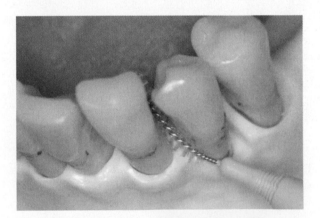

C. By changing the angle of insertion, the bristles can be adapted to the mesial surface of the first premolar. Slight pressure with the brush against the gingiva allows the bristles to clean slightly beneath the gingival margin.

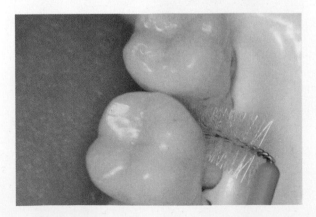

D. For posterior areas, advise the patient to close his or her mouth slightly to relax the cheek. The brush may be bent to facilitate insertion between posterior teeth.

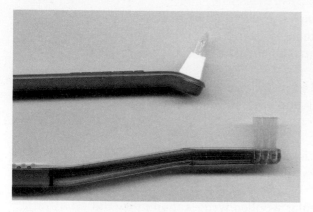

Figure 25-12. End-Tuft Brushes. End-tuft brushes are used to clean areas that are difficult to access with a standard brush.

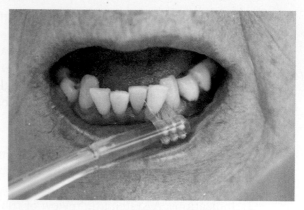

Figure 25-13. Use of End-Tuff Brush. End-tuff brush used around crowded anterior teeth. (Courtesy of Dr. Deborah Milliken, South Florida Community College.)

D. End-Tuft Brush
1. Description. An end-tuff brush is similar to a standard toothbrush except that the brush head has only a small tuft of bristles (Fig. 25-12). A standard toothbrush easily can be modified to create a customized end-tuft brush by removing some of the bristles.
2. Indications
   a. Effectively reaches sites around teeth that are difficult for patients to clean, such as the distal surface of the last tooth in the arch, lingual surfaces of mandibular teeth, and crowded or misaligned teeth (Fig. 25-13).
   b. Works well to remove biofilm from type III embrasure spaces.
   c. Useful in removing biofilm from an exposed furcation area since the small size of the bristle tufts allows them to partially enter the furcation site.
3. Technique
   a. The end of the tuft is directed into the embrasure space or furcation area. Gentle circular strokes are used to clean the area.
   b. For difficult-to-reach mandibular lingual tooth surfaces, the brush is used like a standard brush with a sulcular brushing technique.

E. Wooden Toothpick in a Holder
1. Description. This device consists of a round toothpick in a plastic handle.
2. Indications
   a. The toothpick in a holder has been shown to reduce biofilm and bleeding as effectively as dental floss.[11]
   b. It can be used gently along or slightly below the gingival margin or directed into exposed furcation areas for biofilm removal.
   c. Effective in type II embrasures if the toothpick is easily inserted between the teeth; however, this aid is not effective in cleaning root concavities unless the teeth are widely spaced.
3. Technique for Use of a Wooden Toothpick in a Holder
   a. A toothpick is secured in the holder and the long end is broken off flush with the holder so that it will not scratch the inside of the cheek (Fig. 25-14).
   b. The end of toothpick is moistened with saliva.

c. The toothpick tip is applied at right angles to the tooth or directed just beneath the gingival margin at a less than 45-degree angle. The tip should not be directed against the epithelial attachment. The tip is used to trace the gingival margin around each tooth.

d. Where space permits, the tip is angled into embrasure spaces or exposed furcation areas and moved gently back and forth to remove accumulated biofilm.

F. Wooden Wedge

1. Description. This aid is a short wooden stick usually made of soft wood. These wedges are triangular, wedge-shaped sticks and should not be confused with round or rectangular toothpicks.

2. Indications. A systematic review of triangular wooden wedges found they did not increase the amount of visible biofilm removal beyond toothbrushing but they did improve interdental inflammation better than brushing alone.[12] To use a wedge there must be sufficient interdental space available to allow easy placement of the wooden wedge. Long-term use of wooden wedges in type I embrasures may cause a permanent loss of the papillae.

3. Technique for Use of Wooden Wedge

a. The wooden wedge should be moistened thoroughly in the mouth to soften the wood prior to use.

b. The wedge is inserted between the teeth with the *flat side next to the gums* (Fig. 25-15).

c. The wedge is used with a gentle in and out motion to clean between the teeth. The wedge should not be forced into tightly spaced teeth. The wedge should be discarded as soon as the first signs of splaying are evident.

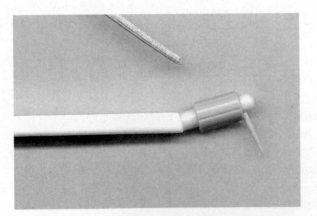

Figure 25-14. Toothpick Holder. To prepare this aid for use, secure a toothpick in the holder and break off the long end so that it is flush with the plastic holder.

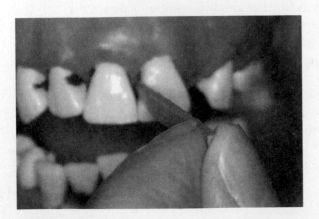

Figure 25-15. Use of Wooden Wedge. The wedge is held between the thumb and index finger with the flat side toward the gingiva. In the upper arch the flat surface faces up, and in the lower arch the flat surface faces down.

Section 3
Tongue Cleaning as an Adjunct

Many patients have coated tongues that make it difficult to maintain fresh breath and cause a lessened sense of taste. ***Periodontal patients have been shown to have significantly higher prevalence of tongue coating.***[13] Daily tongue cleaning controls halitosis and may help to maintain a healthy periodontal environment.

1. **Tongue Coating and the Role of Volatile Sulfur Compounds in Halitosis.** The tongue coating is made up of bacteria and other putrefied debris that produces hydrogen sulfide and methyl mercaptan.
   A. **Volatile sulfur compounds (VSC)** are a family of gases that are responsible for halitosis.
      1. Two members of the VSC family of gases, hydrogen sulfide and methyl mercaptan, are principally responsible for mouth odor. Methyl mercaptan is produced primarily by periodontal pathogens. Some studies have suggested that low concentrations of these gases may be toxic to tissues; however, the research in this area is limited.[14]
      2. Most patients are concerned about controlling halitosis and therefore are receptive to the introduction of tongue cleaning to their self-care routine.
      3. Tongue coating can contribute to a lessened sense of taste. Tongue cleaning should be recommended to geriatric patients who have a low desire to eat due to depressed taste sensation.
   B. Tongue cleaning is recommended because the bulk of bacteria and debris—especially the periodontal pathogens that produce methyl mercaptan—accumulate mostly within the filiform papillae and on the back of the tongue. The practice of tongue cleaning may not only make a patient feel more confident, but actually may help in maintaining a healthy periodontal environment.
2. **Technique for Use of Manual Tongue Cleaners.** Manual tongue cleaners come in a variety of styles. The two most common types are specialized toothbrushes and tongue scrapers (Fig. 25-16).
   A. The tongue brush or scraper is positioned as far back on the tongue as possible.
   B. Once the brush or scraper is in position, it is pulled forward gently over the tongue. This procedure is repeated two or three times or until the tongue is clean.
   C. When first learning tongue cleaning, some individuals gag and find the process unpleasant. In the beginning, encourage the patient to place the cleaner wherever it is most comfortable on the tongue. With regular use, most patients become accustomed to the sensation of the tongue brush or scraper and are able to clean further back on the tongue. Over time, most patients become skilled at tongue cleaning.

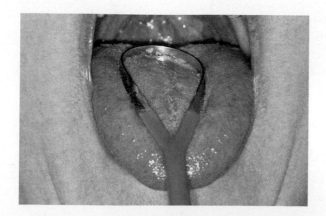

Figure 25-16. Manual Tongue Scraper. Daily tongue cleaning controls halitosis and may help to maintain a healthy periodontal environment.

Chapter Summary Statement

The patient's efforts at self-care are critical to the control of periodontitis. Since the importance of mechanical biofilm control is quite high for the patient with periodontitis, the dental hygienist should be knowledgeable about biofilm control measures and be prepared to recommend appropriate aids based on the individual needs of each patient.

Due to attachment loss, the dentition of an individual with periodontitis often presents anatomical challenges to effective biofilm control, such as recession of the gingival margin, type II or III embrasure spaces, and exposed root concavities. Interdental aids that are especially useful for patients with type II or III embrasure spaces include interdental brushes and end-tuft brushes. Daily tongue cleaning results in reduced amounts of tongue coating and improvements in breath freshness.

Section 4
Focus on Patients

Clinical Patient Care

CASE 1

A patient with periodontitis has generalized recession of the interdental gingival papillae. What options would you have for training this patient in interdental plaque biofilm control?

CASE 2

You are discussing self-care for biofilm removal with a patient with periodontitis. You point out to the patient how the biofilm control on the facial and lingual surfaces of his teeth is greatly improved and praise him for this success. The patient comments that he likes using his powered toothbrush and has been brushing longer. Unfortunately, you note that there is heavy plaque biofilm on the proximal surfaces of most teeth. The patient tells you that there is "No way that I am going to use that string. It is just too hard to use." The patient has type II embrasure spaces throughout his mouth. What suggestions might you make for interdental biofilm control?

CASE 3

A patient with periodontitis has generalized bone loss and gingival recession so that the cervical-thirds of the roots are exposed to the oral cavity. What interdental aid would you recommend to clean interproximally (between the roots)?

Evidence in Action

You recently began working as the dental hygienist in an established periodontal practice. The previous hygienist retired after a 20-year career in dental hygiene.

Today is Mrs. J.'s first maintenance appointment with you. Mrs. J. has had periodontal surgery and has type III embrasure spaces throughout her dentition. She also has extensive restorative work in her dentition. According to her patient record, at the past several maintenance visits, Mrs. J. has had very little plaque biofilm on the facial and lingual surfaces of her teeth, but moderate biofilm accumulation on the mesial and distal surfaces of her teeth. Today, your assessment reveals a similar pattern of plaque biofilm formation.

You ask Mrs. J. about her current self-care program and she explains that she has been instructed to use an electric toothbrush and dental floss daily. She says that she really likes the electric toothbrush, but simply cannot use the floss. She complaints that the floss breaks when she tries to get it between her "fillings" and that it is just simply too frustrating to use.

Based on what you know about plaque biofilm control with type III embrasure spaces what suggestions might you offer to Mrs. J as other options for her self-care regimen?

Ethical Dilemma

As a 50-year-old woman who runs a home day care center, you have been referred to Dr. Rogers' periodontal practice by your general dentist Dr. Patel. You now alternate your periodontal maintenance appointments between the two offices, with appointments every 3 months.

Six months ago, the hygienist at Dr. Rogers' office, Khoa, a recent graduate, recommended that you use an interdental brush, due to the recession and large spaces between your teeth. He spent much time educating you in the proper technique, and even watched you use it effectively in your own mouth. However, at home, you find it difficult to use, and due to the osteoarthritis in your fingers, find changing the small nylon brushes on the handle almost impossible. As a result, you have not been using the aid.

You are sitting in front of Khoa again today, and he reviews your medical history and home care regime. You explain that it has been difficult for you to be compliant with the interdental brush, and ask for an alternative periodontal aid. Khoa feels that the interdental brush is the best device for mechanical biofilm control in your situation.

1. You feel very frustrated and do not think that Khoa is being sensitive to your needs.
2. How should this ethical dilemma be handled?
3. What ethical principles are in conflict in this dilemma?

References

1. Kennedy A, Rogers A, Bower P. Support for self-care for patients with chronic disease. *BMJ.* 2007;335(7627):968–970.
2. Ferreira MC, Dias-Pereira AC, Branco-de-Almeida LS, Martins CC, Paiva SM. Impact of periodontal disease on quality of life: a systematic review. *J Periodontal Res.* 2017;52:651–665.
3. Lang WP, Ronis DL, Farghaly MM. Preventive behaviors as correlates of periodontal health status. *J Public Health Dent.* 1995;55(1):10–17.
4. Asadoorian J. Flossing: Canadian dental hygienists' association position statement. *Can J Dent Hyg.* 2006;40(3):1–10.
5. Graves RC, Disney JA, Stamm JW. Comparative effectiveness of flossing and brushing in reducing interproximal bleeding. *J Periodontol.* 1989;60(5):243–247.
6. Berchier CE, Slot DE, Haps S, Van der Weijden GA. The efficacy of dental floss in addition to a toothbrush on plaque and parameters of gingival inflammation: a systematic review. *Int J Dent Hyg.* 2008;6(4):265–279.
7. Sambunjak D, Nickerson JW, Poklepovic T, et al. Flossing for the management of periodontal diseases and dental caries in adults. *Cochrane Database Syst Rev.* 2011;(12):CD008829.
8. Hujoel PP, Cunha-Cruz J, Banting DW, Loesche WJ. Dental flossing and interproximal caries: a systematic review. *J Dent Res.* 2006;85(4):298–305.
9. Kleber CJ, Putt MS. Formation of flossing habit using a floss-holding device. *J Dent Hyg.* 1990;64(3):140–143.
10. Poklepovic T, Worthington HV, Johnson TM, et al. Interdental brushing for the prevention and control of periodontal diseases and dental caries in adults. *Cochrane Database Syst Rev.* 2013;(12):CD009857.
11. Lewis MW, Holder-Ballard C, Selders RJ, Jr., Scarbecz M, Johnson HG, Turner EW. Comparison of the use of a toothpick holder to dental floss in improvement of gingival health in humans. *J Periodontol.* 2004;75(4):551–556.
12. Hoenderdos NL, Slot DE, Paraskevas S, Van der Weijden GA. The efficacy of woodsticks on plaque and gingival inflammation: a systematic review. *Int J Dent Hyg.* 2008;6(4):280–289.
13. Bolepalli AC, Munireddy C, Peruka S, Polepalle T, Choudary Alluri LS, Mishaeel S. Determining the association between oral malodor and periodontal disease: a case control study. *J Int Soc Prev Community Dent.* 2015;5(5):413–418.
14. Calenic B, Yaegaki K, Kozhuharova A, Imai T. Oral malodorous compound causes oxidative stress and p53-mediated programmed cell death in keratinocyte stem cells. *J Periodontol.* 2010;81(9):1317–1323.

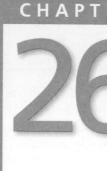

26 Supragingival and Subgingival Irrigation

Clinical Application. This chapter addresses the role of patient-applied and professional irrigation in the treatment of periodontal diseases. The primary objective of ***patient-applied home irrigation*** is to diminish gingival inflammation by physically disrupting bacterial biofilms and reducing the number of bacteria in the periodontal pocket. The goal of ***professional irrigation*** in the dental office is to enhance the outcome of periodontal instrumentation and home care by reducing the number of bacteria in the periodontal pocket.

Learning Objectives

* Discuss the oral health benefits of a water flosser for the patient with periodontal disease.
* Distinguish the depth of the delivery between the water flosser, a toothbrush, dental floss, and other interdental aids.
* Name the types of agents that can be used in a water flosser.
* In a clinical setting, be able to educate a patient how to use a water flosser.
* Summarize research findings that relate to using professional irrigation to deliver chemicals to periodontal pockets.

Key Terms

Water flosser
Oral irrigation
Hydrokinetic activity
Impact zone

Flushing zone
Standard irrigation tips
Subgingival irrigation tips
Orthodontic irrigation tips

Filament-type irrigation tips
Professional subgingival
   irrigation

Section 1
Patient-Applied Home Irrigation

1. **What is a Water Flosser?** The water flosser is a generic term for a device that safely delivers a pulsating stream of water or other solution around and between teeth above the gingival margin (supragingivally) and into the gingival sulcus or periodontal pocket (subgingivally). This process is commonly referred to as home or oral irrigation. A water flosser may also be referred to as a dental water irrigator, home irrigator, or dental water jet.

   A. **Mechanism of Action of a Water Flosser**

      1. A water flosser creates a pulsating fluid stream to flush an area with water or an antimicrobial agent. Figure 26-1 shows examples of devices used for home oral irrigation.

         a. The pulsating fluid delivered by a water flosser incorporates a compression and decompression phase that efficiently displaces biofilm, bacteria, and debris.[1,2]

         b. The pulsating fluid creates two zones of fluid movement termed hydrokinetic activity (Fig. 26-2).

            1) The area of initial fluid contact to the portion of the tooth near the gingival margin is called the impact zone.

            2) The depth of fluid penetration within a subgingival sulcus or pocket is called the flushing zone.[3]

      2. Hydrokinetic fluid movement results in movement (or penetration) of the fluid into the subgingival and interdental areas.

   B. **Fluid Penetration**

      1. A water flosser produces subgingival fluid penetration regardless of the type of tip or attachment used.[4,5]

      2. A water flosser has the greatest potential for reaching deeper into a sulcus or pocket compared to other types of oral hygiene aids such as toothbrushes and interdental devices.[4,5] Table 26-1 shows a comparison of the depth of delivery of common self-care products.

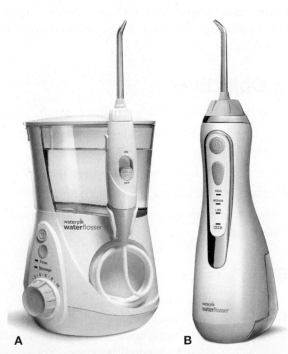

                    A   B

Figure 26-1. Water Flossers. A. A countertop dental water jet that plugs into an electrical outlet. **B.** A portable dental water jet that works off of a rechargeable battery. (Courtesy of Water Pik, Inc., Fort Collins, CO, USA.)

2. **Benefits of Home Oral Irrigation.** Studies demonstrate that the water flosser is clinically proven to remove biofilm and reduce bleeding, gingival inflammation, periodontal pathogens, and inflammatory mediators.[6–21]
   A. **Removal of Biofilm.** A water flosser used in combination with manual toothbrushing has been shown to remove 29% more biofilm than traditional brushing and flossing.[15]
   B. **Reduction in Bleeding.** Studies consistently show that the water flosser is a valuable tool for helping patients reduce bleeding.[6–10,12,13,16,17,19,20]
      1. Daily irrigation with water significantly reduced bleeding in 14 days.[10]
      2. Daily irrigation with water was significantly better than rinsing with 0.12% chlorhexidine at reducing marginal bleeding and bleeding on probing.[13]

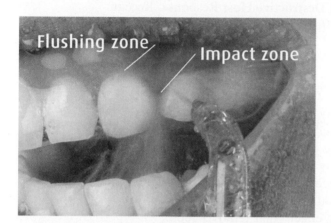

Figure 26-2. The Impact and Flushing Zones. A water flosser creates a pulsating stream of water to flush an area with fluid. The area of the tooth and gingival margin where the fluid initially contacts is called the impact zone. The depth of fluid penetration within the subgingival sulcus or pocket is called the flushing zone. (Courtesy of Water Pik, Inc., Fort Collins, CO, USA.)

TABLE 26-1	DEPTH OF DELIVERY OF VARIOUS SELF-CARE PRODUCTS	
Oral Hygiene Aid	**Penetration**	**Comments**
Toothbrush	1–2 mm	No manual or power toothbrush has clinically proven subgingival access
Oral rinsing	2 mm	Can reach less accessible areas, but penetrates subgingival areas minimally.[4]
Toothpick/wooden wedge	Depends on embrasure size	Effectiveness depends on sufficient interdental space
Interdental brush	Depends on embrasure size	Most effective with an open interdental space
Dental floss	3 mm	Cannot reach into deeper pockets
Waterpik water flosser	6 mm and beyond.[4,5]	Clinically proven to remove supra- and subgingival plaque biofilm and bacteria[15,19]

Courtesy of Water Pik, Inc., Fort Collins, CO, USA.

C. **Reduction in Gingival Inflammation.** The water flosser has been shown to reduce the clinical signs of gingivitis.[6–8,10,12,13,17]

  1. A water flosser used in combination with manual toothbrushing is more effective in the reduction of gingivitis than manual toothbrushing and flossing.[7]

  2. Daily irrigation with water significantly reduces the clinical signs of gingivitis.[8]

D. **Reduction of Periodontal Pathogens.** Studies show the dental water jet can reduce subgingival bacteria.[3,8,11,18]

  1. The water flosser has demonstrated the ability to reduce periodontal pathogens up to a 6-mm level within a periodontal pocket.[3,11]

  2. Daily irrigation with either water or 0.04% chlorhexidine significantly reduces subgingival bacteria compared to toothbrushing and 0.12% chlorhexidine rinsing.[8]

E. **Reduction in Inflammatory Mediators and Destructive Host Response.** Recent studies show that home oral irrigation is effective in significantly reducing inflammatory cytokines IL-1β and PGE_2.[6,10] These cytokines have been implicated in attachment loss and alveolar bone loss.[22,23]

F. **Purported Mode of Action.** The exact mode of action of a water pick has yet to be determined. However, various hypotheses have been put forward:

  1. The hydrokinetic movement of fluid may physically disrupt the biofilm, interfere with plaque maturation, or alter the pathogenic effects of key periodontal pathogens, thereby reducing gingival inflammation.[12]

  2. The hydrokinetic movement of fluid may alter the host inflammatory response to the subgingival biofilm, thereby reducing the level of gingival inflammation irrespective of changes in plaque removal.[8]

  3. The water pick may provide a "flushing effect" that removes loose, nonadherent plaque biofilm, food deposits, debris, and dead bacterial cells.[24]

  4. The initial contact of the irrigant at the impact zone may mechanically stimulate the gingiva.

  5. The mode of action may be a combination of all the above actions.

3. **Indications for Recommending Home Oral Irrigation**

  A. **Individuals on Periodontal Maintenance.** Studies have shown that daily use of the water flosser may be beneficial for patients with gingivitis or for those in periodontal maintenance.[6–10,12,13,17,21] Patients with 5-mm pockets and gingival bleeding who included daily oral irrigation as part of their home care regimen achieved significant reductions in gingival inflammation and bleeding on probing when compared to patients using only traditional self-care methods.[17]

  B. **Individuals Noncompliant With Dental Floss.** While previously considered an adjunctive to brushing *and* flossing, new information indicates that home oral irrigation can be considered an effective *alternative* to daily flossing for those who cannot floss at a level to achieve a health benefit or who are not interested in using string floss.

    1. The addition of a water flosser once daily with plain water to either a manual or power brushing routine was an effective alternative to dental floss for the reduction of bleeding, gingivitis, and biofilm.[7,16,19,20]

    2. The water flosser and a manual toothbrush were 29% more effective at plaque removal than a manual toothbrush and floss.[15]

  C. **Individuals With Special Needs.** Home irrigation has been shown to be safe and effective for patients with special needs. Use of a water pick may simplify interdental cleaning, especially in situations where an individual with special needs experiences limited manual dexterity.

D. **Individuals With Dental Implants.** For improving the health of peri-implant tissues, daily irrigation using a tip with three soft filaments and water at medium pressure was significantly more effective at reducing bleeding than manual brushing and flossing.[16]

E. **Individuals With Diabetes.** For individuals living with diabetes, twice daily water irrigation using the soft rubber tip provided a 44% better reduction in bleeding over routine oral hygiene.[6]

F. **Individuals With Orthodontic Appliances.** For those with orthodontic appliances, the dental water jet with the orthodontic tip provided 3.76 times better biofilm removal and 26% better bleeding reduction than flossing using a floss threader.[20]

4. **Patient Instruction**

A. **Considerations for Irrigator Use: Product Safety**

1. Water flossers have been extensively studied on thousands of people for more than five decades. More than 70 studies have been conducted on the water flosser and none have reported adverse effects. A recent review of the literature pertaining to the safety of the water flosser found no detrimental effects on the attachment, junctional epithelium, or pocket depth.[25]

2. The incidence of bacteremia from a dental water jet is similar to other health care devices.[25]

   a. The American College of Cardiology/American Heart Association 2008 Guideline Update on Valvular Heart Disease: Focused Update on Infective Endocarditis states "Maintenance of optimal oral health and hygiene may reduce the incidence of bacteremia from daily activities and is more important than prophylactic antibiotics for a dental procedure to reduce the risk of infective endocarditis."[26]

   b. Before recommending a water flosser or any device to a patient who is at high risk for infective endocarditis, it is important that dental health care providers exercise caution and consider both the patient's overall medical and oral health status. Consultation with a physician may be advisable to assess the patient's overall health status.

B. **Irrigant Solutions.** Most solutions can be used in a water flosser. The most effective agent is one that is acceptable to the patient.

1. Water

   a. Simple tap water has been demonstrated as highly effective in numerous clinical trials.[6,7,10,12,14–16,19–21] Therefore, the addition of any antimicrobial agent for home oral irrigation should be considered carefully.

   b. Water has several advantages; it is readily available, cost-effective and has no side effects.

2. Antimicrobial Solutions

   a. Chlorhexidine (CHX)

      1) For home irrigation, chlorhexidine can be diluted with water. Use of diluted solutions of chlorhexidine has been studied in concentrations from 0.02% to 0.06%.[8,13,18]

      2) Because of better interproximal and subgingival penetration with irrigation compared to rinsing, a diluted solution of chlorhexidine is acceptable for daily irrigation. In some cases, dilution can minimize staining.

      3) CHX is available by prescription only. In the United States, the maximum strength is 0.12%. In Europe, it is available at 0.2%.

   b. Essential Oils

      1) For home irrigation, the effectiveness of an essential oil mouth rinse has been demonstrated only when used at full-strength.[9]

      2) Essential oil mouth rinses are available over-the-counter in both brand name and generic forms.

C. **Criteria for Equipment Selection.** Selection of an irrigation device may be confusing because there are many types on the market. The commercial and scientific claims of some devices have yet to be evaluated. Only pulsating water flossers have clinical research supporting safety and efficacy. As each device operates differently in respect to pressure and pulsation, outcomes from studies on one brand of product cannot be transferred to another product brand. Therefore, before recommending any device, it is important to evaluate the pertinent research unique to that brand of product.

5. **Technique for Use of Irrigation Tips**
   A. **General Instructions**
      1. It is important for both dental health care providers and patients to read all instructions thoroughly before using a water flosser.
      2. The fluid reservoir can be filled with water, a solution of water and mouthwash, or a solution of an antimicrobial and water. The irrigating solution should be at warm temperature for maximum patient comfort.
      3. The unit should be flushed after using any solution other than water. After using a diluted solution, such as diluted chlorhexidine, the unit is cleaned by filling the reservoir with warm water and running the unit while holding the handle in the sink until the reservoir is empty.
      4. Most patients seem to comply with recommendations to use a water flosser and find a standard irrigation tip easy to use for supragingival irrigation.[12] For subgingival irrigation, it is important to provide patients with clear instructions on its use including the specific areas where the tip should be used.
   B. **Irrigation Tips.** Irrigation is accomplished using a standard irrigation tip, a subgingival soft rubber tip, a soft tapered brush orthodontic tip, or a tip with three fine filaments.
      1. **Standard irrigation tips** are usually made of a plastic material (Fig. 26-3A).
         a. This type of tip is recommended for generalized, full-mouth irrigation.
         b. Water flosser devices with standard irrigation tips may deliver solution that penetrates a depth of 50% or more of the pocket.[5]

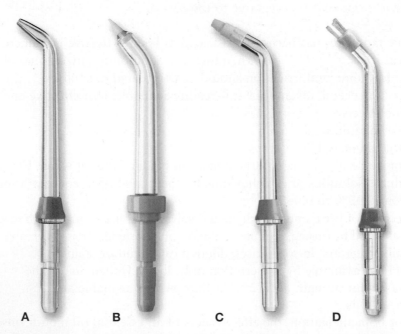

A   B   C   D

Figure 26-3. Irrigation Tips. Four examples of irrigation tip designs. **A.** Standard irrigation tip. **B.** Subgingival tip. **C.** Orthodontic tip. **D.** Filament type-tip.

2. **Orthodontic irrigation tips** have a soft tapered brush end that enhances biofilm removal and provides for simultaneous irrigation (Fig. 26-3C).
   a. Orthodontic tips can be used for full-mouth irrigation and are recommended for people with orthodontic appliances, implants, or who need additional help with biofilm removal.
   b. The bristles should come in light contact with the tooth or orthodontic appliances to facilitate biofilm removal.
      1) The orthodontic tip when used in conjunction with toothbrushing was 3.76 times as effective as dental floss at removing plaque.
      2) When compared to toothbrushing only, the toothbrushing and orthodontic tip combination was 5.83 times as effective.[20]
3. **Filament-type irrigation tips** have three soft filaments surrounding a standard jet tip. This can enhance plaque removal and is safe for use around dental implants (Fig. 26-3D).
   a. The filament-type tip has also been shown to remove plaque biofilm.[14]
   b. The filament-type tip used around an implant was better at reducing bleeding than manual brushing and flossing.[16]
4. **Subgingival irrigation tips** usually have a soft rubber-tipped end (Fig. 26-3B).
   a. Subgingival irrigation tips are not cleansing tips. They are to be used to deliver a medicament in areas such as deep pockets, furcation areas, dental implants, or areas that are difficult to access with a standard tip.
   b. The subgingival irrigation tip should be used after full-mouth irrigation with either the standard irrigation tip, orthodontic tip, or filament-type tip.
   c. Subgingival placement of the tip allows the water or antimicrobial agent to penetrate deeper into a pocket.
      1) In periodontal pockets 6 mm or less in depth, the subgingival tip may deliver water that penetrates up to 90% of the pocket depth.[4]
      2) In deeper pockets—7 mm or more—depth of penetration is somewhat less at 64% of the depth of the pocket.[4]

C. **Procedure for the Use of a Standard Tip**
   1. Initially, the pressure setting should be adjusted to its lowest setting. Over time as the condition of the gingival tissue improves, pressure should be increased to at least the medium setting as this setting is where clinical efficacy has been demonstrated.[1,2]
   2. The water spray is used to "trace" along the gingival margin with the tip positioned at a 90-degree angle almost touching the gingiva (Fig. 26-4). The tip should be held briefly at each interproximal area.

D. **Procedure for the Use of an Orthodontic and Filament Tips**
   1. Initially, the pressure setting should be adjusted to its lowest setting. Over time as the condition of the gingival tissue improves, pressure should be increased to at least the medium setting as this setting is where clinical efficacy has been demonstrated.[1,2]
   2. The water spray is used to "trace" along the gingival margin with the tip positioned at a 90-degree angle touching the gingiva (Figs. 26-5 and 26-6). The tip should be held briefly in each interproximal area.
   3. This tip can also be placed around orthodontic brackets or wires, or implants to enhance cleaning.

E. **Procedure for the Use of a Subgingival Irrigation Tip**
1. The dental clinician should instruct the patient on the areas of his or her mouth where use of a subgingival irrigation tip would be beneficial, such as pockets, dental implants, or furcation areas.
2. The pressure setting is adjusted to its lowest setting. *However, regardless of the pressure setting of the unit, due to the design of the tip, the exit pressure from the subgingival irrigation tip will always be 20 psi.*
3. The tip should be placed at the site prior to starting the irrigation unit. The subgingival tip is directed at a 45-degree angle and placed at the gingival margin or slightly beneath the gingival margin as recommended by the manufacturer (Fig. 26-7).
4. Once the tip is in place, the irrigation unit is turned on and the fluid is allowed to flow briefly in the area.
5. After a site has been irrigated, the unit is paused and the subgingival tip is repositioned in the next area of the mouth.

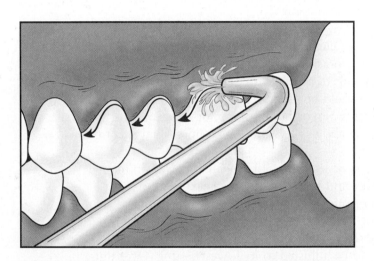

Figure 26-4. Placement of the Standard Irrigation Tip. The water spray is used to "trace" along the gingival margin with the tip positioned at a 90-degree angle almost touching the gingiva.

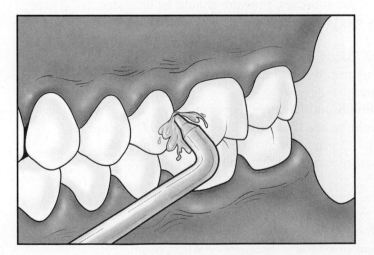

Figure 26-5. Placement of the Subgingival Irrigation Tip. The tip should be placed at the site prior to starting the irrigation unit. The subgingival tip is directed at a 45° angle and placed at the gingival margin or slightly beneath the gingival margin as recommended by the manufacturer.

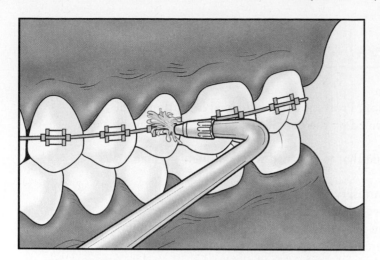

Figure 26-6. Placement of the Orthodontic Tip. The special orthodontic tip is used with the tip positioned at a 90-degree angle.

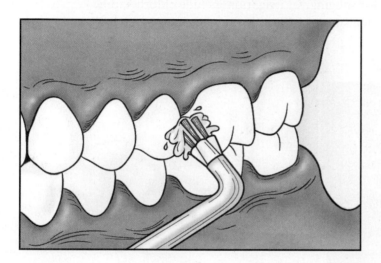

Figure 26-7. Placement of the Filament-type Tip. The filament type tip is used with the tip positioned at a 90-degree angle.

Section 2
Professional Subgingival Irrigation

1. **Introduction to Professional Irrigation**
   A. **Description of Subgingival Irrigation.** Professional subgingival irrigation is the in-office flushing of pockets performed by the dental hygienist or dentist using one of three systems:
      1. A blunt-tipped irrigating cannula that is attached to a handheld syringe (Fig. 26-8)
      2. Ultrasonic unit equipped with a reservoir (Fig. 26-9)
      3. A specialized air-driven handpiece that connects to the dental unit airline
   B. **Goal of Subgingival Irrigation.** The purpose of subgingival irrigation is to enhance the outcome of periodontal instrumentation by disrupting and diluting the bacterial biofilm and bacterial products from within the periodontal pocket.
   C. **Irrigant Solutions.** Solutions used for subgingival irrigation include chlorhexidine gluconate, povidone-iodine and water, stannous fluoride oral rinse, tetracycline dilutions, or Listerine.

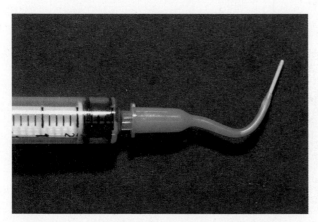

Figure 26-8. Handheld Syringe. Close-up view of the tip of a handheld syringe used for subgingival irrigation. The tip is positioned subgingivally for delivery of an antimicrobial solution.

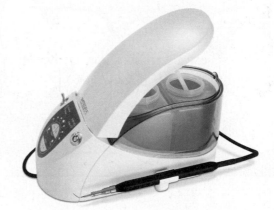

Figure 26-9. Reservoir for Ultrasonic Unit. This ultrasonic device has an optional reservoir system for dispensing irrigant solutions—such as chlorhexidine gluconate—to an ultrasonic tip. (Courtesy of Parkell, Inc.)

2. **Effectiveness of Professional Subgingival Irrigation**
   A. **Single Professional Application**
      1. *A systematic review that included nine studies representing a study population of 129 subjects found that the use of <u>professional irrigation</u> in addition to nonsurgical periodontal therapy provided <u>no additional benefit</u> to nonsurgical periodontal instrumentation alone.*[27]
         a. Very little research on this subject has been conducted in recent years.
         b. *There is no long-lasting substantivity of the antimicrobial agent in the periodontal pocket due to the continuous flow of gingival crevicular fluid from the pocket, and the presence of serum and proteins in the pocket.* A substantive antimicrobial agent, such as chlorhexidine gluconate, would have to be retained in the pocket and be released slowly over a period of time to interfere with the repopulation of bacteria within the pocket. Yet, the rapid elimination of chlorhexidine gluconate from the periodontal pocket renders its antimicrobial substantivity ineffective.
         c. Depth of the periodontal pocket and presence of calculus may impede the depth of solution penetration.
   B. **Multiple Professional Applications.** Additionally, there is a lack of evidence that multiple in-office irrigation applications will provide substantial benefits compared to nonsurgical therapy alone.[28]
   C. **Conclusions Regarding Professional Irrigation**
      1. There is weak evidence to support the use of professional irrigation as a means to enhance the outcome of nonsurgical periodontal instrumentation.[27]
      2. Subgingival irrigation performed before periodontal instrumentation may reduce the incidence of bacteremia and reduce the number of microorganisms in aerosols.

Chapter Summary Statement

When used daily with a traditional home care regimen, oral irrigation via a water flosser can be beneficial for periodontal patients. A well-established body of evidence indicates that pulsating devices have the ability to remove biofilm and reduce bleeding, gingival inflammation, periodontal pathogens, and inflammatory mediators. Irrigation via a water flosser also benefits patients with special oral health needs and considerations including those who are in a periodontal maintenance program or with implants, crowns, bridges, orthodontic appliances, and diabetes.

On the other hand, the evidence for professional subgingival irrigation in the treatment of periodontal disease is weak. In-office subgingival irrigation with an antimicrobial agent has been shown to have only limited or no beneficial effects compared to nonsurgical periodontal instrumentation alone.

Section 3
Focus on Patients

Clinical Patient Care

CASE 1

You have just recommended a water flosser to your patient, and he has accepted, but he has no idea how to use the product. The patient is in periodontal maintenance, has two 5-mm pockets (maxillary right first molar, mesial surface, and mandibular left third molar, distal surface), one 6-mm pocket (maxillary left first molar, mesial surface) and a furcation area on mandibular right first molar. He also has an implant replacing mandibular left first molar. What type of instructions would provide for the patient?

Evidence in Action

A new patient comes to your practice from another state. She has had periodontal therapy in the past. The patient uses a power toothbrush and flosses irregularly. Supragingival plaque control looks good but several areas of the mouth bleed upon probing. The medical history indicates that the patient has had Type 2 diabetes for 7 years. How would you make a recommendation for the water flosser to this patient?

Ethical Dilemma

Your next patient is Darren, a 26-year-old male, who just recently returned from a 3-year stint in the Peace Corps. Prior to his Peace Corps experience, Darren had received routine and regular dental care, but has not been to a dentist in the last 3 years. As you review his medical history, he states that he thinks that he might have suffered from a bout of "infective endocarditis" while away, but as he was working in an underdeveloped third world country, his definitive diagnosis was unclear.

You start your periodontal assessment and discover that his periodontal probe readings have significantly increased from 1 to 3 mm at his last appointment, to generalized 4- to 5-mm probe readings. His tissues appear moderately inflamed, as he presents with substantial supragingival biofilm and subgingival calculus. However, his radiographs show no signs of bone loss.

You recently attended a continuing education course on the use of "water flossers," and feel that this will be an ideal adjunctive periodontal aid for Darren, based on your clinical findings. You start explaining the device and demonstrating its use to Darren, who becomes quite agitated and says that he absolutely refuses to use it. While working in the Peace Corps, clean water was extremely scarce and considered a luxury. There is no way, he states, that he will "waste water" in this fashion. You are not sure how to proceed.

1. What ethical principles are in conflict in this dilemma?
2. What is the best way for you to handle this ethical dilemma?
3. Do you have an ethical obligation to treat this patient?

References

1. Bhaskar SN, Cutright DE, Gross A, Frisch J, Beasley JD, 3rd, Perez B. Water jet devices in dental practice. *J Periodontol.* 1971;42(10):658–664.
2. Selting WJ, Bhaskar SN, Mueller RP. Water jet direction and periodontal pocket debridement. *J Periodontol.* 1972;43(9):569–572.
3. Cobb CM, Rodgers RL, Killoy WJ. Ultrastructural examination of human periodontal pockets following the use of an oral irrigation device in vivo. *J Periodontol.* 1988;59(3):155–163.
4. Braun RE, Ciancio SG. Subgingival delivery by an oral irrigation device. *J Periodontol.* 1992;63(5):469–472.
5. Eakle WS, Ford C, Boyd RL. Depth of penetration in periodontal pockets with oral irrigation. *J Clin Periodontol.* 1986;13(1):39–44.
6. Al-Mubarak S, Ciancio S, Aljada A, Mohanty P, Ross C, Dandona P. Comparative evaluation of adjunctive oral irrigation in diabetics. *J Clin Periodontol.* 2002;29(4):295–300.
7. Barnes CM, Russell CM, Reinhardt RA, Payne JB, Lyle DM. Comparison of irrigation to floss as an adjunct to tooth brushing: effect on bleeding, gingivitis, and supragingival plaque. *J Clin Dent.* 2005;16(3):71–77.
8. Chaves ES, Kornman KS, Manwell MA, Jones AA, Newbold DA, Wood RC. Mechanism of irrigation effects on gingivitis. *J Periodontol.* 1994;65(11):1016–1021.
9. Ciancio SG, Mather ML, Zambon JJ, Reynolds HS. Effect of a chemotherapeutic agent delivered by an oral irrigation device on plaque, gingivitis, and subgingival microflora. *J Periodontol.* 1989;60(6):310–315.
10. Cutler CW, Stanford TW, Abraham C, Cederberg RA, Boardman TJ, Ross C. Clinical benefits of oral irrigation for periodontitis are related to reduction of pro-inflammatory cytokine levels and plaque. *J Clin Periodontol.* 2000;27(2):134–143.
11. Drisko CL, White CL, Killoy WJ, Mayberry WE. Comparison of dark-field microscopy and a flagella stain for monitoring the effect of a Water Pik on bacterial motility. *J Periodontol.* 1987;58(6):381–386.
12. Flemmig TF, Epp B, Funkenhauser Z, et al. Adjunctive supragingival irrigation with acetylsalicylic acid in periodontal supportive therapy. *J Clin Periodontol.* 1995;22(6):427–433.
13. Flemmig TF, Newman MG, Doherty FM, Grossman E, Meckel AH, Bakdash MB. Supragingival irrigation with 0.06% chlorhexidine in naturally occurring gingivitis. I. 6 month clinical observations. *J Periodontol.* 1990;61(2):112–117.
14. Gorur A, Lyle DM, Schaudinn C, Costerton JW. Biofilm removal with a dental water jet. *Compend Contin Educ Dent.* 2009;30 Spec No 1:1–6.
15. Goyal CR, Lyle DM, Qaqish JG, Schuller R. Evaluation of the plaque removal efficacy of a water flosser compared to string floss in adults after a single use. *J Clin Dent.* 2013;24(2):37–42.
16. Magnuson B, Harsono M, Stark PC, Lyle D, Kugel G, Perry R. Comparison of the effect of two interdental cleaning devices around implants on the reduction of bleeding: a 30-day randomized clinical trial. *Compend Contin Educ Dent.* 2013;34 Spec No 8:2–7.
17. Newman MG, Cattabriga M, Etienne D, et al. Effectiveness of adjunctive irrigation in early periodontitis: multi-center evaluation. *J Periodontol.* 1994;65(3):226–229.
18. Newman MG, Flemmig TF, Nachnani S, et al. Irrigation with 0.06% chlorhexidine in naturally occurring gingivitis. II. 6 months microbiological observations. *J Periodontol.* 1990;61(7):427–433.
19. Rosema NA, Hennequin-Hoenderdos NL, Berchier CE, Slot DE, Lyle DM, van der Weijden GA. The effect of different interdental cleaning devices on gingival bleeding. *J Internat Acad Periodontol.* 2011;13(1):2–10.
20. Sharma NC, Lyle DM, Qaqish JG, Galustians J, Schuller R. Effect of a dental water jet with orthodontic tip on plaque and bleeding in adolescent patients with fixed orthodontic appliances. *Am J Orthod Dentofacial Orthop.* 2008;133(4):565–571; quiz 628 e1–e2.
21. Genovesi AM, Lorenzi C, Lyle DM, et al. Periodontal maintenance following scaling and root planing. A randomized single center study comparing minocycline treatment and daily oral irrigation with water. *Minerva Stomatologica.* 2013;62(Suppl 1 to No12):1–9.
22. Offenbacher S, Heasman PA, Collins JG. Modulation of host PGE2 secretion as a determinant of periodontal disease expression. *J Periodontol.* 1993;64(5 Suppl):432–444.
23. Tsai CC, Ho YP, Chen CC. Levels of interleukin-1 beta and interleukin-8 in gingival crevicular fluids in adult periodontitis. *J Periodontol.* 1995;66(10):852–859.
24. Frascella JA, Fernandez P, Gilbert RD, Cugini M. A randomized, clinical evaluation of the safety and efficacy of a novel oral irrigator. *Am J Dent.* 2000;13(2):55–58.
25. Jolkovsky DL, Lyle DM. Safety of a water flosser: A literature review. *Compendium.* 2015;36(2):146–149.
26. Nishimura RA, Carabello BA, Faxon DP, et al. ACC/AHA 2008 guideline update on valvular heart disease: focused update on infective endocarditis: a report of the American College of Cardiology/American Heart Association Task Force on Practice Guidelines: endorsed by the Society of Cardiovascular Anesthesiologists, Society for Cardiovascular Angiography and Interventions, and Society of Thoracic Surgeons. *Circulation.* 2008;118(8):887–896.
27. Hallmon WW, Rees TD. Local anti-infective therapy: mechanical and physical approaches. A systematic review. *Ann Periodontol.* 2003;8(1):99–114.
28. Greenstein G; Research, Science and Therapy Committee of the American Academy of Periodontology. Position paper: The role of supra- and subgingival irrigation in the treatment of periodontal diseases. *J Periodontol.* 2005;76(11):2015–2027.

🖰 STUDENT ANCILLARY RESOURCES

A wide variety of resources to enhance your learning is available online:

- Audio Glossary
- Book Pages
- Chapter Review Questions and Answers

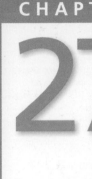

CHAPTER

27 Chemical Agents in Periodontal Care

Clinical Application. As discussed in other chapters of this textbook, it is clear that periodontal diseases are caused by bacterial infections and that bacteria found in dental plaque biofilm is the primary causative agent in these diseases. Many bacterial infections that have affected mankind have been brought under control using various chemical agents to attack bacteria that cause those diseases. It is quite natural for researchers and clinicians alike to search for chemical agents or medications to help in the difficult task of controlling periodontal diseases. This chapter discusses some of the more important chemical agents that can be used in biofilm control. This chapter will also examine the alleged claims and the current scientific evidence behind some unconventional dental products/remedies that have recently gained headlines in the media.

Learning Objectives

- Describe the difference between systemic delivery and topical delivery of chemical agents.
- Define the term systemic antibiotic and explain why systemic antibiotics are not used routinely in the treatment of patients with plaque-induced gingivitis and patients with periodontitis.
- Describe three examples of mouth rinse ingredients that can help reduce the severity of gingivitis.
- List three antimicrobial agents that can be delivered using controlled-release delivery devices.
- Explain why toothpastes are nearly ideal delivery mechanisms for chemical agents.
- List two toothpaste ingredients that can reduce the severity of gingivitis.
- Be able to explain the current scientific evidence behind charcoal-based dental products and oil pulling.

Key Terms

Systemic delivery
Topical delivery
Microbial reservoir
Systemic antibiotics

Antibiotic resistance
Conventional mechanical
  periodontal therapy
Controlled-release delivery device

Therapeutic mouth rinses
Substantivity
Unconventional dentistry

Section 1
Introduction to Chemical Agents in Biofilm Control

As discussed in other chapters of this textbook, it is clear that periodontal diseases are caused by bacterial infections, and that bacteria found in dental plaque biofilm is the primary causative agent in these diseases. Research indicates 1,000 species of bacteria have been found in dental plaque biofilm. Many bacterial infections that have affected mankind have been brought under control using various chemical agents to attack bacteria that cause those diseases.

1. **Delivery of Chemical Agents in Periodontal Patients.** Chemical agents useful in biofilm control can be delivered by using either systemic delivery or topical delivery.
   A. **Systemic Delivery**
      1. In dentistry, systemic delivery usually refers to administering chemical agents in the form of a tablet or capsule. When a tablet is taken by the patient, the chemical agent contained is released as the tablet dissolves, and the agent subsequently enters the blood stream—thus, the chemical agent is circulated "systemically" throughout the body.
      2. As the chemical agent circulates throughout the body in the blood stream, it enters into the periodontal tissues and is subsequently incorporated into the gingival crevicular fluid where it comes into contact with the periodontal microorganisms.
      3. An example of systemic delivery of a chemical agent would a patient who takes the antibiotic penicillin in tablet or capsule form. The penicillin passes through the wall of the gastrointestinal tract and enters the body's tissues. In medical care, systemic delivery of chemical agents can also be administered by injection into a muscle or blood vessel, although this mode of systemic delivery has little to do with the control of dental biofilm.
   B. **Topical Delivery**
      1. In dentistry, topical delivery usually refers to the intraoral placement of a chemical agent or local delivery using controlled-release devices into a periodontal pocket where the chemical agent then comes into contact with biofilm forming either on the teeth or in the periodontal pocket.
      2. Examples of topical delivery in dentistry would be using a mouth rinse or toothpaste that contains a chemical agent that can kill bacteria growing in dental biofilm. In this instance, the chemical agent would come into contact with the teeth, oral mucous membranes, and the surface of dental biofilm.
      3. It should be noted that when chemical agents come into contact with oral mucous membranes, some of the agent enters the blood stream by passing through the mucous membranes, but the bulk of the agent contacts the bacteria topically. See Table 27-1 for an overview of topical and systemic delivery mechanisms for chemical agents used in dental biofilm control.
2. **Considerations for Use of Chemical Agents in Periodontal Patients**
   A. **Resistance of the Biofilm to the Delivery of Chemical Agents.** Research shows that the surface of dental plaque biofilm is covered by a layer—known as the extracellular protective matrix. The extracellular protective matrix acts as a barrier preventing some chemical agents from contacting the bacteria in the plaque biofilm.

TABLE 27-1	DELIVERY MECHANISMS FOR CHEMICAL AGENTS	
Delivery Type	**Specific Mechanisms**	**Possible Patient Benefits**
Topical	Therapeutic mouth rinses	Reduce the severity of gingival inflammation
Topical	Therapeutic dentifrices	Reduction in dentinal hypersensitivity Reduction in gingival inflammation Reduction of supragingival calculus Reduction in surface stains
Topical	Subgingival irrigation	Disruption and dilution of bacteria within the dental biofilm
Topical	Controlled-release delivery devices	Subject subgingival bacteria to therapeutic levels of a drug for a period of a week or longer
Systemic	Tablets, capsules	Help control more aggressive forms of periodontitis Fight acute oral infections

Box 27-1. Microbial Reservoirs for Periodontal Pathogens

- Bacterial plaque biofilm in protected sites such as furcation areas
- Bacteria in residual calculus deposits that are not removed during nonsurgical therapy
- Bacteria living within the epithelial layers and connective tissue adjacent to a periodontal pocket
- Bacteria that have penetrated dentinal tubules
- Bacteria protected by irregularities in tooth surfaces after mechanical treatment
- Bacteria protected by poorly defined restoration margins

B. **Microbial Reservoirs for Periodontal Pathogens.** In the oral cavity, there are a variety of microbial reservoirs that can lead to rapid repopulation of bacterial pathogens in a treated periodontal patient.
   1. A microbial reservoir is a niche or secure place in the oral cavity that can allow periodontal pathogens to live undisturbed during routine therapy and subsequently repopulate periodontal pockets quickly.
   2. An example of a microbial reservoir would be a residual calculus deposit following periodontal instrumentation. Living bacteria found within the calculus deposit can reproduce in periodontal pockets and continue to promote disease even after what appears to be thorough nonsurgical therapy.
   3. Box 27-1 provides an overview of some of the many microbial reservoirs for periodontal pathogens in the oral cavity.
3. **Criteria for Effective Chemical Agents.** For chemotherapy to be effective, it must meet three requirements: (1) reach the sites of disease activity, namely the base of the pocket, (2) be delivered at a bacteriostatic or bactericidal concentration, and (3) remain in place long enough to be effective.[1] See Table 27-2 for a comparison of the effectiveness of common drug delivery systems for management of periodontitis.

4. **Chemical Agents Effective Against Periodontitis.** Periodontal instrumentation is an effective mechanical therapy for periodontitis.[2,3] In deep or tortuous pockets or sites that do not respond to nonsurgical periodontal therapy, however, it may be beneficial to use adjunctive chemical agents.[4,5] At this point, there is no biofilm control chemical agent that can halt periodontitis, but there are a number of different chemical agents that can be used as part of comprehensive treatment for patients with periodontal diseases. An overview of chemical agents that have been suggested for use in biofilm control in periodontal patients is presented in Table 27-3.

TABLE 27-2	COMPARISON OF DRUG DELIVERY SYSTEMS FOR MANAGEMENT OF PERIODONTITIS		
	Adequate Drug Concentration	**Reaches Sites of Disease Activity**	**Adequate Time in Place to Be Effective**
Mouth Rinsing	Good	Poor	Poor
Subgingival Irrigation	Good	Good	Poor
Systemic Delivery	Fair	Good	Fair
Controlled-Release Delivery	Good	Good	Good

TABLE 27-3	OVERVIEW OF SOME OF THE CHEMICAL AGENTS USED IN BIOFILM CONTROL	
Type of Agent	**Example of Agent**	**Means of Administration**
Antibiotics	Tetracyclines	Tablet/capsule Local delivery mechanism
Bisbiguanide antiseptics	Chlorhexidine	Mouth rinse Local delivery mechanism
Fluorides	Stannous fluoride	Mouth rinse Toothpaste
Metal salts	Tin/zinc	Mouth rinse Toothpaste
Oxygenating agents	Hydrogen peroxide	Mouth rinse
Phenolic compounds	Essential oils	Mouth rinse
Quaternary ammonium	Cetylpyridinium chloride	Mouth rinse
Tertiary amine surfactant	Delmopinol	Mouth rinse

Section 2
Use of Systemic Antibiotics to Control Biofilm

1. **Overview of Systemic Antibiotics**
   A. **Definitions**
      1. Antibiotics are medications used to help fight infections either because they kill bacteria or because they can inhibit the growth of bacteria.
      2. Systemic antibiotics refer to those antibiotics that can be taken orally or that can be injected. Worldwide, antibiotics are in widespread use in fighting bacterial infections. In North America, health care providers, such as physicians and dentists, have access to a broad range of antibiotic for use in patients with infections. These drugs have been used for many years to help the body fight certain bacterial infections and have undoubtedly been responsible for saving countless lives.
   B. **Systemic Antibiotics Studied for Use in Periodontal Diseases.** Systemic antibiotics have also been studied for their use in controlling periodontal diseases. Box 27-2 lists examples of systemic antibiotics that have been studied by researchers for use in periodontal patients.
   C. **Plaque-Induced Gingivitis and Periodontitis**
      1. For most patients with the more common forms of periodontal diseases, current recommendations are for clinicians to avoid the routine use of systemic antibiotic drugs to control these diseases. There are two major reasons for recommendations to avoid their routine use in these patients.
         a. One reason dentists do not use systemic antibiotics routinely to control the more common forms of periodontal diseases is antibiotic resistance.[6–8] Antibiotic resistance refers to the ability of a bacterium to withstand the effects of an antibiotic by developing mechanisms to protect the bacterium from the killing or inhibiting effects of the antibiotic. Most species of subgingival bacteria are considerably more resistant in biofilms than in planktonic cultures. Resistance appears to be age-related because biofilms demonstrated progressive antibiotic resistance as they matured with maximum resistance coinciding with the steady-state phase of biofilm growth.[9]
            1) According to the National Science Foundation and the Centers for Disease Control, antibiotic resistance is a serious public health problem throughout the world, and the problem is increasing in scope. When antibiotic resistant strains of bacteria develop, they are generally not affected by the antibiotic and continue to cause more damage.
            2) An example of how antibiotic resistance can be a public health problem is the high incidence of penicillin-resistant microorganisms that have already limited the usefulness of this important drug. As more and more bacteria develop resistance to the antibiotic penicillin, the usefulness of this antibiotic as a life-saving drug will decline.
         b. Another reason dentists do not use systemic antibiotics routinely to control periodontal diseases is that studies indicate that in most patients, these diseases respond to conventional mechanical periodontal therapy just as well as they respond to the systemic administration of antibiotics.

Box 27-2. Examples of Systemic Antibiotics Studied for Use in Periodontal Care

- Penicillin and amoxicillin
- Tetracyclines
- Erythromycin
- Metronidazole
- Clindamycin

Conventional mechanical periodontal therapy is a term that refers to self-care, periodontal instrumentation, surgical interventions, and control of local contributing factors.

2. When antibiotics are being considered for use in periodontal patients, careful patient selection is necessary.

   a. When tempted to use systemic antibiotics to control either plaque-induced gingivitis or periodontitis, dental health care providers must weigh potential benefits and risks. At this point, most clinicians have decided that the potential harm outweighs the benefits.

   b. In patients with periodontitis, the efficacy of using antibiotic therapy is not completely clear, and antibiotic therapy in these patients should usually be limited to those patients that have continued periodontal breakdown after thorough conventional mechanical periodontal therapy.

   c. It should be noted that even though systemic antibiotics are rarely indicated for routine treatment of patients with plaque-induced gingivitis or periodontitis, they are frequently indicated in the treatment of patients with more aggressive forms of periodontitis.

3. Patient Education. Even though systemic antibiotics are not normally used for patients with plaque-induced gingivitis or periodontitis, systemic antibiotics are discussed here because periodontal patients can ask why antibiotics are not being recommended for them.

   a. This question may arise when the patient learns that periodontitis is a bacterial infection. This is a natural question for a patient to ask given the widespread use of antibiotics in fighting infections of all sorts.

   b. When confronted with a question from a patient about why antibiotics are not being recommended, the dental hygienist can explain the following facts:

      1) Most cases of gingivitis and periodontitis can be readily controlled with conventional mechanical treatments that do not require the use of systemic antibiotics.

      2) Overuse of systemic antibiotics often results in the development of antibiotic-resistant strains of bacteria, thereby compounding a complex dental problem. This is a major public health concern, since many antibiotics can be rendered useless for life-saving measures through the development of antibiotic resistant strains of bacteria.

D. **More Aggressive Forms of Periodontitis (previously known as Aggressive Periodontitis)**

   1. The use of antibiotics in conjunction with mechanical therapy was the recommended treatment regimen for what was previously known as aggressive periodontitis.[10]

   2. However, because the 2017 AAP/EFP Disease Classification scheme eliminated aggressive periodontitis as a distinct periodontal disease entity, knowing when to combine systemic antibiotics with the standard conventional treatment regimen is now unclear and murky. So, the dental clinician must rely on his/her own experience, judgment, and treatment philosophy when assessing each individual periodontitis case to determine if systemic antibiotics is necessary as part of the individualized periodontal therapy.

   3. When antibiotics are being considered for use, microbiologic analysis is a wise clinical step. Microbiologic analysis involves sampling the bacteria associated with the disease process and testing cultures of the bacteria for specific antibiotic susceptibility. Utilizing microbiologic analysis can avoid prescribing inappropriate antibiotics that can lead to a poor clinical response.

   4. The flowchart in Figure 27-1 can assist the clinician in evaluating which type of periodontitis case would benefit from systemic antibiotics. However, before reviewing the diagram, it is important for the reader to understand that the recommendations illustrated in Figure 27-1 are neither mandatory rules nor

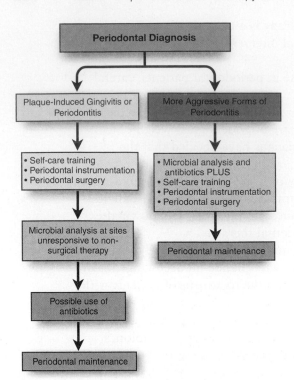

Figure 27-1. The Relationship Between Periodontal Diagnosis and the Use of Systemic Antibiotics.

considered as part of the standards of care. Rather, this figure is designed to illustrate the thought processes that should be in a clinician's mind when evaluating if a specific periodontitis case warrants systemic antibiotics as an adjunct to conventional therapy. Ultimately, it is left to the clinician to determine if systemic antibiotics are warranted on a case-by-case basis.

2. **Use of Tetracyclines in Periodontal Patients.** One of the antibiotic groups, the group of drugs called tetracyclines, has received special attention by researchers because it has some specific properties that make it attractive to consider for use in selected periodontal patients.

A. **Tetracyclines tend to be concentrated in the gingival crevicular fluids.** When tetracyclines are administered orally, the drugs permeate body tissues and reach a certain concentration in the blood serum. The level of tetracycline drugs, however, is more concentrated within the gingival crevicular fluids flowing into periodontal pockets than the level found in the blood serum. This results in a higher concentration of the drug in exactly the sites it might be needed in a periodontal patient.

B. **The tetracyclines are effective against most strains of *Aggregatibacter actinomycetemcomitans*.** *Aggregatibacter actinomycetemcomitans* is one of the periodontal pathogens thought to be a primary player in many patients with periodontitis.

C. **The tetracyclines have other effects in addition to their antimicrobial properties.**
   1. Tetracyclines inhibit the action of collagenase—one of the enzymes responsible in part for the breakdown of the periodontium in periodontitis patients.
   2. Any drug that can inhibit the action of collagenase can be expected to slow the progress of the tissue breakdown caused by periodontitis.

D. **Certain tetracyclines are effective in subantimicrobial doses.**
   1. A subantimicrobial dose of the doxycycline (20 mg twice a day) significantly improved clinical parameters associated with periodontal health in patients with periodontitis when used as an adjunct to a maintenance schedule of periodontal instrumentation.[11–13]
   2. Several studies assessed whether a long-term subantimicrobial dose of doxycycline produces doxycycline-resistant oral microflora in adults with periodontitis. These studies found no evidence of antibiotic resistance in the subantimicrobial doxycycline treatment groups.[12,13]

Section 3
Use of Topically Delivered Chemical Agents

1. **Controlled Release of Antimicrobial Chemicals**
   A. **Overview of Controlled-Release Mechanisms**
      1. Controlled-release delivery device usually consists of an antibacterial chemical that is embedded in a carrier material. It is designed to be placed directly into the periodontal pocket where the carrier material attaches to the tooth surface and dissolves slowly, producing a steady, sustained release of the antimicrobial agent over a period of several days within the periodontal pocket.[14]
      2. The earliest version of these products involved coating carrier fibers with chemical agents that would be released following placement of the fibers within periodontal pockets. Use of these non-dissolvable fibers required the patient to return to the dental office for removal of the fibers.
      3. The latest versions of these products involve embedding antimicrobial agents into carrier materials which dissolve slowly over approximately 1 week. The carrier material can be placed into a periodontal pocket, and as it dissolves, it slowly releases the antimicrobial agent. Unlike early examples of controlled-release devices, the newer types are dissolvable and do not require the patient to return for removal.
      4. Antimicrobial agents currently used in controlled-release delivery devices include chlorhexidine and some of the antibiotic drugs such as the tetracyclines. In the future, other drugs may be used for this purpose.
   B. **Rationale for Use.** The goal of the use of these controlled-release delivery devices is to subject subgingival bacteria to therapeutic levels of an antibacterial drug for a sustained period. Most of these controlled-release devices continue to deliver chemicals into the pockets for approximately 1 week.
   C. **Benefits of Controlled-Release Delivery Devices**
      1. Use of controlled-release delivery devices has been shown to result in a small increase in attachment level in a periodontal pocket (about a 0.5 to 2 mm reduction found in probing depths compared to conventional periodontal instrumentation).
      2. Controlled studies are available to guide dental health care providers in the appropriate use of these new devices.
         a. Controlled-release devices may be indicated for use in localized periodontal pockets that are nonresponsive after thorough nonsurgical and surgical periodontal therapy or sites with disease recurrences. In addition, this therapy will be beneficial for patients who are not good candidates for surgical therapies such as patients who are medically compromised, smokers, and those with inadequate plaque control.
         b. When used along with periodontal instrumentation, these products can result in both an improvement in probing depth reduction and a clinical attachment gain. The clinical significance of the small amount of improvement is unclear at this point. Routine use of controlled-release delivery devices, as an adjunct to periodontal instrumentation and periodontal maintenance, may show improved results in future phase III designed clinical studies.
         c. Current guidelines support the use of controlled-release devices in combination with periodontal instrumentation.[3–5,15–18]

D. **Controlled-Release Mechanisms.** Several controlled-release delivery products have been introduced in the United States over the last few years, and it is likely that more will be available within the next few years. The chemical agents that have been incorporated into these devices and marketed over the past few years are outlined next.

1. Minocycline Hydrochloride Microspheres
   a. Marketed under the brand name Arestin.
   b. Arestin is a controlled-release mechanism that delivers the antibiotic minocycline hydrochloride in a powdered microsphere form. Minocycline hydrochloride is a broad-spectrum, semisynthetic tetracycline derivative that is bacteriostatic.
   c. Application
      1) A cannula tip is used to expel the microspheres into the pocket (Fig. 27-2) where it binds to the tooth surface because of the sticky nature of the carrier material.
      2) Over 5 to 7 days, the powdered microspheres dissolve releasing the embedded minocycline, so there is nothing to remove from the pocket.
   d. Studies demonstrate that repeated subgingival administration of minocycline microspheres in the treatment of adult periodontitis is safe and is more effective than periodontal instrumentation alone in reducing probing depths in periodontitis patients.[19,20]
   e. Adverse Reactions. Possible adverse reactions include oral candidiasis or an allergic response. In addition, the use of antibiotic preparations may result in the development of resistant bacteria.
   f. Contraindications for Use. This product is a tetracycline derivative, and should not be used in patients who are hypersensitive to any tetracycline or in women who are pregnant or nursing.

2. Doxycycline Hyclate Gel
   a. Marketed under the brand name Atridox.
   b. This product is a gel system that delivers the antibiotic doxycycline (also a tetracycline derivative) to the periodontal pocket.
   c. Application of Doxycycline Hyclate Gel
      1) The gel is expressed into the pocket with a cannula (Fig. 27-2), and after placement the gel solidifies into a wax-like substance.
      2) The cannula tip is placed near the pocket base and gel is expressed using a steady pressure until the gel reaches the top of the gingival margin.
      3) A limitation to this delivery system is that the gel tends to cling to the cannula when withdrawn from the pocket, which can be reduced by using a moistened dental hand instrument to hold the gel in place while slowly withdrawing the cannula tip from the pocket.
      4) The gel is biodegradable (it dissolves) so there is nothing to remove from the pocket.
   d. In a 6-month multicenter trial, results indicate that periodontal instrumentation combined with local application of doxycycline in deep periodontal sites can be considered as a justified approach for nonsurgical treatment of chronic periodontitis.[21]
   e. Adverse Reactions to Doxycycline Hyclate Gel
      1) Possible adverse reactions include oral candidiasis or an allergic response.
      2) The use of antibiotic preparations may result in the development of resistant bacteria.

    f. Contraindications for Use. This product is a tetracycline derivative, and should not be used in patients who are hypersensitive to any tetracycline or in women who are pregnant or nursing.

3. Chlorhexidine Gluconate Chip

    a. Marketed under the brand name PerioChip.

    b. Another example of a controlled-release device is a tiny gelatin chip containing the antiseptic chlorhexidine that is inserted into a periodontal pocket that is 5 mm or greater in depth (Fig. 27-3).

    c. Investigations indicate that the chlorhexidine gluconate chip, when used as an adjunct to periodontal instrumentation, significantly reduces loss of alveolar bone.[22]

    d. Application

        1) The gelatin chip is inserted into the periodontal pocket.

        2) The gelatin chip can be difficult to insert into some pockets due to the size and shape of the chip.

        3) The gelatin chip is bioabsorbed so there is no need to have it removed after placement.

    e. Since chlorhexidine is not an antibiotic, there is no risk of antibiotic resistance with use of the chlorhexidine gluconate gelatin chip.

    f. A 1-year clinical trial by Henke and colleagues suggests that a chlorhexidine chip may reduce periodontal surgical needs at little additional cost.[23]

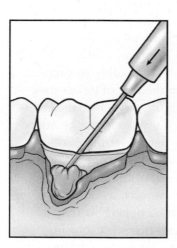

Figure 27-2. Antimicrobial Agents Locally Expressed Into the Pocket. Some local delivery mechanisms involve placing the carrier material into a periodontal pocket with a cannula tip. Minocycline hydrochloride–containing microspheres and doxycycline gel are examples of such products. These carrier materials adhere to the tooth surfaces and dissolve slowly—releasing the antimicrobial agents incorporated in the carrier material.

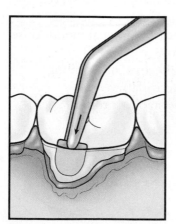

Figure 27-3. Gelatin Chip Inserted Into Pocket. The gelatin chip is inserted into periodontal pockets 5 mm or greater in depth. The gelatin chip adheres to the tooth surface and dissolves slowly—releasing the chlorhexidine antimicrobial agent trapped in the gelatin.

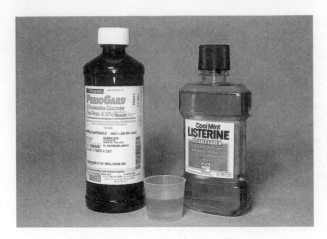

Figure 27-4. Therapeutic Mouth Rinses. Two examples of therapeutic mouth rinses used to aid in dental biofilm control. The mouth rinse pictured on the left contains chlorhexidine gluconate as its active ingredient. The mouth rinse pictured on the right contains essentials oils as the active ingredient and is available over-the-counter.

2. **Mouth Rinses as Aids in Biofilm Control**
    A. **Introduction to Mouth Rinses**
        1. Many mouth rinses available today are therapeutic mouth rinses. Therapeutic mouth rinses are mouth rinses that have some actual benefit (provide some therapeutic action) to the patient in addition to the simple goal of breath freshening and halitosis reduction.
            a. In the context of this chapter, therapeutic mouth rinses would be rinses that decrease dental biofilm enough to also decrease the severity of gingivitis. Figure 27-4 pictures two examples of therapeutic mouth rinses.
            b. Clinical studies support the effectiveness of therapeutic mouth rinses used in addition to proper home care for the reduction of dental biofilm and the control of gingivitis. Insufficient evidence, however, is available to support the claim that therapeutic mouth rinses can reduce the risk of developing periodontitis or the rate of progression of periodontitis.[24,25] Over the last few decades, researchers are still searching for chemicals that can be added to mouth rinses that might actually reduce or halt periodontitis.
        2. It should be noted that in addition to therapeutic mouth rinses that can aid in the control of biofilm and gingivitis, there are other therapeutic mouth rinses available that can benefit the patient in a variety of ways such as decreasing the risk of developing dental caries and treatment of dentinal hypersensitivity.
    B. **Characteristics That an Ideal Mouth Rinse Should Possess.** Investigations into chemical biofilm control have not yet produced a biofilm control mouth rinse that can be used as a total substitute for mechanical biofilm control. However, these investigations have indeed produced mouth rinses that can be effective components of a comprehensive program of patient self-care. An ideal mouth rinse would possess four characteristics that are described below.
        1. **Efficacy.** The active ingredient in the rinse should be effective in inhibiting (bacteriostatic) or killing periodontal pathogens (bactericidal).
        2. **Stability.** The ingredients in the mouth rinse should be stable at room temperature and have a reasonable shelf life.

3. Substantivity (sub-stan-tiv-ity). The active ingredient in the rinse should display the property of substantivity. This means that the active ingredient would be retained in the oral cavity for a while following rinsing and would be released slowly over time (usually several hours), resulting in a continuing antimicrobial effect against periodontal pathogens.
   a. Substantivity is an important characteristic, since dental biofilm grows and matures continuously.
   b. An active ingredient that displays the property of substantivity would continue to kill periodontal pathogens over an extended number of hours following rinsing.
4. Safety. The ingredients in the mouth rinse should not produce any harmful effects to the tissues in the oral cavity or systemically to the patient.

C. Ingredients of Mouth Rinses
   1. Products such as mouth rinses contain both active ingredients and inactive ingredients.
      a. An active ingredient is a component that produces some benefit for the patient (such as a reduction in the severity of gingival inflammation associated with gingivitis).
      b. All mouth rinses also contain inactive ingredients.
         1) Inactive ingredients are included in mouth rinse formulations simply to add other properties such as color enhancement, taste improvements, increase in shelf life, or to keep components in a liquid state.
         2) Though these ingredients are called "inactive," there can be associated side effects with some of these ingredients in certain patients. It is important for clinicians to be familiar with the inactive ingredients of rinses as well as the active ingredients.
   2. Many chemicals that might be placed in mouth rinses have been investigated for their effect against both biofilm and gingivitis.
      a. Chemicals that reduce biofilm formation to only a minor degree usually have little or no clinically significant effect against gingivitis, and therefore may not be very useful in controlling a disease, such as gingivitis. Many mouth rinses marketed today fall into this category.
      b. Among the many ingredients tested for efficacy against gingivitis, four mouth rinse ingredients that have some effect against gingivitis have been studied extensively. These ingredients are listed below.
         1) Chlorhexidine gluconate
         2) Essential oils
         3) Cetylpyridinium chloride
         4) Delmopinol

D. Mouth Rinses Containing Chlorhexidine Gluconate
   1. One group of mouth rinses currently available contains chlorhexidine gluconate as the active ingredient. These rinses are only available through prescriptions in the United States, but they can be purchased over-the-counter in some other countries.
      a. Mouth rinses containing chlorhexidine gluconate as the active ingredient have been demonstrated to reduce the severity of gingivitis in numerous clinical studies.
      b. In the United States, the concentration of chlorhexidine gluconate used in prescription mouth rinses is 0.12%, but it should be noted that a higher concentration is used in mouth rinses in some other countries.

2. At this point, chlorhexidine is the most effective antimicrobial agent for long-term reduction of biofilm and gingivitis. For this reason, it is often regarded as the standard against which all other topical chemical biofilm control agents are judged.[26,27] The effectiveness of chlorhexidine gluconate mouth rinses is due to the following characteristics.

   a. Chlorhexidine is bactericidal agent that is effective against both gram-positive and gram-negative bacteria.

   b. Chlorhexidine binds with oral tissues in the mouth and is slowly released over time (several hours) in a concentration that will continue killing bacteria. Thus, these rinses display the property of substantivity.[27]

   c. Chlorhexidine has a very low level of toxicity and shows no permanent retention in the body.

3. The primary mechanism of action for chlorhexidine gluconate is disruption of the integrity of the cell walls of bacteria.

4. Chlorhexidine-containing mouth rinses are useful adjuncts to biofilm control in many patients. Current recommendations for use of this mouth rinse (0.12% chlorhexidine gluconate) are to rinse with one-half ounce for 30 seconds twice daily, 30 minutes after tooth brushing.

5. There are several groups of patients that should be considered for use of chlorhexidine gluconate mouth rinse. Some of these are outlined below:

   a. Special Needs Patients. The use of a chlorhexidine mouth rinse is suggested for specific groups of patients who have special needs. Two examples of such patients are those with immunodeficiencies that might be more susceptible to infections in general and patients who are unable to perform biofilm control because of some impairment.

   b. Postsurgical Care Patients. Following periodontal surgery, it is frequently difficult for patients to perform adequate mechanical biofilm control during the healing period without damaging the surgical site. In these patients, chlorhexidine mouth rinses can be used for postsurgical rinsing as a temporary adjunct to mechanical biofilm control. Use of a chlorhexidine mouth rinse following periodontal surgery for 4 to 6 weeks can be effective in many patients to promote healing.

   c. Patients with Candida Infections. It should be noted that a variety of medications are used to control Candida infections, but chlorhexidine mouth rinses can be used as a disinfectant for dental appliances such as complete dentures or partial dentures in patients with these infections.

   d. Patients with High Caries Risk. Chlorhexidine is also effective against the bacteria responsible for dental caries. Rinsing with chlorhexidine mouth rinses has been used to reduce the counts of caries-causing bacteria in certain patients.

   e. Patients with Oral Piercings or Dental Implants. Chlorhexidine mouth rinses have also been recommended for use by patients for aftercare of oral piercings and dental implants.

   f. Chlorhexidine rinsing is recommended for patients who have xerostomia to prevent caries and periodontal diseases. Many studies have shown that some medications reduce salivary flow and cause dry mouth conditions. One example of a patient that may experience severe xerostomia is a person who has been treated with head and neck radiation therapy.

6. Chlorhexidine mouth rinses do have their limitations.[27–29]
   a. Chlorhexidine is an antiplaque agent that can prevent plaque formation but its mode of action does not allow it to remove plaque already present on tooth surfaces efficiently. In a randomized split-mouth study, Zanatta and colleagues found that a 0.12% chlorhexidine gluconate mouth rinse had little antiplaque and antigingivitis effect on previously plaque-covered surfaces. These results confirm the diminished effect of chlorhexidine on structured biofilm and reinforce the necessity of mechanical biofilm disruption before the initiation of chlorhexidine mouth rinse.[29]
   b. Also, the chlorhexidine molecule reacts with anionic surfactants (sodium lauryl sulphate) present in certain toothpaste formulation, thus reducing the effectiveness of the chlorhexidine.[26]
   c. The most common side effects of long-term usage of chlorhexidine mouth washes are taste alterations, calculus formation, and extrinsic staining of tooth surfaces and restorations.
7. Chlorhexidine mouth rinses have been evaluated related to their effectiveness as a preprocedural rinse for dental office procedures producing aerosols. Studies suggest that a preprocedural chlorhexidine rinse eliminates the majority of bacterial aerosols generated by the use of an ultrasonic unit.[30,31]

E. **Mouth Rinses Containing Essential Oils**
1. Chemicals referred to as essential oils have been used as active ingredients in some mouth rinses for many years. Chemical agents included in the group of chemicals called essential oils include thymol, menthol, eucalyptol, and methyl salicylate.
2. Mouth rinses containing essential oils are available over-the-counter (i.e., available without a prescription). Listerine mouth rinse is one example of a rinse containing essential oils, but there are other products on the market with similar ingredients.
3. There are numerous investigations related to the efficacy of essential oils in controlling gingivitis published in the literature.
   a. This group of chemicals can indeed help control biofilm, and they have received the Seal of Acceptance from the American Dental Association (ADA) for their effect against *gingivitis*.
   b. A 6-month controlled clinical study demonstrated that the essential oil mouth rinse and the chlorhexidine mouth rinse had comparable antiplaque and antigingivitis activity.[32]
   c. Several investigations found no significant difference with respect to reduction of gingival inflammation between an essential oil mouth rinse and a chlorhexidine mouth rinse. In long-term use, the essential oil mouth rinse appears to be a reliable alternative to chlorhexidine mouthwash with respect to parameters of gingival inflammation.[33,34]
   d. The mechanism of action of essential oils appears to be disruption of the integrity of the cell wall and inhibition of certain bacterial enzymes.
   e. Essential oil mouth rinses are much less expensive than chlorhexidine mouth rinses and can be purchased without a prescription. Insofar as the side effects associated with chlorhexidine mouth rinses—staining, taste alteration—may limit patient compliance, essential oil mouth rinses can have a distinct role in the management of patients with periodontal diseases.

F. **Mouth Rinses Containing Quaternary Ammonium Compounds**
   1. Some mouth rinses currently marketed contain the quaternary ammonium compound cetylpyridinium chloride as the active ingredient.
   2. This surface active agent also kills bacteria by disrupting bacterial cell walls.
   3. This chemical agent binds to oral tissues, but is released so rapidly that it has very limited substantivity, limiting its effectiveness in controlling dental biofilm.
   4. Investigations have shown that cetylpyridinium chloride can reduce the severity of gingivitis and supragingival biofilm, but the level of reduction is less than either chlorhexidine gluconate or essential oils.[35,36]

G. **Mouth Rinses Containing Delmopinol**
   1. Some mouth rinses currently marketed contain delmopinol as the active ingredient, which is a third-generation morpholinoethanol derivative and tertiary amine surfactant.
   2. This chemical agent forms a barrier preventing biofilm from adhering to the tooth surface and gingiva. Delmopinol interferes with the enzymes responsible for the formation of biofilm and inhibits biofilm.
   3. Tooth and tongue staining side effects have been reported with delmopinol, but were not found to be comparable with the staining associated with chlorhexidine gluconate.
   4. Investigations have shown that delmopinol effectively reduces the severity of gingivitis and biofilm when used adjunctively with mechanical biofilm removal and is a good alternative to chlorhexidine gluconate for some patients that cannot tolerate the associated side effects and allergies.[37,38]

H. **Problems With Mouth Rinse Ingredients**
   1. No chemicals are completely safe for all patients, and most mouth rinses have produced unwanted side effects in some patients. Reported side effects for some of the active ingredients discussed above are outlined in Table 27-4.
   2. As already discussed, in addition to the active ingredients, mouth rinses contain inactive ingredients such as flavoring agents and preservatives that can create problems for some patients. Two of these ingredients are listed below.
      a. Alcohol. Some mouth rinses have rather high levels of alcohol content, and these should be avoided in patients addicted to alcohol.
      b. Salt. Some mouth rinses have rather high levels of sodium, making them questionable for use in certain patients with hypertension (high blood pressure).

TABLE 27-4	POSSIBLE SIDE EFFECTS OF MOUTH RINSES
Essential Oils Rinses	**Chlorhexidine Gluconate Rinses**
• Burning sensation in the mouth • Bitter taste • Drying out of mucous membranes	• Allergic reaction • Extrinsic staining of teeth • Discoloration of tongue • Alterations of taste • Increase in calculus formation • Transient anesthesia

3. Toothpastes as Delivery Mechanisms for Biofilm Control Agents. Dentifrices, such as toothpastes and gels, would appear to be nearly ideal delivery mechanisms for chemical agents that might benefit patients, since most patients use these products daily.

   A. Categories of Toothpastes. The ADA loosely classifies toothpastes into one of the following categories:

      1. Antitartar activity

      2. Caries prevention

      3. Cosmetic effects

      4. Gingivitis reduction

      5. Biofilm formation reduction

      6. Reduction of tooth sensitivity

   B. Active Chemical Ingredients. This ADA classification of toothpastes underscores the broad range of benefits that can be derived from active ingredient chemical agents added to some toothpastes.

      1. Some of these chemical agents are added to impart special benefits to periodontal patients. See Table 27-5 for some examples of the chemical agents that can be used as active ingredients in toothpastes for their periodontal benefits.

      2. Stannous fluoride has been used successfully as an anticaries agent for many years. Studies indicate that stannous fluoride also affects dental biofilm and can also reduce the severity of gingivitis when used as an active ingredient in toothpastes.

      3. Triclosan is a topical antimicrobial agent used in many products and is now available as the active ingredient in a toothpaste.

         a. Triclosan can be combined with copolymers to enhance its substantivity (binding and subsequent slow release), which has been found to be retained in the oral cavity for 12 hours.

         b. Studies indicate that when combined with copolymers, triclosan (when delivered in toothpaste form) can decrease the severity of gingivitis more than dentifrice with stannous fluoride.[39,40] Triclosan can also be combined with zinc citrate to reduce dental calculus formation.

   C. The Future. Toothpastes appear to be ideal delivery mechanisms for chemical agents that might be expected to control certain periodontal conditions, such as gingival inflammation. It is reasonable to expect that additional research in this area will result in additional toothpaste formulations that target periodontal conditions, such as gingivitis.

TABLE 27-5	EXAMPLES OF ACTIVE INGREDIENTS IN TOOTHPASTE THAT HAVE PERIODONTAL BENEFITS
Ingredients	**Actions**
Pyrophosphates	Reduces *supra*gingival calculus
Stannous fluoride	Reduces *supra*gingival biofilm Reduces gingival inflammation
Triclosan	Reduces *supra*gingival calculus Reduces gingival inflammation
Zinc citrate	Reduces *supra*gingival calculus

Section 4
Educating Patients on the Use of Unconventional Dental Products/Remedies

The ADA defines the term "unconventional dentistry" as "*encompassing scientifically unproven practices and products that do not conform to generally accepted dental practices or "conventional" methods of evaluation, diagnosis, prevention and/or treatment of diseases, conditions and/or dysfunctions relating to the oral cavity and its associated structures.*"[41]

Today's consumers are being inundated with a wide variety of unconventional dental products/remedies that are backed by unproven claims, questionable effectiveness, and dubious safety. As a result, all members of the dental team must be able to help the patient filter out all the hyperbole and exaggeration associated with some of these unconventional, commercially available products. Equally important, dental clinicians must be prepared to educate the patient that not all over-the-counter dental products have earned the ADA-Seal of Acceptance (which is the gold standard for all dental products that demonstrate safety and efficacy according to the requirements developed by the ADA Council on Scientific Affairs).

Two unconventional, non-ADA approved products/remedies that have made recent headlines are (1) charcoal/charcoal-based products and (2) oil-pulling.

1. **Charcoal/Charcoal-Based Dental Products**
    A. **Historical Overview of Charcoal/Charcoal-Based Dental Products**
        1. The first-recorded use of charcoal for oral hygiene dates back to ancient Greece. Since then, the use of charcoal for oral hygiene—in the form of charcoal paste or charcoal powder—has spread worldwide.
        2. In the 1930s and 1940s, the use of charcoal dental products was twice evaluated by The Council of Dental Therapeutics.[42,43] At the time, no evidence was provided to the Council that would support charcoal's safety and effectiveness. Furthermore, there was a lack of evidence to counter the possibility that charcoal products could be a potentially harmful substance. Thus, at each time, the Council judged charcoal-based dental products to be "not acceptable" for patient use.
    B. **Current Evidence Related to Charcoal/Charcoal-Based Dental Products**
        1. Currently, much of the claims supporting the use of charcoal is based on anecdotal evidence. To date, there remains a lack of controlled clinical trials and laboratory investigations of charcoal-based dentifrices to substantiate its purported benefits (Fig. 27-5).
        2. In the most comprehensive review of the safety and effectiveness of charcoal-based dental products, Brooks et al. found several health risks that may be associated with the use of charcoal-based dental products.[44] First, they found that only 8.0% of charcoal-based products contain fluoride, which may put the patient more at risk of developing caries. Second, they raised the concern that since charcoal is an abrasive material, it may cause damage to the teeth (tooth abrasion) and/or gingiva (gingival recession). Thus, the authors concluded that much of the health benefits, cosmetic, and safety claims made by manufacturers of charcoal-based dental products cannot be verified at this time.

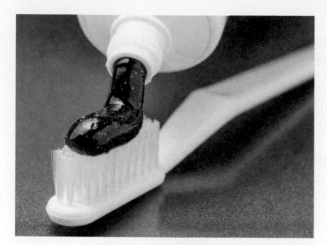

Figure 27-5. Charcoal Toothpaste.

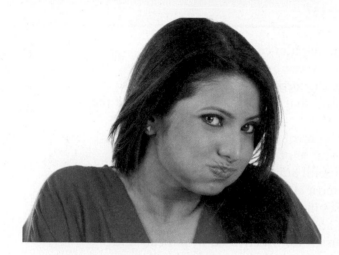

Figure 27-6. Oil Pulling. A teenage girl doing oil pulling.

C. **Purported Mechanism of Action of Charcoal/Charcoal-Based Dental Products.** Charcoal is highly porous, which conceivably gives charcoal the ability to "trap" chemicals. In industrial applications, some gas masks have charcoal filters which help "trap" and filter out noxious substances. In medicine, charcoal is administered in drug overdose cases and acute poisoning cases since its porosity binds to these toxic substances and decreases the body's absorption of these harmful agents. Thinking along the same lines, manufacturers of charcoal-based dental products use this rationale to make the claim that charcoal can be used in the mouth to "trap" and remove toxins and "lift" stains off teeth (tooth-whitening claim).

2. **Oil Pulling**
   A. **Historical Overview of Oil Pulling.** Oil pulling is an ancient Indian folk remedy also known as "Kavala Graha" or "Gandusha." Original practitioners of oil pulling used sunflower and sesame oils as a way to prevent gingival bleeding, caries, and oral malodor. Other oils that have been used as part of this remedy include coconut oil, palm oil, and olive oil (Fig. 27-6).

B. **Current Evidence Related to Oil Pulling.**
1. Like charcoal-based dental products, all existing claims to support oil pulling is purely anecdotal. To date, there has not been any reliable scientific analysis performed to either support or disprove oil pulling as part of the regular oral hygiene regimen.
2. Consequently, both the ADA and Canadian Dental Association (CDA) can neither recommend nor reject oil pulling due to the lack of scientific evidence at this time.

C. **Purported Mechanism of Action of Oil Pulling.**
   Oil is placed in the mouth and either swished or held in the mouth for 10 to 20 minutes, then spit out. Proponents of this remedy claim the prolonged time that the oil stays in the mouth draws (or "pulls") out all the bacteria and toxins that build up in the mouth.

Chapter Summary Statement

Chemical agents that can be used to control dental biofilm can be delivered both systemically and topically. Since dental biofilm is covered by a protective slime layer, chemical agents will not necessarily contact all of the targeted bacteria, and their use must be accompanied by mechanical biofilm control that can disrupt the structure of the biofilm.

Systemic antibiotics are not normally used to control dental biofilm in patients with the most common periodontal conditions because of the high risk of developing antibiotic resistant strains. Mouth rinses can be useful adjuncts in the treatment of patients with periodontal diseases. Thus far, the most effective ingredients to control biofilm that can be incorporated into mouth rinses include chlorhexidine and the essential oils. Controlled-release delivery devices are also available to help control bacterial biofilm in periodontal patients. Toothpastes are widely used by patients and appear to be an ideal mechanism for delivery of chemical agents to aid in biofilm control. In selecting the appropriate delivery system, the clinician has to weigh the efficacy of the products, ease of use, availability, and cost. Although local delivery systems do not replace existing periodontal therapies, they do have a place in the treatment of periodontitis and offer the dental team additional methods to aid in the control of periodontal diseases.

When drugs or remedies fail to perform as intended or patients do not receive sufficient education about chemotherapeutic agents, the consequences can lead to unintended or, even worse, potentially harmful outcomes. Therefore, it is essential that the dental clinician clearly appreciates the rationale for using chemical agents and keeps abreast of the emerging scientific evidence that either support or disprove present day and future chemotherapeutic agents.

Section 5
Focus on Patients

Clinical Patient Care

CASE 1

A patient shows you a bottle of mouth rinse and asks you if it would be all right to use this mouth rinse instead of brushing and flossing so frequently. You study the label on the bottle of mouth rinse and find that the active ingredients are the essential oils. How should you respond to this patient about substituting this rinse for other self-care efforts such as brushing and flossing?

CASE 2

A patient being treated by the members of your dental team has generalized periodontitis. Following your thorough explanation of the nature of periodontitis and your emphasis that this disease is indeed a bacterial infection, the patient asks this question, "If periodontitis is an infection, can you ask the dentist to give me a prescription for an antibiotic?" How should you respond to this patient's question?

CASE 3

A new patient being seen by your dental team has recently moved into your city. She has previously been treated for periodontitis and has been on periodontal maintenance for several years. She is now having trouble with mechanical biofilm control because of increasing dexterity problems. What chemical agents can you recommend that might help reduce the patient's gingival inflammation?

CASE 4

A patient returns to the office for a periodic oral examination. She recalls that she recently watched an internet documentary about charcoal-based dental products. She wonders if there is any benefit to using charcoal toothpaste instead of conventional toothpaste. She also asks if the scientific evidence supports the routine use of charcoal toothpaste. How would you respond to her inquiry?

Ethical Dilemma

Your patient, Sandy L., is a 24-year-old woman who has come to your office for a second opinion. Her chief complaint is that she feels that her periodontal health is not improving, and if anything, getting worse.

You review her health history, and she states that she has been under the care of her uncle, who is a 70-year-old periodontist. She has been taking tetracycline for the last 5 years and is concerned with her periodontal and overall health. She did not bring any radiographs, as she doesn't want her uncle to know about this appointment.

Your examination reveals that Sandy has relatively good oral hygiene, with slight supragingival visible calculus between her mandibular anterior teeth. However, she presents with generalized severe gingival recession, and her attachment level readings range from 3 to 6 mm, with localized 7 mm readings on her posterior teeth.

It is hard to get a full picture due to the lack of radiographs. Sandy's periodontal status is troubling and you are not sure if the antibiotics that she is taking are actually helping her. You ask if she ever had a microbiologic analysis, to sample her oral bacteria susceptibility. She is not sure of any procedures, as she "just left all of that stuff to her uncle, the periodontal expert."

1. What do you think is the possible cause of the patient's generalized recession?
2. What factors may have contributed to the patient's disease progression?
3. What ethical principles are in conflict in this dilemma?

References

1. Finkelman RD, Polson AM. Evidence-based considerations for the clinical use of locally delivered, controlled-release antimicrobials in periodontal therapy. *J Dent Hyg.* 2013;87(5):249–264.
2. Cobb CM. Clinical significance of non-surgical periodontal therapy: an evidence-based perspective of scaling and root planing. *J Clin Periodontol.* 2002;29 Suppl 2:6–16.
3. Drisko CL, Cochran DL, Blieden T, et al. Position paper: sonic and ultrasonic scalers in periodontics. Research, Science and Therapy Committee of the American Academy of Periodontology. *J Periodontol.* 2000;71(11):1792–1801.
4. Hanes PJ, Purvis JP. Local anti-infective therapy: pharmacological agents. A systematic review. *Ann Periodontol.* 2003;8(1):79–98.
5. Greenstein G. The role of local drug delivery in the treatment of chronic periodontitis. Things you should know. *Dent Today.* 2004;23(3):110–115.
6. Mah TF, O'Toole GA. Mechanisms of biofilm resistance to antimicrobial agents. *Trends Microbiol.* 2001;9(1):34–39.
7. Rams TE, Degener JE, van Winkelhoff AJ. Antibiotic resistance in human chronic periodontitis microbiota. *J Periodontol.* 2014;85(1):160–169.
8. Walker CB. The acquisition of antibiotic resistance in the periodontal microflora. *Periodontology 2000.* 1996;10:79–88.
9. Sedlacek MJ, Walker C. Antibiotic resistance in an in vitro subgingival biofilm model. *Oral Microbiol Immunol.* 2007;22(5):333–339.
10. Slots J, Research S, Therapy C. Systemic antibiotics in periodontics. *J Periodontol.* 2004;75(11):1553–1565.
11. Caton JG, Ciancio SG, Blieden TM, et al. Treatment with subantimicrobial dose doxycycline improves the efficacy of scaling and root planing in patients with adult periodontitis. *J Periodontol.* 2000;71(4):521–532.
12. Ciancio S, Ashley R. Safety and efficacy of sub-antimicrobial-dose doxycycline therapy in patients with adult periodontitis. *Adv Dent Res.* 1998;12(2):27–31.
13. Thomas J, Walker C, Bradshaw M. Long-term use of subantimicrobial dose doxycycline does not lead to changes in antimicrobial susceptibility. *J Periodontol.* 2000;71(9):1472–1483.
14. Ciancio SG. Site specific delivery of antimicrobial agents for periodontal disease. *Gen Dent.* 1999;47(2):172–178, 181.
15. Finkelman RD. Re: role of controlled drug delivery for periodontitis (position paper). The American Academy of Periodontology (2000;71:12-40). *J Periodontol.* 2000;71(12):1929–1933.
16. Greenstein G. Local drug delivery in the treatment of periodontal diseases: assessing the clinical significance of the results. *J Periodontol.* 2006;77(4):565–578.
17. Greenstein G, Tonetti M. The role of controlled drug delivery for periodontitis. The Research, Science and Therapy Committee of the American Academy of Periodontology. *J Periodontol.* 2000;71(1):125–140.
18. Killoy WJ. The clinical significance of local chemotherapies. *J Clin Periodontol.* 2002;29 Suppl 2:22–29.
19. van Steenberghe D, Rosling B, Soder PO, et al. A 15-month evaluation of the effects of repeated subgingival minocycline in chronic adult periodontitis. *J Periodontol.* 1999;70(6):657–667.

20. Williams RC, Paquette DW, Offenbacher S, et al. Treatment of periodontitis by local administration of minocycline microspheres: a controlled trial. *J Periodontol.* 2001;72(11):1535–1544.

21. Wennstrom JL, Newman HN, MacNeill SR, et al. Utilisation of locally delivered doxycycline in non-surgical treatment of chronic periodontitis. A comparative multi-centre trial of 2 treatment approaches. *J Clin Periodontol.* 2001;28(8):753–761.

22. Jeffcoat MK, Palcanis KG, Weatherford TW, Reese M, Geurs NC, Flashner M. Use of a biodegradable chlorhexidine chip in the treatment of adult periodontitis: clinical and radiographic findings. *J Periodontol.* 2000;71(2):256–262.

23. Henke CJ, Villa KF, Aichelmann-Reidy ME, et al. An economic evaluation of a chlorhexidine chip for treating chronic periodontitis: the CHIP (chlorhexidine in periodontitis) study. *J Am Dent Assoc.* 2001;132(11):1557–1569.

24. Barnett ML. The role of therapeutic antimicrobial mouthrinses in clinical practice: control of supragingival plaque and gingivitis. *J Am Dent Assoc.* 2003;134(6):699–704.

25. Osso D, Kanani N. Antiseptic mouth rinses: an update on comparative effectiveness, risks and recommendations. *J Dent Hyg.* 2013;87(1):10–18.

26. Jones CG. Chlorhexidine: is it still the gold standard? *Periodontol 2000.* 1997;15:55–62.

27. Mathur S, Mathur T, Shrivastava R, Khatri R. Chlorhexidine: The gold standard in chemical plaque control. *Natl J Physiol Pharm Pharmacol.* 2011;1(2):45–50.

28. Li W, Wang RE, Finger M, Lang NP. Evaluation of the antigingivitis effect of a chlorhexidine mouthwash with or without an antidiscoloration system compared to placebo during experimental gingivitis. *J Investig Clin Dent.* 2014;5(1):15–22.

29. Zanatta FB, Antoniazzi RP, Rosing CK. The effect of 0.12% chlorhexidine gluconate rinsing on previously plaque-free and plaque-covered surfaces: a randomized, controlled clinical trial. *J Periodontol.* 2007;78(11):2127–2134.

30. Gupta G, Mitra D, Ashok KP, et al. Efficacy of preprocedural mouth rinsing in reducing aerosol contamination produced by ultrasonic scaler: a pilot study. *J Periodontol.* 2014;85(4):562–568.

31. Klyn SL, Cummings DE, Richardson BW, Davis RD. Reduction of bacteria-containing spray produced during ultrasonic scaling. *Gen Dent.* 2001;49(6):648–652.

32. Charles CH, Mostler KM, Bartels LL, Mankodi SM. Comparative antiplaque and antigingivitis effectiveness of a chlorhexidine and an essential oil mouthrinse: 6-month clinical trial. *J Clin Periodontol.* 2004;31(10):878–884.

33. Stoeken JE, Paraskevas S, van der Weijden GA. The long-term effect of a mouthrinse containing essential oils on dental plaque and gingivitis: a systematic review. *J Periodontol.* 2007;78(7):1218–1228.

34. Van Leeuwen MP, Slot DE, Van der Weijden GA. Essential oils compared to chlorhexidine with respect to plaque and parameters of gingival inflammation: a systematic review. *J Periodontol.* 2011;82(2):174–194.

35. Haps S, Slot DE, Berchier CE, Van der Weijden GA. The effect of cetylpyridinium chloride-containing mouth rinses as adjuncts to toothbrushing on plaque and parameters of gingival inflammation: a systematic review. *Int J Dent Hyg.* 2008;6(4):290–303.

36. Versteeg PA, Rosema NA, Hoenderdos NL, Slot DE, Van der Weijden GA. The plaque inhibitory effect of a CPC mouthrinse in a 3-day plaque accumulation model—a cross-over study. *Int J Dent Hyg.* 2010;8(4):269–275.

37. Addy M, Moran J, Newcombe RG. Meta-analyses of studies of 0.2% delmopinol mouth rinse as an adjunct to gingival health and plaque control measures. *J Clin Periodontol.* 2007;34(1):58–65.

38. Moran J, Addy M, Wade WG, et al. A comparison of delmopinol and chlorhexidine on plaque regrowth over a 4-day period and salivary bacterial counts. *J Clin Periodontol.* 1992;19(10):749–753.

39. Ciancio S, Panagakos FS. Superior management of plaque and gingivitis through the use of a triclosan/copolymer dentifrice. *J Clin Dent.* 2010;21(4):93–95.

40. Haraszthy VI, Zambon JJ, Sreenivasan PK. Evaluation of the antimicrobial activity of dentifrices on human oral bacteria. *J Clin Dent.* 2010;21(4):96–100.

41. ADA Association. ADA policy statement on unconventional dentistry. Available from: https://www.ada.org/en/about-the-ada/ada-positions-policies-and-statements/unconventional-dentistry. Accessed May 28, 2018.

42. Gordon SM. Kramer's original charcoal dental cream: Not acceptable for A.D.R. *J Am Dent Assoc.* 1932;19(5):868–869.

43. Council on Dental Health. Reports of councils and committees: Peter Paul's charcoal gum—not acceptable for A.D.R. *J Am Dent Assoc.* 1946;33(13):912–913.

44. Brooks JK, Bashirelahi N, Reynolds MA. Charcoal and charcoal-based dentifrices: A literature review. *J Am Dent Assoc.* 2017;148(9):661–670.

STUDENT ANCILLARY RESOURCES

A wide variety of resources to enhance your learning is available online:

- Audio Glossary
- Book Pages
- Chapter Review Questions and Answers

28 Host Modulation Therapy

Clinical Application. Host modulation therapy is currently one of the most exciting areas of research related to periodontal diseases. Although few host modulating agents currently are approved for the treatment and management of periodontal disease, dental practitioners will have greater exposure to this type of therapy as more studies are devoted to this topic. To interpret emerging evidence correctly, dental hygienists will need to understand how host modulation therapy works and prepared to accept this modality as a valid part of patient care. This chapter provides an outline of the topic of host modulation therapy.

Learning Objectives

- Define the term host modulation therapy.
- Discuss the potential importance of host modulation therapy.
- Name some anti-inflammatory mediators.
- Name some pro-inflammatory mediators.
- List three types of drugs that have been studied for use as possible host modulating agents.
- Explain why low-dose doxycyclines are useful as host modulating agents.
- Explain the term sub-antibacterial dose.
- Make a list of treatment strategies for a periodontitis patient that includes host modulation.

Key Terms

Host modulation therapy
Osteoporosis
Biochemical mediators
Anti-inflammatory mediators

Pro-inflammatory
  mediators
Doxycycline
Sub-antibacterial doses

Nonsteroidal anti-inflammatory
  drugs (NSAIDs)
Bisphosphonates

Section 1
Introduction to Host Modulation Therapy

For several decades, the focus of therapy for patients with inflammatory periodontal diseases has been directed toward controlling the microbial etiology of these diseases; minimizing the bacterial challenge to the periodontium has been a successful strategy for the treatment of many patients with both gingivitis and periodontitis. Beyond any doubt, plaque biofilm control strategies will continue to play a major role in the therapy for patients with periodontal disease.

Based upon current knowledge of the underlying pathology involved in periodontal diseases, additional therapeutic strategies are emerging that may also be employed for patients with inflammatory periodontal diseases. One of these additional strategies relates to the concept of host modulation therapy.[1–4]

1. **Host Modulation Therapy Defined.** Host modulation therapy can be defined as modifying a patient's (i.e., the host's) defense responses to help the body's defenses limit damage caused by a disease. In dentistry, the concept of host modulation therapy focuses on how the body responds to the bacterial challenge rather than simply reducing that bacterial challenge posed by plaque biofilm.

2. **Examples of Host Modulation Therapy in Medicine**
   A. Host modulation therapy is *not* a new concept in medicine, and it has been a part of the medical care for patients with a variety of systemic diseases for many years. One example of a common systemic disease for which physicians frequently use host modulation is osteoporosis.
   B. Osteoporosis is a progressive bone disease that is characterized by a decrease in both bone mass and bone density that can lead to an increased risk of bone fractures. Osteoporosis affects millions of patients in the United States.
   C. Treatments for osteoporosis can be broadly divided into two categories based upon how the treatment medications affect bone. One group of medications *reduces bone resorption*, while the second group of medications *stimulates bone formation*.
      1. Anti-resorptive agents, which include medications such as estrogen, selective estrogen receptor modulators and bisphosphonates, reduce bone resorption and help to preserve bone mineral density.
      2. Bone-forming agents, such as teriparatide (Forteo), stimulate bone formation, thereby increasing overall bone mineral density.
   D. Patients who receive the types of medications discussed above are said to be receiving host modulation therapy; that is, the host response to the disease (loss of bone mass and density) is modulated to minimize the effects of the disease to prevent bone fractures.

3. **Importance of Host Modulation Therapy in Dentistry.** The potential importance of host modulation as one strategy in managing periodontitis patients is huge.
   A. Many adults show signs of periodontal disease, with periodontitis affecting approximately 65 million adults in the United States, according to the most recent national estimates. Because so many patients have inflammatory periodontal diseases, there is a continuing need for cost-effective strategies that can be combined with conventional periodontal treatment for managing periodontitis patients.
   B. As the population in the United States ages, it is reasonable to expect the prevalence of periodontitis to increase, making the need for the most cost-effective therapy even greater.

C. In addition, there is mounting evidence that periodontal health and several systemic conditions (such as diabetes and cardiovascular disease) are linked, again making it likely that the demand for periodontal therapy will increase over the upcoming decades.

4. **Review of Host Responses That Can Be Modulated**

A. The fundamental pathologic processes for periodontitis have been outlined in other chapters of this book, including:

1. Bacteria (and bacterial products) that are a part of the plaque biofilm initiate an inflammatory response in the periodontium. The bacteria stimulate the immune cells to produce **biochemical mediators** (i.e., biologically active compounds) that activate this inflammatory response.

2. The inflammatory response functions as a protective mechanism that keeps the bacterial infection from doing serious harm to the periodontium in many patients partly through the production of chemicals called anti-inflammatory mediators. **Anti-inflammatory mediators** are biochemical mediators that are protective and limit the bacterial-induced inflammatory response from doing serious harm to the periodontium. These anti-inflammatory mediators include the cytokines IL-4 (interleukin-4) and IL-10 (interleukin-10).

3. Box 28-1 shows an overview of some of the anti-inflammatory biochemical mediators that have been discussed in other chapters.

4. If the bacterial challenge is great enough, however, the nature of the protective responses changes, resulting in the production of excessive biochemical mediators that can lead to actual damage within the periodontium.

   a. Some biochemical mediators (referred to as **pro-inflammatory mediators**) can damage the periodontium. These pro-inflammatory biochemical mediators include chemicals such as matrix metalloproteinases (MMPs), certain cytokines, prostanoids, and other less well-understood mediators.[5-9]

   b. Specific examples of these pro-inflammatory mediators include prostaglandin E_2, IL-1α (interleukin-1 alpha), IL-1β (interleukin-1 beta), IL-6 (interleukin-6), and tumor necrosis factor alpha.

   c. For example, one of the MMPs is an enzyme called collagenase that can actually break down collagen. Collagen is one of the major building blocks in the periodontium, and its breakdown is part of the fundamental pathology in periodontitis.

   d. Box 28-2 shows some of the pro-inflammatory biochemical mediators.

5. In the periodontium, these altered host defense responses can result in both breakdown of connective tissue fibers and resorption of alveolar bone (the precise types of tissue destruction seen in periodontitis).

6. Much of the destruction of the periodontium that accompanies periodontitis is thought to be a result of these altered processes that occur as part of the host defenses (the host inflammatory and immune responses).

B. Fundamentally, the concept of host modulation therapy as a strategy in treating periodontitis patients is to limit the damaging effect of the altered host responses by modifying (or modulating) the effect of these destructive biochemical mediators. Modulation of host defenses is currently an important focus for periodontal research, and host modulation therapy will undoubtedly play a far larger part in periodontal therapy in the future.

Box 28-1. Examples of Anti-Inflammatory Biochemical Mediators

These biochemical mediators play a key role in limiting the tissue-damaging effects of the pro-inflammatory response.

- IL-4 (interleukin-4)
- IL-10 (interleukin-10)
- IL-1ra (receptor antagonist)
- TIMPs (tissue inhibitors of matrix metalloproteinases)

Box 28-2. Examples of Pro-Inflammatory Biochemical Mediators

These biochemical mediators are produced by the host immune cells in response to microbial invasion. Elevated levels of these mediators can lead to tissue destruction.

- IL-1 (interleukin-1)
- IL-6 (interleukin-6)
- *PGE$_2$* (prostaglandin E$_2$)
- *TNFα* (tumor necrosis factor alpha)
- *MMPs* (matrix metalloproteinases)

Section 2
Potential Host Modulating Therapies in Periodontal Patients

1. Use of Tetracycline Medications
   A. Doxycycline
      1. Doxycycline is a tetracycline-class antibiotic drug that has been used to treat a variety of infections.
         a. As with other antibiotic medications, doxycycline must be given in doses high enough to affect the targeted bacteria to help the body fight an infection.
         b. Antibiotic doses high enough to inhibit or kill bacteria are sometimes called antibacterial doses. A typical antibacterial dose for doxycycline would be 50 to 100 mg every 12 hours.
      2. Doxycycline has other benefits besides its antibiotic effect that is seen with the higher doses described above.
         a. If this medication is given even at low doses (*below that needed for any antibacterial effect*), it inhibits the effects of the enzyme collagenase (one of the matrix metalloproteinases or MMPs).
         b. As already discussed, MMPs (such as collangenase) are released by host "cells as" part of the inflammatory response. Elevated levels of MMPs cause the tissue breakdown that typically occurs in periodontitis. Prevention of the action of collagenase can inhibit the progress of periodontal tissue breakdown.
         c. Doses of an antibiotic that are below the normal bacterial killing or inhibiting doses are referred to as sub-antibacterial doses.
         d. Since doxycycline at low doses (or sub-antibacterial doses) alters the body's defenses by inhibiting part of the destruction that can occur in periodontitis, it is considered one example of a host modulating agent.[10–22]

e. The FDA (U.S. Food and Drug Administration) has approved sub-antibacterial doses of doxycycline (20-mg tablets) for use in treating patients with periodontitis.

1) Low doses of doxycycline must be taken twice daily in tablet form to be effective in periodontitis patients.

2) No antibacterial effect on the oral bacteria or bacteria in other parts of the body have been found with the use of low-dose doxycycline.

3) Studies of this drug have also shown a clinical benefit when used as an adjunct to periodontal instrumentation.

4) Though tetracyclines used at antibacterial doses can have side effects (including nausea, vomiting, photosensitivity, and hypersensitivity reactions), doxycycline at low doses appears to be accompanied by a very low incidence of adverse effects.

3. Studies have shown reductions in probing depths and gains in clinical attachment levels, as well as, the prevention of periodontal disease progression with the use of sub-antibacterial doses of doxycycline in periodontitis patients.

B. **Use of Chemically Modified Tetracyclines**

1. Chemically modified tetracyclines are derivatives of tetracycline group of drugs that lack antimicrobial action but have potent host modulating affects.

2. Though these drugs lack antimicrobial action, they can inhibit elevated MMPs, pro-inflammatory cytokines, and other destructive chemical mediators.[23]

3. Bone resorption also can be suppressed by reducing the effects of inflammation with these medications.

4. Development of resistant bacteria and gastrointestinal toxicity seen with antibacterial doses of the tetracyclines is *not* produced by chemically modified tetracyclines.[23]

5. Chemically modified tetracyclines are currently being investigated as potential host modulation therapeutic agents in the management of chronic diseases like periodontitis, but only further research may demonstrate their efficacy and safety in periodontal patients.

2. **Use of Nonsteroidal Anti-Inflammatory Drugs**

A. Nonsteroidal anti-inflammatory drugs (NSAIDs) have been used for many years in medical care to treat pain, acute inflammation, and chronic inflammatory conditions.

1. Box 28-3 shows examples of drugs included in the group called NSAIDs.

2. NSAIDs can reduce tissue inflammation by inhibiting the action of prostaglandins, such as PGE_2.

B. In periodontal studies, systemically administered NSAIDs have been evaluated for their effect on periodontitis (a disease intimately associated with inflammation).

1. In the periodontium, NSAIDs can both reduce inflammation and inhibit osteoclast activity.

2. Some NSAIDs, when administered daily over 3 years, have been shown to slow the rate of alveolar bone loss associated with periodontitis.

3. More research is needed in this area to clarify the efficacy and safety of using NSAIDs as host modulating agents in periodontal patients.

C. Long-term use of NSAIDs in periodontitis patients is not recommended because of significant systemic side effects that can develop with the use of these drugs.

1. Side effects from NSAIDs can include gastrointestinal problems, hemorrhage (bleeding), and kidney or liver impairment.

2. In addition, when a patient with periodontitis stops taking daily doses of NSAIDs, there can be an acceleration of the bone loss seen prior to taking the drugs.
3. At present, no NSAIDs are approved for the treatment of periodontal disease.

Box 28-3. Examples of NSAID Medications

- Salicylates (aspirin)
- Indomethacin
- Ibuprofen
- Flurbiprofen
- Naproxen

D. Even though NSAIDs are not currently recommended for use in host modulation in periodontitis patients, they have been discussed here because of the extensive dental research that has involved these drugs.
E. In addition to systemically administered NSAIDs, topically applied NSAIDs have been studied for their possible benefits to periodontitis patients.
   1. Topical NSAIDs have also been shown to reduce PGE_2 (prostaglandin E_2) in gingival crevicular fluid in periodontitis patients.[24–27]
   2. Topically administered NSAIDs have not been approved for the management of periodontitis, but more study of the possible use of topical NSAIDs is warranted.

3. **Use of Bisphosphonate Medications**
A. Bisphosphonates are drugs that can inhibit the resorption of bone by altering osteoclastic activity, though the mechanism of action for these drugs is not fully understood.
B. Early research indicates there may be some benefit to periodontitis patients from the ability of bisphosphonates to alter osteoclastic activity (bone resorption activity).[25,28]
C. Some of the bisphosphonates have side effects that may limit their use in periodontitis patients, but they are discussed in this section because of the interest that has been shown in these drugs over the last few years.
D. One of the possible side effects of these drugs is osteonecrosis of the jaws following their extended use.[29] Osteonecrosis is the destruction and death of bone tissue, in this case the bone tissue of the jaw. Studies are underway to clarify the precise risk and etiology of this serious side effect of bisphosphonates.
E. *At present, there are no bisphosphonate drugs that are approved for the treatment of periodontal disease.*

4. **Use of Statin Medications**
A. Recently, it has been suggested that statin drugs that are normally used to control elevated cholesterol levels may have an effect upon periodontitis.
B. There are quite a few statin medications available, but only a few such as simvastatin and atorvastatin have been suggested as possible host modulation agents in periodontal patients.
C. Statin medications have several effects including offering some protection against systemic inflammation.[30]
D. At this point, the efficacy of these drugs in periodontal patients needs to be clarified with additional research studies.

5. **Dietary Supplementation**
   A. Dietary supplementation is another avenue that may hold promise for developing strategies to modify the host response to periodontitis, especially if it is possible to enhance the resolution of inflammation through dietary supplements.
   B. The possibility of supplementing the diet with specific biomolecules, such as essential fatty acids, is currently being investigated for its effect upon periodontitis.[31–33]
   C. Using supplements of omega-3 fatty acids to modify the host response to periodontitis and reduce the tissue-destructive impact of periodontitis would certainly be a straightforward strategy for host modulation therapy if studies demonstrate the efficacy of such supplements.
   D. Resolvins are anti-inflammatory mediators derived from omega-3 fatty acids, and work to resolve inflammation to reduce the risk of tissue breakdown and attachment loss. Topical application of resolvins has been shown to prevent bone loss and attachment loss from periodontitis in animal models.[34] Currently, human trials are underway to test the resolvins. In the near future, resolvin-based materials to treat periodontitis might be commercially available.

6. **Use of Other Types of "Host Modulation Agents"**
   A. Several potential agents have been investigated for use as adjuncts to periodontal surgical procedures.
   B. These drugs do not produce the same types of effects discussed for the other potential host modulating agents, but they are mentioned here because some authors have referred to them as "host modulating agents."
   C. These agents are generally applied topically during periodontal surgical procedures and have been suggested for use for possible enhancement to wound healing or possible enhancement of regeneration of periodontal tissues following the surgery.
   D. Some agents of this type that have been investigated are enamel matrix proteins, bone morphogenetic proteins (BMP-2, BMP-7), and certain growth factors.
   E. Currently, the only local host modulation agent approved for adjunctive use during periodontal surgery is an enamel matrix protein called Emdogain, and this agent is under continuing study.
   F. Members of the dental team should expect additional host modulation products to be investigated and to appear on the market; careful evaluation of each of the products will be needed.[2]

Section 3
Host Modulation Therapy as a Part of Comprehensive Periodontal Patient Management

1. Periodontal therapy based upon minimizing the bacterial challenge has been a primary therapeutic modality for many years, and this therapy has proved to be successful in many patients.
   A. Studies indicate, however, that markers of periodontal disease in patients with periodontitis undergo little change following conventional mechanical periodontal therapy, in spite of its successful outcomes.
   B. It appears that even though conventional periodontal therapy based upon minimizing the bacterial challenge is usually successful, the underlying disease processes may indeed be diminished in severity, but they may remain fundamentally unchanged.
   C. These observations should not distract from a clinician's enthusiasm for recommending conventional periodontal therapy, but they should make clinicians eager for more therapies to be developed and to be added to those currently available.
2. Employing host modulation therapy in the comprehensive management of some periodontal patients seems to be a promising strategy to employ in the future.
   A. It should be reemphasized that at present, the only host modulation therapy agent currently FDA-approved is the low-dose doxyclines, but as discussed, investigations have indicated that at least theoretically other possible host modulation therapies may one day be employed in periodontal patients.
   B. It must also be noted that when used in periodontitis patients, sound clinical practice dictates that the use of low-dose doxycycline therapy be accompanied by all of the usual treatment strategies such as risk factor reduction (i.e., smoking cessation counseling) and bacterial challenge reduction (i.e., self-care training and periodontal instrumentation).
3. Box 28-4 lists the array of therapeutic strategies that can be employed when managing a patient with periodontitis to illustrate that host modulation therapy may be viewed as another therapy among the long list of options available for a patient with periodontal disease.
4. Figure 28-1 shows some theoretical possibilities for host modulation as a part of overall management of periodontitis patients.

Box 28-4. Therapeutic Options for a Periodontitis Patient

1. Patient education and training in self-care.
2. Employment of motivational strategies for patient self-care.
3. Reduction of the bacterial challenge by periodontal instrumentation.
4. Use of local delivery systems for antimicrobial agents.
5. Elimination of local contributing factors.
6. Systemic risk factor reduction.
7. Host modulation therapy.
8. Periodontal surgery.
9. Periodontal maintenance.

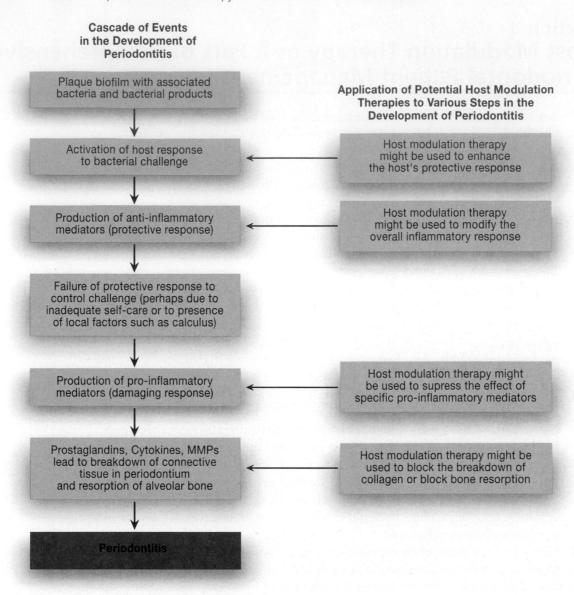

Figure 28-1. Application of Potential Host Modulation Therapies. Potential host modulation therapies can be applied to a cascade of events starting with plaque biofilm and ending with periodontitis. This figure shows the wide range of potential applications that research may make possible in the future.

Chapter Summary Statement

Host modulation therapy in periodontal patients (i.e., modifying the body's defense mechanisms to limit damage from the oral bacterial challenge) is an interesting and ongoing line of investigation. Host modulation therapy has been suggested as an additional therapeutic strategy in periodontitis patients. At this point, low-dose doxycycline has been approved for use as a host modulating agent in humans with periodontitis. When used in sub-antimicrobial doses, this drug can help inhibit the progress of periodontitis. Members of the dental team will undoubtedly encounter much research activity related to additional host modulating therapies over the next several decades.

Section 4
Focus on Patients

Evidence in Action

CASE 1

A new patient in your dental team's office has a periodontal diagnosis of generalized Stage III, Grade B periodontitis. Explain how host modulation therapy might be included among other treatment strategies used to help control the damage to the periodontium that normally accompanies periodontitis.

Ethical Dilemma

Tammy is a 60-year-old artist, who you see every 3 months for periodontal maintenance, as she suffers from generalized periodontitis. As you review her health history today, she states that she is now taking Fosamax, which was prescribed by her primary care physician, Dr. James. She states that she has been diagnosed with osteoporosis, and has been taking Fosamax for the last 2 months. Dr. James also told Tammy that the medication would be helpful in stabilizing her periodontal disease, which was a side benefit. He assured her that there is no downside in taking the medication.

Tammy has done some research on line, and has found some disturbing evidence of the possible side effects of Fosamax. She asks for your thoughts and opinion.

1. Are bisphosphonate drugs approved for the treatment of periodontal disease?
2. What would tell Tammy about the possible side effects of the use of bisphosphonate drugs?
3. Are there ethical principles in conflict with this dilemma?

References

1. Bhatavadekar NB, Williams RC. New directions in host modulation for the management of periodontal disease. *J Clin Periodontol.* 2009;36(2):124–126.
2. Gokhale SR, Padhye AM. Future prospects of systemic host modulatory agents in periodontal therapy. *Br Dent J.* 2013;214(9):467–471.
3. Salvi GE, Lang NP. Host response modulation in the management of periodontal diseases. *J Clin Periodontol.* 2005;32 Suppl 6:108–129.
4. Tonetti MS, Chapple IL; Working Group 3 of Seventh European Workshop on Periodontology. Biological approaches to the development of novel periodontal therapies—consensus of the Seventh European Workshop on Periodontology. *J Clin Periodontol.* 2011;38 Suppl 11:114–118.
5. Birkedal-Hansen H. Role of matrix metalloproteinases in human periodontal diseases. *J Periodontol.* 1993;64(5 Suppl): 474–484.
6. Deo V, Bhongade ML. Pathogenesis of periodontitis: role of cytokines in host response. *Dent Today.* 2010;29(9):60–62, 64–66; quiz 68–69.
7. Golub LM, Lee HM, Greenwald RA, et al. A matrix metalloproteinase inhibitor reduces bone-type collagen degradation fragments and specific collagenases in gingival crevicular fluid during adult periodontitis. *Inflamm Res.* 1997;46(8):310–319.
8. Kornman KS. Host modulation as a therapeutic strategy in the treatment of periodontal disease. *Clin Infect Dis.* 1999;28(3):520–526.
9. Offenbacher S, Heasman PA, Collins JG. Modulation of host PGE2 secretion as a determinant of periodontal disease expression. *J Periodontol.* 1993;64(5 Suppl):432–444.
10. Caton J, Ryan ME. Clinical studies on the management of periodontal diseases utilizing subantimicrobial dose doxycycline (SDD). *Pharmacol Res.* 2011;63(2):114–120.
11. Choi DH, Moon IS, Choi BK, et al. Effects of sub-antimicrobial dose doxycycline therapy on crevicular fluid MMP-8, and gingival tissue MMP-9, TIMP-1 and IL-6 levels in chronic periodontitis. *J Periodontal Res.* 2004;39(1):20–26.

12. Emingil G, Atilla G, Sorsa T, Luoto H, Kirilmaz L, Baylas H. The effect of adjunctive low-dose doxycycline therapy on clinical parameters and gingival crevicular fluid matrix metalloproteinase-8 levels in chronic periodontitis. *J Periodontol*. 2004;75(1):106–115.

13. Golub LM, McNamara TF, Ryan ME, et al. Adjunctive treatment with subantimicrobial doses of doxycycline: effects on gingival fluid collagenase activity and attachment loss in adult periodontitis. *J Clin Periodontol*. 2001;28(2):146–156.

14. Golub LM, Suomalainen K, Sorsa T. Host modulation with tetracyclines and their chemically modified analogues. *Curr Opin Dent*. 1992;2:80–90.

15. Gu Y, Walker C, Ryan ME, Payne JB, Golub LM. Non-antibacterial tetracycline formulations: clinical applications in dentistry and medicine. *J Oral Microbiol*. 2012;4.

16. Novak MJ, Dawson DR, 3rd, Magnusson I, et al. Combining host modulation and topical antimicrobial therapy in the management of moderate to severe periodontitis: a randomized multicenter trial. *J Periodontol*. 2008;79(1):33–41.

17. Novak MJ, Johns LP, Miller RC, Bradshaw MH. Adjunctive benefits of subantimicrobial dose doxycycline in the management of severe, generalized, chronic periodontitis. *J Periodontol*. 2002;73(7):762–769.

18. Preshaw PM, Hefti AF, Bradshaw MH. Adjunctive subantimicrobial dose doxycycline in smokers and non-smokers with chronic periodontitis. *J Clin Periodontol*. 2005;32(6):610–616.

19. Preshaw PM, Hefti AF, Jepsen S, Etienne D, Walker C, Bradshaw MH. Subantimicrobial dose doxycycline as adjunctive treatment for periodontitis. A review. *J Clin Periodontol*. 2004;31(9):697–707.

20. Subramanian S, Emami H, Vucic E, et al. High-dose atorvastatin reduces periodontal inflammation: a novel pleiotropic effect of statins. *J Am Coll Cardiol*. 2013;62(25):2382–2391.

21. Thomas JG, Metheny RJ, Karakiozis JM, Wetzel JM, Crout RJ. Long-term sub-antimicrobial doxycycline (Periostat) as adjunctive management in adult periodontitis: effects on subgingival bacterial population dynamics. *Adv Dent Res*. 1998;12(2):32–39.

22. Walker C, Preshaw PM, Novak J, Hefti AF, Bradshaw M, Powala C. Long-term treatment with sub-antimicrobial dose doxycycline has no antibacterial effect on intestinal flora. *J Clin Periodontol*. 2005;32(11):1163–1169.

23. Agnihotri R, Gaur S. Chemically modified tetracyclines: Novel therapeutic agents in the management of chronic periodontitis. *Indian J Pharmacol*. 2012;44(2):161–167.

24. Howell TH, Williams RC. Nonsteroidal antiinflammatory drugs as inhibitors of periodontal disease progression. *Crit Rev Oral Biol Med*. 1993;4(2):177–196.

25. Reddy MS, Geurs NC, Gunsolley JC. Periodontal host modulation with antiproteinase, anti-inflammatory, and bone-sparing agents. A systematic review. *Ann Periodontol*. 2003;8(1):12–37.

26. Salvi GE, Lang NP. The effects of non-steroidal anti-inflammatory drugs (selective and non-selective) on the treatment of periodontal diseases. *Curr Pharm Des*. 2005;11(14):1757–1769.

27. Williams RC, Jeffcoat MK, Howell TH, et al. Altering the progression of human alveolar bone loss with the non-steroidal anti-inflammatory drug flurbiprofen. *J Periodontol*. 1989;60(9):485–490.

28. Thumbigere-Math V, Michalowicz BS, Hodges JS, et al. Periodontal disease as a risk factor for bisphosphonate-related osteonecrosis of the jaw. *J Periodontol*. 2014;85(2):226–233.

29. Weinreb M, Quartuccio H, Seedor JG, et al. Histomorphometrical analysis of the effects of the bisphosphonate alendronate on bone loss caused by experimental periodontitis in monkeys. *J Periodontal Res*. 1994;29(1):35–40.

30. Price U, Le HO, Powell SE, et al. Effects of local simvastatin-alendronate conjugate in preventing periodontitis bone loss. *J Periodontal Res*. 2013;48(5):541–548.

31. Dawson DR, 3rd, Branch-Mays G, Gonzalez OA, Ebersole JL. Dietary modulation of the inflammatory cascade. *Periodontol 2000*. 2014;64(1):161–197.

32. Elkhouli AM. The efficacy of host response modulation therapy (omega-3 plus low-dose aspirin) as an adjunctive treatment of chronic periodontitis (clinical and biochemical study). *J Periodontal Res*. 2011;46(2):261–268.

33. Sculley DV. Periodontal disease: modulation of the inflammatory cascade by dietary n-3 polyunsaturated fatty acids. *J Periodontal Res*. 2014;49(3):277–281.

34. Chee B, Park B, Fitzsimmons T, Coates AM, Bartold PM. Omega-3 fatty acids as an adjunct for periodontal therapy—a review. *Clin Oral Investig*. 2016;20(5):879–894.

STUDENT ANCILLARY RESOURCES

A wide variety of resources to enhance your learning is available online:

- Audio Glossary
- Book Pages
- Chapter Review Questions and Answers

CHAPTER

29 Periodontal Surgical Concepts for the Dental Hygienist

Clinical Application. As members of the dental team, dental hygienists must understand fundamental concepts related to periodontal surgery so that they can discuss this important topic with both patients and with other health care providers. In addition, hygienists often play a primary role in the management and maintenance of patients following periodontal surgery. A basic understanding of periodontal surgical procedures can provide the framework for improved patient care during critical stages of healing of periodontal surgical wounds. This chapter provides foundational information about basic periodontal surgical concepts.

Learning Objectives

- List objectives for periodontal surgery.
- Explain the term relative contraindications for periodontal surgery.
- Define the terms repair, reattachment, new attachment, and regeneration.
- Explain the difference between healing by primary intention and healing by secondary intention.
- Explain the rationale, indications, and advantages of elevating a periodontal flap.
- Explain two methods for classifying periodontal flaps.
- Describe two types of incisions used during periodontal flaps.
- Describe healing following flap for access and open flap debridement.

- Describe the typical outcomes for apically positioned flap with osseous surgery.
- Define the terms ostectomy and osteoplasty.
- Define the terms osteogenesis, osteoinductive, and osteoconductive.
- Explain the terms autograft, allograft, xenograft, and alloplast.
- Name two types of materials available for bone replacement grafts.
- Explain why a barrier material is used during guided tissue regeneration.
- Explain the term periodontal plastic surgery.
- List two types of crown lengthening surgeries.
- List some disadvantages of gingivectomy.
- Explain what is meant by biological enhancement of periodontal surgical outcomes.
- Name two broad categories of materials used for suturing periodontal wounds.
- Explain the term interrupted interdental suture.
- List general guidelines for suture removal.
- Describe the technique for periodontal dressing placement.
- List general guidelines for periodontal dressing management.
- Explain the important topics that should be covered in postsurgical instructions.
- List steps in a typical postsurgical visit.

Key Terms

Resective
Osseous defect
Relative contraindications
Repair
Reattachment
New attachment
Regeneration
Primary intention
Secondary intention
Tertiary intention
Periodontal flap
Flap elevation
Full-thickness flap
Blunt dissection
Partial-thickness flap
Sharp dissection
Nondisplaced flap
Displaced flap
Horizontal incision

Crevicular incision
Internal bevel incision
Vertical incision
Flap for access
Open flap debridement
Osseous resective surgery
Ostectomy
Osteoplasty
Apically positioned flap with
    osseous resective surgery
Bone replacement graft
Osteogenesis
Osteoconduction
Osteoinduction
Autograft
Allograft
Xenograft
Alloplast
Guided tissue regeneration

Periodontal plastic surgery
Mucogingival surgery
Free soft tissue autograft
Subepithelial connective tissue
    graft
Laterally positioned flap
Coronally positioned flap
Semilunar coronally repositioned
    flap
Frenectomy
Crown lengthening surgery
Functional crown lengthening
Esthetic crown lengthening
Gingivectomy
Gingivoplasty
Periodontal microsurgery
Nonabsorbable suture
Absorbable suture
Periodontal dressing

Section 1
Introduction to Periodontal Surgery

The primary goals for any periodontal procedure—whether it be of nonsurgical or surgical nature—are (1) to eliminate the pathologic changes in the pocket and (2) to create a stable and easily maintainable healthy state of the periodontium throughout the life of the patient. However, in instances where the severity of periodontitis becomes more advanced, arresting disease progression with nonsurgical therapy alone becomes increasingly daunting. Thus, the need for periodontal surgery as part of comprehensive patient care becomes ever more apparent.

EVOLUTION OF CONCEPTS RELATED TO PERIODONTAL SURGERY

1. **Historical Perspective for Periodontal Surgery.** For many years, various types of periodontal surgical procedures have been recommended for dental patients with periodontitis and other periodontal conditions to control and eliminate the disease.
   A. Until the middle of the 20th century, the aims of periodontal surgery was (1) to intentionally sever or remove what was thought to be dead or infected tissue in the periodontium and (2) to reshape gingival and osseous tissues to attain a harmonious topography. These early periodontal surgical techniques are referred to as resective procedures. The term resective surgery refers to those procedures that simply cut away and remove some of the periodontal tissues.
   B. The concept of periodontal resective surgery (cutting away tissues) is still done today in clinical practice, however, it shares little in common with other periodontal surgical procedures that focus on regenerating periodontal tissues.
2. **Move Toward Modern Periodontal Surgical Techniques**
   A. Since the late 20th century, as our understanding of basic sciences and regenerative medicine has advanced, an evolution of both the objectives and techniques for periodontal surgery has taken place.
   B. The emphasis in periodontal surgery has shifted away from the resective types of periodontal surgery to periodontal surgical procedures that rebuild or regenerate periodontal tissues damaged or lost because of disease.

INDICATIONS AND CONTRAINDICATIONS FOR SURGERY

1. **Indications for Periodontal Surgery.** A periodontist can employ an array of surgical techniques that are directed toward different outcomes. The most common indications for periodontal surgery are outlined below and in Box 29-1.
   A. **To Provide Access for Improved Periodontal Instrumentation of Root Surfaces**
      1. Periodontal surgery provides enhanced access and visualization to the root surfaces for more thorough periodontal instrumentation. Since nonsurgical instrumentation of root surfaces in the presence of deep periodontal pockets is challenging, the improved access that is provided by periodontal surgery can be a huge advantage for clinicians.

2. Even though clinicians can select from a wide array of hand and ultrasonic instruments; as probing depths in the dentition increase, it becomes more and more difficult to reach root surfaces for thorough periodontal instrumentation.

Box 29-1. Indications for Periodontal Surgery

- To provide access for improved periodontal instrumentation of root surfaces
- To reduce pocket depths
- To provide access to periodontal osseous defects
- To resect or remove tissue
- To regenerate the periodontium lost due to disease
- To graft bone or bone-stimulating materials into osseous defects
- To improve the appearance of the periodontium
- To enhance prosthetic dental care
- To allow for the placement of a dental implant

---

3. Periodontal surgery involving carefully planned incisions through the gingiva can allow for temporary lifting of the soft tissue off the tooth surface. More details about this type of surgery are presented under *flaps for access* in the following descriptions of periodontal surgery.

B. **To Reduce Pocket Depths**
   1. As pocket depth increases, it can become increasingly difficult for patients to perform effective self-care techniques, and plaque biofilms that thrive in the protected environment of the deep pocket can make it impossible to stop the progress of periodontitis.
   2. Periodontal surgical procedures can reduce the pocket depths so that a combination of daily self-care and periodic professional periodontal maintenance improves the chance of maintaining the periodontium in health throughout the life of the patient.

C. **To Provide Access to Periodontal Osseous Defects**
   1. An osseous defect is a deformity in the tooth-supporting alveolar bone usually resulting from periodontitis. Figure 29-1 shows an example of an osseous defect as viewed during a periodontal surgical procedure.
      a. As periodontitis advances, alveolar bone loss results in changes in the normal contour and structure of the supporting alveolar bone.
      b. The pattern of bone loss can vary from one tooth to the next and even on different aspects of the same tooth, creating an array of defects in alveolar bone contours referred to as osseous defects.
   2. Periodontal surgery to modify the alveolar bone level or contour is called periodontal osseous surgery.
      a. Bone defects can be managed surgically through a variety of techniques discussed later in this chapter.
      b. Information about how osseous defects can be managed using periodontal surgery is presented under the topics *osseous resective surgery*, *apically positioned flap with osseous surgery*, *bone replacement graft*, and *guided tissue regeneration* in other sections of this chapter.

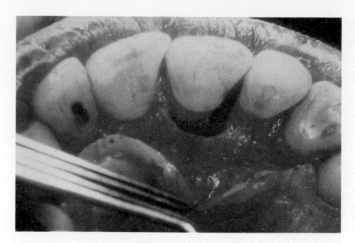

Figure 29-1. Periodontal Osseous Defect Exposed During Surgery. The soft tissues have been incised and temporarily lifted away from the teeth to reveal the bone contour. Note the extensive alveolar bone loss around one of the central incisor teeth creating a moat-like defect around this tooth. This type of bone defect would be an ideal site for bone replacement graft discussed later in the chapter.

D. **To Resect or Remove Tissue**
1. Enlarged gingival tissues can be unsightly and can also interfere with proper self-care; in some patients, enlarged gingiva can even interfere with comfortable mastication.
2. Even though the focus of most modern periodontal surgery is *not* resection of tissues, this surgical approach can still be indicated in some instances.
3. Periodontal surgery can be used to remove and reshape enlarged gingiva; additional information on this type of periodontal surgery is found in the chapter section that discusses the *gingivectomy*.

E. **To Regenerate the Periodontium Lost due to Disease**
1. One of the ultimate goals in periodontics is to be able to regenerate periodontal tissues that were damaged by disease. The term "regenerate" describes the reconstitution of new tissue. Likewise, in periodontal regeneration, the objectives are to form new cementum, new functionally aligned periodontal ligament fibers, and new alveolar bone.
2. Although it is not possible to regenerate the periodontium in all instances, it is possible to achieve this regeneration in many sites using some sophisticated periodontal surgical techniques; information on regenerative periodontal surgery is presented under *guided tissue regeneration* in another section of this chapter.

F. **To Graft Bone or Bone-Stimulating Materials Into Osseous Defects**
1. Some periodontal osseous defects offer the opportunity for the periodontist to graft either bone or bone-stimulating materials into the defects.
2. Although this surgery may seem quite similar to periodontal regeneration surgery, grafting bone does not necessarily imply regeneration of other parts of the periodontium, such as cementum and periodontal ligament. More information on this interesting topic is located under *bone replacement graft* in another section of this chapter.

G. **To Improve the Appearance of the Periodontium**
1. Some patients have gingival levels or gingival contours that result in an unattractive smile; periodontal surgery also includes a variety of techniques for improving the appearance of the gingiva and improving the quality of a patient's smile.

2. There are, of course, many restorative techniques for improving the appearance of the teeth themselves, however for many patients, alteration of the appearance of the gingiva must be coordinated with restorative dentistry and orthodontics to achieve a truly pleasing appearance. More information on this topic is found in the other sections of this chapter under *periodontal plastic surgery* and *crown lengthening surgery*.

H. To Enhance Prosthetic Dental Care

1. Modern prosthetic dental care has created the need for a variety of periodontal surgical procedures such as altering alveolar ridge contours, lengthening tooth crowns, augmenting the amount of gingiva, or augmenting the bone in an edentulous site prior to implant placement.

2. Modern periodontal surgery includes many procedures directed toward enhancing some aspect of restorative dentistry and enhancing prosthetic dental care. These surgical procedures may involve combinations of all types of periodontal surgery.

I. To Allow for the Placement of a Dental Implant

1. Replacement of missing teeth with a dental implant is an option that must be considered when natural teeth are lost. The topic of dental implants is discussed in Chapter 9, but is listed here as one of the indications for periodontal surgery for completeness.

2. Periodontal surgery can also be used to prepare sites for dental implants.

   a. One of the basic tenets of dental implant placement is that the implant must be surrounded by sound alveolar bone.

   b. It is not at all unusual for edentulous sites—where implants are to be placed—to be deficient in the amount of alveolar bone needed to surround the implant. Such sites will require some type of bone grafting procedure prior to implant placement.

2. **Contraindications for Periodontal Surgery**

   A. **The Concept of Relative Contraindications.** A contraindication is a condition which makes a particular treatment or procedure potentially inadvisable. A contraindication may be absolute or relative. Most contraindications for periodontal surgery are relative contraindications rather than absolute contraindications.

   1. A relative contraindication is a condition that *may* make periodontal surgery inadvisable. When a condition or situation is severe or extreme, periodontal surgery may be inadvisable, but a condition may not be a contraindication if the condition is mild. An absolute contraindication, on the other hand, is a situation that makes a particular treatment *absolutely* inadvisable. An example of an absolute contraindication for periodontal surgery might be a patient with full-blown AIDS.

   2. An example of a relative contraindication for periodontal surgery might be a patient with hypertension (high blood pressure).

      a. A patient with uncontrolled severe hypertension would not be a candidate for periodontal surgery as long as the blood pressure remained *severely* elevated.

      b. At the same time, a patient with only mildly elevated blood pressure may be a suitable candidate for periodontal surgery.

   B. **Common Relative Contraindications for Periodontal Surgery.** Common *relative contraindications* for periodontal surgery are outlined below.

   1. **Patients Who Have Certain Systemic Diseases or Conditions**

   a. Systemic diseases or conditions that can be relative contraindications for periodontal surgery include conditions such as the following:
1) Uncontrolled hypertension
2) Recent history of myocardial infarction (heart attack)
3) Uncontrolled diabetes
4) Certain bleeding disorders
5) Kidney dialysis
6) History of radiation to the jaws
7) HIV infection

   b. It should be noted that consultation with a patient's physician is always indicated if there is any doubt about the patient's health status or if there is any doubt about how that status might affect planned periodontal surgical intervention.

2. Patients Who Are Totally Noncompliant With Self-Care

   a. The outcomes of many types of periodontal surgery are at least in part dependent upon the level of plaque biofilm control maintained by the patient's daily efforts at self-care following the surgical procedure.

   b. Lack of compliance with self-care instructions can be a relative contraindication for some types of periodontal surgery if that lack of compliance is so poor that it precludes the possibility of achieving acceptable periodontal surgical outcomes.

3. Patients Who Have a High-Risk for Dental Caries

   a. Some types of periodontal surgery result in exposure of portions of tooth roots. In a patient with uncontrolled dental caries where the risk for dental caries will remain quite high, it may not be wise to perform the types of periodontal surgery that increase root exposure due to the potentially devastating effect of root caries.

   b. Most often a high risk for dental caries can be altered, but when bringing the caries risk to an acceptable level is impossible, this risk can be a relative contraindication for some types of periodontal surgery.

4. Patients Who Have Totally Unrealistic Expectations for Surgical Outcomes

   a. Periodontitis damages the tissues that support the teeth, and surgical correction of that damage does not always result in a perfectly restored periodontium even when performed by the most skilled periodontist.

   b. If a patient cannot understand the nature of periodontal surgery and cannot develop realistic expectations for the outcomes of any planned periodontal surgery, it would not be wise to proceed with a plan for periodontal surgery. Thus, patient expectations can also be a relative contraindication for periodontal surgery.

POSSIBLE OUTCOMES FOR PERIODONTAL SURGERY

Table 29-1 (Fig. 29-2A–D) illustrates possible outcomes that may result from successful periodontal surgery:

1. Formation of a long junctional epithelium (as can be seen in response to nonsurgical therapy)
2. Resolution of inflammation and the associated periodontal pocket (as can be seen in response to nonsurgical therapy)
3. Regeneration (which is an expectation for periodontal regenerative surgery but not expected as a result of nonsurgical therapy alone).

TABLE 29-1	**POSSIBLE OUTCOMES FROM SUCCESSFUL PERIODONTAL SURGERY**

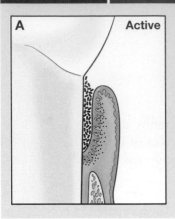

Figure 29-2A. Periodontal Pocket Prior to Therapy. The periodontal pocket with plaque biofilm and inflammation within the tissues prior to therapy.

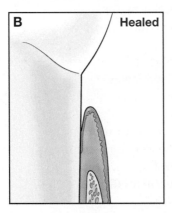

Figure 29-2B. Healing by Long Junctional Epithelium. Healing in the area of the former pocket at the site by formation of a long junctional epithelium. As noted in Chapter 2, the junctional epithelium attaches to the tooth at a level that is slightly coronal to the CEJ. When healing by long junctional epithelium occurs following periodontal surgery, however, the junctional epithelium closely attaches to the cementum (root surface).

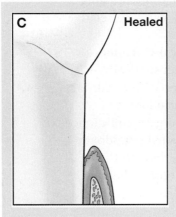

Figure 29-2C. Healing With Tissue Shrinkage. Healing at the site by resolution of the inflammation in the tissues will result in shrinkage of the tissues.

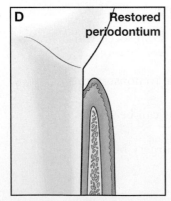

Figure 29-2D. Healing by Regeneration. Healing at the site by regeneration of the periodontal tissues.

TERMINOLOGY USED TO DESCRIBE HEALING AFTER SURGERY

Two sets of terminology are frequently used to describe healing of periodontal surgical wounds. One set of terms attempts to describe the various types of wound healing that can result from the surgery, and the second set of terms describes the degree of wound closure achieved at the time of surgery. The dental hygienist needs to have an understanding of both sets of terms, since all members of the dental team are likely to use both sets of terms when communicating with other dental health care practitioners.

1. **Terminology Describing Types of Wound Healing.** All periodontics textbooks present four terms that are used to describe the types of healing of the periodontium following periodontal surgery: *repair, reattachment, new attachment,* and *regeneration.* These terms are used to convey very specific wound healing concepts when describing the results of periodontal surgery.

   A. **Healing by *REPAIR***
      1. Repair is *healing of a wound by formation of tissues that do not fully restore the original architecture or original function of the body part.*
         a. An example of healing by repair would be the formation of a scar during the healing of an accidental cut involving a finger.
         b. Certainly, the healing of the finger wound is complete following formation of the scar, but the scar tissue is not precisely the same type of tissue in appearance form, or function that existed on that part of the finger before the cut.
      2. Repair is a perfectly natural type of healing for many types of wounds, including some wounds created during periodontal surgery.
         a. An example of repair in the periodontium is the healing that occurs following periodontal instrumentation (scaling and root planing).
            1) The usual healing of the wound created by periodontal instrumentation results in a close adaptation of epithelium to the tooth root.
            2) This adaptation of epithelium to the tooth root has been referred to as formation of a long junctional epithelium and has been discussed and illustrated in Chapter 24.
            3) Healing by long junctional epithelium occurs because the rate of mitosis and migration of epithelial cells across a debrided root surface is faster than other cell types. Thus, if cells of the epithelium make contact with the root surface before other cell types, then a long junctional epithelium will form.
         b. A long junctional epithelium is an acceptable outcome of healing, but it does not fully reconstitute the original periodontal tissues that were lost due to disease.
         c. To summarize, periodontal repair is characterized by *the formation of a long junctional epithelium, however there is no reconstitution or regeneration of new periodontal tissues.*

   B. **Healing by *REATTACHMENT***
      1. Reattachment means to "attach again." It is simply the *healing of a periodontal wound by the reunion of the connective tissue and roots where these two tissues have been separated by surgical incision or physical injury, but **not** by disease.*[1]
      2. Frequently, in periodontal surgery, it is necessary to elevate (gently separate) *healthy tissue* away from the underlying tooth root or bone temporarily during some types of periodontal surgery. For example, elevating the tissue may be necessary to allow access in removing healthy bone for the purposes of increasing the clinical crown height (surgical crown lengthening) of a tooth prior to restorative therapy. The expected type of healing is referred to as "healing by reattachment."

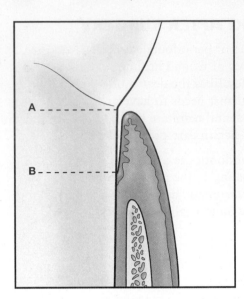

Figure 29-3. Area of the Tooth Root Involved in New Attachment. This drawing shows a site on a root where attachment loss has occurred as a result of disease.

- The region on the root from label **A** to label **B** represents the attachment loss that has occurred as a result of periodontitis.
- If the epithelium or connective tissue is attached to the root surface starting at label **B**, then healing by new attachment has occurred.

C. **Healing by *NEW ATTACHMENT***
   1. **New attachment** is *a term used to describe the union of a pathologically exposed root with connective tissue or epithelium*. This should not be confused with healing by reattachment.
   2. Healing by new attachment occurs when the epithelium and connective tissues are newly attached to a tooth root *where periodontitis had previously destroyed this attachment* (i.e., where attachment loss has occurred).[2,3]
   3. New attachment differs from reattachment because new attachment only occurs in an area formerly *damaged by disease*, whereas reattachment occurs when tissues are separated in the *absence of disease* (frequently as a result of the surgical procedure).
   4. Figure 29-3 illustrates the specific area on a tooth that must have newly attached epithelium and connective tissue for the healing to be called new attachment.

D. **Healing by *REGENERATION***
   1. **Regeneration** is the biologic process by which the architecture and function of lost tissue is *completely* restored.
   2. Unlike healing by new attachment which is characterized by the union of epithelium or connective tissue with a root surface that has been deprived of its original attachment apparatus, healing by regeneration results in the re-establishment of the *original* tissues that were present before the disease or damage occurred.
   3. For healing of the periodontium to be described as regeneration, the healing would have to result in the reformation of new cementum, new functionally oriented periodontal ligament fibers, and new alveolar bone.
   4. Regeneration of the periodontium is indeed possible with modern periodontal surgical procedures, but unfortunately the periodontium cannot be regenerated *predictably* in all sites with current periodontal regenerative approaches. Research is ongoing to improve the predictability of periodontal regenerative approaches.

2. **Terminology Describing the Degree of Wound Closure.** A second set of terms has also been used to describe events following periodontal surgery. These terms describe the degree of wound closure (i.e., how the margins or edges of the surgical wound relate to each other following the surgery but prior to the healing).

A. Healing by Primary Intention

1. Healing by primary intention occurs when the wound margins or edges are closely adapted to each other. The term **wound approximation** is used in medicine and dentistry to describe the lightly pulling together of wound edges from opposite sides so that they appear touching.

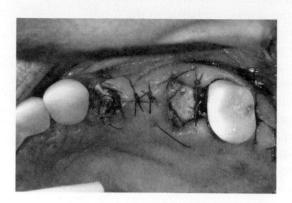

Figure 29-4. Healing by Primary and Secondary Intention. Healing by primary intention will occur across the incision line because the wound edges are closely adapted together. On the other hand, healing by secondary intention will occur in the extraction socket regions because the wound edges are not able to be brought together.

2. An example of primary intention healing would be seen in a small wound in a finger that required stitches. A physician places stitches to bring the margins of the wound closely together.
3. Healing by primary intention is usually faster than the other types of healing, but it is not always possible for wound margins to be closely adapted following periodontal surgery.
4. It should be noted that intraoral healing by primary intention in the periodontium may pose challenges that differ from the healing by primary intention that takes place in other sites in the body—such as healing of a cut finger. One edge of a surgical wound in the periodontium may be a tooth root that is avascular and cannot contribute any living cells to facilitate the wound healing process. This differs from healing by primary intention for a wound on a cut finger since both edges of the wound in the finger would be able to contribute living cells to the healing process.

B. Healing by Secondary Intention

1. Healing by secondary intention takes place when the margins or edges of the wound are not closely adapted (i.e., the two wound edges are not in close contact with each other).
2. When healing by secondary intention takes place, granulation tissue must form to close the space between the wound margins prior to growth of epithelial cells over the surface of the wound.
3. Healing by secondary intention is generally slower than healing by primary intention, since more vascular and cellular events are required in this type of healing.
4. Ideally, all wounds created during periodontal surgery are wounds that would be expected to heal by primary intention, but in reality many of the wounds created during surgery involve some wound healing by secondary intention. The healing of a tooth extraction socket (where the wound edges cannot be approximated together) is a classic example of healing by secondary intention (Fig. 29-4).

C. Healing by Tertiary Intention

1. In this type of healing, the wound is first cleaned by the surgeon and left open deliberately to ensure no infection is apparent before it is closed at a later date.
2. An example of tertiary intention is healing of a wound from a dog bite.
3. Healing by tertiary intention is not normally a type of healing that applies to healing of periodontal surgical procedures and is mentioned here only for completeness.

Section 2
Understanding the Periodontal Flap

Many modern periodontal surgical techniques begin by performing a periodontal flap, and the periodontal flap is an important step in most periodontal surgical procedures. As periodontitis progresses, it damages the attachment of the connective tissue to the tooth roots and destroys the surrounding alveolar bone. Treating patients with periodontitis and repairing damage done to the underlying periodontium requires gaining access both to tooth roots and to alveolar bone. As attachment loss associated with periodontitis progresses, access to tooth roots with conventional nonsurgical periodontal therapy becomes difficult if not impossible. Elevating a periodontal flap provides the means for gaining access to the underlying periodontal structures and to the tooth roots affected by the disease. Any overview of periodontal surgery requires some understanding of the techniques involved in performing a periodontal flap. This chapter section discusses the techniques and the associated terminology related to performing some of the many variations of a periodontal flap.

1. **Introduction to Periodontal Flaps**
   A. **Description of Procedure**
      1. A periodontal flap is a surgical procedure in which incisions are made in the gingiva or mucosa to allow for separation of the surface tissues (epithelium and connective tissue) from the underlying tooth roots and alveolar bone.
      2. Separating the surface tissues from the underlying tooth root and alveolar bone is commonly referred to as **flap elevation** or **reflection** (raising of the flap). The term "elevation" conveys the concept of gently lifting the gingival tissues away from the tooth roots and the alveolar bone.
      3. Once the gingiva or mucosa is elevated off the underlying roots and bone, it can be returned and sutured to its original position (known as a nondisplaced flap), or it can be displaced to different locations (known as a displaced flap). These two types of flaps will be discussed in upcoming sections under some of the specific types of surgery.
      4. Table 29-2 (Fig. 29-5A–C) shows a series of drawings that illustrate a typical periodontal flap surgical procedure used to gain access to the underlying tooth roots and alveolar bone.
   B. **Indications for a Periodontal Flap**
      1. Most modern periodontal surgical procedures require performing periodontal flaps as a part of the procedure.
      2. Basically, the flap elevation is done to provide access for treatment either to tooth roots or to the alveolar bone, or to both of these structures.
         a. Periodontal flaps can be elevated simply to provide access to tooth root surfaces for completion of meticulous periodontal instrumentation (scaling and root planing) that was begun as a part of nonsurgical periodontal therapy. Use of a periodontal flap for improved access to tooth roots is discussed in more detail later in this chapter under the heading *flaps for access*.

TABLE 29-2	TYPICAL PERIODONTAL FLAP SURGICAL PROCEDURE USED TO GAIN ACCESS TO UNDERLYING TOOTH ROOTS AND ALVEOLAR BONE
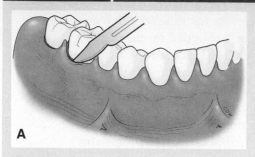	**Figure 29-5A.** Making an incision to allow for separation of the soft tissue from the roots and alveolar bone.
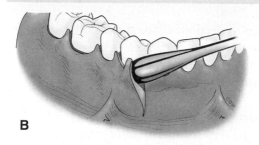	**Figure 29-5B.** Elevating (or raising) the soft tissue flap away from the roots of the teeth and alveolar bone.
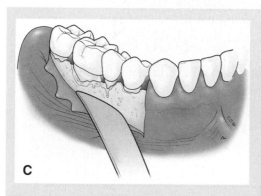	**Figure 29-5C.** Improved visualization of both the tooth roots and alveolar bone contours with the flap elevated.

Box 29-2. Common Terminology Used to Classify Periodontal Flaps

Based on Alveolar Bone Exposure
- Full-thickness flap
- Partial-thickness flap

Based on Location of Flap Margin
- Nondisplaced flap
- Displaced flap

2. **Classification of Periodontal Flaps.** There are several classification schemes used to describe periodontal flaps. Two of the most common include (1) the degree of bone exposure after flap elevation and (2) the location of the margin (or edge) of the flap when it is sutured back into place. Box 29-2 provides an overview of common terminology used to classify periodontal flaps.
   A. **Classification by Degree of Bone Exposure.** One method of classifying periodontal flaps is to describe the flap based upon the degree of exposure of alveolar bone following flap elevation. Using this method of classification, flaps would be categorized as either full-thickness or partial-thickness (Fig. 29-6).

1. The **full-thickness flap** provides complete access to underlying bone when bone replacement grafting or periodontal regeneration procedures are anticipated.
2. The full-thickness flap is elevated with what is generally referred to as a **blunt dissection**.
   a. Blunt dissection means that the tools used to elevate (or raise) the flap are not sharpened on the edge (i.e., blunted or slightly rounded on the edge); blunt dissection minimizes the chance of accidental damage to the flap.
   b. In this type of flap elevation, the flap is lifted or pried up using surgical tools called periosteal elevators, and it is elevated in a manner quite similar to lifting the peeling off an orange. Figure 29-7 illustrates a full-thickness flap (or mucoperiosteal flap) elevated during a periodontal surgical procedure.
3. A **partial-thickness flap**, or split-thickness flap, describes elevation of only the epithelium and a thin layer of the underlying connective tissue rather than the entire thickness of the underlying soft tissues (Fig. 29-8).
   a. The partial-thickness flap is elevated with **sharp dissection**; sharp dissection requires incising the underlying connective tissue in such a manner as to separate the epithelial surface plus a small portion of the connective tissue from the periosteum. *Use of this technique would leave the periosteum covering the bone.*
   b. To perform the sharp dissection needed in a partial-thickness flap, a surgeon uses a sharp scalpel blade to separate the flap from the underlying periosteum. The surgeon must also limit this approach to areas of gingiva that are relatively thick. If sharp dissection is attempted in areas of thin gingiva, then there is a risk of perforating (tearing) through the flap which can lead to flap necrosis.
   c. Research data indicates that when alveolar bone is exposed during a flap procedure there is a potential loss of a very small surface layer of the bone following the procedure. Whereas this change in the surface of the alveolar bone does not affect final healing, this fact can make use of a full-thickness flap inadvisable in certain instances.

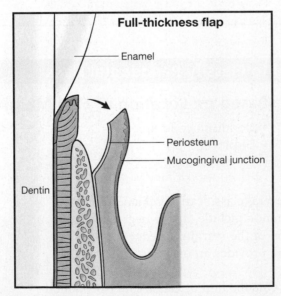
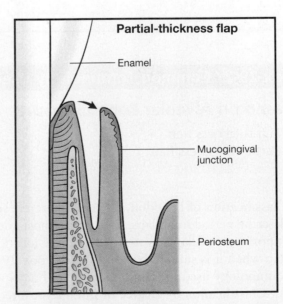

Figure 29-6. Flap Classification by Degree of Bone Exposure. The illustration on the left depicts a full-thickness flap to obtain access to the underlying alveolar bone. The illustration on the right depicts a partial-thickness flap in which the alveolar bone is not exposed.

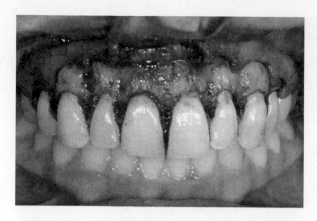

Figure 29-7. Full-Thickness Flap. This photo taken during a typical periodontal flap surgery shows a full-thickness, or mucoperiosteal flap (i.e., a flap of soft tissue that includes epithelium, underlying connective tissue, and the periosteum elevated off the teeth and alveolar bone). Note the exposure of the underlying alveolar bone margin.

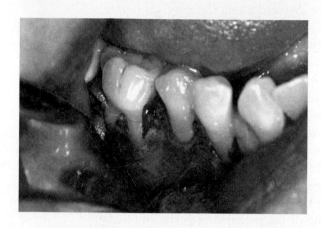

Figure 29-8. Partial-Thickness Flap. In a partial-thickness flap, the bone is not exposed and remains covered by the periosteum. (Case courtesy of Dr. Hawra Al Qallaf, Indianapolis, IN.)

B. **Classification by Location of the Soft Tissue Margin.** Another method of classifying periodontal flaps is to describe flaps based upon the location of the margin of the soft tissue when it is sutured back in place. Using this method of classification, flaps would be described as being either nondisplaced or displaced.
   1. A nondisplaced flap is a flap that is sutured with the margin of the flap at its original position in relationship to the CEJ on the tooth.
   2. A displaced flap is a flap that is sutured with the margin of the flap placed at a position other than its original position in relationship to the CEJ of the tooth. Note that a displaced flap can be positioned either apically, coronally, or laterally in relationship to its original position.
      a. For a displaced flap to be moved to a new position (such as apically, coronally, or laterally), the surgeon must perform the flap elevation in such a manner that the base of the flap extends into the moveable mucosal tissues. To achieve this, vertical incisions are made (discussed below).
      b. Displaced flaps are generally not possible to perform on the palatal gingiva because of the absence of movable mucosa in the maxillary posterior palatal region.
      c. Both a full-thickness flap and a partial-thickness flap can either be displaced or nondisplaced.
   3. **Types of Incisions Used During Periodontal Flap Surgeries.** Most of the incisions made prior to elevation of a periodontal flap are made with surgical scalpel blades, there are a wide variety of different types of incisions that can be made with these surgical scalpel blades. Some familiarization with terminology related to flap incisions

Box 29-3. Types of Incisions Utilized During Periodontal Flaps

Horizontal Incisions

- Crevicular incision
- Internal bevel incision

Vertical Incisions

- Vertical releasing incision

could be useful to the dental hygienist in understanding specific types of periodontal surgery. These incisions can be broadly classified as either horizontal or vertical incisions. Box 29-3 provides an overview of the types of incisions utilized during periodontal flaps.

A. **Horizontal Incisions.** Horizontal incisions are directed along the gingival margins in a mesiodistal direction.

1. One type of horizontal incision commonly employed during flap surgery is the crevicular incision.

2. In the crevicular incision, the surgical scalpel blade is carefully placed into the gingival crevice (also known as the sulcus) and directed apically to bone.

3. A second type of horizontal incision is the internal bevel incision.

4. In an internal bevel incision, the surgical scalpel blade enters the marginal gingiva, but is not placed directly into the crevice. Instead, the scalpel blade enters the gingiva approximately 0.5 to 1.0 mm away from the margin and follows the general contour of the scalloped marginal gingiva.

5. Using an internal bevel incision results in leaving a small collar of soft tissue around the tooth root (including the lining of the preexisting periodontal pocket); this collar of tissue is subsequently removed with hand instruments following flap reflection.

6. Terminology related to these incisions can be quite confusing.

   a. The internal bevel incision has also been referred to as a "reverse bevel incision" or the "initial incision" since it is usually made as a first step during a routine periodontal flap procedure. It is also known as "extrasulcular incision" or "extracrevicular incision" because the scalpel blade enters the gingiva *outside* of the sulcus.

   b. The crevicular incision has also been referred to as the "second incision" since it is usually made as the second step during a routine flap procedure. Another term for this type of incision is "sulcular incision" because the scalpel blade enters the gingiva *inside* the sulcus. Figure 29-9 shows both an internal bevel incision and crevicular incision.

B. **Vertical Incisions.** Vertical incisions run perpendicular or obliquely to the gingival margin in an apico-occlusal direction (Fig. 29-10).

1. Vertical incisions are primarily used to allow for the elevation of the flap without stretching or damaging the soft tissues during the surgical procedure.

2. The vertical incisions also are referred to as "vertical releasing incisions," since once this incision extends apical to the mucogingival junction, the flap is "released" and can be displaced (moved) apically, laterally, or coronally (Fig. 29-11).

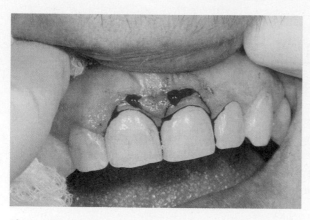
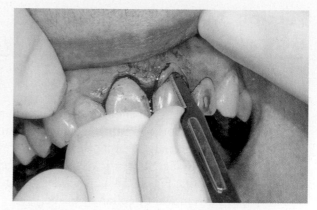

Figure 29-9. Horizontal Incisions. The photo on the left shows the initial incision is the inverse bevel incision. Note how the inverse bevel incision is made from a distance from the marginal gingiva. The right-hand photo shows the second incision is the crevicular incision. Note the location and direction of the scalpel blade in relation to the marginal gingiva when the crevicular incision is made.

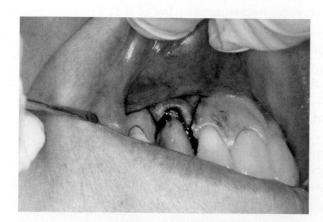

Figure 29-10. Vertical Incision. A vertical incision starts at the line angles of the tooth and extends apically into the alveolar mucosal tissues. Each vertical incision connects to one end of the horizontal incision.

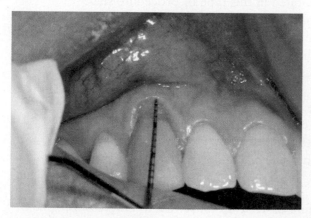
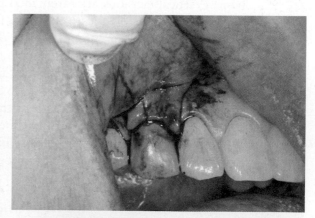

Figure 29-11. Coronal Displacement of Flap. The photo on the left is a presurgical photograph. Note the presurgical location of the gingival margin on the maxillary right canine. The photo on the right is an intraoral surgical photo. Note the "new" location of the gingival margin as a result of the two vertical incisions. The vertical incisions "released" the flap, thereby allowing the clinician to coronally displace the flap and cover the recession defect.

Section 3
Descriptions of Common Types of Periodontal Surgery

1. **Flap for Access**
   A. **Procedure Description**
      1. Flap for access (or modified Widman flap surgery) is used to provide access to the tooth roots for improved root preparation.[1,4–6] In this surgical procedure, both an internal bevel incision and a crevicular incision are made in the gingival tissues. The soft tissue is then gently elevated (lifted away) from the tooth roots. Figure 29-12 shows a flap for access with the flap elevated and partial removal of collar of tissue.
      2. There are two main advantages of flap for access.
         a. Flap for access surgery provides excellent access to the tooth roots for thorough instrumentation in sites where deep pocket depths may have hindered periodontal instrumentation during nonsurgical therapy.
         b. Flap for access surgery also provides an intimate adaptation of healthy connective tissues to the debrided tooth roots following suturing of the wound to allow for healing by primary intention.
      3. The tissues are elevated only enough to allow good access for periodontal instrumentation of the tooth roots. Following root treatment, the gingival tissue is replaced at its original position (i.e., a nondisplaced flap) and stabilized with sutures.
   B. **Steps in a Typical Flap for Access.** The usual steps followed during flap for access surgery are outlined below.
      1. An internal bevel incision is begun through the surface of the gingiva surrounding the teeth; the incision is made approximately 0.5 to 1.0 mm away from the gingival margin and follows the scallop of the marginal gingiva.
      2. The internal bevel incision that was begun as the first incision through the surface gingiva is retraced and extended apically all the way to the alveolar bone. (Vertical incisions are rarely incorporated in this type of procedure since the flap will ultimately return to its original location.)
      3. The flap is elevated far enough to provide good access to the tooth roots.
      4. A crevicular incision is then made from the base of the pocket to the bone to facilitate removal of the small collar of tissue remaining around the necks of the teeth.
      5. If needed, an incision may be made at the base of remaining tissue collar to completely free this tissue, and the tissue collar is removed with a hand curette.
      6. With the flap elevated, tooth roots are instrumented to remove remaining plaque biofilm, calculus deposits, root contaminants, and root irregularities.

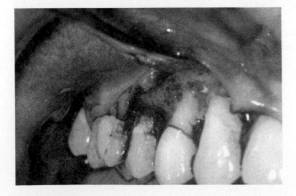

Figure 29-12. Flap for Access in Progress. This photo was taken during a flap for access. In the photo, the flap has been incised and elevated. Partial removal of the collar of tissue has been performed.

While performing the debridement, residual periodontal ligament fibers adhering to the tooth root near the base of the pocket are left undisturbed.

7. The flaps may be thinned if needed to allow for intimate adaptation of the gingiva to the necks of the teeth; alveolar bone contour is not altered unless minor recontouring is needed to allow for proper adaptation of the flap.

8. The flap is repositioned and sutured at its original position (nondisplaced); special effort is made to ensure that the tips of the facial and lingual papillae are in actual contact to promote healing by primary intention at this critical interdental site.

C. **Healing After Flap for Access**

1. The type of healing expected from flap for access surgery is *healing by repair* and usually involves formation of a *long junctional epithelium*.

2. Research shows that flap for access surgery can result in a stable dentogingival unit that can be maintained in health with periodic periodontal maintenance by the dental team and proper self-care by the patient.

D. **Special Considerations for the Dental Hygienist**

1. During routine nonsurgical periodontal instrumentation, it may not be possible to perform thorough subgingival biofilm and calculus removal if the pocket depths are deeper than 5 mm.[7] Flap for access surgery provides greatly improved access to root surfaces in areas of deeper pockets where the effectiveness of conventional nonsurgical periodontal instrumentation alone would be limited.

2. Even in patients where flap for access surgery is part of the treatment plan, every effort should be made to minimize the inflammation associated with periodontitis by performing complete nonsurgical therapy prior to the surgical intervention.

   a. The dental hygienist plays a critical role in promoting patient understanding of how nonsurgical and surgical treatment are related—first, nonsurgical therapy followed by surgical therapy, if needed.

   b. Thorough and meticulous nonsurgical periodontal instrumentation even in areas of deep pockets can reduce the extent of any planned periodontal surgical treatment and is always an important part of patient care.

2. **Open Flap Debridement**

A. **Procedure Description**

1. Open flap debridement is a term that describes a periodontal surgical procedure quite similar in concept and execution to flap for access surgery. In the periodontal literature, another term that has been used interchangeably with open flap debridement is open curettage.

2. Historically, the term open flap debridement was used to describe some of the original flap procedures that were first developed by periodontists many years ago.

3. Today open flap debridement (or flap curettage) is usually performed with steps quite similar to flap for access with the following exceptions:

   a. Exception #1. Open flap debridement usually includes more extensive flap elevation than flap for access—providing access not only to the tooth roots but also to all of the alveolar bone defects. Remember that during flap for access surgery, the flap is elevated only far enough to provide good access to the tooth roots.

   b. Exception #2. Whereas flap for access is considered to be a nondisplaced flap, open flap debridement may involve displacing the flap margin to a new location (i.e., during an open flap debridement, the flap margin may be sutured in a position more apical to its original position).

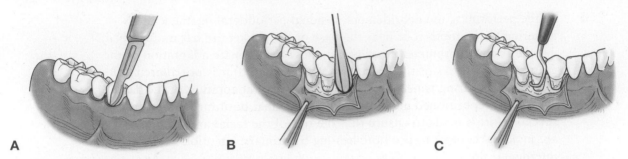

A **B** **C**

Figure 29-13. Critical Steps During a Typical Open Flap Debridement. A. Incisions being made to bone from within the crevice or pocket base. **B.** Flap elevation to expose tooth roots and alveolar bone. **C.** Periodontal instrumentation of the roots of the teeth.

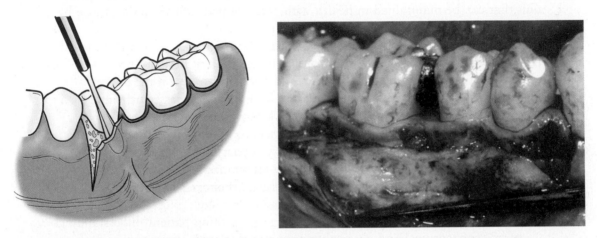

Figure 29-14. Open Flap Debridement. The illustration on the left shows a blunt instrument being used to elevate the overlying soft tissue away from the underlying bone. This type of flap elevation is classified as a full-thickness flap. The right-hand photo is a clinical photograph taken after flap elevation. Note the remaining tissue collar around the necks of the teeth. This tissue collar will be removed with a curette. Also note the extensive flap reflection to expose the underlying bone. (Illustration and photo courtesy of Dr. Donald Newell, Indianapolis, IN.)

B. Steps in Typical Open Flap Debridement

1. Figure 29-13 illustrates critical steps in a typical open flap debridement. The procedure begins with horizontal incisions that can be either crevicular or internal bevel incisions. The decision to use either crevicular incision or internal bevel incision is based on the amount of keratinized tissue. If there is a sufficient band of keratinized tissue available, both a crevicular incision and an internal bevel incision will be employed. However, if there is insufficient keratinized tissue, then only a crevicular incision will be used so as to preserve the tissue. Vertical releasing incisions can be included as needed to allow for atraumatic flap elevation.

2. Full-thickness (mucoperiosteal) flaps are elevated to provide access both to tooth roots and to the underlying alveolar bone defects (Fig. 29-14).

3. Granulation tissue is removed from existing osseous defects and from interdental areas. Tooth roots are instrumented to remove remaining plaque biofilm, calculus deposits, root contaminants, and root irregularities. Osteoplasty, which is not normally included in open flap debridement, is performed only if it is needed to allow for readaptation the tissues to the tooth roots.

4. Flaps are sutured either at their original level (nondisplaced) or at a level more apical to their original position (displaced).

C. Healing Expected After Open Flap Debridement
   1. Healing from open flap debridement is typically resolution of much of the existing inflammation within the periodontal tissues.
   2. The formation of a long junctional epithelium can occur along with slight remodeling of some of the osseous bone defects caused by periodontitis.
   3. Periodontal regeneration is not an outcome that occurs following open flap debridement. Instead, healing following open flap debridement is characterized by periodontal repair (previously discussed in the *Surgical Wound Healing* section).
   4. It is common for residual periodontal pockets to remain in some sites following this procedure—thus, complicating both patient self-care and professional periodontal maintenance.

3. **Osseous Resective Surgery.** The word "osseous" is defined as "having to do with bone." Thus, periodontal osseous surgery is surgery involving the alveolar bone.
   A. Description of Procedure
      1. Periodontal osseous resective surgery (or periodontal osseous surgery) is a term used to describe periodontal surgery employed to correct many of the irregular deformities of the alveolar bone that often result from periodontitis.[8,9]
      2. The fundamental goal for this type of periodontal surgery is to eliminate periodontal pockets, and this goal can be achieved when osseous surgery is combined with an apically displaced flap as discussed in the next section.
   B. Rationale for Periodontal Osseous Surgery
      1. Gingiva has a tendency to follow its natural architecture with or without the support of underlying alveolar bone; the natural architecture of gingiva is a scalloped contour where the level of the facial and lingual gingival margins is apical to the level of the interdental papillae.
      2. As periodontitis progresses, the contours of alveolar bone are altered by the formation of osseous defects referred to by names such as osseous craters, one-walled, two-walled, three-walled, and circumferential osseous defects which have been discussed in other chapters of this textbook (Fig. 29-15). In areas where these osseous defects form, attachment loss accompanies the alveolar bone contour changes and periodontal pockets form.
      3. The objectives of osseous surgery are twofold: (1) to reestablish normal alveolar bone contours that are in harmony with the natural contours of the gingiva following healing from periodontal surgery and (2) to recontour bone so that it resembles the bony contours undamaged by periodontitis. Thus, periodontal osseous surgery minimizes the discrepancy between the bone contour and the gingival contour to eliminate periodontal pockets following complete healing (Fig. 29-16).
      4. Periodontal osseous resective surgery is commonly performed in patients with mild periodontitis or moderate periodontitis where the bone defects created by the periodontitis are primarily osseous craters.
      5. However, osseous surgery is contraindicated in patients with severe periodontitis. Since this is a resective procedure, the intentional removal of bone in a severe periodontitis case may further compromise the support around the tooth.

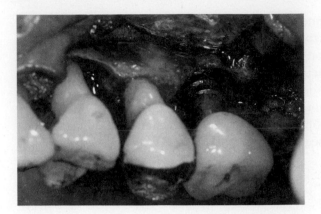

Figure 29-15. Irregular Bone Morphology Caused by the Progression of Periodontitis. After elevation of a full-thickness flap, two types of bony defects are apparent. The first bony defect is the one-wall angular defect on the distal of the maxillary first premolar; the second bony defect is the circumferential (moat-like) defect around the implant.

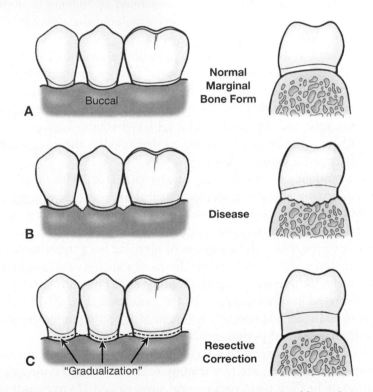

Figure 29-16. Osseous Resection. A. Ideal osseous form. The interproximal bone is consistently more coronal to the marginal bone. Note that the ideal form of the marginal bone has a gradual curved, scalloped configuration in between the interdental peaks. **B.** Diseased osseous form. Note the irregular crestal deformities in the interproximal regions and the loss of the scalloped marginal bone configuration. **C.** Resective correction. Note that osseous surgery has eliminated the irregular crestal deformities and re-established ideal bony contours that will be in harmony with the overlying gingival tissues.

Box 29-4. Special Terminology Associated With Periodontal Osseous Surgery

- Ostectomy—removal of tooth-supporting bone
- Osteoplasty—reshaping of the surface bone contours without removing tooth-supporting bone

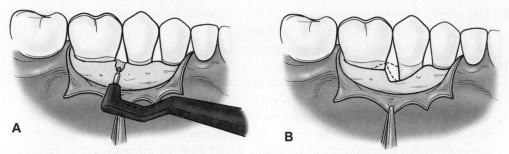

Figure 29-17. Ostectomy Technique. A. Following exposure of the interdental osseous crater, one of the crater walls (facial wall in this illustration) is being removed with a special surgical bur. **B.** Based upon the newly established bone level at the site, the surrounding bone is contoured in an attempt to reestablish a more natural bone contour.

C. **Special Terminology Associated With Osseous Surgery—Ostectomy and Osteoplasty.** Osseous surgery is frequently employed in the treatment of patients with mild periodontitis or moderate periodontitis, and this topic is discussed in detail in all periodontal textbooks. Two terms frequently arise during discussions of osseous surgery, and these terms can be a bit confusing. Box 29-4 summarizes the key difference between ostectomy versus osteoplasty.
1. One of these terms is ostectomy. Ostectomy or osteoectomy refers to the removal of tooth-supporting bone (also known as *alveolar bone proper*).
   a. Ostectomy results in the immediate loss of a small amount of attachment at certain sites, and for that reason ostectomy must be used with appropriate caution by the surgeon.
   b. In spite of the slight attachment loss that occurs during ostectomy, osseous resective surgery is the most predictable method of eliminating periodontal pockets. The removal of small amounts of supporting bone is justified by the attainment of the physiologic form and contours of alveolar bone that is compatible with the natural contours of the overlying gingiva.
   c. Figure 29-17 illustrates technique for ostectomy that might be performed during periodontal osseous resective surgery.
2. The second of these terms is osteoplasty. Osteoplasty refers to reshaping the surface of alveolar bone without actually removing any of the tooth-supporting bone.
3. In reality, most periodontal osseous resective surgery involves a combination of both ostectomy and osteoplasty. When performed with precision, these procedures can result in alveolar bone contours that mimic the contours of the gingiva following complete healing.
D. **Steps in Periodontal Osseous Resective Surgery**
1. Incisions are made and flaps are elevated to provide access to the osseous defects and to the surrounding alveolar bone; these incisions typically are done on both the facial and lingual surfaces of the teeth and typically include both horizontal and vertical releasing incisions.
2. Granulation tissue associated with the osseous defects is thoroughly debrided to allow full visualization to the extent and shape of the osseous defects.
3. All remaining soft tissue tags in the surgical site are identified and removed usually using a combination of hand and ultrasonic instrumentation.
4. Tooth root surfaces are debrided to remove all plaque biofilm, calculus, root contaminants, and root irregularities.
5. Osteoplasty is performed to remove thick bone ledges where they exist on the facial and lingual surfaces of the alveolar bone.
6. Ostectomy is performed to eliminate interproximal osseous defects.
7. Bone contours are refined with hand instruments and surgical burs.

8. The gingiva is sutured into place (usually at a more apical position than the original level as discussed in the next section).

E. Healing After Periodontal Osseous Resective Surgery

1. When periodontal osseous resective surgery is performed in areas of the dentition where osseous craters exist, it is normally possible for the surgeon to recreate a natural contour to the alveolar bone.

2. When this osseous resective surgery is combined with the apically positioned flap (as discussed in the next section of this chapter), it is frequently possible to reestablish a normal crevice or sulcus depth without the presence of residual periodontal pockets following the surgery.

3. For most patients who are treated with this type of surgical procedure, it is possible to maintain a healthy periodontium provided that the patient performs reasonable self-care and complies with their periodontal maintenance regimen.

4. Apically Positioned (or Displaced) Flap With Osseous Resective Surgery

A. Procedure Description

1. An apically positioned flap with osseous resective surgery is a periodontal surgical procedure involving a combination of a displaced flap (displaced in an apical direction) plus resective osseous surgery.

   a. As already discussed, correction of altered alveolar bone contours to mimic the contours of healthy alveolar bone is usually referred to as periodontal osseous resective surgery.

   b. Following contouring of the alveolar bone, the flap in this procedure is sutured at a position that is more apical to its original position in relationship to the tooth CEJs (apically positioned or apically displaced flap).

2. This periodontal surgical procedure is ideal for minimizing periodontal pocket depths in patients with osseous craters caused by moderate periodontitis.

   a. An apically displaced flap can result in a gingival margin that is apical to the CEJ of the tooth. This new position of the gingival margin means that more of the root of the tooth is visible in the mouth.

   b. The reduced pocket depth can facilitate both self-care by the patient and periodontal maintenance by the dental team.

B. Steps in an Apically Positioned Flap With Osseous Resective Surgery. Table 29-3 (Fig. 29-18A–F) illustrates the critical steps in an apically positioned flap with osseous resective surgery.

1. This procedure normally begins with an internal bevel incision. The internal bevel incision can preserve the width of keratinized tissue that is important to the overall procedure, because this width of keratinized tissue will be displaced apically as a final step.

2. The internal bevel incision is followed by flap elevation and crevicular incision prior to removal of the collar of tissues around the necks of the teeth.

3. Vertical releasing incisions are made as needed to avoid damage to the flap.

4. Granulation tissues are debrided, and osseous defects are exposed as discussed in the previous section.

5. Periodontal osseous resective surgery is performed to mimic the contours of healthy alveolar bone; this osseous surgery normally includes both ostectomy and osteoplasty.

6. The flap is sutured at a position apical to its original position (usually near the tooth—bone junction). The surgical site is covered with periodontal dressing to stabilize the flap at its apical location.

TABLE 29-3	CRITICAL STEPS IN AN APICALLY POSITIONED FLAP WITH OSSEOUS RESECTIVE SURGERY

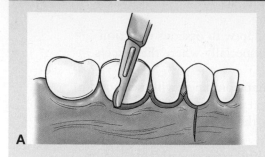

Figure 29-18A. Internal bevel incision and vertical releasing incision being made around the teeth.

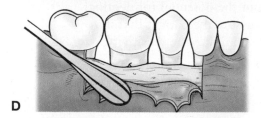

Figure 29-18B. Removal of the collar of soft tissue following flap elevation.

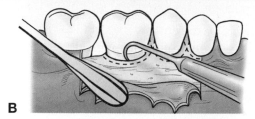

Figure 29-18C. Ostectomy being performed after identification of osseous defects.

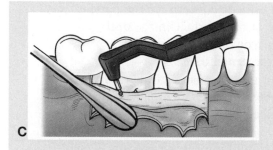

Figure 29-18D. Inspection of the final bone contours after ostectomy and osteoplasty.

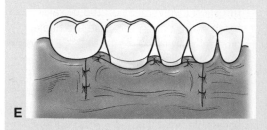

Figure 29-18E. Suturing of both the flap margins and the vertical releasing incisions. Note that the level of the flap margin is displaced in an apical position compared to its original position.

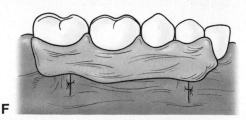

Figure 29-18F. Placement of periodontal dressing to stabilize the flap at its new position during the early phase of healing.

C. **Healing of an Apically Positioned Flap With Osseous Resective Surgery**
   1. Final healing of this type of surgery results in a normal attachment (both junctional epithelium and connective tissue attachment) at a position more apical on the tooth root.
   2. It should be emphasized that apically positioned flap with osseous resection cannot eliminate all periodontal osseous defects, especially where the defects are quite severe.
   3. Research has shown that an apically positioned flap combined with periodontal osseous surgery can result in a stable dentogingival junction that can be maintained in health with reasonable self-care by the patient and periodic periodontal maintenance by the dental team.
   4. Figure 29-19 illustrates the results of a healed apically positioned flap used to treat a furcation involvement on a molar tooth.

D. **Special Considerations for the Dental Hygienist**
   1. During surgery to minimize periodontal pockets, it is common for the gingival margin to be positioned at a more apical level to the CEJ than it originally occupied.
      a. This apical positioning results in exposure of a portion of the root to the oral cavity.
      b. Visibility of a portion of the root may be an esthetic concern for the patient.
      c. In a patient with a high caries risk, exposure of root surface in the oral cavity can lead to root caries. Therefore, this type of surgery may be contraindicated in patients with a high risk for dental caries.
   2. Temporary dentinal hypersensitivity is a frequent patient postsurgical complaint following this type of surgery. As discussed in other chapters, dentinal hypersensitivity usually diminishes over time if the patient maintains good biofilm control.
   3. Before surgery, the members of the dental team should inform the patient about anticipated changes in appearance and about the potential for dentinal hypersensitivity. The dental hygienist should also assure the patient that if sensitivity does occur, measures could be taken to minimize the sensitivity.

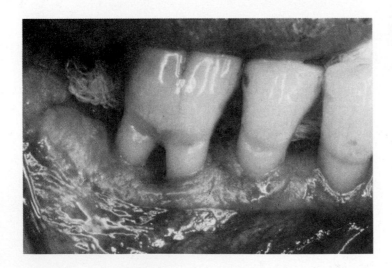

Figure 29-19. Results of an Apically Positioned Flap. This apically positioned flap was performed to treat a large furcation involvement on the molar tooth. Note that in this case the healed gingival margin is apical to the CEJ and the furcation entrance. This is known as "furcation tunneling." The objective of furcation tunneling is to create an "open tunnel" through the furcation that is more accessible and cleansable for a patient using an interdental brush.

5. **Bone Replacement Grafts**
    A. **Procedure description**
        1. **Bone replacement graft** is a broad class of implantable materials that are used in medicine and dentistry to induce the body to augment and/or regenerate tissue that has been lost as a result of disease, trauma, or injury.
        2. Bone grafting has been commonplace in medicine for many years, but transplanting bone replacement graft materials into the periodontium offers some unique challenges different from bone grafting in medicine.
            a. Bone grafts placed into periodontal defects are subject to constant contamination from bacteria and saliva traveling along existing tooth roots adjacent to the graft site; the possibility for bacteria contamination would not be the case in many bone grafts in medicine (such as a bone graft done during a hip replacement).
            b. In addition, the healing of bone grafts in periodontal defects can be disrupted by the apical downgrowth of the epithelium into the wound that can lead to graft failure; this potential disruption by the growth of epithelium would also not be the case in most medical bone graft surgical procedures.
    B. **Terminology Associated With Bone Replacement Grafts**
        1. Bone replacement graft materials are implantable materials that support or promote bone healing through an osteogenic, osteoinductive, and/or osteoconductive mechanisms.
            a. **Osteogenesis** is the term used to describe the formation of new bone by viable, living cells that are contained in the graft material.[10] Examples of bone replacement graft materials that have osteogenic potential are bone harvested from the patient's own tuberosity or ramus.
            b. **Osteoinduction** refers to a chemical process whereby molecules contained in the graft material—known as bone morphogenetic proteins (BMPs)—have the ability to recruit and attract host bone-forming cells (osteoblasts) to the site of implantation to form new bone.
            c. **Osteoconduction** is a physical, passive process whereby the graft material itself acts as a scaffold for host bone-forming cells (existing outside the graft) to migrate, attach, and grow on.
        2. Using this terminology, the ideal bone replacement graft material would be one that has osteogenic, osteoinductive, and osteoconductive potentials.
    C. **Broad Categories of Materials Used for Bone Replacement Grafting.** In general, bone grafting materials fall into one of four broad categories: autografts, allografts, xenografts, and alloplasts. These four categories of bone graft material have widely varying degrees of success in regenerating lost periodontal tissues. Box 29-5 provides an overview of materials used for bone replacement grafts.
        1. **Autografts** are bone replacement grafts taken from the patient that is receiving the graft. Periodontal autografts can be taken from intraoral sites, such as the ramus or tuberosity, or occasionally from extraoral areas of the patient's body, such as the hip.
        2. **Allografts** are bone replacement grafts taken from individuals that are genetically dissimilar to the donor (i.e., another human). An allograft may be either obtained from a living donor or from a cadaveric donor. Because of the source of this type of graft, allografts must undergo a rigorous screening and sterilization process to eliminate the potential for rejection and/or disease transmission.

Box 29-5. Materials Used for Bone Replacement Grafts

- Autograft—bone harvested from patient's own body
- Allograft—bone harvested from another human
- Xenograft—bone harvested from another species
- Alloplast—synthetic (man-made) bone-like material

3. Xenografts are bone replacement grafts taken from another species, such as bovine (cow) bone replacement graft material which can be placed in a human. Like allografts, xenografts must also undergo a rigorous screening and sterilization process to eliminate the potential for rejection and/or disease transmission.

4. Alloplasts are bone replacement grafts that are synthetic materials or inert foreign materials. Unlike autografts, allografts, and xenografts, an alloplast is unique because it is considered to be a nonbone graft material. Examples of alloplast include, but are not limited to sclera, dura, plaster of Paris, coral-derived materials, and ceramics.

5. Autografts have the highest osteogenic potential, and alloplasts have the least osteogenic potential. Allografts and xenografts have an osteogenic potential that is in between those two extremes.

6. Though autografts have the most osteogenic potential, it is not always possible to procure enough autogenous bone from a patient to fill all of the osseous defects that need grafting. This creates the need during many periodontal surgical procedures for a bone graft material from a source other than the patient being treated.

7. In some instances, these grafting materials can be used in combinations such as mixing autogenous bone with an allograft material to obtain the needed volume of grafting material for a particular grafting site.

D. **Examples of Specific Materials Used for Bone Replacement Grafting.** Numerous materials have been studied for use for bone replacement grafting over the past several decades. None of the materials is ideal, but many of them have been shown to have some osteogenic potential. The discussion below describes some examples of the types of bone replacement graft materials that have been studied.

1. Autogenous bone grafts (Autografts) from intraoral sites
   a. As already discussed, autografts are graft materials taken from the patient's own body.
   b. Autografts from intraoral sites have been used in periodontics for many years, and currently these autogenous grafts are considered the gold standard when comparing other grafting materials due to their high osteogenic potential.
   c. It should not be surprising that autogenous bone is the most effective grafting material, since it already contains living bone cells and viable bone growth factors from the patient—in contrast to alloplasts which neither have living viable cells nor growth factors.
   d. Intraoral sources for the autograft material can be harvested from sites such as from bone removed during ostectomy or osteoplasty, from exostoses removed during surgery, from bone removed from edentulous ridges, from bone taken from healing extraction sites, from bone taken from the chin, and from bone harvested from the jaws distal to the most terminal tooth in a dental arch.
   e. A variety of techniques for harvesting the graft material and ensuring its osteogenic potential have been advocated. These techniques usually involve

exposing the alveolar bone by elevating a periodontal flap, removing granulation tissue associated with an osseous defect, treating the tooth root adjacent to the defect, placing the graft material into the defect, and closing the flap by suturing it to its original level on the teeth.

f. In addition to harvesting particles or larger pieces of bone, autogenous bone grafts include the use of materials such as osseous coagulum. Osseous coagulum is a mixture of bone dust and blood taken from the patient and mixed with blood from the surgical site.

g. One technique for collecting autogenous graft material from a patient during a periodontal surgical procedure involves the bone blend technique. This technique involves collecting bone in a plastic capsule and pestle and triturating the material into a workable mass of plastic-like bone graft that can be used to fill an osseous defect.

h. Though small particles or pieces of cortical bone are usually selected as autogenous grafting material, cancellous bone marrow may also be used. One common intraoral site to harvest bone marrow is from a maxillary tuberosity.

i. One *disadvantage* to using autogenous bone grafts is that when they are used, they frequently require a second surgical site for harvesting the graft material, increasing the potential for postsurgical problems. Another disadvantage is that it may be difficult to procure adequate amounts of this type of graft material to treat large periodontal defects.

2. Autogenous bone from extraoral sites

a. Iliac (or hip) cancellous marrow has been studied as an autogenous bone replacement graft material.

b. When used in periodontal defects, this material results in bone formation in osseous defects. Today, marrow from the hip is rarely used for autogenous grafting into periodontal defects because of the potential for root resorption adjacent to the grafting site, the potential for postoperative problems associated with the donor site, the difficulty in surgically obtaining this type of donor material, and the difficulty in procuring adequate amounts of this material for large defects.

3. Freeze-dried bone allografts. Bone allografts (harvested from another human and processed) are attractive surgical options as bone replacement graft materials. There has been a lot of interest in periodontics in identifying an ideal bone allograft. If the ideal bone allograft could be identified for use in periodontal patients, there would be no need for a second surgical site. In addition, if the ideal bone allograft could be identified, there would be no concerns about the limited availability of the amount of graft material needed to treat large osseous defects.

a. As already discussed, allografts are graft materials that are either harvested from another living individual of the same species or from another human who is recently deceased.

b. Freeze-dried bone allografts (both calcified and decalcified) have been used successfully as bone replacement allografts, and bone allograft products have been available commercially for some time.[11–17]

1) Bone allograft materials are obtained from the cortical bone of a donor within a few hours of death, defatted, washed in alcohol, frozen, and vacuum sealed into sterile vials until used in a clinical setting. This type of freeze-dried bone allograft is known as mineralized freeze-dried bone allograft.

2) A second type of freeze-dried bone allograft is known as decalcified freeze-dried bone allograft. This graft material is processed along the same lines as freeze-dried bone allografts, however the outer cortical

layer of decalcified freeze-dried bone allograft is demineralized (decalcified) so as to expose the underlying BMPs and improve its osteogenic potential.

   c. Since allografts are materials that are foreign to the body of the patient receiving the graft and since potential donors may have diseases that could be transmitted to the patient being treated, steps must be taken to maximize the safety of this type of grafting material. These steps usually include:

      1) Excluding potential donors that are members of disease high-risk groups,

      2) Testing of cadaver tissues to exclude donors with infection or malignant disease, and

      3) Treating the allograft with chemical agents or with other techniques to inactivate viruses.

   d. Whereas the risk of disease transmission using allograft materials is not zero, the risk of viral transmission by the use of allograft bone replacement material has been reported to be highly remote.

   e. As mentioned above, allograft products are available in two types based on how they are processed: FDBAs and DFDBAs.

4. Bovine-derived bone

   a. Bovine-derived bone is an example of a xenograft material; xenografts are materials taken from another species.

   b. Xenografts, such as bovine-derived bone, have been used as bone replacement grafts in periodontal defects.[18]

   c. An anorganic bovine bone has been tested and marketed, and studies have shown successful regrowth of some bone with this material.

      1) Anorganic bovine bone is cow bone that has been treated to remove all of its organic components to eliminate the risk of rejection.

      2) Removing the organic components from bovine bone leaves a porous structure, similar in structure to human bone.

      3) It has been suggested that the porous structure of anorganic bovine bone can act as scaffolding for new bone. As such, anorganic bovine bone acts as an osteoconductive material.

5. Plaster of Paris

   a. Plaster of Paris has been used as an alloplastic bone replacement grafting material.[19] When placed in a periodontal defect, Plaster of Paris acts as a scaffold, and only has an osteoconductive potential.

   b. Plaster of Paris is actually calcium sulfate, which is porous and biocompatible when placed in periodontal wounds; when calcium sulfate is placed in a periodontal wound, it resorbs within a few weeks.

   c. Though this material has been studied and used in humans as a bone replacement graft material, its efficacy related to osteogenic potential has yet to be proven.

6. Bioactive glass

   a. Bioactive glass ceramics have been studied and used as alloplastic bone replacement grafting materials.[20–22]

   b. This ceramic material consists of calcium salts, phosphates, and silicone dioxide; when used as an alloplastic bone replacement graft, bioactive glass is used in particulate form.

   c. When bioactive glass comes in contact with periodontal tissues, the particulate surfaces can incorporate proteins and can attract osteoblasts that can subsequently form bone.

7. Calcium phosphate
   a. Calcium phosphate biomaterials have been used as alloplastic grafting materials for several decades. Calcium phosphate is osteoconductive and is well tolerated by body tissues.
   b. Two types of calcium phosphate materials have been used: hydroxyapatite and tricalcium phosphate.
   c. Though these materials can result in some clinical repair of periodontal defects, they are either poorly resorbable (tricalcium phosphate) or not resorbable at all (hydroxyapatite) and can remain encapsulated by collagen within the periodontal tissues.

E. **Healing After Bone Replacement Grafting**
   1. Final healing expected from bone replacement grafting usually includes a partial rebuilding of alveolar bone lost because of periodontitis.
      a. It is not known, however, if successful bone grafting always results in the complete reformation of cementum and periodontal ligament in addition to the alveolar bone.
      b. In spite of what appears to be good radiographic and clinical healing, it is difficult to ascertain if the regenerated bone is actually attached to the cementum by functionally oriented periodontal ligament fibers.
      c. The only way to conclusively prove that periodontal regeneration has occurred is through histological assessment of the defect after the healing phase.
   2. Research has shown that a successful bone graft combined with reasonable self-care by the patient and periodic periodontal maintenance by the dental team can result in retaining a severely periodontally compromised tooth over time.

F. **Special Considerations for the Dental Hygienist**
   1. The site of a bone replacement graft should be left undisturbed for many months and should not be probed until an appropriate interval has elapsed. The dental hygienist should consult with the dentist to determine when a grafted site may be probed safely.
   2. Meticulous plaque control in any grafted site is critical. In the early stages of the healing, the dental team maintains some of the responsibility for biofilm control at the site, because the patient may either be temporarily unable to perform adequate self-care or the patient may have been instructed by the dentist to temporarily refrain from performing self-care during the initial 1 to 2 weeks after surgery to avoid disturbing the grafted site.

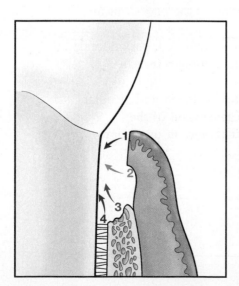

Figure 29-20. Potential Sources of Cells in Healing a Periodontal Surgical Wound. There are four potential sources of cells that can contribute to the healing of a periodontal surgical wound: (1) gingival epithelial cells, (2) gingival connective tissue cells, (3) bone cells, and (4) periodontal ligament cells. Of these four types of cells, gingival epithelial cells proliferate into the healing periodontal wound the fastest. If their downward migration is unimpeded, the gingival epithelial cells will be the first cell type to populate the treated root surface. When this occurs, a long junctional epithelial attachment will adhere to the root and interfere with periodontal regeneration.

6. Guided Tissue Regeneration
   A. Procedure Description
      1. Guided tissue regeneration (GTR) is a periodontal surgical procedure employed to encourage regeneration of lost periodontal structures (i.e., to regrow lost cementum, lost periodontal ligament, and lost alveolar bone) by "guiding" the movement of progenitor cells toward the treated root surface while excluding the migration of the gingival epithelial cells and fibroblasts. The fundamental tenant of GTR is based on classic regeneration studies which demonstrated that *only cells from the periodontal ligament have the potential to induce periodontal regeneration.*[23,24] All other cells—gingival epithelial cells, gingival fibroblasts, and osteoblasts—do not have this potential.
         a. When a periodontal surgical wound is created, such as the elevation of a flap, the healing of the wound may involve cells from multiple sources surrounding the wound.
         b. Figure 29-20 illustrates the potential sources of cells that could contribute to healing tissues within a periodontal surgical wound. They are, namely, gingival epithelial cells, gingival fibroblasts, bone-forming cells (osteoblasts), and cells from the periodontal ligament space.
         c. GTR techniques involve the use of a physical barrier membrane to impede the normally rapid downgrowth of epithelial cells into a healing periodontal wound; the rapid growth of epithelium into the wound can interfere with the slower growth of other cells critical to the regenerative process.
         d. Figure 29-21 illustrates how a barrier membrane might be placed under a periodontal flap at the time of surgery to physically impede the downgrowth of unwanted types of cells into the healing periodontal wound and create an environment that favors repopulation of the area by cells from the periodontal ligament space.
         e. Impeding the downgrowth of epithelial cells into a healing periodontal wound will theoretically allow for undifferentiated cells from the periodontal ligament to populate the root area and differentiate into the tissues that normally comprise the periodontium (i.e., cementum, PDL, and alveolar bone). At the same time, the membrane barrier will exclude cells from the epithelium and connective tissue from populating the root surface during the regenerating phase.
         f. The barrier membranes used during a GTR procedure can also be used in conjunction with bone graft materials in some instances (Fig. 29-22).
         g. As the name implies, GTR facilitates true regeneration of the periodontium.
      2. Goal of GTR
         a. When the entire array of types of periodontal surgery is viewed, periodontal regeneration is the ultimate goal, and there is much ongoing research related to GTR.
         b. Yet while regeneration of the cementum, periodontal ligament, and alveolar bone is the ultimate goal of periodontal therapy, regeneration of the periodontium is not completely predictable with techniques in use today.

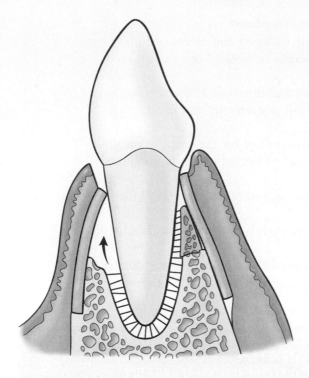

Figure 29-21. Use of Barrier Material to Inhibit the Rapid Growth of the Gingival Epithelial Cells. Note that the barrier has been placed under the flap margin to block the downgrowth of the epithelial cells. As a consequence, the undifferentiated cells from the periodontal ligament have a chance to proliferate into the healing periodontal wound, attach to the decontaminated root surface, and contribute to the new formation of new cementum, new functionally oriented PDL fibers, and new bone.

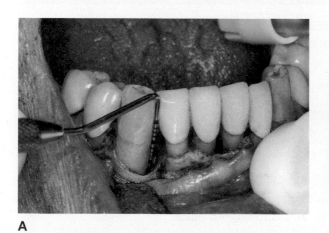

A

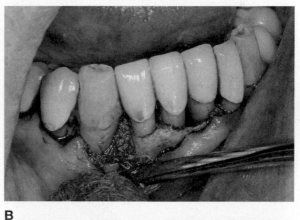

B

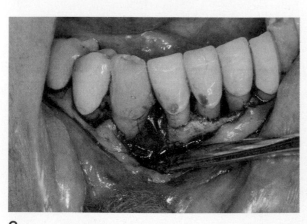

C

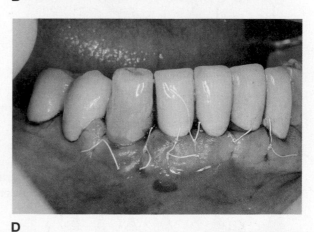

D

Figure 29-22. Guided Tissue Regeneration on Mandibular Right Canine. A. Note the deep angular defect on the mesial aspect of the mandibular right canine. **B.** Following thorough root debridement and degranulation of the osseous defect, an allograft was used to fill the osseous defect. **C.** A resorbable membrane was then placed over the bone graft to exclude epithelial migration into the wound. **D.** Flap was coronally positioned to ensure complete closure of the grafted site.

B. Steps in a Typical Guided Tissue Regeneration Procedure

1. The first step in GTR is to make appropriate incisions and elevate a full-thickness flap. In this procedure, the flap usually is elevated one to two teeth beyond the site of the osseous defects.

2. The osseous defects are thoroughly debrided and the roots in the site are instrumented with a combination of ultrasonic instruments and hand instruments.

3. The selected membrane is trimmed to the size needed for the site; during this membrane trimming, the membrane is allowed to extend several millimeters beyond the defect in all directions.

4. The membrane is sutured into place with a sling suture placed around the tooth.

5. The flap also is sutured into place (frequently slightly coronally) so that the flap covers the membrane completely.

6. Table 29-4 (Fig. 29-23A–C) illustrates the use of a barrier membrane during a GTR procedure for treatment of furcation involvement in a molar tooth.

TABLE 29-4	USE OF BARRIER MATERIAL DURING GUIDED TISSUE REGENERATION IN THE TREATMENT OF A MOLAR TOOTH WITH DEEP FURCATION INVOLVEMENT

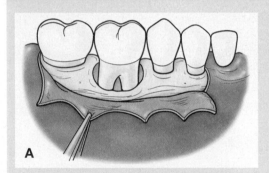

Figure 29-23A. Flap is incised and elevated prior to debridement of the osseous defect and the tooth root.

A

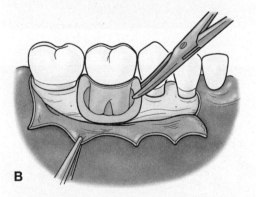

Figure 29-23B. A barrier is selected, custom trimmed to size, and sutured into place.

B

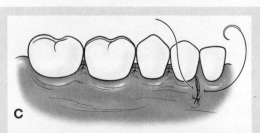

Figure 29-23C. Flap is sutured into place completely covering the barrier material.

C

C. Barrier Materials Used During Guided Tissue Regeneration

1. Some of the barrier materials in current use require removal following healing of the wound, so their use necessitates a second surgical procedure to remove the barrier material.
   a. Dense polytetrafluoroethylene is the most commonly used nonresorbable membrane material.
   b. These nonresorbable membranes are embedded with titanium strips to prevent collapse of the membrane into larger osseous defects (Fig. 29-24).
2. Other barrier materials in current use are resorbable and thus do not require removal at some later date; bioresorbable membranes are preferred by many clinicians for most surgical applications.
   a. There are several types of bioresorbable membranes; these types include polyglycoside synthetic polymers, bovine and porcine collagen, and calcium sulfate (Fig. 29-25).
   b. One disadvantage of bioresorbable membranes is that they lack the same degree of rigidity offered by titanium-reinforced membranes.

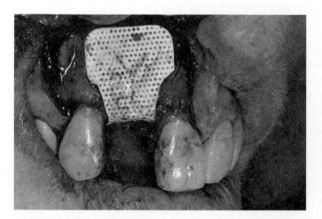
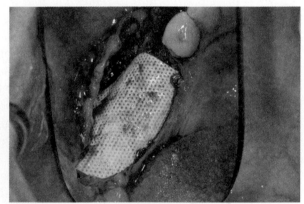

Figure 29-24. Titanium-Reinforced Membranes. Both clinical photos show the surgical placement of titanium-reinforced membranes. Note the embedded metallic titanium strip in each of the membranes. The embedded titanium strip adds stiffness to the membrane. This prevents the membrane from collapsing into the defect and maintains the space during the regenerating phase. (Case courtesy of Dr. Yusuke Hamada, Indianapolis, IN.)

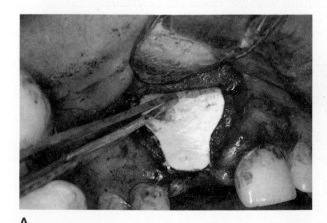
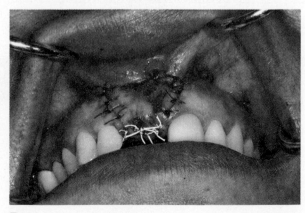

A   B

Figure 29-25. Resorbable Membrane. A. A stiff bovine-derived resorbable membrane is trimmed to fit over the grafted site. **B.** Primary closure is obtained to cover the entire surgical site.

D. Use of Guided Tissue Regeneration With Bone Replacement Grafts

1. The simultaneous use of barrier membranes to promote regeneration along with bone replacement grafts is one clinical option. Figure 29-22 shows an example of use of a barrier membrane.

2. At this point, most of the studies have been directed toward the use of barrier materials combined with either DFDBA or with calcium sulfate.

3. Available studies suggest that regeneration efforts can be improved by the combined use of both barrier materials and bone replacement grafting.

E. Healing Following Guided Tissue Regeneration

1. The healing expected from GTR is *regeneration* of part or all of the periodontium that was destroyed by periodontitis.

2. As already mentioned, GTR requires the use of a barrier material.

   a. During surgery, a barrier material is placed under the flap to stop the rapidly proliferating epithelium from migrating along the root surface and interfering with the connective tissue regrowth on the root. (It is the connective tissue components from the periodontal ligament space that actually provide the cells needed to regrow cementum, periodontal ligament, and alveolar bone.)

   b. *It is important to remember that if a barrier material were not used, the epithelial tissue would proliferate very rapidly, covering the tooth root and blocking access to the root by the slower growing connective tissue and undifferentiated cells of the periodontal ligament. The epithelial growth covering the root blocks the undifferentiated cells of the periodontal ligament from making contact with the root surface, thereby decreasing the likelihood of periodontal regeneration.*

F. Special Considerations for the Dental Hygienist

1. During the GTR surgical procedure, every effort is made to close the wound to cover the barrier material completely.

   a. If exposure of part of the barrier material is noted at any of the post-surgical visits, corrective measures should be instituted to minimize bacterial contamination of the barrier material.

   b. For example, a patient with exposed barrier membrane may need to be instructed to carefully apply a topical antimicrobial agent (such as chlorhexidine) over the surgical site on a daily basis to minimize post-surgical infection.

2. Sites treated by GTR should not be probed for several months following the procedures. The dental hygienist should consult with the dentist to determine when each individual site can be probed safely.

Box 29-6. Overview of Procedures Commonly Included in Periodontal Plastic Surgery

- Free soft tissue autograft (previously called the "free gingival graft")
- Subepithelial connective tissue autograft
- Laterally positioned flap
- Coronally positioned flap
- Semilunar coronally repositioned flap
- Frenectomy
- Crown lengthening surgery

7. **Periodontal Plastic Surgery**
   A. **Description**
      1. Periodontal plastic surgery is the term most commonly used in modern dentistry to describe periodontal surgical procedures that are directed toward correcting or eliminating deformities associated with the gingiva or alveolar mucosa. Examples of periodontal plastic surgery include, but are not limited to, root coverage procedures, esthetic crown lengthening procedures, vestibuloplasty (a surgical procedure used to increase the depth of the vestibule), and frenectomy. On the other hand, bone grafting procedures and surgical implant procedures are not covered under the broad category of periodontal plastic surgery.
      2. The term periodontal plastic surgery includes an array of periodontal surgical procedures that can be used to improve esthetics of the dentition and to enhance prosthetic dentistry as well as to deal with damage resulting from periodontitis.[25–30]
      3. Some of these procedures include techniques that have been used in medical plastic surgery for many years. Periodontal plastic surgery can be used to alter the tissues surrounding both natural teeth and dental implants.
   B. **Terminology Related to Periodontal Plastic Surgery**
      1. Readers of periodontal literature can sometimes be confused by the terminology associated with periodontal plastic surgery, since some other terms have also been used to describe procedures currently included under this term.
      2. The term mucogingival surgery has been used in the past to describe periodontal surgical procedures that correct any deformity associated with the gingiva and mucosa. Some of the periodontal plastic surgical procedures utilized in modern dentistry were previously described as mucogingival surgical procedures, and this older terminology can still be encountered.
      3. Another term that has been used to describe some of these types of procedures is reconstructive surgery; the term reconstructive surgery underscores that the goal of some of these procedures is to reconstruct (or rebuild) periodontal tissues such as gingiva.
   C. **Goals of Periodontal Plastic Surgery**
      1. Many periodontal plastic surgical procedures are designed to alter components of the attached gingiva, and this type of procedure can dramatically alter the appearance of the tissues. Most patients want a pleasing smile, and because the gingiva is readily visible in many patients, patients frequently seek improvements in the appearance of the gingiva.
      2. In addition to altering the appearance of the tissues, some periodontal plastic surgical procedures improve function. Function can be compromised when lack of attached gingiva on a tooth limits the restorative options.
      3. This chapter part includes an overview of some of the more common types of procedures included under the heading periodontal plastic surgery. Box 29-6 provides an overview of the types of procedures commonly included in periodontal plastic surgery.
8. **Free Soft Tissue Autograft**
   A. **Description of a Free Soft Tissue Autograft**
      1. A free soft tissue autograft is a type of periodontal plastic surgery that was one of the first procedures used to augment the width of attached gingiva. This procedure previously was called the "free gingival graft."

2. In the free soft tissue autograft procedure, epithelial and subepithelial soft tissues (connective tissue), from the same patient, are transplanted from one area of the mouth to another. As such, there are two intraoral wounds that are created during this surgery: the donor site and the recipient site.

   a. The donor tissue for a free soft tissue autograft includes both the *surface epithelium and some of the underlying connective tissue.*

   b. Harvesting the tissue from the donor site leaves an open wound that can be discomforting and painful for the patient if left exposed during the healing phase (Fig. 29-26). To minimize adding postoperative pain and discomfort to the donor site, the clinician will typically protect the donor site with a dressing material or with a plastic stent. Over several weeks, the donor site will eventually heal by secondary intention.

3. Figure 29-27 shows a free soft tissue autograft sutured in place on the facial surface of a mandibular incisor tooth roots.

4. The free soft tissue autograft may be indicated in cases that require root coverage over exposed root surfaces or in cases that require augmentation of the width of attached gingiva, without the need for obtaining root coverage.

5. One complicating factor of the free gingival autograft is that the graft is completely severed from its blood supply and at least a portion of the graft is then placed over an avascular root surface; special care is required to encourage diffusion of nutrients to the graft to maintain its viability during the early stages of healing.

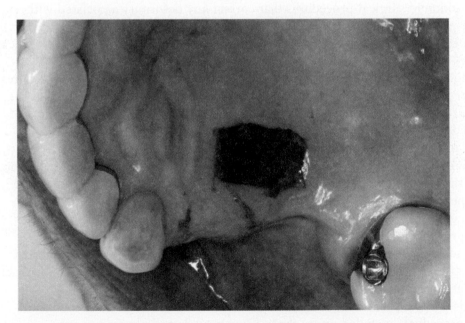

Figure 29-26. Donor Site of a Free Soft Tissue Autograft. This donor site on the palate will heal as an open wound (since the epithelium has been removed as part of the donor tissue). The donor site should be covered with a plastic stent or dressing material to minimize patient discomfort, aid in bleeding control, and protect the wound from the tongue, food, and drink. If the donor site remains covered during the healing phase, the open wound will eventually heal by secondary intention. (Case courtesy of Dr. Jennifer Chang, Indianapolis, IN.)

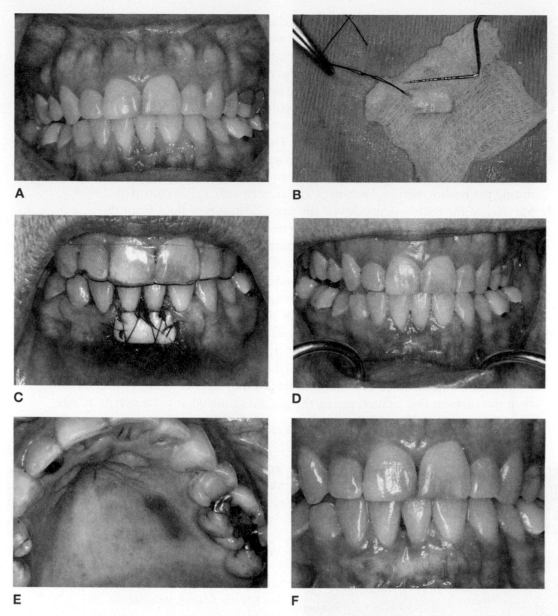

Figure 29-27. Free Soft Tissue Autograft. A. Presurgical (pre-grafting) photo. Note the gingival recession on the mandibular central incisors. **B.** Donor tissue obtained from palate. **C.** Donor tissue sutured over the recipient site. **D.** 1-month healing recipient site. **E.** 1-month healing donor site. **F.** 12-month healing of recipient site. Note the increase in root coverage obtained and maintained after 1 year. (Case courtesy of Dr. Jennifer Chang, Indianapolis, IN.)

B. Steps in Performing a Free Soft Tissue Autograft Procedure

1. The root surfaces in the area of gingival recession are instrumented to remove plaque biofilm, calculus, root contaminants, and root irregularities.
2. Horizontal and vertical incisions are made at the recipient site after determining the precise location of the needed graft; using sharp dissection, surface epithelium is removed to prepare a firm connective tissue bed to receive the graft material.
3. A template (frequently made from foil) is prepared to provide a pattern for the exact size and shape of the donor graft that will be needed.
4. Using the template as a guide for the size and shape, the graft is obtained from the donor site (usually the palate) by incising through the epithelium and through a thin layer of connective tissue beneath the epithelium; the graft is removed from the site using sharp dissection.

5. The graft is sutured to the recipient site; during suturing, care is taken to prevent a blood clot from forming between the graft and the recipient vascular bed. A clot in between the graft and recipient site may interfere with vascularization of the donor tissue and may lead to graft necrosis.

6. Both the donor site and recipient site are protected with periodontal dressing; in some instances, the donor site on the palate is covered with a previously prepared acrylic retainer to hold the dressing over the donor site.

C. **Healing Expected With a Typical Free Soft Tissue Autograft**

1. Successful healing of a free soft tissue autograft depends upon the survival of the connective tissue part of the graft. In most instances, the epithelium sloughs off during the healing period, later to be replaced by new epithelium (Fig. 29-28).

2. Survival of the tissues depends initially upon diffusion of fluid from the vascular recipient bed, followed by growth of new blood vessels into the grafted material. Immobilization of the autograft during the healing phase is a critical element in allowing the diffusion of nutrients, reconnection of existing blood vessels, and formation of new blood vessels.

3. Successful augmentation of gingiva as well as successful root coverage has been reported following the use of the free soft tissue autograft.

4. Unfortunately, in some cases, following complete healing of the free soft tissue autograft, the esthetic results may be less than ideal. For example, there may be a less than ideal color match between the healed graft and the adjacent gingiva. Moreover, the healed free soft tissue autograft may appear "lumpy" and bulkier than the surrounding tissues, giving the grafted tissue what is known as a "tire-patch" appearance (Fig. 29-29).

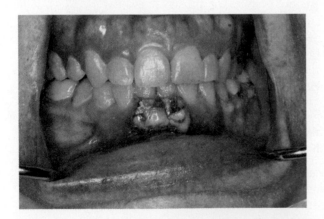

Figure 29-28. Autograft at 1-Week Post-Surgical Period. This clinical photograph shows the fate of the free soft tissue autograft from Figure 29-27 at 1 week after surgery. Note the whitish-yellow irregular layer of tissue covering the surface of the autograft. While it may appear as if the autograft is failing, this is actually a typical appearance of the free soft tissue autograft 7 to 10 days after placement. (Courtesy of Dr. Jennifer Chang, Indianapolis, IN.)

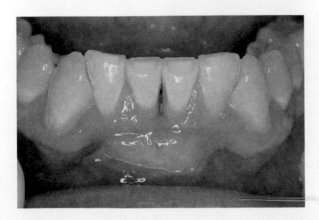

Figure 29-29. "Tire-Patch" Appearance of Free Soft Tissue Autograft. A 12-week post-surgical photo. From an esthetic standpoint, the graft is bulbous and irregular. This is termed as a "tire-patch" appearance. The surgical site will need to be followed up by a gingivoplasty at a later date to make the grafted tissue appear more uniform with the neighboring gingival tissues and give it a more esthetically pleasing appearance.

9. Subepithelial Connective Tissue Graft
   A. Description of Subepithelial Connective Tissue Graft
      1. The subepithelial connective tissue graft is another type of periodontal plastic surgical procedure that can also be used to augment the width of attached gingiva and to cover areas of gingival recession.
      2. In addition to gingival augmentation, the subepithelial connective tissue type of graft can be used to alter the contour of alveolar ridges to improve the esthetics of some types of dental prostheses.
      3. Unlike a free soft tissue autograft, this procedure utilizes autogenous donor tissue that is solely composed of connective tissue without epithelium. A subepithelial connective tissue can be harvested from a variety of intraoral sites but is usually taken from the patient's palate.
   B. Steps in Performing a Subepithelial Connective Tissue Autograft Procedure
      1. A partial-thickness flap is elevated at the recipient site using sharp dissection; the flap normally extends one half to one tooth to the mesial and distal of the site of recession to be covered.
      2. The exposed tooth root is thoroughly instrumented to remove plaque biofilm, calculus, root contaminants, and root irregularities.
      3. The connective tissue graft is obtained by incising through the epithelium of the palate and excising a segment of connective tissue from beneath the epithelium using sharp dissection. The surface tissues at the donor site can then be sutured to allow for healing by primary intention (Fig. 29-30). This facilitates improved healing compared to the type of healing that occurs in the palate from a free soft tissue autograft procedure.
      4. The graft tissue is placed over the denuded tooth root and under the partial-thickness flap at the recipient site. The outer portion of the partial-thickness flap is placed over the graft and sutured into place, making sure that at least half of the graft is covered by the outer portion of the flap.
      5. Periodontal dressing is placed to protect the grafted site; since the donor site will heal by primary intention, normally no dressing is needed at the donor site.
   C. Healing Expected After a Subepithelial Connective Tissue Autograft
      1. When root coverage is attempted with the subepithelial connective tissue graft, it is reasonable to expect coverage, though not all sites result in complete root coverage.
      2. The subepithelial connective tissue graft results in excellent esthetics since the color of the healed tissues often mimics the natural preexisting tissue color precisely (Fig. 29-31).

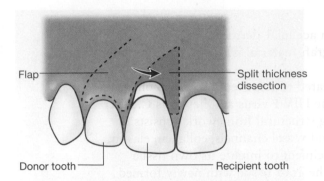

Figure 29-34. Laterally Positioned Flap. The flap is rotated to "slide" over from the donor site to the neighboring recipient site.

10. **Laterally Positioned Flap**
    A. **Description of a Laterally Positioned Flap**
       1. The **laterally positioned flap** is a periodontal plastic surgery technique that can be used to cover root surfaces with gingiva in isolated sites of gingival recession.
       2. The laterally positioned autograft involves a displaced flap (displaced laterally in this case) that "slides" over to cover a neighboring recession defect (Fig. 29-34). Another term to describe this type of flap is a lateral displaced pedicle flap.
       3. The primary prerequisite of this technique is that the donor site must be adjacent to the recipient site so that the flap can "slide" over to cover the recipient site.
       4. A secondary prerequisite is that the donor site itself must have a thick, healthy layer of gingiva covering it to prevent post-surgical recession *at the donor site*.
    B. **Steps in a Typical Laterally Positioned Flap**
       1. The recipient site is prepared by thoroughly planing the exposed tooth root and by removing epithelium from the surface of the gingiva surrounding the area of recession, thus exposing some connective tissue to serve as a vascular recipient bed for the displaced flap.
       2. A partial-thickness flap is elevated from the donor site using a series of carefully planned vertical incisions to provide mobility in the flap after elevation.
       3. The elevated flap is rotated laterally so as to cover the recipient site including both the prepared bed of connective tissue and the prepared tooth root.
       4. The flap is stabilized at its new location using a combination of interrupted sutures and sling sutures.
       5. If the surgery was extensive, the clinician may decide to cover the surgical site with aluminum foil and/or periodontal dressing to protect the healing wound.
    C. **Expected Healing of a Laterally Positioned Flap**
       1. With careful selection of donor sites and skillful manipulation of the tissues, little recession will occur on the donor site.
       2. The laterally positioned flap can result in excellent root coverage in many instances since the flap maintains part of its own blood supply (unlike the free soft tissue auto graft which is completely severed from its blood supply).
11. **Coronally Positioned Flap**
    A. **Description of a Coronally Positioned Flap**
       1. The **coronally positioned flap** is a periodontal plastic surgical procedure that can be used to repair gingival recession if the recession is not severe.
       2. As the name implies the coronally positioned flap is a displaced flap; the coronally positioned flap is advanced coronally to cover the gingival recession defect.[31] For an example, refer to Figure 29-11.

3. One advantage to this procedure compared to a free soft tissue autograft or a subepithelial connective tissue graft is that it does not require a second surgical site to provide the donor tissue (in other words, the donor site is the recipient site). Another advantage of this procedure compared to other periodontal plastic surgical procedures is that it is simple and predictably provides 2 to 3 mm of root coverage.

4. One disadvantage to this procedure is that it can be difficult to stabilize and secure the flap with sutures at a more coronal position. Another disadvantage is that there must be a sufficient band of thick keratinized tissue to avoid post-surgical gingival recession.

B. **Steps in a Typical Coronally Positioned Flap**

1. Exposed tooth roots are instrumented to remove plaque biofilm, calculus, root contaminants, and root irregularities.

2. Internal bevel and vertical releasing incisions are made at the site so that the flap can be coronally positioned; the vertical releasing incisions extend into the alveolar mucosa to allow for mobility of the flap margin in a coronal direction.

3. The flap is elevated; the elevation can be full-thickness or split-thickness or a combination of the two depending upon the overall thickness of the tissues being elevated.

4. The flap is advanced in a coronal direction and sutured using a combination of interrupted and sling sutures.

5. Periodontal dressing is placed to prevent movement of the flap during healing.

C. **Healing Expected with a Typical Coronally Positioned Flap.** The coronally positioned flap can be used successfully to cover areas of gingival recession when the gingival recession is not severe.

12. **Semilunar Coronal Repositioned Flap**

A. **Description of a Semilunar Coronal Repositioned Flap.** Tarnow proposed a procedure known as the semilunar coronally repositioned flap to cover gingival recession where the recession is not far advanced and where the keratinized tissues have an adequate thickness (Fig. 29-35). The semilunar flap is a variation of a coronally positioned flap.[32]

B. **Steps in a Typical Semilunar Coronally Repositioned Flap**

1. The level of the alveolar bone is located (sounded) to ensure that coronal positioning of the semilunar flap does not inadvertently expose alveolar bone at the base of the flap.

2. A semilunar, curved incision is made from one interdental area to the adjacent interdental area over the tooth root. The interdental sites for the incisions are selected to be slightly coronal to the position anticipated for the flap advancement. This incision begins in the gingiva and arcs into the mucosa and then back into the gingiva.

3. A split-thickness flap is performed using sharp dissection to free the surface of the flap from the underlying connective tissue.

4. The semilunar flap is displaced coronally and stabilized with gentle pressure for several minutes; if needed, the flap can be stabilized with interrupted sutures, but sometimes suturing is not required.

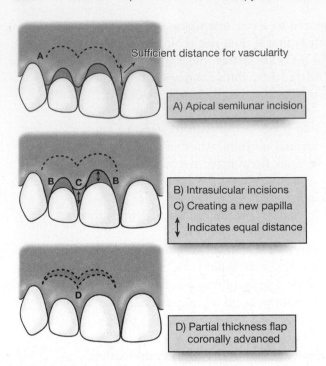

A) Apical semilunar incision

B) Intrasulcular incisions
C) Creating a new papilla
↕ Indicates equal distance

D) Partial thickness flap coronally advanced

Figure 29-35. Semilunar Coronally Positioned Flap. A semilunar coronally repositioned flap is used to cover gingival recession where the recession is not far advanced and where the keratinized tissues have an adequate thickness.

13. **Frenectomy**
    A. **Description of a Frenectomy**
       1. **Frenectomy** is a periodontal plastic surgical procedure that results in removal of a frenum, including removal of the attachment of the frenum to bone (Fig. 29-36).
          a. Some authors use the term frenotomy to indicate a variation of the frenectomy.
          b. The frenotomy includes only incision of the frenum but does not remove the attachment of the frenum from the bone surface.
          c. A frenum is a fold of mucosal tissue that contains muscle fibers. It attaches the lips and cheeks to the alveolar mucosa.
       2. If a frenum is attached too close to the gingival margin, it will act as a cable that constantly pulls the gingival margin away (apically) from the tooth when the enclosed muscle fibers in the frenum tense up. This can contribute to a buildup of plaque biofilm around the exposed root surface and marginal gingiva and eventually lead to persistent inflammation. In addition, a frenum too close to the gingival margin can interfere with daily self-care as it may be discomforting every time the bristles of the toothbrush contact the exposed root surface and movable frenum.
          a. An aberrant frenum position that requires a frenectomy occurs most often in the frenum between the maxillary central incisors and mandibular central incisors.
          b. An aberrant frenum position can also occur in other locations such as on the facial surface of premolar and canine teeth and on the lingual surface of the mandibular central incisors.
       3. If a frenum is present in a fully edentulous patient who is planned to receive a denture, a frenectomy may need to be performed prior to fabrication of the denture. This is because the movable frenum can affect the retention of the future denture (Fig. 29-37).

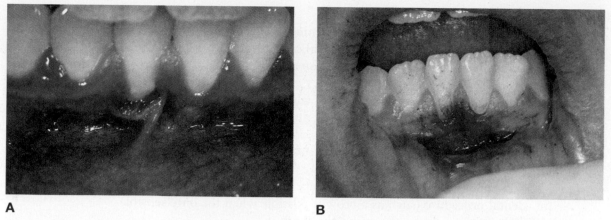

A   **B**

Figure 29-36. Frenectomy of Mandibular Frenum. A. Note the plaque-induced inflammation around the mandibular central incisors. The frenum is interfering with proper home care. **B.** Frenum is resected and removed to expose the fibrous attachment to the bone. These fibrous attachments will need to be severed with blunt dissection to the bone.

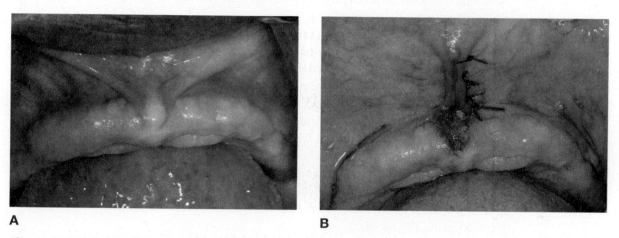

A   **B**

Figure 29-37. Frenectomy in Fully-Edentulous Patient. A. Note the broad maxillary labial frenum. Since movement of a frenum can displace the future seating of a denture, a frenectomy is indicated. **B.** Note complete removal of the frenum including its attachment to the underlying bone.

B. **Steps in a Typical Frenectomy**
   1. The frenum is grasped with a hemostat placed to the depth of the vestibule.
   2. Incisions are made through the tissues on both the under surface and the upper surface of the beaks of the hemostat.
   3. The triangular piece of tissue held by the hemostat is removed exposing connective tissue over the surface of the bone.
   4. The fibrous attachment covering the bone is incised and dissected with a blunt instrument.
   5. Periodontal dressing is applied to the wound.
C. **Alternative Techniques for the Frenectomy**
   1. Frequently, the frenectomy is performed in conjunction with other types of periodontal surgery, and a variety of techniques have been described.
   2. Other techniques for performing a frenectomy include removing the tissue of the frenum with electrosurgery or with a laser.
D. **Healing following a Frenectomy.** Expected healing following a frenectomy is elimination of the gingival margin movement caused by the frenum.

14. **Crown Lengthening Surgery**
   A. **Description of Procedure.** Crown lengthening surgery refers to periodontal plastic surgery designed to create a longer clinical crown for a tooth by removing some of the gingiva and usually by removing some alveolar bone from the necks of the teeth.
   B. **Terminology.** Two terms frequently used when describing crown lengthening surgery are functional crown lengthening and esthetic crown lengthening
      1. Functional crown lengthening refers to crown lengthening performed on a tooth where the remaining tooth structure is inadequate to support a needed restoration.
         a. Functional crown lengthening surgery can be used to make a restorative dental procedure (such as a crown) possible when the only sensible alternative might be to remove the tooth.
         b. Crown lengthening surgery may be necessary when a tooth is decayed or broken below the gingival margin.
            1) When a badly damaged tooth is to be restored, the dentist will evaluate the tooth and surrounding tissues to determine if the final restoration of the tooth will damage the soft tissue attachment (i.e., encroach upon the biologic width).
            2) If such damage can be expected, crown lengthening surgery is usually indicated prior to the placement of the final restoration.
      2. Esthetic crown lengthening refers to crown lengthening performed on teeth to improve the appearance of the teeth where there is excessive gingiva or a "gummy smile" as it is sometimes called.
         a. Crown lengthening surgery can be used to improve the esthetics of the gingiva, especially on anterior teeth with short clinical crowns.
            1) An individual's smile may be unattractive because of the height or lack of symmetry of the gingiva surrounding the teeth.
            2) In some cases, tooth crowns are actually the correct length, but they appear too short in the mouth because there is an excess of gingival tissue covering the teeth.
         b. During esthetic crown lengthening, the gingival tissues are incised and reshaped to expose more of the natural crown of the tooth; frequently some of the alveolar bone must also be removed to ensure healing of the tissues at a more apical position (Fig. 29-38).
   C. **Surgical Procedure.** The actual surgical procedure during crown lengthening surgery usually involves an apically positioned flap (displaced flap) with osseous resective surgery much like that already discussed.
      1. Unlike the typical indications for an apically positioned flap with osseous surgery, esthetic crown lengthening surgery is indicated in the presence of a perfectly healthy periodontium simply to allow for improved esthetics or exposure of more tooth structure prior to restoration.
      2. Also, unlike the typical apically positioned flap with osseous surgery, esthetic crown lengthening frequently requires the use of a surgical template prepared to guide the surgeon in positioning the tissues during the surgery and to determine the final, most esthetically pleasing apical location of the gingival margin (Fig. 29-39).
      3. Occasionally, esthetic crown lengthening may require only a gingivectomy type procedure to be discussed later in this chapter, but most often, esthetic crown lengthening requires some alveolar bone removal, so an apically positioned flap with osseous surgery is most often indicated instead of a gingivectomy.

D. Healing After Crown Lengthening Surgery
1. Healing of crown lengthening surgery is similar to that described for the apically positioned flap with osseous surgery.
2. Final healing of crown lengthening surgery results in a normal attachment (both junctional epithelium and connective tissue attachment) at a position more apical on the tooth root.

E. Special Considerations for the Dental Hygienist
1. Since crown lengthening surgery usually involves exposure of root surface to the oral environment, temporary dentinal hypersensitivity may be a common outcome of this type of periodontal surgery; it is imperative for the dental team to warn patients in advance that they may experience temporary dentinal hypersensitivity following crown lengthening surgery (Fig. 29-40).
2. As already discussed, when dentinal hypersensitivity results, the dental hygienist may need to institute measures to help the patient deal with the sensitivity.
3. Control of dentinal hypersensitivity requires meticulous plaque control during the healing phase, and this can be a problem since mechanical plaque control must be restricted following most surgical procedures.
4. It is the responsibility of the members of the dental team to aid the patient in plaque control until healing allows the patient to resume routine self-care.

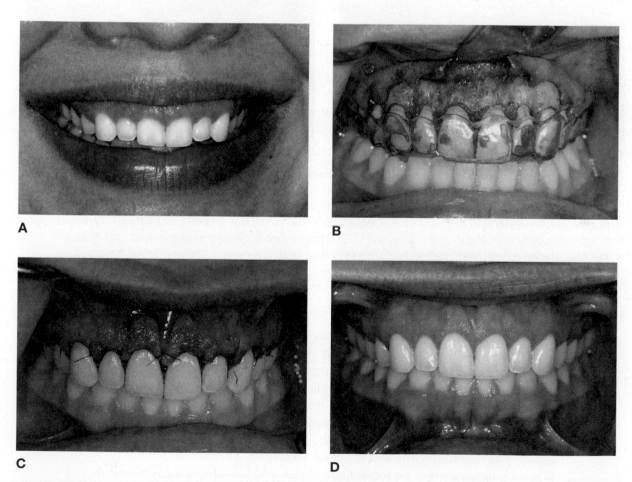

A

B

C

D

Figure 29-38. Esthetic Crown Lengthening. A. The clinical crowns from maxillary right premolar to maxillary left premolar appear short. **B.** Following the appropriate incisions and flap elevation, osseous recontouring was performed to expose more of the clinical crown length. **C.** Final suturing of the flap. Note the apical repositioning of the gingival margin. **D.** 3-month post-surgical clinical photograph. Note the increased clinical crown lengths of the maxillary teeth. (Courtesy of Dr. Hawra Al Qallaf, Indianapolis, IN.)

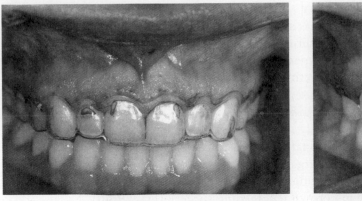
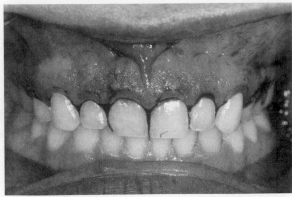

A   **B**

Figure 29-39. Purpose of the Surgical Template in Esthetic Crown Lengthening. A. Prior to esthetic crown lengthening surgery, a transparent, acrylic surgical template was made off of this patient's diagnostic casts. **B.** The surgical template is used as a guide to help the surgeon position the tissues during surgery.

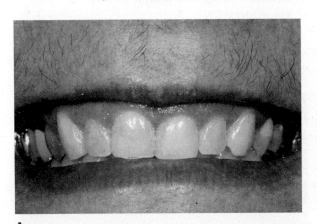
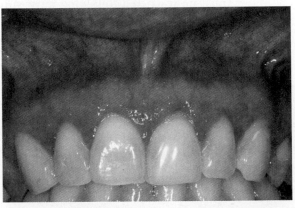

A   **B**

Figure 29-40. Root Exposure Following Esthetic Crown Lengthening. A. Pre-esthetic crown lengthening photograph. Note the gingival asymmetry and the short lengths of the clinical crown of the maxillary anterior teeth. **B.** 2-week post-esthetic crown lengthening photograph. At this time, the patient experienced slight dentinal hypersensitivity due to 1 mm of root exposure on the facial aspect of the maxillary left central incisor. The hypersensitivity subsided within several weeks and the patient is pleased with the outcome. Note the meticulous plaque control that is achieved by the efforts of both the patient and her dental hygienist.

15. **Gingivectomy**
    A. **Description of a Gingivectomy**
       1. The gingivectomy is a surgical procedure designed to excise and to remove some of the gingival tissue. Historically the gingivectomy was used for many years in periodontics as a primary treatment modality. In modern dentistry, the gingivectomy now has a reduced role because this procedure has a higher rate of surgical relapse (the soft tissue may grow back), slower wound healing, greater postsurgical discomfort and bleeding compared to surgical procedures that heal by primary intention. Also, the gingivectomy procedure fails to conserve keratinized tissue and maintain esthetics.
       2. When a gingivectomy is performed, the tissues are excised (cut away), removing some of the gingiva that would normally be attached to the tooth surface. Thus, the gingivectomy is a resective procedure. It is important to keep in mind that the gingivectomy procedure does not involve any removal of bone.
       3. The gingivectomy results in a more apical position of the marginal gingiva in relationship to the CEJ of the tooth.

4. Terminology related to gingivectomy can be confusing because of the overlapping use of two terms: gingivectomy and gingivoplasty.
   a. In contrast to the gingivectomy described above, gingivoplasty is a term used to describe a surgical procedure that simply reshapes the surface of the gingiva to create a natural form and contour to the gingiva.
   b. Unlike the gingivectomy, gingivoplasty implies reshaping the surface of the gingiva without removing any of the gingiva actually attached to the tooth surface.
   c. In reality, most gingivectomy type procedures, a certain amount of gingivoplasty is also performed, so the precise distinction between these two companion terms can be a bit cloudy.
5. There is still a limited place in modern dentistry for the gingivectomy procedure.
   a. Periodontal diseases can produce deformities of the gingiva including conditions such as gingival enlargements, gingival craters, and gingival clefts.
   b. Occasionally, even in the absence of periodontal pockets these deformities occur and need to be altered to allow for improved esthetics, improved mastication, or enhanced ease of patient self-care.
6. Figure 29-41 illustrates the types of incisions involved when performing a gingivectomy.

B. **Disadvantages of Gingivectomy**
   1. In modern periodontal therapy, the gingivectomy is usually limited to removing enlarged gingiva to improve esthetics or to allow for better access for self-care in isolated sites.
   2. Though gingivectomy can be used to reshape more extensive areas of enlarged gingiva as might be seen in gingival overgrowth in response to certain medication use, periodontists have other more effective surgical options today.
   3. As a surgical technique, gingivectomy has several *disadvantages*:
      a. One disadvantage to gingivectomy is that it leaves a large open connective tissue wound that results in a somewhat slower surface healing than most other periodontal surgical procedures; this generally results in the expectation of more discomfort for the patient during the healing phase.
      b. Figure 29-42 depicts the type of connective tissue wound that occurs following a gingivectomy.
      c. Another disadvantage of gingivectomy is that following healing, it invariably results in a longer appearing tooth because of the excision of some of the gingiva.
      d. A third disadvantage to the gingivectomy is that it does not provide access to the underlying alveolar bone. So, when access to the alveolar bone is needed, the surgeon must select another type of surgical approach.
      e. A fourth disadvantage to the gingivectomy is that it does not conserve keratinized tissue (gingiva); in many surgical sites it is unwise to remove keratinized tissue since it may already be minimal in width.
      f. In spite of these disadvantages, the gingivectomy can be a useful surgical procedure in selected sites.

C. **Steps in Performing a Typical Gingivectomy**
   1. Existing periodontal pockets are explored and the levels of the bases of the pockets are marked on the surface of the gingiva by punching a hole through the surface of the gingiva.
   2. Using special gingivectomy knives (both broad bladed and narrow bladed), gingiva is excised at the levels of the bases of the pockets.

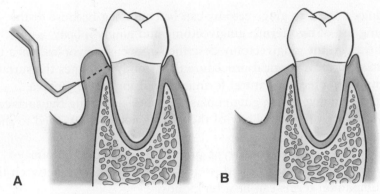

A **B**

Figure 29-41. Gingivectomy Incisions. A. The placement of a special gingivectomy knife to incise the excess gingival tissue. Note that the direction of the tissue bevel being created is approximately 45 degrees to the tooth surface. This type of incision is known as an external bevel incision. **B.** The excess tissue has been excised and removed creating a more natural level and contour of the gingiva on the tooth surface.

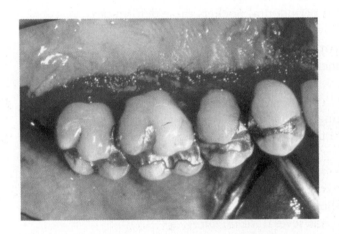

Figure 29-42. Connective Tissue Wound Created by Gingivectomy. Note that the gingivectomy results in a rather large wound that exposes connective tissue. This large wound usually results in protracted healing since the healing requires that the epithelium grows across the wound created by the gingivectomy.

3. As the incision is made, care is taken to produce a 45-degree bevel of the gingiva against the tooth to mimic the natural contour of the surface of the gingiva in relationship to the tooth.

4. The excised portion of the gingiva is removed (which also removes the soft tissue wall of existing periodontal pockets).

5. The wound surface is inspected, remaining tissue tags are removed, and gingival contours are refined as needed.

6. The tooth surfaces are inspected and debrided to remove biofilm, calculus, root contaminants, and root irregularities.

7. The surgical wound is covered with periodontal dressing.

D. **Healing Expected After a Gingivectomy**

1. Healing of the gingivectomy requires healing by secondary intention since the gingivectomy incisions invariably leave an exposed connective tissue surface.

2. The approximate rate that gingiva grows across a connective tissue wound in the oral cavity is 0.5 mm each day; since the gingivectomy normally leaves many millimeters of connective tissue exposed, the healing time can be protracted.

3. The final healing of the wound created by a gingivectomy is a normal attachment of the epithelium and connective tissues to the tooth root at a level that is more apical in position than the original gingival level.

4. Following a gingivectomy, the teeth in the surgical area will appear to be longer since more of the root is exposed where the tissue was excised.
   a. Of course, if more tooth exposure is the desired result of the procedure, this procedure can result in an acceptable outcome.
   b. However, if the exposure of more root structure is not esthetically desirable in a particular site in the oral cavity, another surgical approach would be selected by the surgeon.

E. **Special Considerations for the Dental Hygienist**
   1. As already mentioned, the gingivectomy wound leaves a broad connective tissue surface exposed that can be very uncomfortable for the patient during the healing phase.
   2. Postsurgical discomfort can be managed by placing a periodontal dressing over the wound to provide protection and by prescribing analgesics (pain medications) for use following surgery.
   3. At the time of the dressing removal at the first postsurgical visit following a gingivectomy, the dental hygienist will frequently need to replace the periodontal dressing to enhance wound comfort until total epithelialization of the wound has occurred.
   4. Healing of the wound created by a gingivectomy procedure progresses in a predictable manner.
      a. As already discussed, research studies have shown that oral epithelium grows across the exposed connective tissue at an approximate rate of 0.5 mm per day.
      b. Thus, it is possible for the clinical team to predict approximate healing times by estimating the wound size. This, of course is useful when counseling patients about what to expect during the postsurgical phase.

16. **Dental Implant Placement.** Dental implants are discussed in Chapter 9. They are briefly mentioned in this section to provide an overview of the surgical aspects of implant dentistry. The planning and surgical placement of dental implants is quite complex, and the interested reader is directed toward the many excellent textbooks devoted to that topic.

A. **Description of Dental Implant Placement**
   1. A dental implant replaces a tooth root with a screw-shaped post that is surgically placed into the alveolar bone and is strong enough to hold a replacement crown or prosthesis (denture or bridge).
   2. Most conventional dental implants are categorized as endosseous implants which are implants placed completely within the alveolar bone.
      a. Dental implant placement usually requires exposure of alveolar bone using the principles of periodontal flap surgery, drilling a precise hole (termed the "implant osteotomy site") in the alveolar bone, insertion of a dental implant into the site, and suturing of the surgical site (Fig. 29-43).
      b. Implants may be placed immediately at the time of tooth extraction known as immediate implant placement (Fig. 29-44), *or* they may be placed several months after tooth extraction known as delayed implant placement (Fig. 29-43 is an example of delayed implant placement since the maxillary premolar was extracted several months prior to implant surgery.). Many factors influence the decision to either immediately place the implant or delay the placement of the implant for a particular case, including site-specific factors (i.e., amount of available bone and location of anatomic structures), patient-specific factors (i.e., patient expectations and status of

medical conditions), and technical factors (such as clinician's experience and overall interdisciplinary treatment plan goals). The decision to place the implant either immediately after tooth extraction or several months after tooth extraction is a balance between the aforementioned factors and the risks associated with complications to the patient.

c. Additionally, conventional endosseous implants may be placed utilizing either a one-stage (nonsubmerged) approach or a two-stage (submerged) approach. In the one-stage surgical approach, the implant or abutment emerges from the soft tissue at the time of implant placement (Fig. 29-45). In the two-stage surgical approach, the implant and cover screw are completely covered by the flap (Fig. 29-46). The two-stage surgical approach will require a second surgical procedure following osseointegration to expose the top of the implant. This step is typically performed 3 months after implant placement to allow for sufficient time for osseointegration to take place.

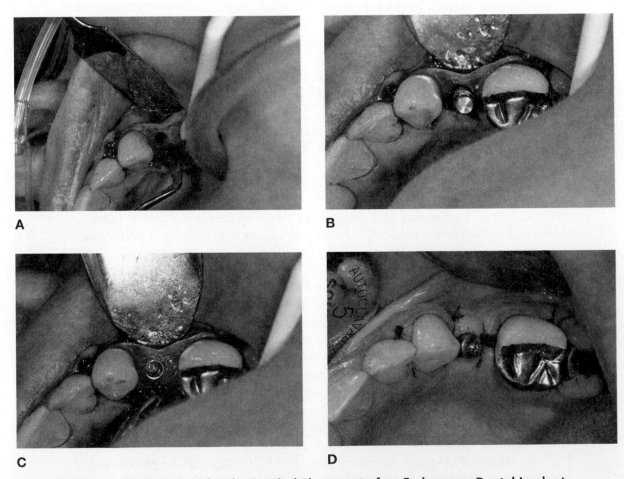

A

B

C

D

Figure 29-43. Standard Protocol for the Surgical Placement of an Endosseous Dental Implant.
A. After a full-thickness flap is elevated, the implant osteotomy site is prepared using a surgical stent and series of implant drills. **B.** Osteotomy site alignment and parallelism with adjacent roots is checked with guide pin and radiograph. **C.** The implant is inserted into the osteotomy site until the head of the implant (collar) is flush with the alveolar bone. **D.** A healing abutment (or a cover screw) is secured to the top of the implant and the flaps are sutured together.

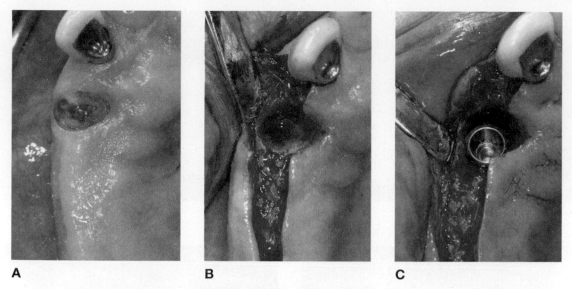

Figure 29-44. Immediate Implant Placement. A. Retained root that is deemed to be nonrestorable. **B.** Extraction of retained root. **C.** Placement of the endosseous implant immediately following extraction of the root.

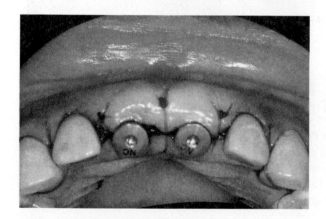

Figure 29-45. One-Stage (Nonsubmerged) Approach. In a one-stage implant protocol, the implant abutment emerges through the gingival tissues at the time of implant placement. Unlike a two-stage implant protocol, employing a one-stage approach does not require a second surgical procedure to uncover the top of the implant. (Case courtesy of Dr. Hawra Al Qallaf, Indianapolis, IN.)

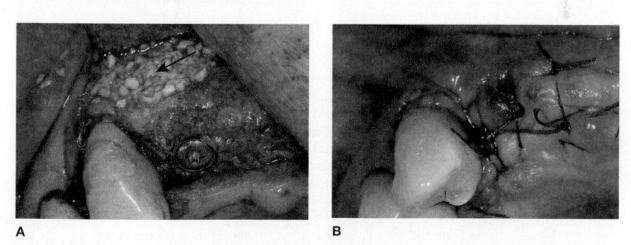

Figure 29-46. Two-Stage (Submerged) Approach. A. Surgical placement of implant with cover screw secured to the head of the implant. Note that the cover screw is flush with the alveolar crest to minimize the chance of exposure. Also note that bone graft material was placed at the time of surgery to minimize the effects of post-surgical resorption of the facial plate (*black arrow*). **B.** Flap closure. Primary closure of the flap is important to ensure that the implant and the bone graft material will remain completely submerged all throughout the healing process.

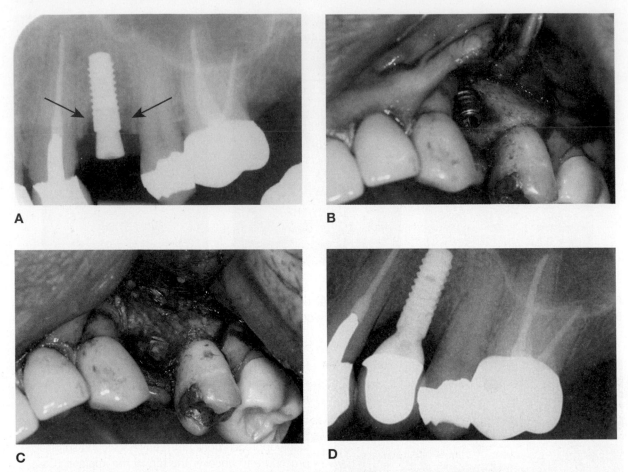

Figure 29-47. Surgical Intervention of Implant With Peri-implantitis. A. Dental radiograph showing alveolar bone loss around a dental implant at the time of periodontal recall visit. **B.** Flap elevated to reveal precise bone contours and to allow for treatment of exposed implant surfaces and grafting of bone defect. **C.** Graft and membrane placement prior to suturing. **D.** Radiograph taken 10 months following surgery showing bone fill. (Case courtesy of Drs. Allison Marlow and Apoorv Goel, Indianapolis, IN.)

3. There are a variety of dental implants with various lengths, diameters, and designs.
4. If there is an inadequate amount of bone and/or keratinized gingiva, then any of the periodontal regenerative procedures previously discussed can be employed *either prior to surgery or at the time of surgery* (refer to the *arrows* in Fig. 29-46A) to compensate for this deficiency.

B. **Healing Expected Following Dental Implant Placement**
1. Healing following placement of a dental implant results in bone growth in such close proximity to the metal implant surface that the implant is stable enough to support a tooth-shaped restoration or a dental prosthetic appliance. Per-Ingvar Branemark (the father of modern dental implants) coined the term **"osseointegration"** to describe the direct structural and functional connection between living bone and the implant surface. Osseointegration is critical for implant stability and is a prerequisite for the long-term success of the dental implant.
2. Although dental implants are not surrounded by cementum and do not have periodontal ligament attached to it (as seen in natural teeth), implants are still subject to the same inflammatory process that affect the

supporting periodontal tissues around a natural tooth. If not arrested, the inflammatory process will lead to subsequent loss of supporting bone around the osseointegrated implant. This is termed as **peri-implantitis**. The eventual outcome, if the peri-implantitis is not appropriately managed, is loss of osseointegration which leads to implant failure. Since peri-implantitis jeopardizes implant survival, periodic monitoring of the peri-implant tissue, probing depth assessments, and radiographic evaluations are the best means to recognize early implant pathology before it becomes more advanced. Therefore, at each recall visit, it is very important for all members of the dental team to spend time and effort in carefully assessing the health of the implant and determine if interventional therapy is warranted (Fig. 29-47).

C. **Special Considerations for the Dental Hygienist**
   1. Patient self-care following placement of a dental implant is as critical as it is following every periodontal surgical procedure, and the members of the dental team must assume responsibility for helping the patient with plaque control during the critical healing period.
   2. Once an implant site heals, the gingiva surrounding the implant can be maintained in health using self-care techniques similar to what is required to keep tissues around a natural tooth healthy.
   3. Implant maintenance and the role played by the dental hygienist are discussed in detail in Chapter 9.

17. **Periodontal Microsurgery.** Periodontal microsurgery is a term used to describe periodontal surgery performed with the aid of a surgical microscope. Principles of microsurgery have had a good deal of influence in medicine and will continue to influence the performance of certain periodontal surgical procedures, especially periodontal plastic surgery. Periodontal surgery performed using microsurgery techniques can result in procedures performed with increased precision on the part of the surgeon.

18. **Laser Therapy.** The use of lasers (light amplification by stimulated emission of radiation) to focus a beam of light of a single wavelength at diseased sites has become an important topic in dentistry and periodontics.
    A. Lasers can incise and coagulate soft tissues with efficiency, and this fact makes the use of lasers during some surgical procedures, such as gingivectomy, gingivoplasty, biopsy of soft tissues, ablation of lesions, vestibuloplasty, and frenectomies useful adjuncts. Figures 29-48 and 29-49 provide several pre-surgical and post-surgical cases that involved the use of laser therapy.
    B. Lasers of varying wavelengths have been proposed to be effective in treating periodontitis and peri-implantitis. It has also been proposed that lasers have the capability to stimulate periodontal regeneration. Some of the proposed benefits of laser therapy are (1) the laser beam is bactericidal against pigmented periodontal pathogens, (2) the laser is able to deliver a precise, intensive energy to the periodontal pocket without damage to the adjacent tissue, and (3) the laser has the ability to seal the pocket orifice with a "thermal fibrin clot" which creates a physical barrier to epithelial downgrowth. However, at this point, due to conflicting studies, it remains inconclusive if laser therapy can effectively and predictably treat periodontitis and induce true periodontal regeneration. Ongoing clinical studies are being conducted to settle this debate.
    C. Current statements by the American Academy of Periodontology and the American Dental Association caution that there is *insufficient evidence to support the use of lasers as a single form of treatment in periodontitis patients at this time.*[33,34]

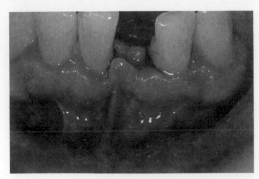

A

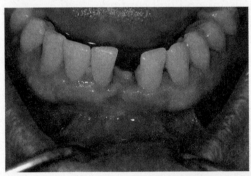

B

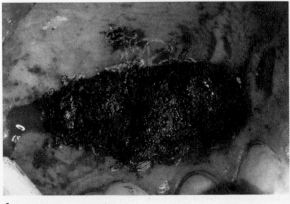

C

Figure 29-48. Application of CO$_2$ laser for a Frenectomy.
A. Clinical photograph showing excessive frenal pull in the mandibular anterior region.

B. Laser incision to remove frenum and to perform vestibuloplasty.

C. Follow-up photograph 10 days after surgery showing excellent healing and minimal inflammation. (Case courtesy of Drs. Vidya Prabhu and Yusuke Hamada, Indianapolis, IN.)

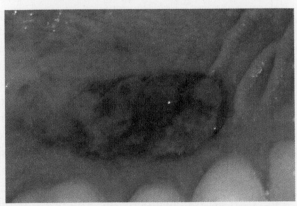

A   **B**

Figure 29-49. Hemostasis at Free Soft Tissue Autograft Donor Site. A. After obtaining a free soft tissue autograft from the palate, a CO$_2$ laser was set on the coagulation setting to gain hemostasis at the donor site. **B.** 7 days after the surgery, note the early signs of healing and re-epithelialization of the donor site. (Case courtesy of Drs. Vidya Prabhu and Yusuke Hamada, Indianapolis, IN.)

Section 4
Biological Enhancement of Surgical Outcomes

Many attempts have been made to enhance the outcomes of periodontal surgery by using chemical or biologic mediators to influence the healing following periodontal surgical procedures. This chapter section provides a brief overview of some of the chemical and biologic mediators that have been studied. There is much ongoing research into this topic, and it is reasonable to expect that this ongoing research will shine more light on the fundamental mechanisms for enhancing periodontal regeneration.

1. **Root Surface Modification**
   A. **Mechanical Root Preparation**
      1. Many years of observation of the healing of periodontal surgical wounds demonstrate that gingival tissues adjacent to tooth roots—that have previously been exposed because of attachment loss—heal better when the roots are free of plaque biofilm, calculus, and root contaminants.
      2. These observations have led to the incorporation of mechanical root preparation as a routine part of most periodontal surgical procedures. Hand and ultrasonic instruments have been used extensively for this purpose.
   B. **Chemical Biomodification Mediators.** Chemical biomodification mediators have been used in attempts to enhance the healing of the gingiva adjacent to the tooth roots beyond what can be achieved by periodontal instrumentation alone. Several chemical biomodification mediators have been studied for possible benefits to the gingival healing process.
      1. Ethylenediaminetetraacetic acid (EDTA) is a gel that is applied to treated root surfaces to modify (condition) the surface of the root following mechanical root preparation (Fig. 29-50).
         a. Possible benefits of using EDTA on roots include removal of the dentin smear layer, exposure of ends of embedded collagen fibers in remaining cemental surface, and removal of endotoxin buried deeper below the root surface.
         b. Though some clinicians have used EDTA to enhance root preparation, most of the evidence indicates that there is a questionable positive effect on the outcomes of any surgery by the use of this chemical to prepare tooth roots.
      2. A second chemical agent that has been referred to as a biologic mediator, again to enhance the outcomes of periodontal root preparation, is tetracycline (Fig. 29-51).
         a. Tetracyclines are a family of antibiotics with varied properties in addition to their antibiotic effects. It has been suggested that tetracyclines applied to roots during surgery may enhance the migration of fibroblasts to the root surfaces during healing in addition to slightly decalcifying the surfaces of the roots.
         b. Most studies indicate that using this biologic mediator on root surfaces during surgery has a questionable effect on the outcomes of the surgical procedures.
      3. Both EDTA and tetracyclines are also known as root conditioning agents.
2. **Growth Factors.** Growth factors are naturally occurring proteins that regulate both cell growth and development. Several growth factors are being studied for their effect in enhancing the predictability of periodontal regeneration.[35,36] These growth factors include platelet-derived growth factor (PDGF) and insulin-derived growth factor (IGF). It is reasonable to expect that continued research into the use of growth factors to improve periodontal surgical outcomes might lead to clinical application of some of these factors in the future.

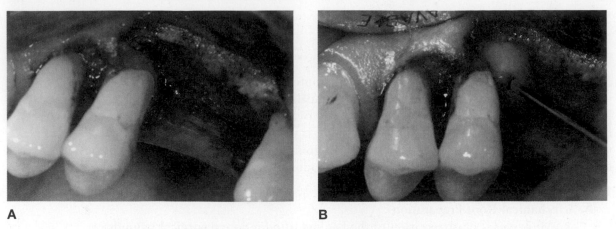

A **B**

Figure 29-50. Application of EDTA to Treat an Intrabony Defect. A. An intrabony defect is exposed on the distal of the maxillary premolar. **B.** Following meticulous root debridement and degranulation of the intrabony defect, the treated root surface is "conditioned" by using EDTA. From a theoretical standpoint, EDTA "biomodifies" the root, thus facilitating attachment of healing connective tissue to the treated root surface. (Case courtesy of Dr. Kelly Hill, Indianapolis, IN.)

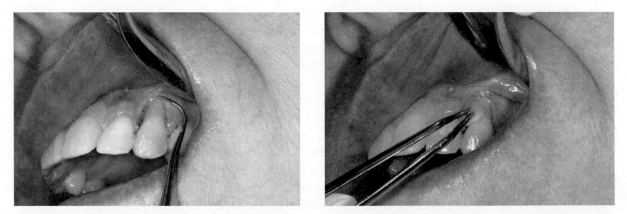

Figure 29-51. Application of Tetracycline. After meticulously instrumenting the exposed root surface, tetracycline is burnished onto the root surface in order to remove the smear layer and to selectively remove mineral from the dentin or cementum surface exposing a collagenous matrix.

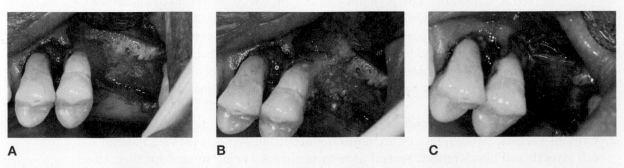

A **B** **C**

Figure 29-52. Application of EMD, Bone Graft, and Resorbable Membrane. This is a continuation of the case shown in Figure 29-50. **A.** After root conditioning with EDTA, EMD gel is placed in the defect. **B.** DFDBA (bone graft) is packed into the defect. **C.** A resorbable barrier membrane is placed to cover and contain the grafted site. (Case courtesy of Dr. Kelly Hill, Indianapolis, IN.)

3. **Enamel Matrix Derivative**
   A. **Periodontal Regeneration Factors**
      1. It is clear that periodontal regeneration depends upon the type of cells that first populate the periodontal surgical wound.
      2. As already discussed, using barrier materials to ensure that cells of the periodontal ligament enter the healing surgical wound without the early interference of epithelium can result in more predictable periodontal regeneration. The use of barriers to ensure periodontal regeneration, however, has not been very successful in all sites of more advanced osseous defects.
   B. **Protein Preparations.** Research into using protein preparations and growth factors to enhance periodontal regeneration by mimicking natural healing processes has shown some promising results.[37–41]
      1. Enamel matrix derivative is a Food and Drug Administration (FDA)-approved therapy that is applied to treated root surfaces to stimulate healing and regeneration through angiogenesis and osteogenesis.
      2. Enamel matrix derivative is a preparation of proteins extracted from porcine tooth buds. Enamel matrix derivative is a preparation of proteins extracted from porcine tooth buds mixed with a propylene glycol alginate carrier.
      3. While it is unclear as to what the exact mechanism of action of enamel matrix derivative is, research has proposed several biological effects of enamel matrix derivative which may potentially promote periodontal regeneration: (1) increased attachment of periodontal ligament to the treated root surface, (2) increased differentiation of periodontal ligament stem cells into cementoblasts and osteoblasts, (3) decreased proliferation of epithelium (blocks the downgrowth of the long junctional epithelium), and (4) stimulation of the release of important growth factors, such as TGF-β.
      4. The major constituents of this extract appear to be proteins called amelogenins and enamelin.
      5. At this point, it appears that enamel matrix derivative may indeed enhance periodontal regeneration and that the effectiveness of this material is quite high when used in conjunction with different types of graft materials and/or barrier membranes (Fig. 29-52).
      6. Enamel matrix derivative is currently being used by clinicians in an attempt to improve outcomes of some types of periodontal surgery.
      7. Studies into the precise constituents in this protein extract that can enhance healing are continuing.

4. **Platelet-Rich Plasma.** Another example of a biologic mediator is platelet-rich plasma. Platelet-rich plasma is classified as a first-generation platelet concentrate. The purported advantages of platelet-rich plasma are that (1) it is derived from an autogenous source (from the patient's own blood), thus eliminating concerns associated with disease transmission or immunogenic reactions and (2) it is a practical source of growth factors needed for periodontal regeneration.[42,43]
   A. **Multistep Process for Platelet-Rich Plasma Development**
      1. Developing platelet-rich plasma is a multistep process (Fig. 29-53). First, blood is drawn from the patient through a process known as venipuncture.
      2. The blood sample is then mixed with an anticoagulant (to prevent spontaneous blood clot formation) and separated through a centrifugation process into three separate fractions: platelet-rich plasma, red blood cells, and platelet-poor plasma.

     a. The red blood cells and platelet-poor plasma fractions have no clinical benefit and are therefore discarded.

     b. The platelet-rich plasma fraction, on the other hand, is a rich source of platelets which have the ability to produce and release a cocktail of multiple growth factors that work synergistically to initiate the wound healing cascade and enhance the regenerative process.

  3. Next, the platelet-rich plasma fraction is mixed with bovine thrombin and calcium to biochemically activate the platelets so that they degranulate and release their growth factors.

  4. Finally, the platelet-rich plasma is ready to be delivered to the surgical site via an applicator.

B. Research on the Regenerative Role of Platelet-Rich Plasma

  1. While some studies indicate a potential enhancement of the healing process following the use of this preparation, it is still unclear if the growth factors are present in high enough concentrations to have much effect on the actual surgical outcomes. Additional studies of this material are underway.

  2. Furthermore, platelet-rich plasma has several undesirable adverse effects that can pose problems. First, the platelet-rich plasma fraction contains anticoagulants that block the full coagulation cascade which plays a critical role in tissue wound healing. Second, platelet rich plasma is mixed with bovine thrombin which can induce an allergic reaction in individuals sensitive to bovine materials.

5. Platelet-Rich Fibrin. Platelet-rich fibrin is a second-generation platelet concentrate which was first developed in France in 2001 by Choukroun et al. Like platelet-rich plasma, platelet-rich fibrin is obtained from the patient's own blood and subjected to centrifugation. Yet, there are several key differences between platelet-rich plasma and platelet-rich fibrin.

- First, anticoagulants and bovine thrombin are *not* added to platelet-rich fibrin, thereby avoiding the potential adverse effects associated with platelet-rich plasma. Collecting blood without anticoagulants allows for the natural coagulation process to take place so that the desired platelet fibrin clot forms.
- Second, is a three-dimensional fibrin matrix that can be used as a scaffold for a variety of procedures including serving the function of a barrier membrane in guided bone regeneration and guided tissue regeneration procedures (Fig. 29-54).
- Third, platelet-rich fibrin has been demonstrated to contain even higher levels of growth factors over an extended period of time compared to platelet-rich plasma.

6. Bone Morphogenetic Proteins. Bone morphogenetic proteins are a group of regulatory glycoproteins that have been studied for possible use in the field of periodontal regeneration because of their known osteoinductive effects. Both purified and recombinant BMPs are currently being studied, and early results indicate possible enhancement of regeneration in some treated sites. Unfortunately, using bone morphogenetic proteins to enhance surgical outcomes has resulted in tooth ankylosis and much further study of this material is indicated. Investigations into the use of bone morphogenetic proteins to enhance periodontal regeneration are continuing.

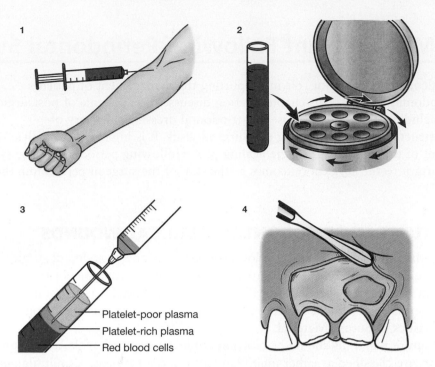

Platelet-poor plasma
Platelet-rich plasma
Red blood cells

Figure 29-53. Process of PRP Therapy. 1. Blood is first drawn from the patient's arm. **2.** Blood is then placed and spun in a centrifuge. The centrifuge separates the platelets from the rest of the blood components. **3.** The platelet-rich plasma is extracted from the glass tube coated with an anticoagulant. **4.** After mixing the prepared platelet-rich plasma fraction with bovine thrombin and calcium which activate the platelets, the platelet-rich plasma gel is now ready to be applied to the periodontal defect.

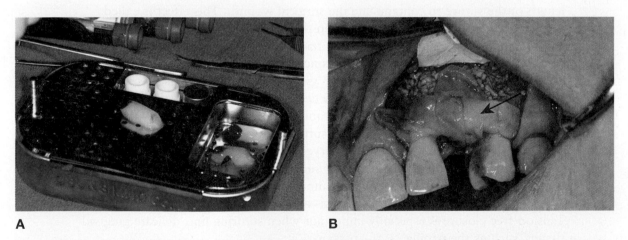

A

B

Figure 29-54. Platelet-Rich Fibrin Therapy for a Periodontal Defect. A. After centrifugation, the PRF clot is removed from the test tube using sterile tweezers and placed on a sterile metal tray. Each platelet-rich fibrin clot releases its serum (PRF-clot exudate) and is ready for compression into the barrier membrane. **B.** The platelet-rich fibrin clot (*arrow*) can be compressed and molded to form a strong fibrin matrix that covers the bone graft and serves as the barrier membrane. The fibrin matrix is remodeled in a way comparable with a natural clot and does not dissolve rapidly after application. (Case courtesy of Drs. Hawra Al Qallaf, Jennifer Chang, and Yusuke Hamada, Indianapolis, IN.)

Section 5
Patient Management Following Periodontal Surgery

The dental hygienist plays a major role in supporting the management of patients following periodontal surgery. This chapter section discusses components of postsurgical management including use of sutures, use of periodontal dressings, delivery of postsurgical instructions, and organizing postsurgical visits. It is important to realize that the management of the patient during the healing phase following periodontal surgery can be as important to the surgical outcomes as the skill of the surgeon performing the surgery.

USE OF SUTURES IN PERIODONTAL SURGICAL WOUNDS

1. **Overview of the Use of Sutures in Periodontal Wounds.** Many periodontal surgical procedures require the placement of sutures to stabilize and secure the position of the soft tissues during the early phases of healing; a suture, or "stitch" as it is sometimes called, is a material placed by a surgeon to hold tissues together during healing.
   A. **Characteristics of Suture Material**
      1. Ideal suture materials should be biocompatible, nontoxic, flexible, and strong.
      2. Sutures are classified as either multifilament or monofilament. A multifilament suture, such as black silk suture, is composed of smaller strands that are braided or twisted together whereas a monofilament suture, such as a polypropylene suture and nylon suture, is composed of a single strand. One undesirable property of multifilament sutures is its capability to absorb and retain fluid and/or bacteria within its suture fibers (i.e., bacteria can accumulate in between the multiple smaller strands and travel down the entire length of the suture to contaminate the surgical wound). This effect is called "wicking" which has a negative effect on the surgical outcomes as it triggers an inflammatory reaction. On the other hand, the "wicking" effect is rarely associated with a monofilament suture since it is composed of a single strand.
      3. When placing sutures, the surgeon takes great care not to put tension on a flap with sutures (i.e., to ensure that the flap lies passively at the intended position prior to suturing); sutures are used to stabilize the flap in its passive position.
      4. If a suture places tension on a flap, the suture material will pull out of the tissues during healing and will fail to serve the purpose of stabilizing the tissues. Another adverse consequence of suturing the flap with tension is that it may traumatize the soft tissue and compromise vascularization to the flap. This will ultimately result in flap necrosis and compromise surgical outcomes. Tension-free closure is especially important when suturing fine, delicate gingival tissues, such as the papilla.
   B. **Types of Suture Material.** In general, two types of suture material are used: nonabsorbable and absorbable. Box 29-7 provides an overview of some of the suture materials available for use in periodontal wounds.
      1. Nonabsorbable suture, also referred to as nonresorbable suture, is a suture made from a material that does not dissolve in body fluids. A clinician must remove the nonabsorbable sutures after some healing of the wound has occurred.
      2. Absorbable suture, also referred to as resorbable suture, is a suture made from a material designed to dissolve harmlessly in body fluids over time; though absorbable sutures do not normally require removal by the dental team, some absorbable sutures do not dissolve particularly well in saliva.

Box 29-7. Examples of Suture Materials

Nonabsorbable

- Braided silk
- Monofilament nylon
- Polytetrafluoroethylene
- Braided polyester
- Polypropylene

Absorbable

- Plain and chromic gut
- Polyglactin 910 (Coated Vicryl)
- Poliglecaprone 25 (Monocryl)

Box 29-8. Overview of General Indications for Common Suture Techniques

1. Interrupted suture: closure of vertical incisions, closure of nondisplaced flaps
2. Sling suture: closure of displaced flaps
3. Continuous sling suture: closure of displaced flaps, closure of nondisplaced flaps

---

2. **Suture Placement Techniques.** Familiarity with some general techniques for suturing can guide the hygienist assigned to the task of suture removal at a postsurgical appointment. Box 29-8 provides an overview of general indications for some of the more common suturing techniques for periodontal surgical wounds. Three of the most common suture placement techniques are discussed and illustrated below.

A. **Interrupted Interdental Suture**

1. In most periodontal flap surgeries, flaps are elevated on both the facial and lingual (or palatal) surfaces of the teeth. At the completion of the surgery, an interrupted interdental suture is typically used to suture the facial and lingual papillae together. This technique is also ideal for closing vertical incisions.
2. When interrupted interdental sutures are placed to close a periodontal flap that involves several teeth, a separate suture is placed and tied in each of the interdental sites. The interrupted suture ensures that the flap remains closed in the event that one suture fails.
3. An interrupted interdental suture that might be utilized during a periodontal flap for access procedure is illustrated in Figures 29-55 and 29-56.
4. When removing interrupted interdental sutures, the clinician must cut each of the interdental sutures prior to pulling out the suture material.

B. **Continuous Sling Suture**

1. The continuous sling suture is preferred by many clinicians for suturing many types of periodontal flaps.
2. When continuous sling sutures are used, following placing the suture material through two interdental papillae, the end of the suture is looped around the teeth to reach the next interdental site rather than being tied at each interdental site; the suture is tied following placement of the loop around the terminal tooth.
3. A continuous sling suture that might be utilized during an apically positioned flap is illustrated in Figures 29-57 and 29-58.
4. Removal of a continuous sling suture can frequently be accomplished with a single cut through the suture near the knot prior to pulling out the suture material.

C. **Sling Suture**

1. Some periodontal surgical wounds require the placement of a sling suture; the sling suture is used to sling or suspend the tissues around the cervical area of a tooth rather than to tie soft tissue to other soft tissue.

2. The sling suture is frequently used when a flap is displaced in an apical direction. Figure 29-59 illustrates a sling suture.
3. It should be noted that when facial and lingual flaps are sutured using the sling suture technique, a separate sling suture must be placed on both the facial and lingual surfaces.
4. Removal of the sling suture only requires locating the individual knots, cutting the suture near the knot, and careful extraction of the suture.

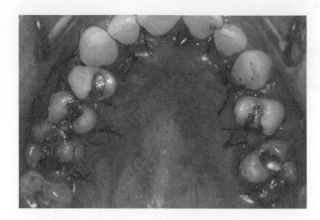

Figure 29-55. Interrupted Interdental Sutures. Interrupted interdental sutures have been placed in each interdental site on the maxillary arch. Note that there is a knot associated with each of these interrupted sutures that would need to be cut prior to removal. (Courtesy of Dr. John S. Dozier, Tallahassee, FL.)

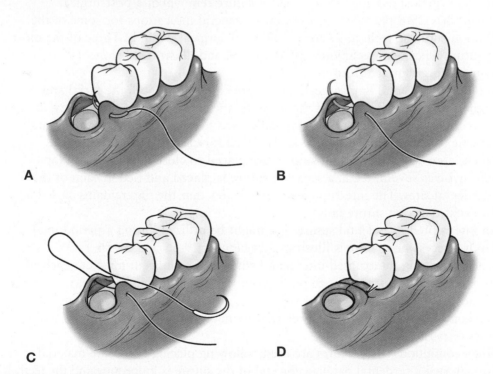

Figure 29-56. Interrupted Interdental Suture. In these drawings, the most mesial tooth has been removed to allow for visualization of the path of the interrupted interdental suture. **A.** Suture placed through papilla on the facial. **B.** Suture placed through the papilla on the lingual. **C.** Suture returned to facial side. **D.** Knot tied in suture on the facial side.

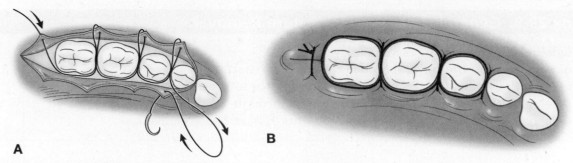

Figure 29-57. Continuous Sling Suture. Note that the suture is looped around each of the cervical areas of the teeth and passed through the tissues associated with each interdental area (**A**), but that it is tied only at the end of the continuous loop (**B**).

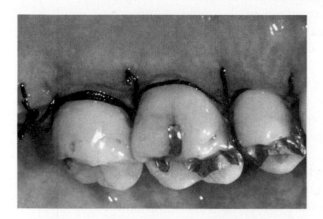

Figure 29-58. Continuous Sling Suture. Continuous loop suture has been placed on the segment of teeth in maxillary arch. Note that the only knot visible is associated with the most distal tooth. (Courtesy of Dr. Don Rolfs, Periodontal Foundations, Wenatchee, WA.)

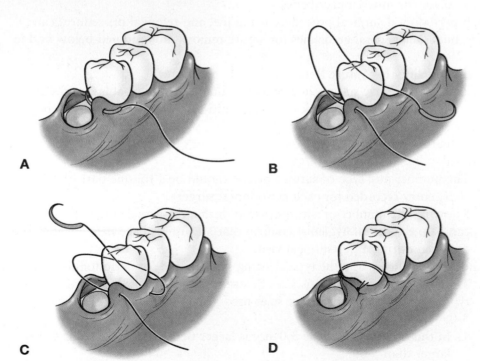

Figure 29-59. Sling Suture. In these drawings, the most mesial tooth has been removed to allow for visualization of the path of the sling suture. **A.** Suture placed through the facial papilla. **B.** Suture looped around the lingual surface of the tooth without engaging the lingual soft tissues. **C.** Suture continues back to the facial surface under the contact and engages the facial papilla on the distal of the tooth. **D.** Suture continues back on same path and is tied on the surface where it first penetrated the facial papilla.

Box 29-9. General Guidelines for Suture Removal

Guideline 1: Remove sutures in a timely manner.
Guideline 2: Read the surgical note in the patient's chart.
Guideline 3: Understand the typical sizing system for sutures.
Guideline 4: Never allow the knot to be pulled through the tissues.
Guideline 5: Always confirm that all of the sutures have been removed.

---

3. **Suture Removal**
   A. **Removal of Sutures**
      1. Nonabsorbable sutures placed during surgical procedures are removed as part of routine postsurgical visits. Frequently, remnants of absorbable sutures can also be removed at the routine postsurgical visits to avoid unnecessary tissue inflammation that can occur if the retained absorbable suture is not dissolved in a timely manner.
      2. Guidelines for timing of removal vary, but in general, sutures should be removed when wound healing has progressed to the point at which the sutures are no longer needed to stabilize the tissues. Many sutures are loose and no longer needed to stabilize the tissues at the time of the 1-week postsurgical visit.
      3. Most periodontal sutures should not be left in place longer than 2 weeks because they can act as irritants if the suture material remains in the tissues too long. It should be noted that sutures in some periodontal wounds are routinely left in place for much longer periods.
      4. Each periodontal surgical procedure is unique, and removal procedures can vary, but some general guidelines for suture removal are outlined below and in Box 29-9.
   B. **General Guidelines for Suture Removal**
      1. Guideline 1: Remove sutures in a timely manner. Nonabsorbable sutures are generally removed after 1 week of healing; most absorbable sutures can be left in place 1 to 3 weeks.
      2. Guideline 2: Read the surgical note in the patient's chart prior to suture removal.
         a. The number and type of sutures placed should be a routine part of the chart entry recorded for each periodontal surgery.
         b. Knowing the number of sutures placed during the actual surgical procedure can help the dental hygienist confirm that all sutures have been located and removed during a postsurgical visit.
      3. Guideline 3: Understand the typical sizing system used for periodontal sutures.
         a. Though there are numerous sizes of sutures used in a medical setting, typical designations for suture sizes used in periodontal surgery are sizes 3-0, 4-0, and 5-0.
            1) In this sizing system, the 3-0 size is larger than the 4-0 size, and 4-0 is larger than 5-0.
            2) In the mouth, 5-0 can be more difficult to locate than a 4-0 size, especially in the posterior part of the mouth.
         b. The dental hygienist should learn the precise abbreviations used in the chart entries in the individual clinical setting. A typical example of an abbreviation would be "4-0 BSS." This would mean the size of the suture is

4-0, and BSS stands for black silk suture, a commonly used nonabsorbable suture material.

c. Table 29-5 outlines designations for typical suture sizes used during periodontal surgery as they might appear in a patient's chart.

4. Guideline 4: Never allow the knot to be pulled through the tissues.

a. Grasp the knot with sterile tissue forceps.

b. Use scissors to cut the sutures under the knot as close as possible to the tissue. This should be done to avoid passage of the plaque-contaminated outer portion of the suture back through the tissue.

c. Gently pull the suture with the sterile forceps away from the tissue.

1) When the suture is gently pulled from the tissue, care should be taken not to force the knot itself through the tissue. This technique is illustrated in Figure 29-60.

2) It should be noted that suture removal is rarely painful for the patient if care is taken not to create unnecessary tissue movement.

5. Guideline 5: Always confirm that all of the sutures have been removed.

a. Following suture removal, it is imperative to visually inspect the wound with care to ensure that all of the sutures have indeed been located and removed.

b. Remember that the patient chart entry made on the day of the surgery usually will contain information about how many sutures were actually placed.

TABLE 29-5	TYPICAL DESIGNATIONS FOR SUTURE SIZES USED IN PERIODONTAL SURGERY	
Suture Size		**Approximate Diameter of Suture**
3-0		0.20 mm
4-0		0.15 mm
5-0		0.10 mm

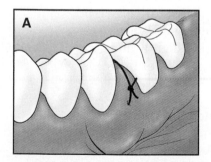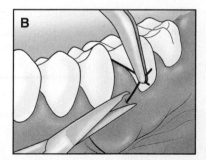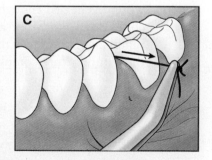

Figure 29-60. Suture Removal. A. Suture in place. **B.** Grasp the suture material with forceps and cut under the knot *as close as possible to the tissue.* **C.** Pull the suture material gently from the tissue taking care not to pull the knot through the tissue.

USE OF PERIODONTAL DRESSING

1. **Purpose of Periodontal Dressing**
   A. Periodontal dressing, or periodontal pack as it sometimes called, is a protective material applied over a periodontal surgical wound (Fig. 29-61). Periodontal dressings are used somewhat like a bandage covering a finger wound. Periodontal dressing provides mechanical protection for the surgical wound and therefore facilitates healing, enhances patient comfort by isolating the area from external irritations or injuries, prevents postsurgical bleeding by maintaining the initial clot in place, and maintains a debris-free area of the protected site.
   B. *Though the placement of periodontal dressings following periodontal surgery used to be routine, modern surgical techniques may or may not require placement of a periodontal dressing.*
      1. The surgical wound created by the gingivectomy procedure leaves a raw connective tissue surface exposed that always requires a periodontal dressing.
      2. Periodontal flaps that are well adapted to the alveolar bone and tooth roots may not always require a periodontal dressing.
      3. Periodontal dressings can be placed to facilitate flap adaptation and are frequently indicated when the surgical procedures have created varying tissue levels or when displaced flaps are used.
      4. The periodontist will determine the need for dressing placement at the time of the surgical procedure.
2. **General Guidelines for Management of Periodontal Dressings**
   A. **Proper Placement**
      1. Periodontal dressing is retained primarily by pushing some of the material into the embrasure spaces to lock the dressing around the necks of the teeth mechanically.
      2. Using less periodontal dressing is better than using more of the material during placement; the proper amount of dressing is only enough to cover the wound. The dressing should be placed so that there is no contact between the dressing and the teeth in the opposing arch when the patient bites down; occlusal contact with teeth in the opposing arch will quickly dislodge the dressing. Table 29-6 (Fig. 29-62A–E) illustrates the proper placement of a periodontal dressing.
      3. Periodontal dressings should be replaced every 5 to 7 days until the surgical wound is healed enough to be exposed. It should be noted that suture material could accidentally become trapped within the periodontal dressing. When removing dressings, it may be necessary to loosen the dressing slightly and cut the suture before completely removing the dressing from the necks of the teeth.

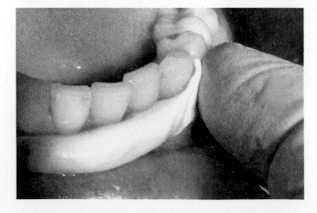

Figure 29-61. Periodontal Dressing. Periodontal dressing is placed over a periodontal surgical site. Note that gentle finger pressure is applied to mechanically push the pack around the necks of the teeth so that it interlocks around each tooth in the interproximal areas.

TABLE 29-6	STEPS IN PERIODONTAL DRESSING PLACEMENT

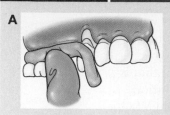

Figure 29-62A. Dressing is pressed into the interdental spaces with gentle finger pressure on the facial.

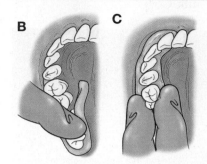

Figure 29-62B. Dressing is looped around the most distal tooth and pressed into the interdental spaces on the palatal.

Figure 29-62C. Gentle finger pressure is continued against the dressing to join it interdentally on the facial and palatal aspects.

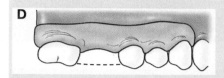

Figure 29-62D. Dressing can be bridged across edentulous areas.

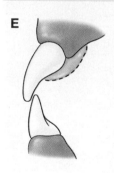

Figure 29-62E. Dressing amount should be minimal to avoid contact of the dressing with the teeth in the opposite arch.

3. **Types of Periodontal Dressing.** There are two types of modern periodontal dressings commonly available for use today. Both types of periodontal dressing are held in place primarily by mechanical retention around the necks of the teeth.
   A. **Chemical Cure Paste.** One type is a two-paste chemical cure material that requires the mixing of paste from two tubes to form a dressing with a putty-like consistency which has a soft texture, but still has enough flexibility to facilitate its placement and adaptation over the surgical wound area.
      1. This type usually contains zinc oxide, mineral oils, and rosin plus a bacteriostatic or fungicidal agent.
      2. Mixing of these two-paste dressings is either by hand (Fig. 29-63) or in an auto-mix cartridge.
      3. Examples of two-paste dressings are Coe-Pak manufactured by GC America, Inc. and PerioCare manufactured by Pulpdent Corp.

B. **Light-Cured Paste.** A second type is a light-cured gel that contains polyether urethane dimethacrylate resin (Fig. 29-64).

1. The dental hygienist must study the manufacturer's instructions with care and must practice placement of the dressing on a typodont (model) before using it in a patient's mouth.

2. This type of dressing is available as a clear, translucent material that is preferred for use by some clinicians in esthetic areas of the dentition.

3. An example of a light-cured gel periodontal dressing is Barricaid VLC periodontal surgical dressing manufactured by Dentsply Caulk Co.

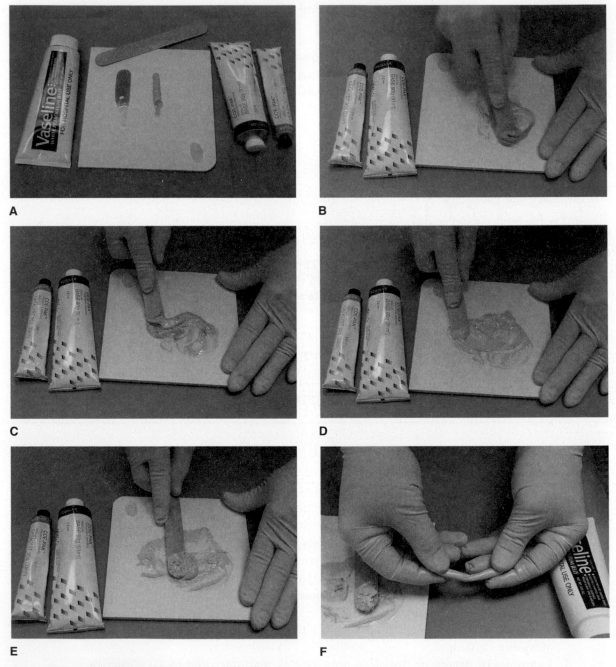

Figure 29-63. Two-Tube Chemical Cure Paste. A. Equal lengths of paste from the catalyst and the base tube are extruded onto the mixing pad. **B–E.** A wooden tongue depressor (or a metal spatula) is used to mix the paste until a thick consistency and uniform color is reached. The setting time can be altered by adding a few drops of warm water during mixing or by immersing the pack into a bowl of warm water just after mixing. **F.** Once the paste loses its tackiness, it can be handled and molded using gloves lubricated with water or petroleum. The pack is then formed into uniform pencil-sized rolls that have a smooth consistency.

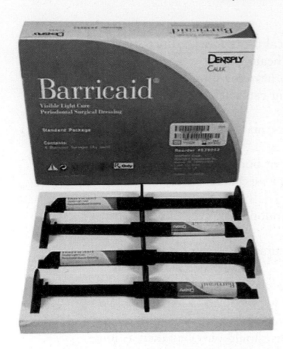

Figure 29-64. Light-Cured Dressing Material. Barricaid by Dentsply is an example of a periodontal dressing available in prefilled syringes. The dressing is applied over the surgical site and light-cured to form an elastic protective covering that is pink, tasteless, and allows for superior esthetics. Unlike chemical-cure pastes, light-cured dressing material eliminates the time-consuming process of mixing pastes together. (Courtesy of Dentsply International.)

POSTSURGICAL INSTRUCTIONS AND FOLLOW-UP VISITS

A member of the dental team should provide postsurgical instructions to the patient following periodontal surgery. Usually the patient is provided with both written and verbal instructions to minimize confusion and to maximize compliance. Typical postsurgical instructions are outlined in Box 29-10. For patients where sedation was required, the companion who accompanied the patient to the office is included when postsurgical instructions are given.

Box 29-10. Typical Postsurgical Instructions

1. If you have questions or concerns, call the office or the office emergency number right away. Office: 555-1111; emergency 555-2222.
2. *Do* take medications as prescribed. Report any problems with the medications immediately.
3. *Do* take it easy for several days. Limit your activity to mild physical exertion.
4. *Expect* some bleeding following the procedure. If heavy bleeding persists, call the office emergency number.
5. *Expect* some swelling. Intermittent use of an ice pack on the face in the area of the surgery during the first 8 to 10 hours following surgery can minimize swelling.
6. Diet Recommendations:
   a. Soft food only on the day of the surgery
   b. No hot beverages on the day of surgery
   c. Avoid chewing on the surgical site
7. Oral Self-Care:
   a. Rinse with recommended mouth rinse starting the day after surgery.
   b. If dressing was placed, it may also be brushed lightly.

1. **Postsurgical Instructions to the Patient**
   A. **Restrictions on Self-Care.** Most periodontal surgical procedures require some restrictions on self-care during the early phase of healing.
      1. It is common practice to prescribe 0.12% chlorhexidine mouth rinse to be used twice daily to aid with self-care until the patient can safely resume mechanical plaque control.
      2. In most cases following any periodontal surgery, manual self-care can be resumed by the patient in 10 to 14 days.
      3. For selected surgical procedures (such as GTR or bone grafting procedures), the surgical sites should not be cleaned with routine mechanical plaque control for up to 4 to 6 weeks.
      4. Areas of the dentition not involved by the periodontal surgery may be cleaned with routine self-care techniques.
   B. **Postsurgical Medications.** Patients should be encouraged to take medications as prescribed.
      1. If systemic antibiotics are prescribed, it is particularly important for the patient to understand that all of this prescribed antibiotic medication should be taken.
      2. Common postsurgical medications include either nonsteroidal or narcotic pain medications, but usually, these pain medications should only be taken as long as needed.
   C. **Dietary Changes.** Chewing frequently must be limited to areas not involved by the surgery until healing has progressed to an acceptable level.
      1. Many of these periodontal procedures require that the surgical site be undisturbed for an extended period of time.
      2. Recommendations for a soft or liquid diet for 24 to 48 hours are routine following most periodontal surgical procedures.
      3. Chewing should be limited to the side of the mouth not involved by the surgery, especially during the early phases of healing.
2. **Postsurgical Complications**
   A. Facial swelling: It is common for the patient to experience some facial swelling following most types of periodontal surgery.
      1. Swelling can arise from the tissue trauma incurred during the procedure and can even occur during the second and third day following the surgery.
      2. Although this swelling can be disconcerting to the patient, it is usually not a sign that healing is compromised.
      3. Swelling can be minimized by the intermittent use of ice packs for the first 8 to 10 hours following the surgery.
   B. Postsurgical bleeding: Some bleeding following periodontal surgery is to be expected.
      1. Patients should be reassured that minor bleeding is not a cause for alarm.
      2. Postsurgical instructions should be clear, however, that if excessive bleeding occurs the emergency number should be contacted immediately.
   C. Smoking: Surgical patients, who have elected to continue smoking, should be cautioned to suspend their habit during the healing phase.
3. **Organizing Postsurgical Visits.** It is the dentist's responsibility to manage postsurgical problems, such as extreme pain or infection. The dental hygienist, however, can perform much of the routine postsurgical patient management. Following periodontal flap surgery, the patient is most often reappointed in 5 to 7 days for the first postsurgical visit. Postsurgical care for the various types of periodontal surgery varies; however, steps to be followed at a typical postsurgical visit are outlined below.

A. Steps Involved in a Typical Postsurgical Visit

1. Step 1. Patient interview: An interview is conducted with the patient to determine what the patient experienced during the days following the surgery. The patient interview should be detailed enough to provide the dental hygienist with an overview of possible problems to investigate and solve at the postsurgical visit. The following are some of the items that would normally be included in this interview. It is imperative that the dental hygienist alerts the dentist if any unusual conditions are reported by the patient or are observed during the postsurgical visit.

   a. Analgesics: Following periodontal surgery, analgesics (pain control medications) are used to control patient discomfort. The patient should be asked about the current level of discomfort and if another prescription is needed.

   b. Antibiotics: If antibiotics were needed following a surgical procedure, remind the patient that all of the antibiotic tablets should be taken. It is also important to find out if the patient experienced any unusual reactions to the antibiotic.

   c. Antimicrobial mouth rinse: An antimicrobial mouth rinse such as 0.12% chlorhexidine gluconate may have been prescribed for the patient to use during healing, since mechanical plaque control must be restricted at the surgical site following periodontal surgery. Ask about the amount of mouth rinse remaining. During the course of the visit, it may be necessary to provide the patient another prescription for this mouth rinse.

   d. Swelling: Following periodontal surgery, it is common for the patient to experience some facial swelling. Remember that although this swelling can be disconcerting to the patient, it is common and usually not a sign that healing is compromised.

   e. Postsurgical bleeding: Inquire about postsurgical bleeding. It is common for patients to experience a little bleeding following periodontal surgery, but heavy bleeding should not have occurred following the procedure. If abnormal bleeding is suspected, the dentist should be alerted prior to planning any additional periodontal surgical intervention.

   f. Sensitivity to cold: Sensitivity to cold following root exposure during many types of periodontal surgery is quite common. Although this is an annoying postsurgical occurrence, the sensitivity normally disappears within the first few weeks following the surgery if excellent plaque control is maintained.

2. Step 2. Vital signs: The patient's vital signs including blood pressure, pulse, and temperature are assessed. An elevated temperature at the first postsurgical visit can indicate a developing infection.

3. Step 3. Periodontal dressing: Any periodontal dressing placed at the time of surgery is removed so that the surgical site can be examined. The surgical site is rinsed with warm sterile saline and cotton-tipped applicators are used to remove any debris adherent to the teeth, soft tissues, or sutures. Suture material can become trapped within the periodontal dressing. When removing dressings, it might be necessary to loosen the dressing slightly and cut the suture before completely removing the dressing from the necks of the teeth. Figure 29-65 shows interrupted interdental sutures ready for removal at the 1-week postsurgical visit.

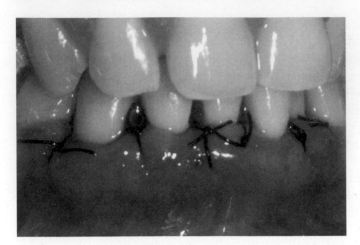

Figure 29-65. Interrupted Interdental Sutures Ready for Removal. At the 1-week postsurgical visit, the periodontal dressing has been removed, the sutures have been cleaned with sterile saline, and the sutures are ready for removal.

4. Step 4. Examination of Surgical Site: Examine the surgical site with care. Tissue swelling or exudate such as pus can indicate a developing infection. Excessive granulation tissue that occasionally forms in the surgical site should be removed with a sharp curette.

5. Step 5. Suture removal: The sutures are cut and removed using sterile scissors and tissue forceps. Remember to pull the suture out of the tissue *without drawing the knot through the tissue.*

6. Step 6. Plaque biofilm removal: All plaque biofilm on the teeth in the area of the surgery is removed. It is typical for patients to be unable to perform good plaque control during the days following periodontal surgery, so plaque accumulation is likely. Part of the responsibility of the dental team is to help the patient with plaque control at each postsurgical visit during the critical stages of healing.

7. Step 7. Replacement of periodontal dressing: If indicated, the periodontal dressing is replaced. For most surgical procedures, the periodontal dressing should be discontinued as soon as the patient can resume some mechanical plaque control. In a few instances, the tissues may not be well adapted to the necks of the teeth, and replacement of the periodontal dressing should be considered to protect the continuing healing of the wound for at least another week.

8. Step 8. Self-care instructions: The patient is instructed in self-care. Mechanical plaque control should be resumed as soon as possible following periodontal surgery, but special instructions may be necessary during the first few weeks following the surgery.

   a. Special self-cleaning aids, such as postsurgical toothbrushes with very delicate and flexible bristles, may be recommended during early stages of healing.

   b. During postsurgical healing, it is frequently necessary to continue to modify the patient's plaque control techniques as the tissues heal and mature. Gingival margin contours usually are altered to some degree by the surgery, and this may necessitate the introduction of additional self-care aids that were not necessary prior to the surgery. Monitoring and modification of the patient's self-care efforts during the healing phase is one of the most important responsibilities of the dental team and can help assure success of the surgical procedure.

9. Step 9. Reappointment: The patient is reappointed for the second postsurgical visit. This second visit should occur 2 to 3 weeks following the surgery.

B. **Follow-up Visits**
  1. Following the initial postsurgical visit, additional postsurgical visits may be scheduled based upon the extent of healing of the surgical wound.
  2. Professional tooth polishing should be performed every 2 weeks until the patient can safely resume routine self-care.
  3. When healing is deemed complete by the dental team, the patient is always placed on a program of periodontal maintenance. Enrolling the patient in a periodontal maintenance program is critical in preserving and sustaining the long-term benefits of periodontal surgery.
  4. Attachment of the flap back to the alveolar bone is usually complete within 3 weeks following the surgery, and for many surgical procedures it is safe to proceed with restorative care in the surgical site after at least 6 weeks of healing. Note that some periodontal surgical procedures (such as bone replacement graft and periodontal regeneration) will require much longer periods of healing prior to restoration placement.
  5. Remodeling of the soft tissue can continue, however, for up to 6 months, so the dentist may wait quite a while prior to final restoration placements in esthetic zones such as on anterior teeth.

Chapter Summary Statement

Periodontal surgery is a critical element in the care of most patients with moderate to severe periodontitis and a critical element in the care of many patients in need of restorative dental procedures. The periodontal flap is a fundamental part of most periodontal surgical procedures, and a basic understanding of the principles of periodontal flap surgery is important to the dental hygienist. The healing of periodontal surgical wounds is a complex process, and the terminology that has been used to describe the various types of healing that can occur in the periodontium can be confusing. A variety of specific types of periodontal surgery are being used; these techniques include procedures such as flap for access, osseous resective surgery, bone replacement grafting, periodontal regeneration, and periodontal plastic surgery among others; the dental hygienist should be familiar with the common types of periodontal surgery employed. Current research into enhancing the outcomes of periodontal surgery by using chemical and biologic mediators is ongoing. Postsurgical care following periodontal surgery is vital to maintaining the successful results of surgical outcomes, and dental hygienists play a key role in the management of patients following periodontal surgery.

Section 6
Focus on Patients

CASE 1

You are assigned the task of providing nonsurgical therapy for a periodontitis patient. During routine nonsurgical periodontal therapy, you encounter multiple sites where the probing depths exceed 6 mm. During periodontal instrumentation, you are unable to instrument the root surfaces thoroughly in the areas of the deepest pockets. What should you tell the patient related to this clinical observation?

CASE 2

During nonsurgical periodontal therapy, a patient with periodontitis informs you that the dentist had previously discussed the possibility of periodontal surgery. The patient expresses deep concern and fear over the thought of agreeing to any periodontal surgery. The patient tells you about an aunt who had periodontal surgery many years ago and had many problems following the surgery. How should you proceed?

CASE 3

At the time of the first-week postsurgical visit, you note that a patient who had undergone flap for access surgery has a temperature of 101.5°F and a pulse rate of 70 beats per minute. Clinical examination of the surgical site reveals that the sutures are in place, but there appears to be a good deal of swelling in one part of flap. How should you proceed?

CASE 4

You are assigned the task of managing the first-week postsurgical visit for a patient who had an apically positioned flap with osseous resective surgery. Following removal of the periodontal dressing and removal of the sutures, you note that there are several areas where the healing is progressing by secondary intention because the flap could not be adapted to the teeth perfectly at the time of surgery. Though healing is progressing satisfactorily, it is apparent that not all of the connective tissue wound around the teeth is completely covered by epithelium yet. How should you proceed?

References

1. Caton J, Nyman S. Histometric evaluation of periodontal surgery. I. The modified Widman flap procedure. *J Clin Periodontol.* 1980;7(3):212–223.
2. Nyman S, Lindhe J, Karring T, Rylander H. New attachment following surgical treatment of human periodontal disease. *J Clin Periodontol.* 1982;9(4):290–296.
3. Polson AM, Ladenheim S, Hanes PJ. Cell and fiber attachment to demineralized dentin from periodontitis-affected root surfaces. *J Periodontol.* 1986;57(4):235–246.
4. Gantes BG, Garrett S. Coronally displaced flaps in reconstructive periodontal therapy. *Dent Clin North Am.* 1991;35(3):495–504.
5. Graziani F, Gennai S, Cei S, et al. Clinical performance of access flap surgery in the treatment of the intrabony defect. A systematic review and meta-analysis of randomized clinical trials. *J Clin Periodontol.* 2012;39(2):145–156.
6. Ramfjord SP, Nissle RR. The modified Widman flap. *J Periodontol.* 1974;45(8):601–607.
7. Waerhaug J. Healing of the dento-epithelial junction following subgingival plaque control. II: As observed on extracted teeth. *J Periodontol.* 1978;49(3):119–134.
8. Caton J, Nyman S. Histometric evaluation of periodontal surgery. III. The effect of bone resection on the connective tissue attachment level. *J Periodontol.* 1981;52(8):405–409.
9. Ochsenbein C. A primer for osseous surgery. *Int J Periodontics Restorative Dent.* 1986;6(1):8–47.
10. Reynolds MA, Aichelmann-Reidy ME, Branch-Mays GL, Gunsolley JC. The efficacy of bone replacement grafts in the treatment of periodontal osseous defects. A systematic review. *Ann Periodontol.* 2003;8(1):227–265.
11. Bowen JA, Mellonig JT, Gray JL, Towle HT. Comparison of decalcified freeze-dried bone allograft and porous particulate hydroxyapatite in human periodontal osseous defects. *J Periodontol.* 1989;60(12):647–654.
12. Guillemin MR, Mellonig JT, Brunsvold MA. Healing in periodontal defects treated by decalcified freeze-dried bone allografts in combination with ePTFE membranes (I). Clinical and scanning electron microscope analysis. *J Clin Periodontol.* 1993;20(7):528–536.
13. Guillemin MR, Mellonig JT, Brunsvold MA, Steffensen B. Healing in periodontal defects treated by decalcified freeze-dried bone allografts in combination with ePTFE membranes. Assessment by computerized densitometric analysis. *J Clin Periodontol.* 1993;20(7):520–527.
14. Mellonig JT. Freeze-dried bone allografts in periodontal reconstructive surgery. *Dent Clin North Am.* 1991;35(3):505–520.
15. Oreamuno S, Lekovic V, Kenney EB, Carranza FA, Jr., Takei HH, Prokic B. Comparative clinical study of porous hydroxyapatite and decalcified freeze-dried bone in human periodontal defects. *J Periodontol.* 1990;61(7):399–404.
16. Rummelhart JM, Mellonig JT, Gray JL, Towle HJ. A comparison of freeze-dried bone allograft and demineralized freeze-dried bone allograft in human periodontal osseous defects. *J Periodontol.* 1989;60(12):655–663.
17. Sanders JJ, Sepe WW, Bowers GM, et al. Clinical evaluation of freeze-dried bone allografts in periodontal osseous defects. Part III. Composite freeze-dried bone allografts with and without autogenous bone grafts. *J Periodontol.* 1983;54(1):1–8.
18. Mellonig JT. Human histologic evaluation of a bovine-derived bone xenograft in the treatment of periodontal osseous defects. *Int J Periodontics Restorative Dent.* 2000;20(1):19–29.
19. Bier SJ, Sinensky MC. The versatility of calcium sulfate: resolving periodontal challenges. *Compend Contin Educ Dent.* 1999;20(7):655–661; quiz 662.
20. Froum SJ, Weinberg MA, Tarnow D. Comparison of bioactive glass synthetic bone graft particles and open debridement in the treatment of human periodontal defects. A clinical study. *J Periodontol.* 1998;69(6):698–709.
21. Lovelace TB, Mellonig JT, Meffert RM, Jones AA, Nummikoski PV, Cochran DL. Clinical evaluation of bioactive glass in the treatment of periodontal osseous defects in humans. *J Periodontol.* 1998;69(9):1027–1035.
22. Low SB, King CJ, Krieger J. An evaluation of bioactive ceramic in the treatment of periodontal osseous defects. *Int J Periodontics Restorative Dent.* 1997;17(4):358–367.
23. Gottlow J, Nyman S, Karring T, Lindhe J. New attachment formation as the result of controlled tissue regeneration. *J Clin Periodontol.* 1984;11(8):494–503.
24. Gottlow J, Nyman S, Lindhe J, Karring T, Wennstrom J. New attachment formation in the human periodontium by guided tissue regeneration. Case reports. *J Clin Periodontol.* 1986;13(6):604–616.
25. Consensus report. Mucogingival therapy. *Ann Periodontol.* 1996;1(1):702–706.
26. Cairo F, Nieri M, Pagliaro U. Efficacy of periodontal plastic surgery procedures in the treatment of localized facial gingival recessions. A systematic review. *J Clin Periodontol.* 2014;41 Suppl 15:S44–S62.
27. Camargo PM, Melnick PR, Kenney EB. The use of free gingival grafts for aesthetic purposes. *Periodontol 2000.* 2001;27:72–96.
28. Harris RJ. Root coverage with connective tissue grafts: an evaluation of short- and long-term results. *J Periodontol.* 2002;73(9):1054–1059.
29. Langer B, Langer L. Subepithelial connective tissue graft technique for root coverage. *J Periodontol.* 1985;56(12):715–720.
30. Miller PD, Jr., Allen EP. The development of periodontal plastic surgery. *Periodontol 2000.* 1996;11:7–17.
31. Bernimoulin JP, Luscher B, Muhlemann HR. Coronally repositioned periodontal flap. Clinical evaluation after one year. *J Clin Periodontol.* 1975;2(1):1–13.
32. Tarnow DP. Semilunar coronally repositioned flap. *J Clin Periodontol.* 1986;13(3):182–185.
33. American Academy of Periodontology statement on the efficacy of lasers in the non-surgical treatment of inflammatory periodontal disease. *J Periodontol.* 2011;82(4):513–514. doi: 10.1902/jop.2011.114001.
34. Abduljabbar T, Javed F, Shah A, Samer MS, Vohra F, Akram Z. Role of lasers as an adjunct to scaling and root planing in patients with type 2 diabetes mellitus: a systematic review. *Lasers Med Sci.* 2017;32(2):449–459.
35. Cochran DL, Wozney JM. Biological mediators for periodontal regeneration. *Periodontol 2000.* 1999;19:40–58.
36. Darby IB, Morris KH. A systematic review of the use of growth factors in human periodontal regeneration. *J Periodontol.* 2013;84(4):465–476.
37. Esposito M, Grusovin MG, Papanikolaou N, Coulthard P, Worthington HV. Enamel matrix derivative (Emdogain) for periodontal tissue regeneration in intrabony defects. A Cochrane systematic review. *Eur J Oral Implantol.* 2009;2(4):247–266.
38. Hammarstrom L. Enamel matrix, cementum development and regeneration. *J Clin Periodontol.* 1997;24(9 Pt 2):658–668.

39. Heijl L, Heden G, Svardstrom G, Ostgren A. Enamel matrix derivative (EMDOGAIN) in the treatment of intrabony periodontal defects. *J Clin Periodontol*. 1997;24(9 Pt 2):705–714.

40. Koop R, Merheb J, Quirynen M. Periodontal regeneration with enamel matrix derivative in reconstructive periodontal therapy: a systematic review. *J Periodontol*. 2012;83(6):707–720.

41. Okuda K, Momose M, Miyazaki A, et al. Enamel matrix derivative in the treatment of human intrabony osseous defects. *J Periodontol*. 2000;71(12):1821–1828.

42. Lynch SE, Williams RC, Polson AM, et al. A combination of platelet-derived and insulin-like growth factors enhances periodontal regeneration. *J Clin Periodontol*. 1989;16(8):545–548.

43. Marx RE, Carlson ER, Eichstaedt RM, Schimmele SR, Strauss JE, Georgeff KR. Platelet-rich plasma: Growth factor enhancement for bone grafts. *Oral Surg Oral Med Oral Pathol Oral Radiol Endod*. 1998;85(6):638–646.

STUDENT ANCILLARY RESOURCES

A wide variety of resources to enhance your learning is available online:

- Audio Glossary
- Book Pages
- Chapter Review Questions and Answers

30 Acute Periodontal Conditions

Clinical Application.
Several periodontal conditions can bring a patient to a dental office on an emergency basis for relief of pain or discomfort. As one of the first members of the dental team to possibly confront acute periodontal conditions, dental hygienists may be called upon to promptly address the patient's immediate chief complaint. Thus, dental hygienists must have a clear understanding of how to recognize, manage, and treat acute periodontal conditions. This chapter outlines some of the more common acute periodontal conditions and offers suggestions for management of the patients with these conditions.

Learning Objectives

- Name and describe the three types of abscesses of the periodontium.
- List the possible causes of abscesses of the periodontium.
- Compare and contrast the abscess of the periodontium and the pulpal abscess.
- Outline the typical treatment steps for a gingival abscess and a periodontal abscess.
- Describe the clinical situation that can result in a pericoronal abscess.
- Outline the typical treatment for a pericoronal abscess (pericoronitis).
- Describe the characteristics of necrotizing gingivitis.
- Outline the typical treatment steps for necrotizing gingivitis.
- Describe the symptoms of primary herpetic gingivostomatitis.

Key Terms

Acute periodontal conditions
Abscess of the periodontium
Pus
Suppuration
Circumscribed
Pulpal abscess
Acute abscess

Chronic abscess
Gingival abscess
Periodontal abscess
Pericoronal abscess
Pericoronitis
Operculum
Trismus

Necrotizing periodontal disease
Necrosis
Punched-out papillae
Pseudomembrane
Sequestrum
Primary herpetic
    gingivostomatitis

Section 1
Introduction to Acute Periodontal Conditions

1. Most periodontal diseases are chronic in nature and progress rather slowly; they can take years or decades to destroy the periodontium and lead to tooth loss. These diseases are rarely painful. On the other hand, there are other types of periodontal diseases that can bring patients to a dental office or hospital emergency room for relief of pain or other more dramatic symptoms. The emergency conditions described in this chapter are considered examples of acute periodontal conditions.

   A. The term "acute periodontal conditions" refers to conditions that are commonly characterized as having a sudden onset and a rapid course of progression. These acute conditions are frequently accompanied by pain and discomfort, and they may be unrelated to the presence of any preexisting gingivitis or periodontitis (Box 30-1).

   B. It is imperative that all members of the dental team, especially the dental hygienist, be alert for these conditions because their prompt recognition and early intervention can limit subsequent permanent damage to the periodontium.[1] On the other hand, if an acute periodontal condition is not promptly diagnosed and treated, then the prognosis of the affected tooth may be jeopardized, or the bacteria within the acute lesion may spread systemically and result in infections in other distant sites in the body.

2. This chapter outlines some of the more common periodontal emergency conditions and briefly describes treatment options that may be recommended and performed by the dentist, dental hygienist, or by other health care providers.

Box 30-1. Characteristics of Acute Periodontal Conditions

- Sudden onset of the condition
- Rapid course of progression
- Accompanied by pain and discomfort
- May be unrelated to preexisting gingivitis or periodontitis
- Intraorally, the acute periodontal lesion may affect a localized site or it may be more widespread in the mouth
- May have systemic manifestations

Section 2
Abscesses of the Periodontium

1. Overview of Abscesses of the Periodontium
   A. Abscesses of the Periodontium Defined
      1. An abscess of the periodontium may be defined as an acute infection involving a circumscribed collection of pus localized within the gingival wall of the periodontal pocket.
      2. Pus (also known as purulence) is a whitish-yellowish exudate that consists primarily of dead and dying neutrophils, bacteria, cellular debris, and fluid leaked from blood vessels; pus can result when the body's defense mechanisms are involved in attempting to control an infection. The process of forming pus is called suppuration.
      3. Abscesses of the periodontium are usually described as being circumscribed. The term circumscribed means that the abscess is localized or confined to a specific site (i.e., the facial surface of a single tooth or perhaps the gingival margin on a specific tooth). Figure 30-1 illustrates a typical example of an abscess of the periodontium.
      4. The precise bacterial etiology of the abscess of the periodontium is not clear, but it is known that most of these lesions contain microflora that are predominantly Gram negative and anaerobic. Most studies indicate that the bacteria seen in these abscesses are similar to bacteria seen in periodontitis patients with deeper pockets.

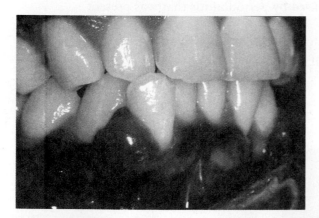

Figure 30-1. Abscess of the Periodontium. Note the localized swelling between the mandibular right canine and lateral incisor. Palpation of the swelling would reveal what feels like a fluid-filled sack. This fluid-filled sack is full of pus.

Box 30-2. Characteristics of an Abscess of the Periodontium

- An acute abscess is characterized by constant and localized pain.
- Typically, a chronic abscess is characterized by no pain. However, it should be noted that in rare cases the chronic abscess may be characterized by dull pain.
- Circumscribed (localized) swelling in the periodontium
- Possible increase in tooth mobility
- Radiographic loss of alveolar bone not involving the tooth apex
- Tooth usually has a vital pulp.

B. Characteristics of an Abscess of the Periodontium

1. Typical patient complaints related to an abscess of the periodontium include dental pain and swelling in the gingiva at a specific location (Box 30-2).
   a. Pain resulting from an abscess of the periodontium is usually described by the patient as a constant pain (as opposed to intermittent). Patients frequently report that the pain is easy for them to localize (i.e., the patient can point to the exact spot that hurts). Note that in some other conditions, a patient can report pain that is not at all localized to a specific location.
   b. In addition to pain and swelling, the patient may report difficulty in mastication and may report a bad taste in the mouth.
2. Oral examination will usually reveal the presence of a circumscribed swelling of the soft tissue. This swelling may involve the gingiva only, or it may involve both the gingiva and the mucosa.
3. In many cases, teeth with an abscess of the periodontium can exhibit a temporary increase in mobility.
4. Dental radiographs of a tooth with an abscess of the periodontium frequently reveal alveolar bone loss in the area of the abscess, but the bone loss does not usually involve the tooth apex (unlike a pulpal abscess). Figure 30-2 shows a radiograph of a tooth with an abscess of the periodontium.
   a. Alveolar bone loss resulting from an abscess of the periodontium can occur extremely rapidly when compared with the rate of alveolar bone loss usually associated with periodontitis.
   b. Although a dental radiograph of an abscess of the periodontium may reveal alveolar bone loss, in a periodontitis patient it is not always possible to tell what part of the missing bone actually resulted from the acute infection and what part of the missing bone was caused by periodontitis that was present before the abscess formed.
5. Teeth affected by an abscess of the periodontium are usually vital (have healthy pulp tissue) and respond positively if pulp testing is performed.

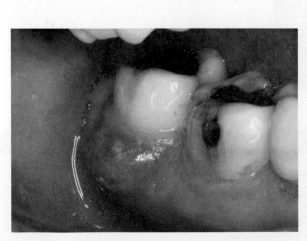
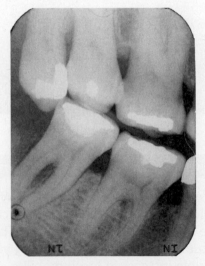

Figure 30-2. Abscess of the Periodontium Involving the Mandibular Second Molar. The clinical photograph shows circumscribed swelling and inflammation of the gingival tissue on the buccal aspect of a mandibular second molar with an abscess of the periodontium. The radiograph of the site reveals loss of bone density between the roots of the molar tooth (the furcation region) affected by the abscess. (Courtesy of Dr. Richard Foster, Guilford Technical Community College, Jamestown, NC.)

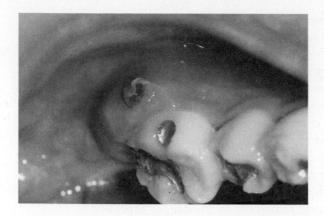

Figure 30-3. Path of Drainage. The abscess of the periodontium shown in this figure has broken through the surface tissues, establishing a path of drainage for the pus on its own. Note the milky, yellowish-whitish fluid exiting from the sinus tract. This is the suppuration being discharged from the abscess.

6. Another possible clinical sign of an abscess of the periodontium can be an elevated body temperature (fever). An elevated body temperature would not normally be present unless the infection (from the abscess of the periodontium) is spreading throughout the body. This would represent a serious sign, if present. Since many abscesses of the periodontium are circumscribed (localized), they frequently are not associated with an elevated body temperature.

7. When there is delay in treating an abscess of the periodontium, there can be additional oral changes.[2] The collection of pus can break through the surface tissues by draining through a sinus tract. This establishes a path of drainage for the pus on its own. Figure 30-3 illustrates an abscess of the periodontium that has drained spontaneously by breaking through the surface tissues.

C. **Causes of Abscesses of the Periodontium.** Several causes of abscesses of the periodontium have been reported.[3] Theories about the origin of the abscess of the periodontium vary, but most investigators attribute formation of this type of abscess to one of the following scenarios.

1. **Blockage of the Orifice of a Pocket.** Blockage of the orifice (or opening) of a preexisting periodontal pocket has been suggested as a cause of some abscesses of the periodontium. Most periodontal pockets have readily accessible openings that give easy access to a periodontal probe. Some authors have theorized that in certain instances, the opening of a periodontal pocket can become restricted in size or may become completely occluded because of temporary improvement of the surface tissue tone. This improvement of tissue firmness could result in trapping bacteria and fluids in a preexisting periodontal pocket, leading to an abscess that begins within this existing periodontal pocket.

2. **Accidentally Forcing a Foreign Object into the Tissues.** It has also been suggested that an abscess of periodontium can be caused by accidentally forcing and lodging a foreign object into the supporting tissues of a tooth.
   a. A variety of foreign objects have been implicated in the formation of some abscesses of the periodontium. For example, an abscess could result when a patient accidentally punctures the gingiva with a toothpick, forcing bacteria into the tissue.
   b. Another common event that can result in an abscess of the periodontium is accidentally forcing some food product like a husk from a kernel of popcorn or a peanut skin into the tissues associated with the tissue inflammation as part of a periodontal pocket. As a result, the foreign object would act as a physical barrier which blocks the orifice of the pocket.

3. **Incomplete Calculus Removal in a Periodontal Pocket.** Incomplete calculus removal in a periodontal pocket has also been suggested as a cause of an abscess of the periodontium.

   a. When this occurs, it is usually thought to be in a site with a very deep probing depth where the calculus deposits are removed only in the most coronal aspects of the pocket near the gingival margin, but the calculus deposits deeper in the pocket are not completely removed because of difficulty of access for instrumentation of the tooth surface.

   b. It is theorized that removal of the more coronal calculus deposits allows the gingival margin to heal somewhat and to tighten around the tooth, like a drawstring of a pouch, preventing drainage of bacterial toxins and other waste products from the pocket. Bacteria remaining in the deeper aspects of the periodontal pocket could result in the formation of an abscess of the periodontium.

2. **Comparison Between the Periodontal Abscesses and the Pulpal Abscesses.** The clinical recognition and diagnosis of a periodontal abscess can be complicated in some instances because of the possible overlap of signs of a periodontal abscess with the signs of a pulpal abscess.

   A. Abscesses affecting the tissues around a tooth can result from two different sources: (1) the periodontium itself which surrounds the tooth or (2) the pulpal tissues that are within the pulp chamber of the tooth.

      1. It is helpful for the dental hygienist to be familiar with the characteristics of these two types of abscesses, since the periodontal abscess and the pulpal abscess sometime appear to have somewhat similar clinical characteristics.

      2. The characteristics of each of these types of abscesses are outlined in Table 30-1.

   B. As already discussed, a periodontal abscess is an abscess that results from an acute infection of the periodontium.

   C. On the other hand, a **pulpal abscess** is an abscess that results from an infection of the tooth pulp that can sometimes extend into the periodontium.

      1. A pulpal abscess can be caused by death of the tooth pulp from trauma to the tooth or from deep dental decay; a dead tooth pulp is frequently referred to as a nonvital pulp.

      2. Management of a patient with a pulpal abscess usually requires root canal treatment and will not be discussed in this chapter.

TABLE 30-1	DIFFERENTIATION OF THE TYPES OF ABSCESS	
Characteristic	**Periodontal Abscess**	**Pulpal Abscess**
Vitality test results:	Usually vital pulp	Usually nonvital pulp
Radiographic appearance:	Bone loss present as an angular defect and/or furcation radiolucency	Bone loss at tooth root apex
Symptoms:	Localized, constant pain	Difficult to localize, intermittent pain

3. **Classification Abscesses of the Periodontium**
   A. **Classification by Course of the Lesion.** One way to classify abscesses of the periodontium is according to the course—progression—of the lesion.
      1. An **acute abscess** has a rapid onset and is characterized by pain and discomfort. It is primarily caused by an exacerbation of a chronic inflammatory periodontal lesion.
         a. Contributing factors to the etiology of an acute abscess may be the lack of spontaneous drainage or inadequate host response.
         b. Unlike a chronic abscess (which will be discussed below), an acute abscess is symptomatic because as it grows, the pressure rapidly builds up within the lesion and has nowhere to escape. As the pressure builds up, the patient will experience mild-to-severe pain that is a distinguishing clinical characteristic of an acute abscess.
      2. A **chronic abscess** grows slowly and is not typically associated with pain. It forms after the spread of infection has been controlled by spontaneous drainage, host response, or therapy.
         a. In most cases, the pus from a chronic abscess is able to drain through an abnormal "channel" (known as a **sinus tract**) in the periodontium and discharge out of the gingiva. Drainage of pus through a sinus tract will relieve the pain and discomfort associated with the pressure.
         b. As a result (of this drainage), some patients may not be aware that they have a chronic abscess. In a limited number of cases, however, members of the dental team should keep in mind that the chronic abscess can also be associated with dull pain.
   B. **Classification Based on Location.** A second way to classify abscesses of the periodontium is based on the location of the abscess: (1) the gingival abscess, (2) the periodontal abscess, and (3) the pericoronal abscess, but there is considerable overlap in this very loose classification system.
      1. **Gingival Abscess.** The **gingival abscess** refers to an abscess of the periodontium that is primarily limited to the gingival margin or to the interdental papilla without involvement of the deeper structures of the periodontium.
         a. The gingival abscess can occur in a previously periodontally healthy mouth when some foreign object is forced into a healthy gingival sulcus. An abscess of the periodontium that is limited to the gingival margin area can follow this traumatic event.
         b. Figure 30-4 illustrates a typical gingival abscess where the swelling is limited to the marginal gingiva of a single tooth.

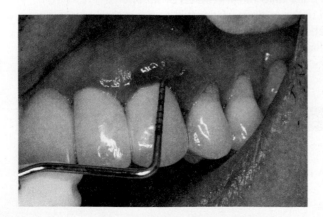

Figure 30-4. Gingival Abscess. Note that this abscess is limited to the gingival margin on the facial surface of this maxillary canine. (Courtesy of Dr. Richard Foster, Guilford Technical Community College, Jamestown, NC.)

2. **Periodontal Abscess.** The true periodontal abscess refers to an abscess of the periodontium that affects the deeper structures of the periodontium as well as the gingival tissues. The abscess in Figure 30-2 is classified as a periodontal abscess. A periodontal abscess usually occurs in a site with preexisting periodontal disease including preexisting periodontal pockets and usually affects the deeper structures of the periodontium and is not limited to the gingiva only.

3. **Pericoronal Abscess.** The pericoronal abscess refers to an abscess of the periodontium that involves tissues around the crown of a partially erupted tooth. The soft tissue inflammation associated with the pericoronal abscess is referred to as pericoronitis.

   a. This type of abscess is seen in teeth where some of the soft tissues surrounding the teeth actually cover part of the occlusal surface of the teeth. Figure 30-5 illustrates a patient with a pericoronal abscess under a soft tissue flap partially covering a third molar tooth.

   b. The pericoronal abscess (or pericoronitis) is most frequently seen around mandibular third molar teeth. Since many third molar teeth do not have space to erupt fully, these teeth can have a flap of tissue covering part of the occlusal surface.

   c. The flap of gingival tissue that covers a portion of the crown of a partially erupted tooth can become infected, and it is this type of infection under this flap of tissue that is referred to as a pericoronal abscess. The flap of soft tissue is called an operculum, and some authors also refer to the pericoronal abscess as an operculitis.

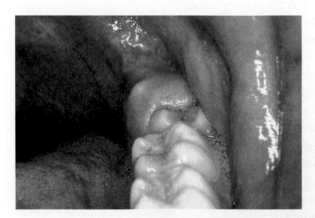 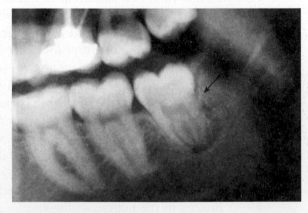

Figure 30-5. Pericoronal Abscess Involving a Mandibular Third Molar. The clinical photograph shows a typical clinical appearance of a partially exposed mandibular third molar covered by an operculum. The radiograph of the site illustrates the position of the third molar in close relationship to the mandibular ramus. Note that the infection associated with the pericoronal abscess has progressed apically to affect the distal support of the third molar (*red arrow*). (Courtesy of Dr. Richard Foster, Guilford Technical Community College, Jamestown, NC.)

Box 30-3. Signs and Symptoms of a Pericoronal Abscess

- Pain at the site
- Swelling of operculum
- Possible trismus (limited mouth opening)
- Possible elevated body temperature
- Possible lymphadenopathy

    d. The operculum can be thought of as a "lid" of soft tissue that entraps plaque biofilm and food debris. Because of the difficulty of keeping the area clean, the operculum leads to soft tissue inflammation which is a characteristic of pericoronitis.

    e. Streptococci milleri group bacteria, well-known for their ability to cause suppurative infections, are most likely involved in the pathogenesis of acute severe pericoronitis of the lower third molar.[4]

    f. The signs and symptoms of the pericoronal abscess are discussed below and outlined in Box 30-3.

    g. Pain is common with the pericoronal abscess. The pain can arise from the tissue swelling itself, but pain can also arise when an opposing tooth occludes with the infected, swollen operculum.

    h. Soft tissue swelling (edema) and redness (erythema) also usually accompany the pericoronal abscess.

    i. As damage to tissue covering the partially erupted tooth progresses and the tissue swelling increases, the opposing tooth can frequently be seen to impinge (press) on the swollen tissue, creating additional tissue trauma and additional patient discomfort.

    j. Limited mouth opening is also seen in some cases of advanced pericoronal abscess; limited mouth opening is referred to as trismus.

    k. Elevated body temperature (fever) and swollen lymph nodes (lymphadenopathy) also can be seen in advanced cases of pericoronitis.

4. Management of Patients With Abscesses of the Periodontium

  A. Treatment of a Gingival or Periodontal Abscess. The treatment of a patient with either a gingival or a periodontal abscess is similar.

    1. Fundamental treatment steps include (1) establishment of a path of drainage for the pus, (2) thorough periodontal instrumentation of the affected tooth surfaces in the area of the abscess, and (3) relief of pain.

    2. Steps commonly followed in treatment of patients with a gingival or a periodontal abscess are discussed below and are outlined in Box 30-4.

      a. It is normally necessary to anesthetize the site to be treated, since manipulation of the tissues involved by an abscess can be quite uncomfortable.

      b. Drainage of the pus from the abscess is critical. The abscess can be drained either through the pocket itself or by performing periodontal surgery (as discussed in Chapter 9). When drainage is established through the pocket, the toe of a *sterile* curette is used to puncture the soft tissue wall of the pocket to allow the drainage. In some cases, drainage can be accomplished by externally incising through the fluctuant surface of the abscess with a surgical scalpel blade and draining the purulent discharge with light digital pressure. This type of procedure is known as an incise and drain procedure.

      c. Since one of the possible etiologies of a gingival or periodontal abscess is incomplete calculus removal, thorough periodontal instrumentation of the affected tooth surfaces in the site of the abscess is important in bringing these types of abscesses under control.

      d. Some adjustment of the tooth occlusion is usually also indicated since inflammation resulting from the abscess can force a tooth to extrude slightly from its socket, leading to trauma from occlusion and pain when masticating.

      e. In more advanced cases of abscesses, antibiotics may also be needed, as with any other serious oral infection.

Box 30-4. Steps in Treatment of a Gingival or Periodontal Abscess

- Administer local anesthesia
- Drain pus
- Thorough periodontal instrumentation
- Adjust occlusion, if needed
- Prescribe antibiotics, if needed
- Recommend warm saline rinses
- Prescribe pain medications, if needed
- Follow-up appointments

---

    f. Some clinicians recommend using warm saline (saltwater) rinses several times each day to help keep the abscess draining until it has healed completely.

    g. A prescription for pain medication should always be considered, but over-the-counter pain medications can be adequate in many patients once the abscess has been drained.

    h. Following emergency treatment of a patient with any abscess of the periodontium, the dental team should appoint the patient for a thorough periodontal assessment, since the abscess of the periodontium frequently occurs in a patient with a preexisting untreated periodontal disease, and routine periodontal therapy may be needed.

B. Treatment of a Pericoronal Abscess. Treatment of patients with pericoronal abscess differs slightly from treatment of patients with other types of abscesses of the periodontium because of the difference in the anatomical location of these abscesses.

    1. Fundamental treatment steps for a patient with pericoronitis include (1) establishment of a path of drainage for the pus, (2) irrigation of the undersurface of the operculum, (3) thorough periodontal instrumentation of the tooth surfaces in the area of the abscess, and (4) relief of pain.[5]

    2. Steps commonly followed in treatment of patients with a pericoronal abscess are discussed below and outlined in Box 30-5.

      a. It is normally necessary to anesthetize the site to be treated, since manipulation of the tissues affected by an abscess can be quite uncomfortable.

      b. Drainage of the pus from the abscess is critical. The abscess can be drained through the pocket itself. Nonsurgical steps to treat a pericoronal abscess are outlined below.

        1) The patient should be adequately anesthetized.

        2) The clinician should use a periodontal probe to gently lift the soft tissue operculum off the occlusal surface of the affected tooth.

        3) The underlying debris can now be removed with hand instruments and gentle irrigation with sterile saline.

        4) The toe of a *sterile* curette can be used to puncture the soft tissue wall of the pocket to allow drainage. Abscesses around the crown of a partially erupted third molar tooth may be difficult to drain because of the anatomy of the region.

        5) If this attempt fails to achieve adequate draining of the abscess, then periodontal surgery is indicated (as discussed in Chapter 29).

c. In more advanced cases of abscesses, antibiotics may be needed, as with any other serious oral infection.

d. Some clinicians recommend using warm saline (saltwater) rinses several times each day to help keep the abscess draining until it has healed completely.

e. A prescription for pain medication should always be considered, but over-the-counter pain medications (NSAIDs) can be adequate in many patients once the abscess is drained.

f. Following emergency treatment of a patient with any abscess of the periodontium, the dental team should appoint the patient for a thorough periodontal assessment, since the abscess of the periodontium frequently occurs in a patient with existing untreated periodontal disease.

g. In some cases, following resolution of the abscess, it is wise to excise the operculum that was involved in the pericoronal abscess. This removal can prevent recurrence of the abscess. In some cases, following resolution of the abscess, the dentist may recommend extraction of malposed third molar teeth if there is inadequate jaw space for the third molar teeth to fully erupt or if the pericoronal abscess continually reoccurs.

Box 30-5. Common Steps in Treatment of Patient With Pericoronal Abscess

- Administer local anesthesia
- Drain pus
- Thorough periodontal instrumentation
- Irrigate under operculum
- Prescribe antibiotics, if needed
- Recommend warm saline rinses
- Prescribe pain medications, if needed
- Evaluate for need for third molar extractions
- Establish follow-up appointments

Section 3
Necrotizing Periodontal Diseases

Necrotizing periodontal diseases (NPD) include necrotizing gingivitis (NG) and necrotizing periodontitis (NP). Studies suggest that necrotizing gingivitis and necrotizing periodontitis may represent different stages of the same disease, because they have similar etiology, clinical characteristics, and treatment.[6,7] Necrotizing periodontal diseases present three typical clinical features: tissue necrosis, bleeding, and pain.[8,9] *They represent the most severe biofilm-related periodontal condition.*

Necrotizing periodontal disease is an inflammatory destructive infection of periodontal tissues that involves tissue necrosis (localized tissue death). Necrotizing gingivitis, necrotizing periodontitis, and necrotizing stomatitis are painful infections with ulceration, swelling and sloughing of dead epithelial tissue from the gingiva, and fetid oral odor. All three of these diseases are acute infections of the periodontium that can bring patients to the dental office for emergency treatment.

1. Necrotizing Gingivitis
   A. Overview of Necrotizing Gingivitis
      1. Necrotizing gingivitis is an acute infection of the periodontium that is limited to gingival tissues.[7,9,10]
         a. Historically, the names for this condition were Vincent infection, trench mouth, ulceromembranous gingivitis, acute necrotizing gingivitis (ANUG), and necrotizing ulcerative gingivitis (NUG). The terminology "ulcerative" was later eliminated because ulceration is secondary to the tissue necrosis that characterizes necrotizing periodontal diseases.[11]
         b. As the name necrotizing gingivitis implies, the clinical hallmark of necrotizing gingivitis is tissue *necrosis* of the gingiva. The term necrosis refers to cell death, in this instance referring to the death of the cells comprising the gingival epithelium.
      2. An impaired host response appears to be associated with the development of necrotizing gingivitis in many patients.[12] This impaired response may be related to any of several factors such as poor nutrition, fatigue, psychosocial factors, systemic disease, alcohol abuse, or drug abuse. It should be noted that necrotizing gingivitis also may be associated with the immunosuppression seen in HIV infection.
      3. It is not known if bacteria are the primary cause of necrotizing gingivitis, but studies indicate that certain bacteria including spirochetal organisms and fusiform bacilli are always associated with the disease. Other organisms have also been reported to be present in necrotizing gingivitis.
      4. Subjects of any age can be affected by necrotizing gingivitis, but the highest prevalence of necrotizing gingivitis is found in patients between 20 and 30 years of age.[13] In developed countries, the reported prevalence of necrotizing gingivitis is lower than that found in developing countries, especially among children.[14,15] The higher prevalence of necrotizing gingivitis found in children in developing countries may be attributed to malnutrition or an underlying systemic condition that may make them more susceptible to acute periodontal conditions.

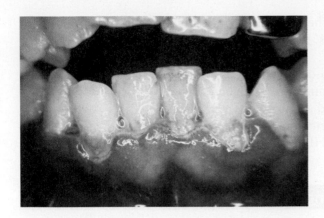

Figure 30-6. Necrotizing Gingivitis. Note that the necrotic areas have extended from the papillae onto the facial surfaces. The necrotic areas of the gingiva are covered with gray-white layer called the pseudomembrane. The necrosis has destroyed the papillae leading to what is called punched-out papillae. In most cases, the punched-out papillae may be visually obscured by the pseudomembrane and gingival inflammation.

5. There are several clinical signs that distinguish necrotizing gingivitis from other forms of gingivitis.
   a. One of those clinical signs is the presence of punched-out papillae (Fig. 30-6). In necrotizing gingivitis, the necrosis associated with this condition can destroy the papillae between the teeth, resulting in the clinical appearance that the papillae are missing or "punched-out." The term "punched-out papillae" is used to describe the gingival craterlike depressions left by the loss of the papillae.
   b. Another clinical sign is the formation of a pseudomembrane covering the surface of the punched-out papillae. The necrotic areas of gingiva are covered by a gray-white slough sometimes referred to as a pseudomembrane.
      1) This pseudomembrane actually consists of dead cells, bacteria, and oral debris; underlying this pseudomembrane is raw connective tissue.
      2) Patients with necrotizing gingivitis may exhibit spontaneous gingival hemorrhage or pronounced bleeding that is elicited by the slightest manipulation of the gingival tissues. This bleeding results from breakage of some of the tiny blood vessels in the connective tissues exposed under the pseudomembrane.
B. **Characteristics of Necrotizing gingivitis.** The characteristics of necrotizing gingivitis are described below and outlined in Box 30-6.
   1. Patients with necrotizing gingivitis experience oral pain and frequently seek emergency care for that oral pain; the gingival ulceration associated with the infection results in exposure of connective tissue, which can be quite uncomfortable for the patients. Because of the exposure of connective tissue, bleeding from the area can appear to be spontaneous.
   2. The tissue necrosis that is characteristic of necrotizing gingivitis can lead to destruction of the interdental papillae, resulting in punched-out papillae; the remaining gingival crater-like defects are normally covered by a collection of dead tissue cells and debris called a pseudomembrane.
   3. Patients with necrotizing gingivitis can display swollen lymph nodes (lymphadenopathy), a vague feeling of discomfort (malaise), and an elevated body temperature. In some cases, the pain may be so disabling that it may limit food and/or liquid intake.

4. Because of the necrosis (death) of cells, there is usually noticeable halitosis or malodor in necrotizing gingivitis patients. Some authors have described this halitosis as a fetid odor.

5. Certain associated behaviors and psychosocial conditions are frequently present in patients who develop necrotizing gingivitis; these include a history of smoking, a history of poor nutrition, and a history of severe stress.

6. It has also been reported that some patients that develop necrotizing gingivitis have a human immunodeficiency virus (HIV)-positive status.

Box 30-6. Characteristics of Necrotizing Gingivitis

- Oral pain
- Necrotic or punched-out gingival papillae
- Spontaneous gingival hemorrhaging or gingival bleeding with even the slightest manipulation of the gingival tissues
- Presence of pseudomembrane layer covering the gingival craters
- Swollen lymph nodes (lymphadenopathy)
- Vague feeling of discomfort (malaise)
- Elevated body temperature
- Extreme halitosis (fetid breath)

C. **Typical Treatment Steps for Necrotizing Gingivitis.** The treatment of patients with necrotizing gingivitis aims to control the disease process, limit its progression, and reduce pain/discomfort for patient. Typical treatment steps are summarized below and outlined in Box 30-7.

1. The first appointment

   a. The pseudomembrane should be removed carefully with irrigation and moist cotton.

   b. Superficial supragingival periodontal instrumentation is performed. Subgingival instrumentation should be avoided because of discomfort elicited by tissue manipulation.

   c. The patient is instructed regarding a gentle self-care regimen. Tooth brushing may need to be restricted to light removal of debris with soft brushes.

   d. The patient is counseled to consume adequate amounts of fluids, get rest, and avoid excessive physical exertion and stress. The patient is also instructed to avoid tobacco and alcohol.

   e. For pain relief, the patient is advised to use nonsteroidal anti-inflammatory agents.

   f. Patients may need to use a regimen of twice daily rinses of chlorhexidine. Some authors have suggested using 3% hydrogen peroxide with equal parts of warm water every 2 to 3 hours. This type of regimen contributes to mechanically cleaning the necrotizing gingivitis lesion and provides an antibacterial effect of oxygen against anaerobic bacteria that may be associated with necrotizing gingivitis.[16]

2. The second visit (first follow-up appointment 2 days after initial visit)

   a. Subgingival periodontal instrumentation usually can be initiated at this appointment.

    b. Further instruction in self-care should be reviewed and reinforced at this visit.

    c. Attention should be paid to control the systemic predisposing factors associated with the onset of necrotizing gingivitis, such as enrolling the patient in a smoking cessation program or treatment of involved systemic conditions.

3. The third visit (second follow-up appointment approximately 5 days after initial visit)

    a. Subgingival instrumentation usually can be completed.

    b. Patient is evaluated for resolution of symptoms. Patient is further counseled on nutrition, smoking cessation, home care, and other factors which may have contributed to the onset of necrotizing gingivitis.

4. In more advanced cases of necrotizing gingivitis that either fail to favorably respond to conventional mechanical therapy or have systemic involvement, systemic antibiotics may be needed. Local antibiotics, on the other hand, are not recommended because the local drug may not achieve adequate subgingival concentration levels to have a significant antibacterial effect.

5. Following the resolution of the infection, the patient should be appointed for a comprehensive clinical assessment to identify any underlying periodontal disease. Figure 30-7A and 30-7B illustrates before and after treatment photographs of a typical patient with early stages of necrotizing gingivitis. Following complete resolution of the infection, some necrotizing gingivitis patients require periodontal surgery to reestablish natural gingival contours.

6. Supportive (Maintenance) Therapy. During the maintenance phase, the clinician should assess the periodontal status, reinforce self-care, control the predisposing factors, and perform the necessary periodontal instrumentation. The clinician should determine compliance with health habits, psychosocial factors, and the interval of subsequent recall visits.

Box 30-7. Typical Treatment Steps for a Patient With Necrotizing Gingivitis

1. At the first appointment.
   - The pseudomembrane should be removed carefully.
   - Supragingival periodontal instrumentation is performed. Instrumentation is limited because of the discomfort elicited by tissue manipulation.
   - The patient is instructed regarding a gentle self-care regimen.
2. At the first follow-up appointment 2 days after initial visit.
   - Subgingival periodontal instrumentation usually can be begun at this appointment.
   - Further instruction in self-care should be included at this visit.
3. At the second follow-up appointment approximately 5 days after initial visit.
   - Subgingival instrumentation usually can be completed.
4. Following the resolution of the infection, the patient should be appointed for a comprehensive clinical assessment to identify any underlying chronic periodontal disease or the possible need for surgical reshaping of the gingiva.
5. Supportive (Maintenance) Therapy—after the disease has resolved, the patient should be enrolled in a supportive (maintenance) program. During each maintenance appointment, the clinician should assess the periodontal status, reinforce oral hygiene, control the predisposing factors, and perform the necessary periodontal instrumentation.

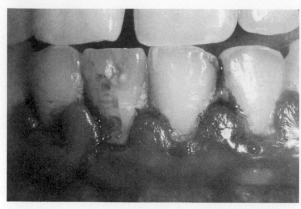

A

Figure 30-7A. Necrotizing Gingivitis: Before Treatment. A clinical photo of a patient with necrotizing gingivitis before treatment. (Courtesy of Dr. Don Rolfs, Wenatchee, WA.)

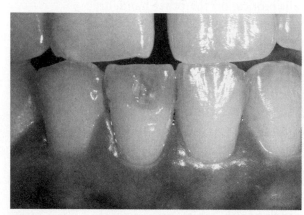

B

Figure 30-7B. Necrotizing Gingivitis: After Treatment. The patient pictured in Figure 30-7A after treatment and resolution of the infection. (Courtesy of Dr. Don Rolfs, Periodontal Foundations, Wenatchee, WA.)

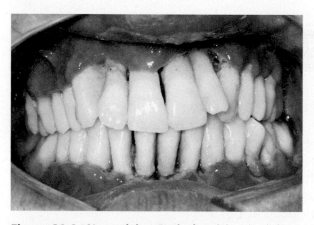
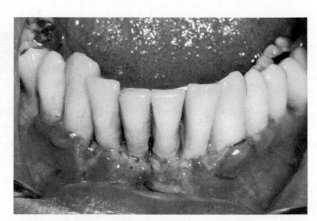

Figure 30-8. Necrotizing Periodontitis. The left-hand photo shows a patient with NP. The right-hand photo is a close-up of the mandibular arch showing bone sequestration. (Courtesy of Dr. Don Rolfs, Periodontal Foundations, Wenatchee, WA.)

2. **Necrotizing Periodontitis**
   A. **Overview of Necrotizing Periodontitis (NP)**
      1. Necrotizing periodontitis (NP) is tissue necrosis of the gingival tissues combined with loss of attachment and alveolar bone loss. The most distinguishing feature of NP is its destructive disease progression which manifests as periodontal attachment loss and bone loss.[9] Necrotizing periodontitis may be an extension of necrotizing gingivitis. As such, NP may occur in patients who previously had necrotizing gingivitis that was left untreated.
      2. One unusual finding in NP is that it can be accompanied by the formation of bone sequestra. A sequestrum is a fragment of necrotic (dead) bone. Sequestration is the process of forming a sequestrum. Figure 30-8 illustrates a patient with NP.
   B. **Typical Treatment of Necrotizing Periodontitis.** Treatment of patients with NP is complex and may require medical consultation since the patients that develop this condition may have serious underlying immunocompromising disorders (i.e., HIV) that must be managed simultaneously with dental therapy.[11] Additionally, when patients with NP are encountered in a general dental office, immediate referral to a periodontist is indicated.
3. **Necrotizing Stomatitis.** Necrotizing stomatitis is an extension of either necrotizing gingivitis or NP where the necrosis progresses to deeper tissues beyond the mucogingival line, such as the lip or cheek mucosa.
   A. **Overview of Necrotizing Stomatitis**
      1. Clinical symptoms are similar to necrotizing gingivitis and NP. But the most distinguishing feature of necrotizing stomatitis is the bone denudation extending to the alveolar mucosa. This may result in an oral-antral fistula and osteitis (inflammation of the bone).
      2. Although it is a rare condition to encounter, necrotizing stomatitis is the most extensive and invasive form of necrotizing periodontal disease. Necrotizing stomatitis is associated with patients who have severe immunocompromised conditions, such as AIDS.
   B. **Typical Treatment of Necrotizing Stomatitis.** Since the disease is the most extensive and most invasive form of the necrotizing periodontal disease family, an immediate consultation and referral to an oral pathologist, oral maxillofacial surgeon, and physician is indicated.

Section 4
Primary Herpetic Gingivostomatitis

1. **Overview of Primary Herpetic Gingivostomatitis**
   A. **Etiology of Primary Herpetic Gingivostomatitis.** Primary herpetic gingivostomatitis is actually a medical condition resulting from a viral infection (herpes simplex). It is listed here as a periodontal emergency condition since patients with this condition may first seek care in a dental office because of the nature of the oral symptoms.
   B. **Characteristics of Primary Herpetic Gingivostomatitis**
      1. **Primary herpetic gingivostomatitis** is a painful oral condition that can result from the initial infection with the herpes simplex virus (HSV).[17-19]
         a. There are two types of herpes simplex virus, oral herpes virus (HSV-1) and genital herpes virus (HSV-2). Primary herpetic gingivostomatitis is usually caused by initial infection with HSV-1, but, in rare cases, may be caused by initial infection with HSV-2.
         b. In the majority of patients, the initial infection with these viruses produces no noticeable clinical signs and can go undetected clinically. In other patients, however, the oral symptoms resulting from this initial infection can be quite severe, and it is these severe oral symptoms that are known as primary herpetic gingivostomatitis (Fig. 30-9).
         c. Primary herpetic gingivostomatitis usually occurs in infants or children who are less than 6 years old. However, individuals may acquire the disease later on when they kiss an infected person during adolescence or adulthood.

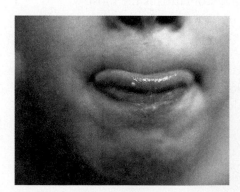 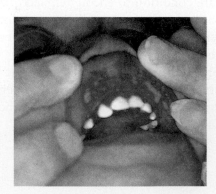 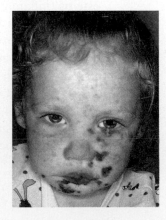

Figure 30-9. Primary Oral Infection With Herpes Simplex Virus. These three children demonstrate the spectrum of primary oral infection with the herpes simplex virus, which ranges from nearly asymptomatic to severe. The patient in the left-hand photo has a single vesicle on his tongue. The patient in the center photo manifests widespread labial and gingival lesions. The parent's fingers are shown in the photograph; however, touching the infected area with bare fingers is *not* recommended. The dental hygienist should inform parents that physical contact with the open sores or saliva infected with HSV1 virus without personal protective equipment (i.e., gloves) can spread the virus. The patient in the right-hand photo shows a severe infection with lesions on the face. (From Fleisher GR, Ludwig W, Baskin MN. *Atlas of Pediatric Emergency Medicine*. Philadelphia, PA: Lippincott Williams & Wilkins; 2004.)

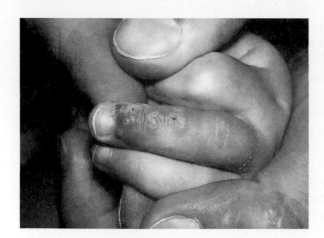

Figure 30-10. Primary Herpes Simplex Virus Infection in Infancy. Finger sucking likely caused the spread of the infection from the mouth to the hand of this infant (herpetic whitlow). The parent's fingers are shown in the photograph, however touching the infected area with bare fingers is not recommended since the parent is at risk of contracting the disease. (From Goodheart HP. *Goodheart's Photoguide of Common Skin Disorders*. 2nd ed. Philadelphia, PA: Lippincott Williams & Wilkins; 2003.)

2. *Primary herpetic gingivostomatitis is contagious and requires careful attention to prevent its spread.*
   a. HSV lesions proceed through several stages before healing. The usual stages are prodrome, macule, papule, vesicle, ulcer, scab, healed area with redness, and complete healing.
      1) Of all the stages of HSV, the two most important stages, from a dental management standpoint, are the vesicle and ulcer stages. The vesicle stage is characterized by fluid-filled blisters that is filled with actively reproducing HSV viral particles. When the vesicle ruptures (the ulcer stage), the HSV-filled fluid can potentially spread to other areas of the patient's mouth or other individuals, such as a dental practitioner.
      2) It is primarily for this reason that the American Academy of Oral Medicine recommends "delaying care until an HSV lesion is scabbed over or completely healed is prudent for minimizing recurrences and spread of the infection, and that the presence of an infectious HSV lesion orally or periorally can be a reason for deferral of care."[20]
   b. HSV-1 is primarily spread by direct contact through kissing, contact with open sores, or by contact with infected body fluids, such as saliva.
   c. HSV-1 can also spread from one part of the body to another, such as from saliva to the fingers, then to the eye. Touching the eye can result in a painful and dangerous herpetic infection of the cornea (herpes keratitis). Herpetic whitlow is a painful herpetic infection of the hands and fingers which is initiated by exposure to HSV-1-infected body fluids (Fig. 30-10).
3. The initial infection with HSV-1 usually occurs in children or in young adults, but it can occur at any age.[21]
4. Primary herpetic gingivostomatitis has a short duration that self-resolves within 2 weeks following onset. Yet, in spite of the self-limiting nature of HSV lesions, procedures that reduce the risk of disease transmission and that provide pain relief for the patient are still essential for the dental hygienist to know.
5. Once a patient is infected with this virus, the virus travels to the trigeminal ganglion where it enters the latent-stage (dormant state). Throughout the lifetime of the patient, the infection may reactivate ("wake up") periodically to cause recurrent HSV infection. Recurrent HSV infections are characterized by either single or multiple vesicles that form on keratinized tissue (i.e., hard palate or gingiva) which rupture quickly to form ulcers. It can be triggered

by a wide variety of factors, such as stress, trauma, sunlight, and fever. The most common manifestation of recurrent HSV-1 infection is herpes labialis (known commonly as the "cold sore"). Treatment protocols for recurrent HSV infections are the same as what is recommended to treat primary herpetic gingivostomatitis.

2. **Clinical Signs and Treatment of Primary Herpetic Gingivostomatitis**
    A. **Clinical Signs.** As already mentioned, the clinical signs of primary herpetic gingivostomatitis can range from subclinical (no noticeable signs at all) to rather severe; the severe clinical signs are discussed below and outlined in Box 30-8.
       1. Severe oral pain can be associated with primary herpetic gingivostomatitis, and this discomfort results in difficulty in eating and drinking.
       2. The gingival tissues appear swollen (edematous), red (erythematous) and bleed quite easily when disturbed.
       3. Primary herpetic gingivostomatitis is accompanied by painful oral ulcers. Careful inspection of the gingival tissue can reveal small clusters of fluid-filled blisters (vesicles) on the tissues that burst, leaving numerous, painful oral ulcers. The ulcers are surrounded by a red halo. It is important to re-emphasize that when the fluid-filled blisters rupture, HSV-1 viral particles are released. This viral-filled fluid can serve as a source of infection and spread the disease to others.
           a. The ulcers can occur on lips, palate, and tongue as well as the gingival tissue.
           b. Pain caused by these ulcers can be such a major problem that it is difficult for the individual to eat and drink. Restricting fluids can even lead to dehydration, and dehydration in a child can be a serious medical emergency.
       4. In the more severe clinical manifestation, this infection is associated with signs and symptoms such as elevated body temperature, a vague feeling of discomfort (malaise), headache, and swollen lymph nodes (lymphadenopathy).
    B. **Treatment.** Treatment of patients with primary herpetic gingivostomatitis is primarily supportive (i.e., designed to keep the patient as comfortable as possible until the viral infection runs its course). Typical steps in the management of a patient with primary herpetic gingivostomatitis are discussed below and outlined in Box 30-9.
       1. *The dental hygienist should keep in mind that primary herpetic gingivostomatitis is contagious*, and any plan for periodontal instrumentation of the teeth should be postponed until the initial infection regresses.[22,23]
       2. In young children, herpes simplex virus is transmitted primarily by contact with infected saliva. Precautions should be taken to protect others in the home, daycare center, or other environment in which the patient may encounter other children. Contact should be avoided with the child's mouth, as a painful cross-infection can occur on the fingers or nail cuticle if infected oral membranes are touched (Fig. 30-10). All members of the dental team must adhere to universal precautions for infection control, and parents or guardians should be informed as well.
       3. Primary herpetic gingivostomatitis usually regresses spontaneously (goes away without treatment) in approximately 2 weeks. Controlling discomfort and ensuring fluid intake are the main focus for supportive treatment.

4. Topical oral anesthetics can be used to control oral discomfort temporarily to allow the patient to eat or to drink fluids. Examples of topical anesthetics that can be used are (1) Lidocaine 2% viscous and (2) Orabase with benzocaine.[24–26]

5. In some patients, treatment will include antiviral medications (acyclovir), medications to reduce fever (antipyretics), and systemic medications to control pain (analgesics).[24,27] Antivirals have their greatest effects when taken within 72 hours of lesion eruption.[20]

6. In 2007, over 20,000 patients had hospital emergency department visits with a diagnosis of herpetic gingivostomatitis. Physicians should be trained to diagnose, manage, and refer patients. Improving access to dental care is crucial to managing this problem.[27]

Box 30-8. Clinical Signs of Primary Herpetic Gingivostomatitis

- Oral pain with difficulty in eating and drinking
- Edematous gingival tissues (swollen gingival tissue)
- Bleeding from gingival tissue
- Vesicles (blisters) and ulceration of the gingival tissue and sometimes the lips, tongue, and palate; ulcerations surrounded by red halo
- Elevated body temperature
- Malaise (vague feeling of discomfort)
- Swollen lymph nodes

Box 30-9. Typical Steps in Management of Primary Herpetic Gingivostomatitis

1. Keep in mind that this disease is highly contagious, especially in its vesicle and ulcer stages. Consequently, all elective dental treatment should be deferred until the HSV-1 lesion is scabbed over or completely healed.
2. Primary herpetic gingivostomatitis regresses spontaneously in about 2 weeks.
3. Control oral discomfort. Topical oral anesthetics can be used for temporary relief of oral discomfort so that the patient can eat and drink fluids.
4. Recommend frequent fluid intake to avoid dehydration.
5. Refer the patient to a physician if systemic symptoms are severe or if the patient is unable to tolerate fluid intake.

Chapter Summary Statement

This chapter discussed some acute periodontal conditions that can bring patients to the office for an emergency visit. All members of the dental team should be on alert for these conditions. The dental hygienist may be the first member of the dental team to confront these types of conditions. Acute periodontal conditions include abscesses of the periodontium, necrotizing periodontal diseases, and primary herpetic gingivostomatitis.

Section 5
Focus on Patients

Clinical Patient Care

CASE 1

During a routine patient visit for periodontal maintenance, you note that there is swelling in the interdental papilla between a patient's two central incisors. The swelling is localized to the area between the incisors. As you manipulate the tissues, you note pus coming from the sulcus of one of the central incisors. You also note some mobility of one of the incisor teeth. When questioned, the patient informs you that she is aware that these tissues are swollen and that she has been flossing more in hope that the swelling would go down. In view of these clinical findings how should you proceed at this maintenance visit?

CASE 2

A patient with necrotizing gingivitis is referred to you by the dentist for calculus removal. Your examination of the patient reveals ulceration of most interdental papillae with the typical punched-out papillae often seen with this disease. The necrotic tissue pseudomembrane is present covering the ulcerations, and heavy calculus deposits are evident. The patient is quite uncomfortable. How should you proceed with the calculus removal?

Evidence in Action

A concerned mother, who is one of your maintenance patients, brings her 3-year-old daughter to the office. An examination reveals that the child has primary herpetic gingivostomatitis.

Her mouth is very painful to the touch and she has an elevated temperature. What patient education would you provide to the child's mother? What treatment recommendations should the dental team make?

Ethical Dilemma

You are in your last semester of dental hygiene school, and the clinic has booked your morning appointment. Your patient is Josh K, a 21-year-old senior pre-med student who attends your university. As you review Josh's health history, he tells you that he is extremely stressed, as he has been studying for his MCATS, for entrance to medical school, as well as completing all of his papers and projects that are due before he graduates. He admits to eating poorly, due to his busy schedule, as well as feeling very fatigued. He is getting very little sleep, only about 3 hours per night, just trying to keep up and get everything done. He has scheduled his appointment today as his gums have become very sore and are bleeding. He tells you that he is just very uncomfortable.

Your clinical exam reveals that Josh's interdental papilla seems to have a "punched out" appearance. There also appears to be a gray-white layer covering his gingival tissue. During your examination, even the slightest manipulation of his gingival tissues causes bleeding. Josh also presents with swollen lymph nodes, an elevated temperature, and extreme halitosis.

Although the clinical dentist is on vacation this week, and did not examine Josh, you remember from your Periodontology class that these classic symptoms and appearance of his tissue appear to be consistent with a necrotizing periodontal disease. You excitedly tell Josh your diagnosis, and once you have finished his assessments, reappoint him for treatment next week.

You meet your roommate Maeve, who is also a dental hygiene student, for dinner in the cafeteria after clinic. You tell her all about Josh, and his classic textbook case of necrotizing gingivitis. You decide to become "Poster Presentation" partners, and necrotizing gingivitis will be your topic. You plan to take before and after photographs of Josh's gingiva for your poster.

1. How would you explain necrotizing periodontal disease to Josh?
2. What are the typical treatment steps for a patient with necrotizing gingivitis?
3. Are there ethical principles in conflict in this dilemma?

References

1. Parameter on acute periodontal diseases. American Academy of Periodontology. *J Periodontol.* 2000;71(5 Suppl):863–866.
2. Silva GL, Soares RV, Zenobio EG. Periodontal abscess during supportive periodontal therapy: a review of the literature. *J Contemp Dent Pract.* 2008;9(6):82–91.
3. Herrera D, Roldan S, Sanz M. The periodontal abscess: a review. *J Clin Periodontol.* 2000;27(6):377–386.
4. Peltroche-Llacsahuanga H, Reichhart E, Schmitt W, Lutticken R, Haase G. Investigation of infectious organisms causing pericoronitis of the mandibular third molar. *J Oral Maxillofac Surg.* 2000;58(6):611–616.
5. Blakey GH, White RP, Jr, Offenbacher S, Phillips C, Delano EO, Maynor G. Clinical/biological outcomes of treatment for pericoronitis. *J Oral Maxillofac Surg.* 1996;54(10):1150–1160.
6. Novak MJ. Necrotizing ulcerative periodontitis. *Ann Periodontol.* 1999;4(1):74–78.
7. Rowland RW. Necrotizing ulcerative gingivitis. *Ann Periodontol.* 1999;4(1):65–73; discussion 8.
8. Herrera D, Alonso B, de Arriba L, Santa Cruz I, Serrano C, Sanz M. Acute periodontal lesions. *Periodontol 2000.* 2014;65(1):149–177.
9. Herrera D, Retamal-Valdes B, Alonso B, Feres M. Acute periodontal lesions (periodontal abscesses and necrotizing periodontal diseases) and endo-periodontal lesions. *J Periodontol.* 2018;89 Suppl 1:S85–S102.
10. Campbell CM, Stout BM, Deas DE. Necrotizing ulcerative gingivitis: a discussion of four dissimilar presentations. *Tex Dent J.* 2011;128(10):1041–1051.
11. Feller L, Lemmer J. Necrotizing gingivitis as it relates to HIV I = infection: A review of the literature. *Periodontal Prac Today.* 200;2:31–37.
12. Hooper PA, Seymour GJ. The histopathogenesis of acute ulcerative gingivitis. *J Periodontol.* 1979;50(8):419–423.
13. Kumar A, Masamatti SS, Virdi MS. Periodontal diseases in children and adolescents: a clinician's perspective part 2. *Dent Update.* 2012;39(9):639–642, 645–646, 649–652.
14. Albandar JM, Tinoco EM. Global epidemiology of periodontal diseases in children and young persons. *Periodontol 2000.* 2002;29:153–176.
15. Barnes GP, Bowles WF, 3rd, Carter HG. Acute necrotizing ulcerative gingivitis: a survey of 218 cases. *J Periodontol.* 1973;44(1):35–42.

16. Wennstrom J, Lindhe J. Effect of hydrogen peroxide on developing plaque and gingivitis in man. *J Clin Periodontol.* 1979;6(2):115–130.
17. Kolokotronis A, Doumas S. Herpes simplex virus infection, with particular reference to the progression and complications of primary herpetic gingivostomatitis. *Clin Microbiol Infect.* 2006;12(3):202–211.
18. Mohan RP, Verma S, Singh U, Agarwal N. Acute primary herpetic gingivostomatitis. *BMJ Case Rep.* 2013;2013. pii: bcr2013200074.
19. Tovaru S, Parlatescu I, Tovaru M, Cionca L. Primary herpetic gingivostomatitis in children and adults. *Quintessence Int.* 2009;40(2):119–124.
20. AAOM Clinical Practice Statement: Subject: Dental Care for the Patient with an Oral Herpetic Lesion. *Oral Surg Oral Med Oral Pathol Oral Radiol.* 2016;121(6):623–625.
21. Chauvin PJ, Ajar AH. Acute herpetic gingivostomatitis in adults: a review of 13 cases, including diagnosis and management. *J Can Dent Assoc.* 2002;68(4):247–251.
22. Browning WD, McCarthy JP. A case series: herpes simplex virus as an occupational hazard. *J Esthet Restor Dent.* 2012;24(1):61–66.
23. Lewis MA. Herpes simplex virus: an occupational hazard in dentistry. *Int Dent J.* 2004;54(2):103–111.
24. Blevins JY. Primary herpetic gingivostomatitis in young children. *Pediatr Nurs.* 2003;29(3):199–202.
25. Stoopler ET, Balasubramaniam R. Topical and systemic therapies for oral and perioral herpes simplex virus infections. *J Calif Dent Assoc.* 2013;41(4):259–262.
26. Faden H. Management of primary herpetic gingivostomatitis in young children. *Pediatr Emerg Care.* 2006;22(4):268–269.
27. Nasser M, Fedorowicz Z, Khoshnevisan MH, Shahiri Tabarestani M. Acyclovir for treating primary herpetic gingivostomatitis. *Cochrane Database Syst Rev.* 2008(4):CD006700.

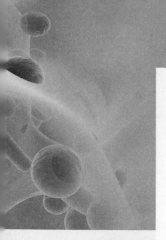

31 Periodontal Disease in the Pediatric Population

Clinical Application. Clinicians must be aware that children and adolescents as well as adults can be affected by gingival and periodontal diseases. Preserving the periodontal structures around deciduous (primary) teeth and during transitional (mixed) dentition stages is important in ensuring normal orofacial development, in promoting general health, in promoting intellectual progression, and in establishing normal social maturation. This chapter will explain the differences in periodontal anatomy associated with deciduous teeth versus that of adult teeth and will outline the common types of gingival and periodontal diseases/conditions that affect the pediatric population. It will also present treatment strategies that can be employed when managing patients with these conditions.

Learning Objectives

- Describe the normal clinical appearance of the periodontal anatomy surrounding the primary dentition and be able to explain how these features differ from the clinical appearance of the periodontium surrounding the permanent dentition.
- Describe the normal radiographic appearance of the periodontal anatomy surrounding the primary dentition and be able to explain how these features differ from the normal radiographic appearance found around the permanent dentition.
- Explain the differences between a "cold sore" and a "canker sore" and be able to describe treatment strategies for each condition.
- Explain the importance of educating pediatric patients and their caretakers about the relationship between periodontal health and oral development.
- Describe the potential implications of untreated periodontal disease in the pediatric patient.
- Describe the common types of acute periodontal conditions that are seen in the pediatric population.
- Recognize the common forms of periodontal diseases that affect the pediatric patient and be able to detail the treatment regimens to manage each of these conditions.

Key Terms

Eruption gingivitis
Pericoronitis
Operculum
Plaque-induced gingivitis
Puberty gingivitis

Drug-influenced gingivitis
Drug-influenced gingival enlargement
Familial aggregation
Episodic
Molar/Incisor pattern

Generalized pattern
Primary herpetic gingivostomatitis
Recurrent herpes simplex labialis
Recurrent aphthous ulcers

Section 1
Periodontal Anatomy of the Primary Dentition

At the heart of the interdisciplinary relationship between periodontics and pediatric dentistry is the complex interconnection between the primary dentition and the surrounding periodontal anatomy. In a clinical setting, understanding this premise is paramount because the dental practitioner must be competent in treating a wide array of different types of pediatric periodontal conditions that are commonly encountered in a dental office. Thus, the clinician must (1) understand how this close interrelationship affects both the periodontal anatomy and the primary dentition and (2) be able to recognize and detect the differences between periodontal health versus periodontal disease in the pediatric population, as some periodontal diseases may start during childhood or adolescence.

The clinical and radiographic characteristics of the periodontium in children and adolescents differ somewhat from those seen in adults. The periodontium during childhood and puberty is in a constant rapid state of change because of the growth of the jaws, the exfoliation deciduous teeth, and the eruption of permanent teeth. This section outlines the important characteristics of pediatric and adolescent periodontium.

1. **Periodontium of the Primary Dentition**
   A. **Clinical Assessment.** The clinical appearance of the oral soft tissues of the primary (deciduous) dentition differs from that of the permanent dentition in several aspects. Figure 31-1 shows a typical clinical appearance of the healthy gingiva of a child. Some of the key differences in the periodontal anatomy of children and adults are listed below and summarized in Table 31-1:
      1. Gingival color appears more reddish because of increased vascularity and a thinner overlying gingival epithelium which makes the underlying blood vessels appear more visible.[1,2] In contrast, the healthy periodontium of an adult has a coral pink color.
      2. Gingival surface texture appears less stippled or smoother than that of an adult. Stippling appears at about 3 years of age and is present in about 56% of children between ages 3 and 10 years.[3]
      3. Gingival contour of a healthy pediatric patient is characterized by a free marginal gingiva that meets the tooth with a rounded margin. The prominence of the bulbous cervical ridge of the crown of the deciduous tooth accounts for the thick rounded form of the overlying free marginal gingiva. In contrast, an adult with a healthy periodontium has a free gingival margin that has a sharp-knifelike edge that is closely adapted around the necks of the teeth.
      4. Gingival consistency of a healthy pediatric patient may have a flabby or loose appearance due to the comparatively less well-developed net of collagen fibers than in adults.
      5. The gingival sulcus (as measured with a periodontal probe) starts off as being shallow at an early age but becomes deeper as the pediatric patients become older. In other words, there is a tendency for the probing depths to increase as the pediatric patient's age increases. In a study that was conducted to evaluate the relationship between age and probing depth in each primary tooth, it was found that the mean probing depth of upper central incisor on the buccal side at 4 years of age was 1.26 mm and at 6 years, 1.55 mm.[4] In addition, in the majority of buccal and lingual sites measured in the same study, mean values increased from anterior to posterior positions in both arches. The mean

probing depths values for all teeth examined showed the highest mean value in lingual sites of mandibular second molars (2.08 mm) and the lowest mean in lingual sites of mandibular central incisors (1.03 mm).[4]

6. The interdental papilla is rounded (saddle-shaped) with a broad facial to lingual dimension and a narrow form from the mesial to distal aspect.

7. The width of the attached gingiva is narrower in the mandible than in the maxilla, and both widths increase with age as children transition from primary to permanent dentition.[5] Several studies confirm that an increase in attached gingiva is correlated with age.[4]

B. **Radiographic Assessment.** Differences in periodontal anatomy are also noted upon radiographic assessment. These include (Figure 31-2):

1. The periodontal ligament in children is wider and has less dense fibers compared to adults.[1,2,6]

2. Alveolar bone in the primary dentition has less trabeculae and calcification with larger marrow spaces.[1,2,6]

3. Lamina dura (the radiopaque lining of an alveolus) is prominent in the primary dentition with a wider periodontal ligament space than in the permanent dentition.

4. Interdental septa of pediatric patients are generally broader and flatter than the interdental septa seen in healthy adults, with bony crests within 1 to 2 mm of the cementoenamel junction.

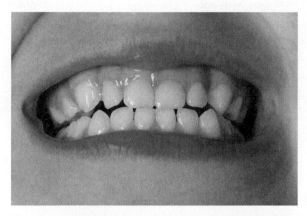

Figure 31-1. A Healthy Pediatric Periodontium. This clinical photograph shows a child with the clinical features characteristics of a healthy periodontium. Note the minimal signs of inflammation, the smooth gingival texture, and the rounded free marginal gingiva.

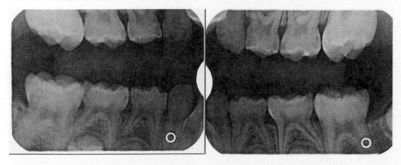

Figure 31-2. Radiographic Characteristics of Healthy Pediatric Patient. Bitewing radiographs of a child illustrating the flattened interseptal bone and bony crests within 2 mm of the cementoenamel junction.

TABLE 31-1	DIFFERING CLINICAL CHARACTERISTICS OF THE HEALTHY PERIODONTIUM IN CHILDREN VERSUS ADULTS	
Features	**Children**	**Adults**
Gingival Color	More reddish	Coral pink
Contour	Rounded free marginal gingiva	Sharp, knife-edged marginal gingiva that is closely adapted to the cervical neck of a tooth
Consistency	Flabby due to less connective tissue density and lack of organized fiber bundles	Firm and resilient
Surface Texture	Stippling absent in infancy; may be seen by age 6 years. However, it should be noted that in many cases the healthy pediatric gingiva may not exhibit any gingival stippling but may appear smooth.	Stippling may be present; however, its pattern and extent varies in different areas of the mouth of the same individual
Interdental Area	Saddle-shaped interdental gingiva	Triangular papillary gingiva
Attached Gingiva	Width increases with age	Width greater in adults

Section 2
Gingival Diseases in Pediatric Patients

There is a high prevalence of gingivitis among children and adolescents, and a small percentage of children exhibit attachment loss and alveolar bone loss. Even though the percentage of children with attachment loss is small, it is clear that clinicians need to examine every child's periodontium with care since failure to identify periodontal conditions early can lead to unnecessary tooth loss. The American Academy of Periodontology and the American Academy of Pediatric Dentistry[7–9] have reported the following points related to gingival and periodontal diseases in children and adolescents:

- Gingivitis of varying severity is nearly universal in children and adolescents.
- In children, the amount of plaque biofilm often does not correlate with the level of inflammation; it is not uncommon to see copious amounts of plaque biofilm with little or no gingivitis.
- Loss of periodontal attachment and supporting bone is uncommon in ages 5 to 11 years but increases in children ages 12 to 17 years.
- The presence of severe attachment loss on multiple teeth among children and young adults has been reported to be approximately 0.2% to 0.5%.
- Children and adolescents should receive periodic periodontal evaluation as a component of routine dental visits. Both the American Academy of Periodontology and the American Academy of Pediatric Dentistry strongly recommend that all patients, regardless of age, receive a comprehensive periodontal evaluation as part of routine dental visits.

ERUPTION GINGIVITIS AND PERICORONAL ABSCESS

1. **Eruption gingivitis** is a short-lived type of gingivitis observed in young children as the primary teeth are erupting. Additionally, eruption gingivitis can occur as the primary teeth are exfoliating (shedding) and as the permanent successors emerge.
   A. **Characteristics of Eruption Gingivitis**
      1. Tooth eruption, by itself, is not a cause of gingivitis. Rather, this type of gingivitis is caused by plaque biofilm accumulation that occurs in areas of primary teeth shedding or permanent teeth erupting (Fig. 31-3). The inflammatory response is further accentuated by the fact that the patient is unable to perform adequate oral hygiene in the eruption area because it is too painful or difficult to access.
      2. Also, as a normal part of exfoliation, the junctional epithelium migrates under the resorbing tooth, thereby increasing pocket depth and creating a niche for further bacteria plaque, food debris, and materia alba collection.[10]
   B. **Treatment.** Eruption gingivitis is quickly reversible and subsides after the tooth has completely emerged into the oral cavity. It can also be managed with improved oral hygiene.
   C. A first and/or second permanent molar that is in the process of tooth eruption may be associated with severe gingival inflammation which can develop into a pericoronal abscess.
2. Pericoronal Abscess (Pericoronitis)
   A. **Disease Characteristics of Pericoronal Abscess (Pericoronitis)**
      1. **Pericoronitis** is a localized purulent infection within the soft tissue surrounding the crown of a partially erupted tooth or a tooth that is in the process of tooth eruption.
      2. As mentioned above, this condition is most frequently seen around erupting permanent molars (Fig. 31-4).

3. The fold of tissue partially covering the erupting tooth is termed an operculum. This enlarged tissue fold acts like a partially enclosed lid that covers the occlusal surface of the partially impacted molar (or tooth that is erupting) and collects and retains bacteria, food debris, and materia alba beneath the operculum. This leads to pericoronitis, which literally means "inflammation around the crown of a tooth."

B. Clinical Manifestations of Pericoronal Abscess (Pericoronitis)

1. Some of the clinical signs and symptoms associated with pericoronitis are bad taste (from the pus that forms underneath the operculum), bad smell (halitosis), and tenderness and redness of the gingiva. The operculum can also be painful if the patient occludes on it.

2. Over time, if acute pericoronitis is left untreated, there is the possibility that it can lead to more serious consequences, especially if the infection does not resolve and spreads to cause trismus (difficulty in jaw opening), dysphagia (difficulty in swallowing), or dyspnea (difficulty in breathing, especially if the infection spreads to the floor of the mouth and results in Ludwig angina).

C. Treatment Pericoronal Abscess (Pericoronitis)

1. The treatment for this condition is typically irrigation of the tissue with gentle debridement or surgical excision of the operculum. Depending on the severity of the case, antibiotic therapy may be required, especially in cases of lymph node involvement, fever, and malaise. Extraction of the involved molar tooth may also be a viable option.

2. Pain may be managed with the use of over-the-counter acetaminophen and/or ibuprofen.

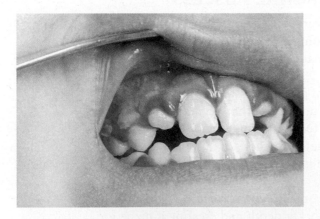

Figure 31-3. Eruption Gingivitis. Inflammation of the gingival margin is clinically evident around the erupting teeth of this child.

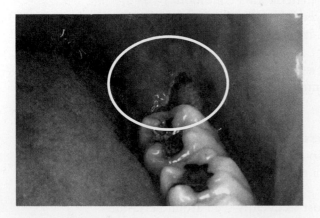

Figure 31-4. Pericoronitis. An adolescent patient with pericoronitis. Note the fold of soft tissue—the operculum—partially covering the occlusal surface of the third molar. The area is too painful for the patient to properly clean. This allows for further plaque accumulation which accentuates the inflammation seen around the operculum. The patient may also be experiencing pain whenever he occludes on it.

PLAQUE-INDUCED GINGIVAL DISEASE

1. **Characteristics of Plaque-Induced Gingivitis in Children and Adolescents.** Plaque-induced gingivitis is characterized by the presence of inflammation limited to the marginal gingiva without detectable loss of clinical attachment or alveolar bone (Figs. 31-5 and 31-6).
   - Gingivitis is extremely common among children and adolescents. As children age, their tendency to develop gingivitis increases.[10] The prevalence is lowest during the preschool years and peaks during puberty. Approximately 60% of teenagers exhibit gingival bleeding on probing.[9]
   - The degree of gingival inflammation generally is less intense than what would be expected in an adult with a similar amount of plaque biofilm formation.[6,10] The junctional epithelium of the primary dentition tends to be thicker than in the permanent dentition and thus, may reduce the permeability of the gingival tissues to bacteria that initiate the inflammatory response.[10]
   - The incidence of gingivitis peaks at ages 9 to 14 years of age and then decreases slightly after puberty.[10] Such gingivitis often is termed puberty gingivitis (Fig. 31-7).
   - Puberty gingivitis is believed to be related to hormonal changes during this developmental stage that intensify the inflammatory response to plaque biofilm.[6,10]
2. **Treatment for Plaque-Induced Gingivitis in Children.**
   - Early gingivitis is quickly reversible with professional care and daily plaque biofilm control.
   - Professional care may involve removal of plaque biofilm (Fig. 31-8). About 9% of 4- to 6-year-old children exhibit calculus deposits. By age 7 to 9 years, 18% of children present with calculus deposits, and by the age of 10 to 15 years, 33% to 43% have some calculus formation.[11]

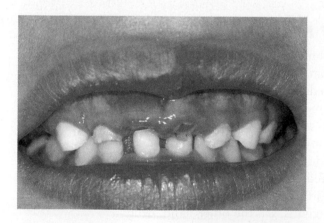

Figure 31-5. Inadequate Self-Care. At his first dental appointment, this young child exhibits plaque-induced gingivitis. Note the accumulation of plaque biofilm at the gingival margins and the presence of exfoliating teeth interfering with self-care efforts.

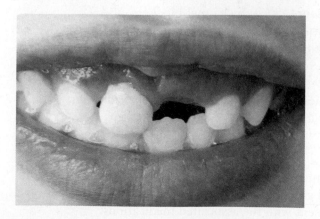

Figure 31-6. Plaque-Induced Gingivitis. This child exhibits gingival erythema and edema associated with moderate plaque biofilm accumulation around the central incisor tooth.

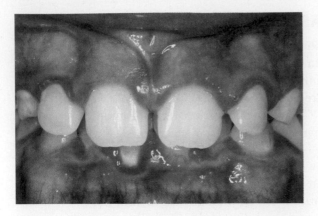

Figure 31-7. Puberty-Associated Gingivitis. Puberty-associated gingivitis is an exaggerated inflammatory response of the gingiva to a relatively small amount of plaque biofilm. The exaggerated response is modulated by hormones released during puberty. (Courtesy of Dr. Richard Foster, Guilford Technical Community College, Jamestown, NC.)

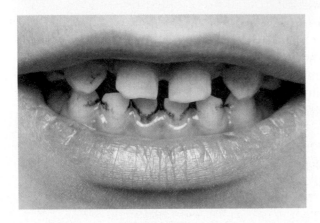

Figure 31-8. Dental Calculus. This young patient exhibits heavy tooth staining and dental calculus.

GINGIVAL DISEASES MODIFIED BY MEDICATIONS

Due to systemic disease, it is necessary for some pediatric patients to take systemic medications which have unwanted side-effects on the periodontium. One of the most common medication side-effects manifested in the periodontal tissues of pediatric population is gingival overgrowth.

With respect to gingival diseases modified by medications, it should be noted that there are two separate and distinct conditions which sound similar but are not the same. Drug-influenced gingivitis results from any systemic medication that causes an exaggerated inflammatory response to plaque biofilm. Oral contraceptives are an example of a drug class that triggers an exaggerated inflammatory response to plaque biofilm; the gingival inflammation that is seen in drug-influenced gingivitis is similar to that seen in pregnancy gingivitis or puberty gingivitis. On the other hand, drug-influenced gingival enlargement is an increase in size of the gingiva resulting from systemic medications, most commonly anticonvulsants, calcium channel blockers, and immunosuppressants. Unlike inflammatory gingivitis and drug-influenced gingivitis, the distinguishing clinical feature of drug-influenced gingival enlargement is that it does not bleed easily and typically appears firm, resilient, and pale pink in color *when uncomplicated by inflammation.* Figure 31-9 shows an example of a child with phenytoin-induced gingival enlargement. Plaque biofilm accumulation is not necessary for the initiation of gingival enlargement, but it will exacerbate the gingival disease. Meticulous plaque biofilm control can reduce but will not eliminate gingival overgrowth so long as the patient remains on the medication.

1. **Characteristics of Drug-Induced Gingival Enlargement**
   - The clinical manifestations of drug-influenced gingival enlargement frequently appear within 1 to 3 months after initiation of treatment with the associated medications.

- Gingival overgrowth first typically affects the facial interdental papillae of anterior teeth and progresses to affect the marginal lingual papilla. The interdental papillae overgrow, forming firm triangular tissue masses that protrude from the interdental area.
- Gradually, the enlarged papilla from one interdental area may unite with the adjacent enlarged papilla to partially cover the anatomical crown with marginal gingiva (Fig. 31-9). Overgrowths are most commonly seen on the facial aspect of the maxillary and mandibular anterior teeth. The gingival overgrowth may serve as plaque-retentive areas.
- Ultimately, the enlargement may transform into a massive tissue fold covering a considerable portion of the crowns.
- In severe cases, the fibrotic enlargement normally may extend coronally and interfere with esthetics, mastication, or speech. The tissue may completely cover the crowns of the teeth making it more difficult to keep the teeth clean and increase the patient's susceptibility to oral diseases, such as caries and periodontal disease.
- In the presence of good biofilm control, the enlarged tissue is pink in color and firm and rubbery in consistency. In the presence of poor biofilm control, the tissue appears red, edematous, and spongy.

2. **Treatment for Drug-Induced Gingival Enlargement in Children and Adolescents**
   - Close collaboration between medical and dental clinical teams is necessary for the joint management of individuals being treated with anticonvulsants, calcium channel blockers, or immunosuppressants.
   - Medication-induced gingival enlargement may resolve either partially or completely when the medication is discontinued. However, if the medication cannot be discontinued, a gingivectomy for surgical elimination of the tissue overgrowth may be required. If plaque biofilm control is inadequate, the re-growth will occur rapidly. The patient should be advised of the likelihood of the recurrence of the gingival overgrowth following surgery.
   - As this condition is somewhat worsened by the level of biofilm accumulation on the teeth, effective oral hygiene measures should be implemented to reduce the severity.
   - Thus, it is important that the dental clinician continually reinforce the importance of stringent home care to the patient with drug-influenced gingival enlargement. Gingival diseases modified by medications are discussed in Chapter 6, Diseases of the Gingiva and Chapter 16, Systemic Risk Factors That Amplify Susceptibility to Periodontal Diseases.

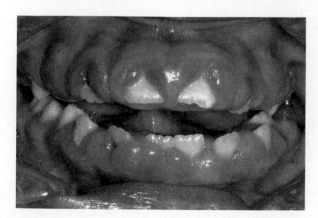

Figure 31-9. Phenytoin-Influenced Gingival Overgrowth. Severe enlargement of the gingiva associated with phenytoin (Dilantin) medication in an individual with epilepsy. (Courtesy of Dr. Ralph Arnold, San Antonio, TX.)

Section 3
Common Types of Periodontitis in Pediatric Patients

PERIODONTITIS

As already discussed, periodontitis is far less common in children and adolescents than in adults.[12] Nevertheless, although it is rare to see this condition in children and adolescents, periodontitis can indeed occur in this subset of the population.[12] When periodontitis occurs in pediatric patients, the disease has a similar etiology and pathophysiology to the adult version of the disease. Figure 31-10 shows a pediatric patient with periodontitis.

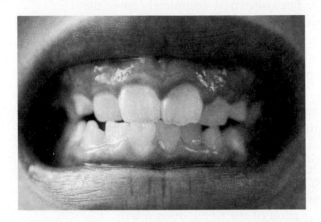

Figure 31-10. Chronic Periodontitis. This adolescent patient has periodontitis. Periodontal probing and radiographs indicated attachment loss and alveolar bone loss. When periodontitis occurs in pediatric patients, characteristics of the disease are similar to the characteristics in adults.

MORE AGGRESSIVE FORMS OF PERIODONTITIS IN THE PEDIATRIC POPULATION

1. **Characteristics of More Aggressive Forms of Periodontitis in Children/Adolescents.** The more aggressive forms of periodontitis seen in children and adolescents (Figure 31-11) has several well-recognized primary and secondary clinical features.[12]
   A. **Primary Features.** The primary features of the more aggressive forms of periodontitis in the pediatric population are[13–15]:
      1. Rapid destruction of periodontal ligament and supporting alveolar bone. Baer estimates that the loss of attachment—in what was previously known as localized juvenile periodontitis—progresses three or four times faster than in periodontitis affecting the adult population.[16]
      2. No obvious signs or symptoms of systemic disease.[17]
      3. Other close family members (parents, siblings) also exhibiting this form of periodontitis.[18–20] **Familial aggregation** refers to the occurrence of more cases of the disease in close family members than can be readily accounted for by mere chance.
   B. **Secondary Features.** Secondary features that are generally but not always present are:
      1. Relatively small amounts of bacterial plaque biofilm; the disease severity seems to be exaggerated given the light amount of plaque biofilm.[13,21]
      2. Elevated proportions of *Aggregatibacter actinomycetemcomitans (Aa)*.[18,22]
      3. Impaired phagocytosis.[23–25]
      4. Hyperinflammatory response to bacterial endotoxins (bacterial lipopolysaccharide).[26,27]
      5. A lack of clinical signs of disease.[14,28]
         a. Affected tissue may have a normal clinical appearance with no signs of inflammation and calculus deposits are minimal.
         b. Probing reveals deep periodontal pockets on affected teeth.[29]

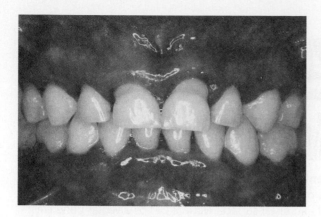

Figure 31-11. Child With a More Aggressive Form of Periodontitis. Periodontitis in a 5-year-old child with attachment loss on all teeth. Note the minimal amount of plaque buildup that is not consistent with the degree and severity of attachment loss.

6. A poor response to periodontal therapy.
7. Episodic Disease Progression
   a. Periodontitis is the adult population is a very slowly progressing disease.
   b. In more aggressive forms of periodontitis, attachment loss is episodic, occurring in a succession of acute destructive phases with intermittent inactive phases.[14]

2. **Two Patterns of the More Aggressive Forms of Periodontitis Affecting the Pediatric Patient**
   A. **The Molar/Incisor Pattern.** The molar/incisor pattern of periodontitis (previously called "localized juvenile periodontitis") is characterized by localized attachment loss affecting the first molars and/or incisors and involving no more than two teeth other than first molars and incisors.[14,16,30–33] It has been generally accepted that this type of periodontitis can affect both the primary and permanent dentition. In fact, a child affected with the molar/incisor pattern of periodontitis may experience severe periodontitis of the permanent dentition later in his/her life.[34]
   1. **Features of the Molar/Incisor Pattern of Periodontitis**
      a. In children, the onset of the molar/incisor pattern of periodontitis can occur in the primary dentition as early as age 4. One early indication is radiographic evidence of bone loss around the primary molars and/or incisors. On the other hand, in young individuals, the onset of this form of periodontitis may occur around the time of puberty. However, based on the amount of periodontal destruction seen at the time of detection, it is assumed that the disease process may have begun earlier.[35]
      b. There is minor tissue inflammation and minimal amounts of plaque biofilm that seem inconsistent with the amount of periodontal destruction.[14,28]
      c. The molar/incisor form frequently is associated with *Aggregatibacter actinomycetemcomitans* (Aa) in combination with *Porphyromonas* spp.[22,36,37] To date, no single microorganism has been found to be the causative agent responsible for this form of periodontitis.
      d. Vertical bone loss around the first molars and incisors is a classic radiographic sign of the molar/incisor form of periodontitis.[38]
      e. Functional defects of neutrophils are suspected as a systemic contributing factor that makes certain patients more susceptible to this form of periodontitis.[39]
   2. **Prevalence of the Molar/Incisor Pattern of Periodontitis.** Less than 1% of the population is affected with this condition. This form of disease may first affect the deciduous dentition but then progress to affect the permanent dentition as the pediatric patient ages, if the disease is left untreated.

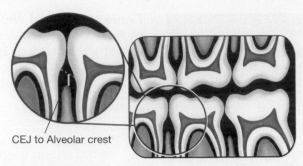

CEJ to Alveolar crest

Figure 31-12. Use of Bitewing Radiographs in Screening for the Molar/Incisor Pattern of Periodontitis. The distance from the CEJ and the alveolar bone crest is measured from a line connecting the CEJs of the two adjacent teeth. Measurements are taken for each mesial and distal surface. Normal CEJ-to-alveolar bone crest distances for 7- to 9-year-old children are less than 2 mm.

3. **Screening of Primary and Mixed Dentitions for the Molar/Incisor Pattern of Periodontitis**
   a. The measurement of attachment loss on primary teeth or partially erupted teeth may be difficult.
   b. Measurement of the distance between the CEJ and the alveolar bone crest on bitewing radiographs is a useful screening approach with children (Fig. 31-12).
   c. The "normal" distance between the CEJ and the alveolar bone crest has been evaluated by recent investigations.[28,40]
      1) The median distance between the CEJ and the alveolar crest of primary molars in 7- to 9-year-old children is 0.8 to 1.4 mm. The CEJ of permanent molars is 0 to 0.5 mm coronal to the alveolar crest in 7- to 9-year-olds.
      2) Greater distances between the CEJ and alveolar crest are seen at sites with caries, restorations, or open contacts. These local intraoral factors may contribute to localized bone loss in children in a similar manner to that seen in adults and are not necessarily indicative of aggressive periodontitis.
      3) A distance of more than 2 mm between the CEJ and alveolar crest, in the absence of local contributing factors, should cause the clinician to suspect periodontitis. If the measurement exceeds this value, periodontitis should be suspected, and a comprehensive periodontal examination should be performed.

4. **Treatment of the Molar/Incisor Pattern of Periodontitis**
   a. The successful treatment includes early diagnosis, surgical or nonsurgical periodontal therapy in combination with systemic antibiotic therapy.[9,41]
   b. According to a number of studies, the most successful antibiotics in the treatment of the molar/incisor pattern of periodontitis are broad-spectrum antibiotics, such as tetracycline alone or with metronidazole.[42,43] However, administering tetracycline to a child should be prescribed with caution as there is the possibility that the antibiotic may discolor and stain the developing dentition.
   c. Since there may be an underlying systemic condition that makes the child more susceptible to the disease, medical consultation with the child's pediatrician is recommended to coordinate medical care with periodontal therapy.
   d. If the primary teeth are affected, then the child must be diligently monitored at subsequent recall visits for the possibility of this form of periodontitis affecting his/her permanent dentition.

    e. More frequent recalls and dental checkups for pediatric patient with this pattern of periodontitis may be recommended to provide maintenance care, reinforce the importance of a good oral hygiene regimen, verify that the disease is arrested, or intercept the disease reoccurrence at its early stages.

B. Generalized Pattern of More Aggressive Forms of Periodontitis. The generalized pattern of the more aggressive forms of periodontitis is characterized by generalized interproximal attachment loss affecting at least three permanent teeth other than the first molars and incisors. Most of the permanent teeth usually are affected in this form of periodontitis.[14,32]

  1. Features of the Generalized Pattern of More Aggressive Forms of Periodontitis

    a. Usually occurs in persons younger than 30 years of age, but patients may be older.[14,44]

    b. Destruction of attachment and alveolar bone is very episodic, occurring in a succession of acute phases rather than in a gradual progression.[14]

    c. The appearance of the gingival tissues varies in this type of periodontitis.

      1) The gingival tissues may be acutely inflamed, ulcerated, and fiery red.[14,44] This tissue response is believed to occur in the destructive phase of disease progression.

      2) The gingival tissues may appear pink and free of inflammation. However, deep pockets can still be detected with conventional periodontal probing. This tissue response may coincide with periods of disease inactivity.[45]

  2. Treatment of the Generalized Pattern of More Aggressive Forms of Periodontitis. In general, the treatment regimen for the generalized pattern of more aggressive forms of periodontitis is similar to that used to treat the molar/incisor pattern of periodontitis.

    a. Medical evaluation of the patient is warranted to determine if any underlying undiagnosed systemic conditions are putting the patient at higher risk of having a refractory or recurrent form of this type of periodontitis.

    b. The generalized pattern does not always respond well to conventional nonsurgical periodontal therapy or to antibiotics commonly used to treat periodontitis.[46–48]

    c. Microbiological assaying may be considered to identify the specific putative pathogen and determine the specific type of antibiotic to prescribe.[43]

NECROTIZING PERIODONTAL DISEASES

Necrotizing periodontal diseases occur with low frequency (less than 1%) in North American and European children.[9] Factors that predispose children to necrotizing periodontal diseases include viral infections (including HIV), malnutrition, emotional stress, lack of sleep, and a variety of systemic diseases.[9] Necrotizing periodontal diseases are discussed in Chapter 8, Other Periodontal Conditions.

Section 4
Common Acute Periodontal Conditions in Pediatric Patients

HERPES VIRUS INFECTIONS AND APHTHOUS ULCERS

1. **Primary Herpetic Gingivostomatitis.** Primary herpetic gingivostomatitis is a severe reaction to the initial viral infection with—first exposure of an individual to the Herpes Simplex Virus Type-I (HSV-1).

    A. **Disease Characteristics**

    1. According to the World Health Organization, approximately 3.7 billion people under the age of 50 are infected with HSV-1.

        a. In most cases, the virus never causes symptoms during the primary HSV-1 infection. This is known as a subclinical—symptom free—infection.

        b. In some individuals, however, this initial infection presents with intensely painful gingival inflammation and multiple vesicles that easily rupture to form painful ulcers. This severe reaction to the initial HSV-1 infection is known as primary herpetic gingivostomatitis (Figs. 31-13 and 31-14).

        c. Once infected, most individuals develop immunity to the virus. In certain individuals, the herpes simplex virus type-1 can remain latent in the trigeminal ganglion and is responsible for recurrent oral herpetic lesions (cold sores).

    2. The initial infection with the HSV-1 usually affects young children—with heightened incidence from 1 to 3 years of age—but may also affect adolescents and adults.

        a. Of children with primary infections, 99% are symptom free or the symptoms are attributed to teething.

        b. The remaining 1% develops significant gingival inflammation and multiple painful ulcerative lesions found on keratinized tissue, such as the lips, gingiva, hard palate, and dorsal side (top) of the tongue.[49]

    3. The infection is contagious during the vesicular stage as the virus is contained in the clear fluid in the vesicles. The virus may be easily spread through transmission of viral-infected saliva from one part of the body to another in the same individual (i.e., perioral involvement or herpetic whitlow) or from one infected individual to another individual.

    4. Primary herpetic gingivostomatitis is associated with severe pain that makes eating and drinking difficult. This may result in nutritional deficiencies during the active stage of the disease.

    5. Systemic symptoms associated with primary herpetic gingivostomatitis are headache, swollen lymph nodes, and sore throat (Fig. 31-15). Because this condition is a viral infection, there may be a low-grade fever usually not above 101°F.

    6. Primary herpetic gingivostomatitis regresses spontaneously within 10 to 20 days without scarring.

    B. **Clinical Manifestations of Primary Herpetic Gingivostomatitis.** Primary herpetic gingivostomatitis may occur anywhere on the free or the attached gingiva.

    1. Primary herpetic gingivostomatitis is characterized by widespread inflammation of the marginal and attached gingiva.

    2. The gingiva exhibits intense gingival inflammation.

3. Small clusters of yellowish-white liquid-filled vesicles rapidly form throughout the mouth.
4. Later, these vesicles burst, forming yellowish ulcers that are surrounded by a red halo.
5. Systemic involvement—such as headache, fever, swollen cervical and submandibular lymph nodes (lymphadenopathy), and sore throat—usually is present.

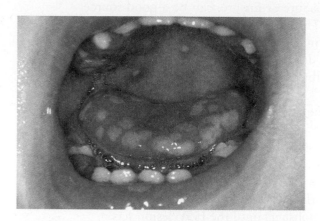

Figure 31-13. Primary Herpetic Gingivostomatitis. This clinical photograph shows a young child with oral lesions associated with primary herpetic gingivostomatitis. Note the oral ulcerations surrounded by red halos. (Courtesy of Mediscan Company.)

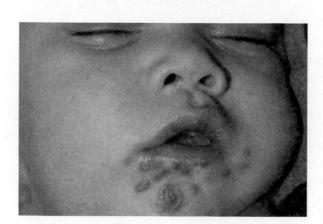

Figure 31-14. Facial Lesions of Primary Herpetic Gingivostomatitis. Oral lesions of primary herpetic gingivostomatitis can occasionally be accompanied by skin lesions. This clinical photograph shows an infant with primary herpetic gingivostomatitis with vesicle formation on the face.

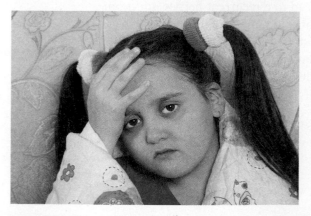

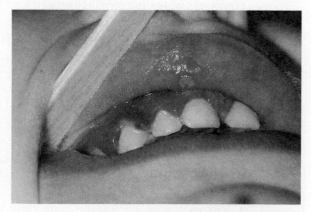

Figure 31-15. Symptoms of Primary Herpetic Gingivostomatitis. This child demonstrates common symptoms of primary herpetic gingivostomatitis including fever and multiple ulcerative lesions of the oral cavity. Other common systemic symptoms associated with primary herpetic gingivostomatitis are lymphadenopathy, sore throat, and general malaise.

C. **Treatment for Primary Herpetic Gingivostomatitis**

1. If possible, treat an outbreak within the first 48 to 72 hours with a systemic antiviral medication such as acyclovir, valacyclovir, or famciclovir.

2. Counsel the child and his/her caregiver that adequate intake of fluids is important. Since eating and drinking are painful, dehydration is a major concern with these individuals. Athletic drinks, such as Gatorade, can be consumed to replenish electrolytes lost due to dehydration.

3. A dietary replacement drink, such as PediaSure or Ensure, can be a good source of nutrition since eating will be difficult. The patient may be able to eat foods processed in a blender. Vitamin supplementation may also be beneficial so as to maintain healthy levels of micronutrients during the course of the disease.

4. Pain may be relieved by acetaminophen, ibuprofen, or viscous lidocaine regimen.

5. An antimicrobial mouthwash like Listerine or Peridex should be recommended to prevent a secondary infection.

6. Precautions should be taken to prevent the spread of the virus to the patient's eyes or transmission from an infected individual (child) to a noninfected individual (parent). The infected patient should wash with soap and water frequently.

7. Avoid any procedure that results in the airborne spread of viral-infected aerosol (i.e., handpiece, ultrasonic scaler, and air polisher) until the HSV lesion has scabbed over.

8. Avoid any procedure that involves the manipulation of soft tissues infected with HSV (i.e., periodontal probing and periodontal instrumentation).

9. Implement strict infection control procedures to reduce the risk of spreading the virus from an infected patient to a dental health care worker.

2. **Recurrent Oral Herpes Simplex Labialis.** Recurrent herpes simplex labialis—commonly referred to as a fever blister or cold sore—is an infection of the mouth area caused by the reactivation of Herpes Simplex Virus Type-I (HSV-1). It's a common and contagious infection that spreads easily. According to the American Sexual Health Association, over half of adults in the United States carry this virus.

A. **Characteristics of Recurrent Oral Herpes Simplex Labialis.**

1. This lesion can occur in patients of all ages, including children. After the primary infection, the virus lays dormant inside the nerve cells of the face for the rest of a person's life. This means that symptoms are not always present. However, certain events can make the virus reawaken and lead to a recurrent herpes infection.

2. Events that trigger a recurrent infection of oral herpes might include excessive exposure to sunlight, physical/emotional stress, lack of sleep, hormonal changes, fever, a weakened immune system, lowered tissue resistance resulting from various types of trauma, or recent dental treatment.

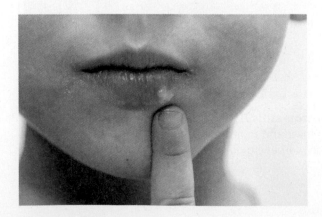

Figure 31-16. Recurrent Oral Herpes. Child with a recurrent oral herpes blister on her lower lip. The fluid-filled blister will eventually rupture and leave superficial ulcers that crust and heal without scaring within 2 weeks.

B. **Clinical Manifestations of Recurrent Oral Herpes.** The majority of recurrent oral herpes occurs on the vermillion border of the lip, hence the condition also being referred to as "recurrent herpes labialis" while only 5% of recurrent oral herpes occurs in intraoral locations, such as nonmovable mucosa (keratinized tissue) of the hard palate and/or the attached gingiva (Fig. 31-16). Like primary herpetic gingivostomatitis, these lesions may spread to perioral areas, such as the nose, cheek, and chin. While recurrent oral herpes is milder than the primary attack, it can be dangerous if the infection spreads to the eyes and causes blisters or sores to form close to the cornea. If such a situation arises, immediate consultation with an ophthalmologist is warranted.

1. Tingling on or near the lips is usually a warning sign that the cold sores of recurrent oral herpes lesions are about to appear in 1 to 2 days.
2. Symptoms of a recurrent episode may include:
   - Blisters or sores on the mouth, lips, tongue, nose, or gums
   - Burning pain around the blisters
   - Tingling or itching near the lips
   - Outbreaks of several small blisters that grow together and may be red and inflamed

C. **Treatment for Recurrent Oral Herpes**

1. Recurrent oral herpes has a spontaneous resolution in 10 to 14 days and therefore, is managed by palliative care.
2. It can be helpful to treat an outbreak within the first 48 to 72 hours with systemic antiviral medications such as acyclovir, valacyclovir, and/or famciclovir.
3. It has been reported that outbreaks which occur on the lip can be treated by over-the-counter medicaments such as Abreva.
4. Milk products are helpful in coating lesions.
5. Parents should be cautioned to monitor the child to prevent him or her from touching ulcerations and spreading the contagious virus to other mucous membranes. Educating the child and the parent of the importance of meticulous hygiene is critical in minimizing disease transmission.

3. **Recurrent Aphthous Ulcers**

A. **Disease Characteristics.** Recurrent aphthous ulcers are recurrent, painful ulcers of the oral mucosa that occur in school-aged children and adults. This condition also is referred to as recurrent aphthous stomatitis.

1. Aphthous ulcers—commonly called "canker sores"—are small recurrent, painful, round or ovoid ulcers with well-defined erythematous margins, like a halo, and a central yellow or gray floor that typically develop on the nonkeratinized tissue such as buccal mucosa, mucobuccal fold, floor of the mouth, ventral side (bottom) of the tongue, and on the soft palate (Fig. 31-17). Unlike oral herpetic lesions, aphthous ulcers are not contagious, are not caused by a virus, and generally are not associated with detectable systemic involvement.
2. The precise cause of aphthous remains unclear, though researchers suspect that a combination of local factors (such as trauma, allergy to toothpaste constituents, or salivary gland dysfunction) and systemic factors (such as autoimmune dysfunction, bacterial or viral infection, nutritional deficiencies) contribute to outbreaks, even in the same person.
3. The peak age is between 10 and 19 years of age.

B. **Aphthous Ulcer Triggers.** Possible triggers for recurrent aphthous ulcers include:
   1. A minor injury to the oral cavity from dental work, overzealous brushing, sports mishaps or an accidental cheek bite
   2. Toothpastes and mouth rinses containing sodium lauryl sulfate
   3. Food sensitivities, particularly to chocolate, coffee, strawberries, eggs, nuts, cheese, and spicy or acidic foods
   4. A diet lacking in vitamin B_{12}, zinc, folate (folic acid) or iron
   5. Emotional stress
C. **Treatment of Aphthous Ulcers**
   1. Ulcers usually heal spontaneously within 4 to 14 days.
   2. Treatment focuses on promoting ulcer healing, reducing ulcer pain, and maintaining the patient's nutritional intake.

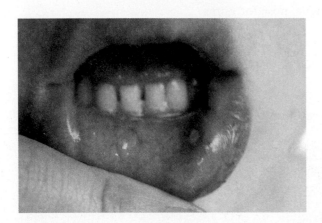

Figure 31-17. Aphthous Ulcer. A young child with an aphthous ulcer on the mucosal lining of the lip. Although it clinically appears to look like an intraoral herpetic lesion, its location on nonkeratinized mucosa (inner lip) is typical of an aphthous ulcer.

Chapter Summary Statement

The landmark U.S. Surgeon General's report titled "*Oral Health in America: A Report of the Surgeon General*" is a profound wake-up call that underscores the extensive toll that has been inflicted on the American population as a result of oral, dental, and craniofacial disorders/diseases. One subset of our population that the report identifies as being vulnerable to what amounts to be a "silent epidemic" is children who present unique challenges, and are at an increased risk for oral infections, delays in tooth eruption, periodontal disease, enamel irregularities, and malocclusion. Their exposure to certain medications and therapies, special diets, and their difficulty in maintaining daily oral self-care further compromises their oral health. According to estimates highlighted in the report, the ramifications of untreated oral diseases account for serious general health problems, significant pain, interference with eating (which affects growth and development), improper utilization of hospital emergency rooms, and lost school time. One of the most critical themes repeatedly emphasized in the report is that effective prevention requires an early start.

To meet this challenge head-on, clinicians, especially dental hygienists, must be ready to take the lead in educating pediatric patients and their caregivers on multiple oral health issues—dental caries, periodontal health, injury prevention, dental development, oral habits, common soft tissue ulcerative lesions, and bite development—as well as promoting the child's complete oral health by performing a comprehensive periodontal examination at each routine dental visit. In cases where preventative therapy has not been effective in suppressing the disease, early interventional therapy makes a big difference in ensuring the greatest chance for success in preserving the dentition and periodontium while maintaining the normal developmental progression and maturation of the child. While it is true that the pediatric population has a lower occurrence of destructive periodontal diseases (i.e., periodontitis) compared to the adult population, it is essential that all participants invested in the care of the pediatric patient—which include the dental practitioner, the child, and the caregiver—not let their guard down in fighting this "silent epidemic."

Section 5
Focus on Patients

Clinical Patient Care

CASE 1

A 28-month-old child is brought to your office for an emergency appointment. The parent informs you that her child has had a fever for the past 2 days, has not been eating well, and barely wants to drink fluids. The parent informs you that the child has no significant medical history and no known drug allergies. The child's immunizations are up-to-date. Examination of the child reveals an elevated temperature, swollen cervical and submandibular lymph nodes, inflammation of the marginal and attached gingiva, small clusters of blisters on lips, tongue, and buccal mucosa, and some ulcers on oral tissues surrounded by red halos.

1. What might be a likely diagnosis for this child's condition?
2. What kind of therapy would be appropriate for this child?
3. What information about this condition should be given to the parent?

CASE 2

A 13-year-old female presents for a routine preventive visit in your office. The patient tells you that she recently had a painful blister form on her lip, and she indicates with her finger that the blister had been on the vermillion border of her upper lip. She explains that the blister lasted about 2 weeks and disappeared after that 2-week period. She also tells you that she has had painful blisters like this before. Examination reveals that there is no evidence of a lip lesion at the time of this visit and no other oral pathology.

1. What might be a likely diagnosis for this blister?
2. What information should be given to the patient about this condition?

Ethical Dilemma

A mother brings her 8-year-old daughter to your office for an examination. The mother explains that Mary woke up 2 days ago with a slight fever and a headache. She explains that she took her daughter to a pediatrician who prescribed amoxicillin and referred Mary to your dental office. The mother explains that Mary's symptoms are not improved after 48 hours. When you examine Mary's oral tissues, you notice small vesicular lesions on her gingiva and on the dorsal surface of her tongue. Her oropharynx appeared clear of lesions. She has palpable cervical lymph nodes that are a bit tender. Mary's temperature is elevated. The mother is frustrated and asks you to tell her if the pediatrician managed her daughter's care properly.

1. How should you respond to the mother's frustration?
2. How should you respond to her question about the care provided by the pediatrician?

References

1. Harokopakis-Hajishengallis E. Physiologic root resorption in primary teeth: molecular and histological events. *J Oral Sci.* 2007;49(1):1–12.
2. Pinkham JR. *Pediatric Dentistry: Infancy Through Adolescence.* 4th ed. St. Louis, MO: Elsevier Saunders; 2005. xv, 750 pp.
3. Bimstein E, Peretz B, Holan G. Prevalence of gingival stippling in children. *J Clin Pediatr Dent.* 2003;27(2):163–165.
4. Gomes-Filho IS, Miranda DA, Trindade SC, et al. Relationship among gender, race, age, gingival width, and probing depth in primary teeth. *J Periodontol.* 2006;77(6):1032–1042.
5. Bosnjak A, Jorgić-Srdjak K, Maricević T, Plancak D. The width of clinically-defined keratinized gingiva in the mixed dentition. *ASDC J Dent Child.* 2002;69(3):266–270, 34.
6. Oh TJ, Eber R, Wang HL. Periodontal diseases in the child and adolescent. *J Clin Periodontol.* 2002;29(5):400–410.
7. Research, Science and Therapy Committee of the American Academy of Periodontology. Treatment of plaque-induced gingivitis, chronic periodontitis, and other clinical conditions. *Pediatr Dent.* 2017;39(6):445–454.
8. Guideline for periodontal therapy. *Pediatr Dent.* 2017;39(6):440–444.
9. Periodontal diseases of children and adolescents. *Pediatr Dent.* 2017;39(6):431–439.
10. Bimstein E, Matsson L. Growth and development considerations in the diagnosis of gingivitis and periodontitis in children. *Pediatr Dent.* 1999;21(3):186–191.
11. Wotman S, Mercadante J, Mandel ID, Goldman RS, Denning C. The occurrence of calculus in normal children, children with cystic fibrosis, and children with asthma. *J Periodontol.* 1973;44(5):278–280.
12. Califano JV; Research, Science and Therapy Committee American Academy of Periodontology. Position paper: periodontal diseases of children and adolescents. *J Periodontol.* 2003;74(11):1696–1704.
13. Armitage GC. Periodontal diagnoses and classification of periodontal diseases. *Periodontol 2000.* 2004;34:9–21.
14. Armitage GC, Cullinan MP. Comparison of the clinical features of chronic and aggressive periodontitis. *Periodontol 2000.* 2010;53:12–27.
15. Lang NP, Bartold M, Cullinan MP, et al. Consensus Report: Aggressive Periodontitis. *Ann Periodontol.* 1999;4(1):53.
16. Baer PN. The case for periodontosis as a clinical entity. *J Periodontol.* 1971;42(8):516–520.
17. Parameter on aggressive periodontitis. American Academy of Periodontology. *J Periodontol.* 2000;71(5 Suppl):867–869.
18. Monteiro Mde F, Casati MZ, Taiete T, et al. Periodontal clinical and microbiological characteristics in healthy versus generalized aggressive periodontitis families. *J Clin Periodontol.* 2015;42(10):914–921.
19. Nibali L, Donos N, Brett PM, et al. A familial analysis of aggressive periodontitis—clinical and genetic findings. *J Periodontal Res.* 2008;43(6):627–634.
20. Vieira AR, Albandar JM. Role of genetic factors in the pathogenesis of aggressive periodontitis. *Periodontol 2000.* 2014;65(1):92–106.
21. Stabholz A, Soskolne WA, Shapira L. Genetic and environmental risk factors for chronic periodontitis and aggressive periodontitis. *Periodontol 2000.* 2010;53:138–153.
22. Aberg CH, Kelk P, Johansson A. Aggregatibacter actinomycetemcomitans: virulence of its leukotoxin and association with aggressive periodontitis. *Virulence.* 2015;6(3):188–195.
23. Fredman G, Oh SF, Ayilavarapu S, Hasturk H, Serhan CN, Van Dyke TE. Impaired phagocytosis in localized aggressive periodontitis: rescue by Resolvin E1. *PLoS One.* 2011;6(9):e24422.
24. Van Dyke TE, Schweinebraten M, Cianciola LJ, Offenbacher S, Genco RJ. Neutrophil chemotaxis in families with localized juvenile periodontitis. *J Periodontal Res.* 1985;20(5):503–514.
25. Van Dyke TE, Zinney W, Winkel K, Taufiq A, Offenbacher S, Arnold RR. Neutrophil function in localized juvenile periodontitis. Phagocytosis, superoxide production and specific granule release. *J Periodontol.* 1986;57(11):703–708.
26. Allin N, Cruz-Almeida Y, Velsko I, et al. Inflammatory response influences treatment of localized aggressive periodontitis. *J Dent Res.* 2016;95(6):635–641.
27. Shaddox LM, Spencer WP, Velsko IM, et al. Localized aggressive periodontitis immune response to healthy and diseased subgingival plaque. *J Clin Periodontol.* 2016;43(9):746–753.

28. Needleman HL, Ku TC, Nelson L, Allred E, Seow WK. Alveolar bone height of primary and first permanent molars in healthy seven- to nine-year-old children. *ASDC J Dent Child.* 1997;64(3):188–196, 165.

29. Dopico J, Nibali L, Donos N. Disease progression in aggressive periodontitis patients. A retrospective study. *J Clin Periodontol.* 2016;43(6):531–537.

30. Manson JD, Lehner T. Clinical features of juvenile periodontitis (periodontosis). *J Periodontol.* 1974;45(8):636–640.

31. Liljenberg B, Lindhe J. Juvenile periodontitis. Some microbiological, histopathological and clinical characteristics. *J Clin Periodontol.* 1980;7(1):48–61.

32. Burmeister JA, Best AM, Palcanis KG, Caine FA, Ranney RR. Localized juvenile periodontitis and generalized severe periodontitis: clinical findings. *J Clin Periodontol.* 1984;11(3):181–192.

33. Saxen L, Murtomaa H. Age-related expression of juvenile periodontitis. *J Clin Periodontol.* 1985;12(1):21–26.

34. Delaney JE, Keels MA. Pediatric oral pathology. Soft tissue and periodontal conditions. *Pediatr Clin North Am.* 2000;47(5):1125–1147.

35. Eres G, Saribay A, Akkaya M. Periodontal treatment needs and prevalence of localized aggressive periodontitis in a young Turkish population. *J Periodontol.* 2009;80(6):940–944.

36. Fine DH, Markowitz K, Furgang D, et al. Aggregatibacter actinomycetemcomitans and its relationship to initiation of localized aggressive periodontitis: longitudinal cohort study of initially healthy adolescents. *J Clin Microbiol.* 2007;45(12):3859–3869.

37. Fine DH, Markowitz K, Fairlie K, et al. A consortium of Aggregatibacter actinomycetemcomitans, Streptococcus parasanguinis, and Filifactor alocis is present in sites prior to bone loss in a longitudinal study of localized aggressive periodontitis. *J Clin Microbiol.* 2013;51(9):2850–2861.

38. Armitage GC. Development of a classification system for periodontal diseases and conditions. *Ann Periodontol.* 1999;4(1):1–6.

39. Page RC, Vandesteen GE, Ebersole JL, Williams BL, Dixon IL, Altman LC. Clinical and laboratory studies of a family with a high prevalence of juvenile periodontitis. *J Periodontol.* 1985;56(10):602–610.

40. Sjodin B, Matsson L. Marginal bone level in the normal primary dentition. *J Clin Periodontol.* 1992;19(9 Pt 1):672–678.

41. Kornman KS, Robertson PB. Clinical and microbiological evaluation of therapy for juvenile periodontitis. *J Periodontol.* 1985;56(8):443–446.

42. Kapoor A, Malhotra R, Grover V, Grover D. Systemic antibiotic therapy in periodontics. *Dent Res J (Isfahan).* 2012;9(5):505–515.

43. van Winkelhoff AJ, Rams TE, Slots J. Systemic antibiotic therapy in periodontics. *Periodontol 2000.* 1996;10:45–78.

44. Loe H, Brown LJ. Early onset periodontitis in the United States of America. *J Periodontol.* 1991;62(10):608–616.

45. Page RC, Baab DA. A new look at the etiology and pathogenesis of early-onset periodontitis. Cementopathia revisited. *J Periodontol.* 1985;56(12):748–751.

46. Asikainen S, Jousimies-Somer H, Kanervo A, Saxen L. The immediate efficacy of adjunctive doxycycline in treatment of localized juvenile periodontitis. *Arch Oral Biol.* 1990;35 Suppl:231S–234S.

47. Gunsolley JC, Califano JV, Koertge TE, Burmeister JA, Cooper LC, Schenkein HA. Longitudinal assessment of early onset periodontitis. *J Periodontol.* 1995;66(5):321–328.

48. van Winkelhoff AJ, de Graaff J. Microbiology in the management of destructive periodontal disease. *J Clin Periodontol.* 1991;18(6):406–410.

49. King DL, Steinhauer W, Garcia-Godoy F, Elkins CJ. Herpetic gingivostomatitis and teething difficulty in infants. *Pediatr Dent.* 1992;14(2):82–85.

Part 6

Health Maintenance in Treated Periodontal Patients

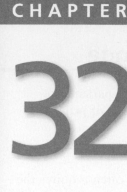

32 Encouraging Patient Behavior Change With Motivational Interviewing

Clinical Application. Behaviors such as effective plaque biofilm removal, adherence to regular professional periodontal maintenance visits, periodontal risk factor reduction, and healthy lifestyle habits, such as smoking cessation, are crucial issues for dental hygienists to address in their patient encounters. Effective management of the periodontal patient requires both knowledge of the disease process and understanding of human behavior and motivation to foster oral self-care behavior change in patients. Motivational interviewing as discussed in this chapter can be a useful tool for hygienists to employ when attempting to enhance behavior change in patients.

Learning Objectives

- Recognize the role of ambivalence in patient behavior change and explain the goal of Motivational Interviewing with respect to ambivalence.

- Describe the primary difference between how hygienists often approach patient education and the Motivational Interviewing approach.

- Identify the four key elements of the Motivational Interviewing.

- Give examples of specific Motivational Interviewing methods and how they are used to enhance patient motivation for change.

Key Terms

Motivational interviewing	Evocation	Engaging
Patient-centered	Open-ended questions	Focusing
Guiding style	OARS	Evoking
Ambivalence	Reflective listening	Planning
Partnership	Affirm	Change talk
Acceptance	Summaries	Sustain talk
Compassion	Elicit, Provide, Elicit	Developing discrepancy

Section 1
Introduction to Human Behavior Change

1. **Improved oral health often requires behavior change.** Working with patients to change their behavior is increasingly recognized as an important part of providing comprehensive health care.
   A. **Behavior change is important for prevention of periodontal diseases and maintenance of the periodontium**
      1. Chronic periodontitis is largely preventable, but prevention often requires the patient to become actively involved in making and maintaining changes in his or her oral self-care and lifestyle habits.
      2. Dental hygienists instruct their patients to change or engage in certain behaviors—use soft tuft-end toothbrushes, floss regularly, or stop smoking.
   B. **Helping patients change behavior can be very challenging**
      1. Dental hygienists often encounter periodontal patients who do not practice effective oral self-care measures or adhere to recommendations for professional periodontal maintenance. In order to persuade patients to improve, dental hygienists usually attempt to educate patients regarding the importance of these behaviors.
      2. Unfortunately, education and expert advice is usually not very effective in getting patients to change their behavior. Patients often do not follow through and may even argue with their hygienist about why they are unable to make the change. Patients can become resistant and hygienists can become frustrated and even convinced that talking about behavior change is pointless (Fig. 32-1).
   C. **There are many reasons why patients do not change behavior**
      1. Although it is tempting to blame the patient for being resistant, a great deal of research has shown there are many understandable reasons why patients struggle with health behavior change.
      2. Patient motivation is affected by such things as past life experiences (e.g., attitudes, beliefs, and habits developed over time), their current circumstances (e.g., lack of time, lack of money, health literacy, and knowledge), and their confidence and skills to make the necessary behavior change.[1,2] These can be very big barriers and probably explain why even dental hygienists do not lead perfectly healthy lives!
      3. The communication style used by the dental hygienist can increase or reduce patient motivation to change.[3,4] Motivation is important because behavior change usually takes energy and time. Patients are asked to make behavior change an important priority even though they may not have decided whether or not it is an important priority.
   D. **Education and advice can reduce patient motivation**
      1. Dental hygienists typically try to persuade their patients to change by offering facts about oral disease and giving advice on what the patient needs to do differently. This "directive" style of communication in which the dental hygienist acts as the "expert" and the patient is the "recipient" often reduces motivation.
      2. When patients are not ready to change, or have struggled with change, being directed to change can often make them feel embarrassed, guilty, or even ashamed. Patients often become defensive, explaining why they cannot or have not been doing the right thing (Fig. 32-2). They may ignore the advice given or delay returning for treatment.[5-8]
      3. Studies have shown that approximately 30% to 60% of health information provided by clinicians is forgotten within an hour! Also, when asked to recall what advice was given and what next steps were agreed to during an encounter,

patients and providers do not agree.[9,10] It is therefore not surprising, that 50% of health recommendations provided by clinicians are not followed.[10]

4. In order to better help patients with behavior change, an alternative to the usual expert-oriented, directive, educational approach is needed. Motivational Interviewing is an alternative that research has shown is effective at increasing behavior change.

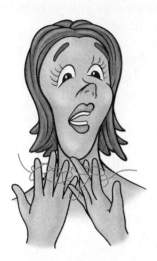

Figure 32-1. The Self-Care Struggle. Patients often struggle with professional recommendations for self-care—such as flossing—leading to frustration or even resistance to oral self-care routines.

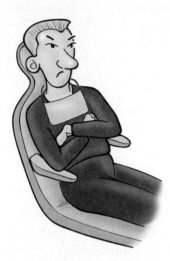

Figure 32-2. Defensive Patient Response. Health education advice alone usually creates defensiveness in the patient.

2. **Motivational Interviewing encourages change through guiding rather than directing.** Motivational Interviewing offers a way of working with patients on behavior change that differs from directive education or advice. Rather than assuming the reason patients do not change their behavior is because they need information and advice, Motivational Interviewing focuses on exploring what the patient thinks about changing their behavior.

A. **Motivational Interviewing is a way of building motivation for change**

   1. Motivational interviewing is a method of counseling or talking with patients to encourage behavior change. The goal is to collaborate with patients to strengthen their *own* (internal) motivation and commitment to change rather than to persuade.[6]

B. **Motivational Interviewing is "patient-centered"**

   1. Being patient-centered means the clinician works to understand the way the patient sees the situation. For example, the clinician may want a patient not to smoke in order to prevent periodontitis. While the patient might like to have healthier gums, s/he may enjoy smoking too much to quit. It is important for the clinician to understand, acknowledge, and be accepting of the fact that the patient finds smoking enjoyable.

   2. Although the approach is patient-centered this does not mean that the clinician does not try to encourage behavior change. In Motivational Interviewing, the clinician DOES influence and guide the patient toward healthy behavior change, but not in a directive, expert-driven way.

   3. The alternative to being "directive" is to use a "**guiding style.**"[11] In the guiding style, a clinician doesn't tell the patient what to do but rather asks the patient what their thoughts are about trying to floss every day.

C. **Patients are ambivalent about change**
1. One of the assumptions of motivational interviewing is that it is normal to have mixed feelings or ambivalence about *ANY* behavior change process. For example, how do *you* feel about recommended health behaviors like eating at least five servings of fruit and vegetables every day, or exercising for 40 minutes 5 to 7 days a week? Almost everyone has experience with struggling to engage in some behavior they know they ought to be doing. When you think about your own behavior, it is usually quite easy to see the reasons why you want to engage in the healthy behavior and reasons why you do not or cannot.
2. Motivational Interviewing also assumes that, when possible, patients *WANT* to be healthy. Even though patients may emphasize why they *are not* able or motivated to make a change, they almost always prefer to be healthy if they can.

D. **Motivational Interviewing focuses on internal motivation**
1. In Motivational Interviewing, the clinician encourages patients to talk about *their reasons* for change because the patient's own reasons for making a change are considered much more likely to lead to behavior change than reasons a clinician might provide.
2. One way to think about this is that patients are more likely to act if they are "internally" rather than "externally" motivated. Specific strategies are used to increase "internal" motivation.

3. **Motivational Interviewing is effective and useful.** Motivational Interviewing is being used more and more in health care because of its effectiveness and usefulness.

A. **Motivational Interviewing is clinically proven.**
1. You may be thinking that Motivational Interviewing sounds quite complicated and wondering if trying to understand it is worth it. One reason you may want to try learning Motivational Interviewing is that research shows it is effective.
2. Studies that combine the results of multiple studies find motivational interviewing is effective for changing many different behaviors including those that improve health.[12–16] Studies with periodontal patients have also had generally good results.[17–24]
3. Patient outcomes also seem to improve in relation to the amount of time or number of sessions of motivational interviewing that are provided.[13] This suggests that hygienists could maximize their impact on periodontal patients if they used motivational interviewing repeatedly during treatment and maintenance phases.

B. **Dental Hygiene students are learning and using Motivational Interviewing.**
1. Motivational interviewing training is increasingly becoming part of the dental hygiene curriculum in the United States and abroad.
2. A recent study found that both dental hygiene faculty and students liked having motivational interviewing as part of the curriculum. Students who received motivational interviewing training also performed better on a standardized patient assessment of their ability to motivate patients.[25]
3. *Although clinicians are often worried about the time it may take to do Motivational Interviewing, as little as 15 minutes has been shown to be effective in the majority of studies.*[12,26]

Section 2
Components of Motivational Interviewing

1. **The "Spirit" of Motivational Interviewing**
   A. **Key Elements.** Motivational interviewing is more than just a set of techniques or strategies. Motivational Interviewing requires clinicians to adopt a particular philosophy or "spirit" of working with their patients. The philosophy or "spirit" of motivational interviewing is captured in four key elements (Fig. 32-3).
      1. The first element is **partnership** between the patient and clinician. In the motivational interviewing approach, the clinician tries to avoid being "the expert." The patient, not the clinician, is viewed as the expert on his or her life and the challenges of behavior change.
      2. The second element is complete **acceptance** of the patient and their choices. Acceptance includes avoiding judgment, supporting the patient's freedom to make their own choices, understanding the patient's perspective, and affirming their strengths and efforts.
      3. The third element is **compassion** which refers to the importance of using motivational interviewing only for the welfare of the patient.
      4. The fourth element is **evocation**, in which the clinician encourages the patient to do the talking. This is how the clinician learns about the way the patient views the situation and finds out about any internal motivation the patient may have. The clinician does not attempt to persuade the patient.
   B. **Responsibility for Change.** Although it is sometimes easy for a health care provider to feel frustrated with the behavior of a patient, in motivational interviewing, the clinician recognizes they are not responsible for their patient's decisions. It is ultimately not the clinician's choice or life.
      1. Patients are far more likely to choose and succeed with behavior change when they have voiced their own reasons for change and made their own decision to commit.
      2. The final decision for change rests with the patient. The clinician may communicate respect for the patient's freedom to choose directly such as "*So how would you like to proceed?*" or indirectly such as at the beginning of the visit by asking permission to talk about oral self-care (Fig. 32-4). Paradoxically, patients who feel their provider is giving them the freedom to choose are more likely to follow the guidance of their provider.

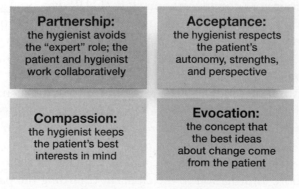

Figure 32-3. Four Key Elements of Motivational Interviewing. The motivational interviewing philosophy integrates four key elements: partnership, acceptance, compassion, and evocation.

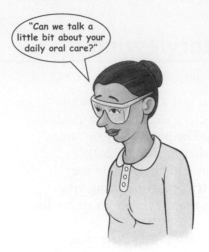

Figure 32-4. Asking Permission. Starting with asking the patient's permission can help foster a collaborative partnership.

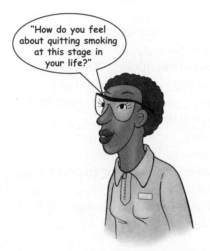

Figure 32-5. Use of Open-Ended Questions. Open-ended questions—that cannot be answered with a simple "yes" or "no" response—encourage the patient to provide additional information.

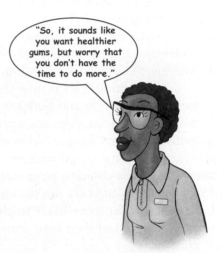

Figure 32-6. Reflecting Listening. By paraphrasing the patient's remarks, the clinician can double check if she understands the meaning of the patient's comments correctly.

2. **Motivational Interviewing Core Skills and Strategies.** Motivational interviewing requires skillful use of four core communication skills. **OARS** is a brief way to remember these four skills: Open-ended questions, Affirmations, Reflections, and Summaries. In health care settings, it is also important to know how to give advice in a patient-centered style (see E below). We have added this as another core skill of MI.

A. **Open-ended questions**
   1. Open-ended questions are inquiries that are framed to avoid a simple yes/no response. For example, "*How do you feel about using dental floss?*" "*How does brushing and flossing fit into your routine*" rather than "*Do you use dental floss?*" or "*Do you brush twice a day?*".
   2. The open-ended style of questioning encourages patients to elaborate and provides much more information to the clinician regarding the patient's perspective (Fig. 32-5).

B. **Reflective Listening**
  1. **Reflective listening** is the process in which the health care provider listens to the patient's remarks and then paraphrases what the clinician heard the patient say. This approach allows the clinician to check if he or she is correctly understanding the meaning of what the patient is saying (Fig. 32-6).
  2. Reflective listening helps patients feel understood and accepted, even if their behaviors are not healthy. Expressing understanding (or empathy) also typically encourages the patient to elaborate so that the clinician can learn more about how the patient sees the situation.
  3. Skilled reflective listening incorporates body language and tone of voice and may also involve inferring what is implied by the patient's remarks. For example, the patient's tone of voice may suggest emotions (such as worry or fear) that are not directly expressed in words (e.g., *"Talking about quitting smoking is difficult because it makes you think about serious health effects that scare you.").*
  4. Through the process of open-ended questioning and reflective listening, the clinician shifts from being a directive expert to using a patient-centered guiding style. Unfortunately, research shows that the average health care provider interrupts patient disclosures after 18 seconds.[10] Interrupting the patient sends a clear message that the patient's input is not respected or seen as relevant.
  5. Inviting patients to explain their view of the situation through open questions and reflective listening increases patients' willingness to honestly express themselves about their ambivalence or mixed feelings about change (Fig. 32-7).

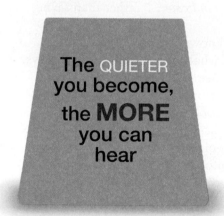

The QUIETER you become, the **MORE** you can hear

Figure 32-7. Listening. As clinicians, we all need to be reminded of how important it is to sometimes just sit back and listen to what our patients have to say.

C. **Affirm**
  1. In motivational interviewing, the clinician should **affirm** (acknowledge, support) the patient's willingness to discuss a difficult topic (i.e., a change about which they may feel embarrassment, guilt, and ambivalence).
  2. The clinician may express appreciation for the patient being willing to discuss their smoking or taking some small steps toward change. Affirming can strengthen the bond between the clinician and the patient and encourage the patient to engage further in the behavior change discussion (e.g., *"Thank you for taking the time to help me understand how busy your days are now that you are caring for your elderly mother in your home.").*

D. **Summarize**

1. Brief summaries are used in motivational interviewing to link and reinforce what has been discussed and provide an opportunity for the clinician to demonstrate empathy (e.g., *"So I think I now have a fairly good picture of how you view your smoking...."*).

2. Summaries can be used to move the conversation in a new direction (e.g., the summary can lead to a statement like *"So given what we've talked about so far, what are your thoughts about the next step..."*

3. Summaries also are used to tie different elements of the conversation together (e.g., after summarizing the patient's perspective on the difficulties of brushing regularly, the clinician might link to an earlier part of the conversation on the patient's dislike of the pain that he is experiencing: *"So it sounds like it's a real challenge to get a good brushing routine but at the same time you are really unhappy with the pain you are experiencing...."*).

E. **Providing Information and Advice in Motivational Interviewing**

1. As discussed, it is very common for clinicians to take on the role of expert and to give their patients advice. Yet there are times when it would be helpful to provide information to a patient. For example, if the patient asks for information, or if new information might help in overcoming obstacles to change. MI offers strategies for giving information that help avoid "taking on the expert role." One strategy is to first ask for permission: *"Would you be interested in hearing some more information about the benefits of quitting smoking for your oral health?"* (Fig. 32-8). When providing information, the clinician can further avoid coming across as the expert by referring to other sources for the information such as *"Many patients tell me..."* or *"Research seems to indicate..."* rather than saying *"I have found..."* or *"I would recommend..."*.

2. Another strategy is to use a three-step process known as **"Elicit, Provide, Elicit."** The first step (Elicit) involves enquiring what the patient already knows. For example, *"What have you heard about the benefits of flossing on a daily basis?"*. The second step (Provide) involves the providing relevant information and advice: *"Yes you are right, those are some good reasons to floss daily. There are also some other reasons dental hygienists encourage flossing for cases like yours, such as..."*. The final step (Elicit) involves checking back with the patient to see what they have taken from the information or advice provided. For example, *"So I'm wondering what you think about that research and how it applies to you?"*.

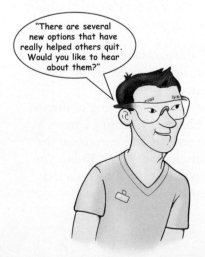

Figure 32-8. Providing Information or Advice. In this example, the clinician supports the patient's autonomy by asking permission before providing information.

3. **The Four Processes of Motivational Interviewing**
   The four processes of MI are the engaging, focusing, evoking, and planning stages. These four processes may not all occur in one appointment or in sequence. Rather, the four processes are employed, as needed, throughout the conversation.
   A. **Engaging: The "connection" process.** The first process upon meeting a patient is to engage the patient in wanting to work together. Engaging establishes the connection or rapport that is the foundation for everything that follows.
      1. Core skills, or OARS, are used in all four stages of MI. Rather than beginning the interaction with a series of closed-ended questions to gather patient information, in motivational interviewing the clinician immediately encourages the patient to talk using the OARS skills:
         a. An open-ended question can be used to initiate the discussion (e.g., *"What kinds of problems have you been having with your teeth lately?"*).
         b. Reflective listening can then be used to encourage the patient to elaborate while at the same time communicating empathy and acceptance (e.g., *"You've noticed your gums are bleeding a lot."*).
         c. During the listening process, the clinician pays attention to any opportunities to affirm the patient for any strengths or efforts (e.g., *"You've really been making an effort to try to brush more regularly."*).
         d. Summaries can be used to tie the conversation together highlighting the most relevant parts of the patient's story.
      2. During this engaging process, the clinician is focused on developing an understanding of the situation as the patient sees it. There is no attempt to provide education or advice.
      3. The clinician should be mindful of the following during engaging:
         a. Am I using open-ended questions to encourage the patient to talk openly?
         b. Am I using reflective listening once the patient starts answering my questions?
         c. Can I summarize the patient's view of the problem?
   B. **Focusing: The "What" Process.** The focusing process is about collaborating with the patient to find a clear direction or goal. At this stage, the OARS skills are used to develop an understanding of patient priorities; as well as, to collaborate with the patient to determine focus for behavior change.
      1. Focusing is the process of clarifying, in collaboration with the patient, what direction the conversation about behavior change should take.
      2. A guiding style can be used to explore the patients' preferences, concerns, and priorities while considering the clinicians' concerns and priorities. For example, the clinician may offer a range of alternative options for discussion (e.g., *"We should decide what is most important to focus on today. We could talk about some of the challenges you're having with your brushing and flossing routine, we could discuss how to go about changing some of your eating habits to protect your teeth and gums, or we could talk about your smoking and how I could perhaps be of some help."*).
      3. During the focusing stage, it may be necessary to provide information to the patient. The clinician can use the "elicit, provide, elicit" method to accomplish this in a motivational interviewing consistent style.

4. The clinician should be mindful of the following during engagement:
   a. What goals for change does this patient have?
   b. Do I have different goals for change for this patient?
   c. Are we working together with a common purpose? Or moving in different directions?

C. **Evoking: The "Why Process".** With the goal in mind, the process of **evoking** is used to encourage the patient to express their motivation and confidence to change. The OARS skills are used to encourage patients to talk about and elaborate on their reasons for change and, as necessary, to acknowledge reasons they do not want to change.

   1. As discussed previously, most patients have mixed feelings about change. In this process, the role of the clinician is to encourage the patient to talk about ambivalent feelings and elicit reasons that he/she has for wanting to change. *The task of the clinician is to evoke, facilitate, and strengthen this patient's own desire for change.*

      a. Statements made by the patient "in the direction" of change are referred to as **change talk** (e.g., *"I know smoking is bad for me; I would like to do a better job with taking care of my teeth."*). Research indicates that the more patients express change talk, the more likely they change their behavior.[6,27]

      b. Change talk can be encouraged with a simple open-ended question such as *"What advantages, if any, do you see of cutting back on sugary foods?"*.

      c. Another approach is to use the "motivation" or "importance ruler" in which the clinician asks, *"On a scale of 0 to 10 with 10 being most important, how important is to you to improve your oral self-care habits?"* (Fig. 32-9). Because patients are generally ambivalent they will rarely answer this question with a zero. This implies that they place at least *some* importance on making a change.

         1) Once the patient identifies the self-rated importance of change (red bar), the clinician encourages change talk by asking, *"What made you pick [number] rather than zero?"*. Asking this open-ended question encourages the patient to express any importance that he or she DOES place on improving oral self-care behaviors even if the number is low. This is change talk.

         2) After asking about and reflecting change talk, barriers to change can also be explored by asking, *"What would it take for you to increase the importance from a [number] to a [higher number]?"* (green bar). This approach can also be used to encourage talk about the patient's confidence (or self-efficacy) to make a change. Having confidence to make a change is a key contributor to an individual's motivation and success in making behavior change.

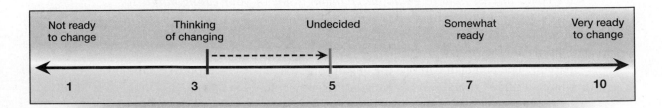

Figure 32-9. A Motivation Ruler. A motivation ruler is a method for facilitating change talk.

2. In general, once the clinician has encouraged the initial expression of change talk, the goal is to encourage even more change talk.
   a. Reflective listening is very effective means of encouraging elaboration of a topic.
   b. For example, a reflection might sound like: "*You want to cut down on sugary foods partly because you want to set a good example to your children*", encourages elaboration by the patient of the desire to set a good example.
3. Because patients are ambivalent, they are also likely to talk about the reasons they do not want to change or why they find it difficult to change. Statements that are against change (or in favor of continuing with their current behavior) are referred to as "**sustain talk**" (e.g., "*I don't have enough time to floss every day.*").
   a. When the patient expresses reasons not to change, this is an ideal opportunity to listen well and acknowledge the patient's perspective rather than attempting to persuade or provide counter arguments.
   b. Acknowledging the patient's mixed feelings can most simply be done with reflective listening (Fig. 32-10). Patients whose concerns or hesitations about change have been validated through reflective listening are usually much readier to also talk about the reasons why they might want to change.
4. As mentioned previously, a key component of motivation for behavior change is having the confidence to overcome obstacles to making the change.[2] It is common for patients to bring up obstacles to change after they have acknowledged the need to change or the desire to change. To help encourage patients to overcome obstacles the clinician can evoke confidence in various ways, including brainstorming possible solutions, providing information and advice, or reviewing past successes.
5. Evoking may also involve "**developing discrepancy**" in which inconsistencies between a patient's values and goals and their current behavior are explored to enhance motivation for change. For example, most patients want to be healthy even though they may miss appointments for periodontal maintenance.
   a. The discrepancy between what would be ideal (e.g., be healthy or have no pain) and the status quo (poor self-care that results in periodontitis) can be elicited through open-ended questions and reflective listening (Fig. 32-11).
   b. For example, the hygienist might highlight the discrepancy with this reflection: "*It sounds like you find it hard to stick with the thorough brushing and flossing each day, but you would really like to have healthy gums.*" Highlighting the discrepancy between the patient's behavior and what he says that he values (healthy gums).
6. The clinician should be mindful of the following during evoking:
   a. What are the patient's reasons for wanting to change?
   b. Is the patient's reluctance due to a lack of confidence in his ability to change or because he feels that the change is not important?
   c. What "change talk" am I hearing?

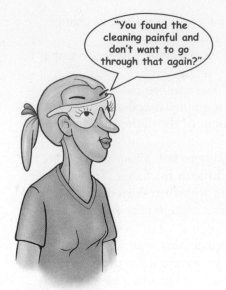

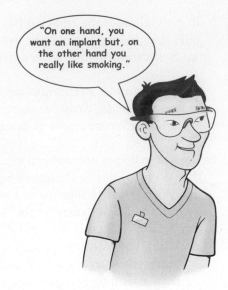

Figure 32-10. Reflecting Sustain Talk. When a patient expresses hesitation about change, the clinician should listen well and explore the patient's point of view rather than attempting to persuade the patient that change is needed.

Figure 32-11. Develop Discrepancy. Open-ended questions and reflective listening can highlight discrepancies between what would be ideal (e.g., improved health) and the status quo (continuing to smoke).

D. **Planning: The "How" Process.** When patients become sufficiently interested in making change, the process of **planning** can begin. The goal is to encourage commitment to change and to develop a specific plan of action for change. The OARS skills are used in this process to ensure the plan for change is developed collaboratively rather than falling into the trap of telling the patient what to do.

1. The planning process can begin when the patient is ready to discuss changing. Signs of readiness include the patient expressing more change talk and less sustain talk, asking questions about change, or taking some small steps toward change. At this stage of the process, the hygienist should remain alert to any renewed patient ambivalence that might call for a return to one of the earlier three processes.

2. The clinician guides the patient to consider whether they want to make a change and how that change will occur.

   a. Effective planning involves discussing with the patient the precise "how?" and "when?" of making the change. For example, rather than simply agreeing with the patient that they will "try to do a better job of brushing" the clinician might help the patient to work out a specific plan that will increase the likelihood of brushing (e.g., to brush right after eating dinner rather waiting until just before going to bed when they feel too tired to do even one more thing).

   b. Once the plan is developed the clinician will attempt to strengthen commitment to the plan by evoking intention and commitment from the patient (e.g., *"What do you think of that strategy?* or *"Does it sound like something you want to try?"*).

3. The clinician should be mindful of the following during planning:

   a. Does the patient seem on board with making a plan?

   b. Are they coming up with the main ideas for the plan?

   c. Once the plan is summarized are they willing to commit to the plan?

Section 3
Implications for Dental Hygiene Practice

Moving from the clinician-centered perspective of oral health education to the patient-centered view of behavior change can enhance the patient's motivation for a healthy behavior change. Using motivational interviewing, the hygienist can engage in a more productive interaction in which he or she no longer feels responsible (and frustrated!) about the patient's decisions. Instead, the hygienist focuses on encouraging the patient to examine his or her attitudes about periodontal disease, healthy oral health behaviors, or the periodontal maintenance schedule.

MOTIVATIONAL INTERVIEWING: EXAMPLE 1

Mrs. J. is a 50-year-old attorney who has been referred to your periodontal dental office for evaluation and treatment. Mrs. J. has type 2 diabetes, a glycosylated hemoglobin value (HbA1c) of 8, and moderately severe chronic periodontitis. Mrs. J. has been sporadic in visiting her regular dentist and the letter from the referring dentist states that after a 1-year absence Mrs. J. presented recently with increased bleeding on probing and evidence of increasing attachment loss. The general dentist is concerned that without periodontal therapy, Mrs. J. will likely lose several teeth.

> **Hygienist:** I see your general dentist has referred you here for periodontal treatment. Can you tell me a little about your past dental care and why you are here today?
>
> **Mrs. J.:** Yes, Dr. Smith thinks if I don't get specialty treatment I'm going to lose some of my back teeth. I take care of my teeth and I think he's over reacting to my gums bleeding a bit more than usual. My gums have always bled.
>
> **Hygienist:** I am very happy you followed up with Dr. Smith and came in to see us. [Affirmation] So if it's okay with you, I'd like to spend a little time talking about the health of your gums. [Getting permission]
>
> **Mrs. J.:** That's fine with me.
>
> **Hygienist:** Good. So, if you would, can you tell me what is a typical day is like for you and how taking care of your teeth fits into your normal day? [Open-ended question]
>
> **Mrs. J.:** Sure. Most days I need to be at my office by 8:30, so I generally get up around 7, shower, have some coffee and toast, check emails, brush my teeth and drive my 20-minute commute to the office. Once I'm at my office, my schedule is really full. I'm currently working on three really difficult cases that take up most of my time. I'm pretty stressed out! I don't eat a regular lunch but will usually snack on a granola bar to hold me over to dinner. I'm usually home around 6:30, have dinner, and then catch up on reading documents for the next day. Sometimes I brush my teeth before bed, but mostly I'm just too exhausted to care at night. I do try, but don't always succeed. The dental hygienist at Dr. Smith's is always on my case about not brushing enough, not flossing enough, and not coming in every 3 months.
>
> **Hygienist:** It sounds like you have a really busy schedule that makes it difficult for you to keep up with recommendations given by Dr. Smith's hygienist. If I understand you, though, you do make a concerted effort to brush at least every morning. [Reflective listening]
>
> **Mrs. J.:** Yes, I am very good about brushing in the morning.
>
> **Hygienist:** That's great. It's important to have a routine that works well for you. [Affirmation] You mentioned that the hygienist at Dr. Smith's office is concerned that you were not flossing enough or coming in every 3 months. Tell me about that. [Open-ended questioning]

Mrs. J.: Shelley, that's her name, says that if I don't floss every day and come in to have my teeth scraped every 3 months that I'll end up losing my teeth. She lectures me every time I go in, and I really dread going to see her. I don't think she understands how busy I am. The only reason I agreed to come here was that Dr. Smith thought you might be able to do something to get rid of my pockets.

Hygienist: So, it sounds like you are interested in improving your gum health but don't like being lectured when you go to the dentist. [Reflective listening]

Mrs. J.: That's right. I also read in a magazine that diabetes might make my gum disease worse, so I figured it's worth finding out. Is that true? Can my diabetes make my gums worse? Can you get rid of my pockets so this gum disease will stop?

Hygienist: There is quite a bit of new information about diabetes and periodontal disease, and there are some things that we can do at our office to reduce pockets. Research has shown that controlling gum disease, especially in diabetics, requires professional care but also requires patients to be actively involved in helping control the disease on a day-to-day basis. We have had many patients who have had very good success using this approach. Would you like to know more about it? [Providing information that was requested/Supporting autonomy]

Mrs. J.: I would like to know more, but I'm skeptical that it's going to be more of the same that I hear from Shelley—"brush—floss—come to see me—brush—floss—come to see me."

Hygienist: Right…you want help but worry that it will still involve more effort on your part than you really have time for. [Reflect]

Mrs. J.: Exactly!

Hygienist: Well, I want to emphasize that how we move forward is up to you. The time and effort you put in brushing and flossing is something you will need to determine based on what's most important to you. [Support autonomy] If it's ok with you [Support autonomy/Ask permission], I'd like to try to go slowly, try to work with your busy schedule, and help you keep your teeth. After I conduct my exam, I'd also like to give you some information on diabetes and gum disease that you can read before your next visit and then we can talk more about how that might be contributing to your gum disease. Are you interested in that? [Support autonomy/Ask permission]

Mrs. J.: That sounds good—the magazine article didn't give much detail, but it did say that diabetes can make gum disease worse. I'll make it a point of adding it to my evening reading tonight.

Hygienist: Excellent! I think you might find the information helpful as we work toward getting your gum disease under control.

MOTIVATIONAL INTERVIEWING: EXAMPLE 2

Mr. A. is a 58-year-old banker who has come to the dental office wanting an implant for a first premolar that was lost due to periodontal disease last year. At the time, he was not interested in discussing a replacement but has made an appointment today, as he wants to get an implant for replacement. Although he contends he brushes and flosses regularly, his oral self-care has only been fair for many years, he has a 30-year tobacco habit, and is currently smoking about 1½ pack of cigarettes a day.

Hygienist: Good morning Mr. A. What brings you in today? [Open ended questioning]

Mr. A.: Well, you know, I have this missing tooth here and when I chew it really bothers me. You know, food gets stuck up in there and on top of that it just doesn't look good when I smile. A buddy at work told me about implants and I'm seriously interested in getting one.

Hygienist: So, where your tooth is missing is causing you some problems and you aren't happy with the appearance of that gap. [Reflective listening]

Mr. A.: Yeah, every time I eat I get food caught. It doesn't hurt but it's gotten really irritating. I know we talked about it when you took the tooth out, but I don't want a partial. I really want the implant.

Hygienist: Your friend told you about dental implants and you think it's the right choice for replacing that tooth. [Reflective listening]

Mr. A.: That's right. I know when I was here before you said that my smoking might be a problem with getting an implant.

Hygienist: Yes, smoking is a major barrier for using implants because it makes it much harder for healing to occur and then maintain the health of tissues around the implant. But it sounds like you are really interested in getting an implant. [Providing information in response to an implied question/Reflective listening]

Mr. A.: I am!

Hygienist: Well, can we spend a few minutes talking about your smoking, and what your thoughts and feelings about smoking are? [Asking permission]

Mr. A.: Sure, I'm a smoker and not ashamed of it.

Hygienist: Okay, let me put it another way. On the one hand you want an implant but on the other hand you really like smoking? [Developing discrepancy]

Mr. A.: Well I've tried to quit before and it wasn't any fun. I'm not sure I could quit if I wanted to.

Hygienist: Okay. You have tried to stop before without any luck so you have the sense that even if you wanted to try to quit again, you don't think you could. It's something that is very hard for you. [Reflective listening]

Mr. A.: I went through that agony before and it didn't work. I don't want to put myself through that again.

Hygienist: Trying to quit would be too painful and it's not important enough to you to stop right now. [Rolling with resistance]

Mr. A.: Yes, I enjoy it and haven't had any ill effects from smoking. I'm pretty happy to continue as I am.

Hygienist: Well, other than the possible disadvantage that smoking has to getting this implant, are there any other disadvantages that you see to smoking? [Evoking change talk]

Mr. A.: Taxes keep going up, and it's an expensive habit, but I'm willing to pay the price. It's one of my luxuries in life.

Hygienist: Anything else? [Evoking change talk]

Mr. A.: Only one thing – my kids really want me to quit. They are afraid I'm going to end up with something bad, but I haven't had any ill effects from smoking.

Hygienist: So, it sounds like the cost of smoking bothers you, but not too much, but you really haven't had any health problems. Your family worries though. [Reflective listening to evoke more change talk]

Mr. A.: Yes, that's right.

Hygienist: I have the sense that you're not ready to quit right now, but I'd like to learn more regarding your thoughts about smoking if that's ok with you. Where would you put yourself on a scale of 0 to 10 where 0 is "no motivation at all to quit" and 10 is "very motivated"? I know you aren't a 10, but where would you be. [Evoking change talk using the motivation ruler]

Mr. A.: Hmmmm. I'd probably put myself at a 2 or 3, somewhere in there.

Hygienist: So, you have some small amount of motivation to quit—what gives you that level of motivation? [Evoking change talk using the motivation ruler]

Mr. A.: Well I know that smoking isn't good for me, I'm not dumb. And like I said before, my family really wants me to quit. It would be a nice gesture to do that for my family. They really do have my best interests in mind.

Hygienist: You mentioned you know smoking isn't good for you and your family worries about your health. Can you tell me what ill health effects worry you? [Evoking change talk]

Mr. A.: Sure—cancer and lung disease.

Hygienist: So, there are some disadvantages besides the implant that you've thought about but you still aren't sufficiently motivated to quit. Earlier, though, you mentioned that you weren't sure that you would be able to quit even if you wanted to. [Reflective listening to explore influence of confidence on motivation] How motivated would you be if you were more confident that you could quit?

Mr. A.: I guess if I knew I could succeed with quitting I'd be more motivated.

Hygienist: If we could help you with improving your confidence in quitting, would you find that helpful? [Evoking change talk/Assess interest before providing information or advice to support autonomy]

Mr. A.: Yes, it might.

Hygienist: There are several options that we could work on to improve your confidence to quit smoking. We could focus on doing that while also discussing the feasibility of the implant. Do you think you might be interested in pursuing this? [Evoke commitment/change talk while supporting autonomy]

Mr. A.: Sure. I guess I don't have anything to lose.

MOTIVATIONAL INTERVIEWING: EXAMPLE 3

Ms. S. is a 35-year-old administrative assistant at the local community college. She has come to the dental office as a new patient and desires tooth whitening for her "yellowed teeth." During the routine dental evaluation, no caries are found; however, there is generalized moderate gingival inflammation with slight bone loss in the interproximal posterior regions. The patient reports that she had a partial "deep cleaning" 2 years ago at her previous dentist but had really sensitive teeth and didn't return for completing treatment.

Hygienist: Hello Ms. S. What brings you to our office? [Open-ended questioning]

Ms. S.: My friend recently came to see you to have his teeth whitened and they look terrific. I haven't been happy with the color of my teeth for a long time, so I thought you could make my smile whiter too.

Hygienist: Okay. Can we first spend a few minutes talking about your mouth and oral health? [Getting permission]

Ms. S.: Sure, that's fine.

Hygienist: Good. Can you tell me a little about problems you have had and how taking care of your teeth fits into your regular day's events? [Open-ended questioning]

Ms. S.: I have really healthy teeth and have never had any cavities. I'm really not happy with the yellow color of my teeth and want to do something about that.

Hygienist: Anything else?

Ms. S.: Well, the last dentist I went to said I had some gum disease. My gums have always bled when I brush, but they made a big deal out of it. I had to see the hygienist for a deep cleaning, but my teeth got so sensitive afterward, I didn't go back.

Hygienist: Tell me a little more about your gum treatment. [Open-ended questioning]

Ms. S.: The dentist and hygienist told me I had to have that deep cleaning or I could lose my teeth. Everyone in my family has gum disease and they still have most of their teeth. I must have inherited it. I'm really only interested in tooth whitening. I don't want to have any more deep cleanings.

Hygienist: It sounds like the deep cleaning you had was unpleasant and your gum disease is not very important to you. [Reflective listening]

Ms. S.: I didn't say it wasn't important—I just want my teeth to look better. My teeth were so sensitive after having half of my mouth deep cleaned, I could barely drink anything with ice in it. If that is what it takes to have healthy gums, I'm happy just as I am.

Hygienist: The effects of the deep cleaning treatment were so bad that you don't want to go through it again even if it means not having healthy gums. [Responding to sustain talk with reflective listening]

Ms. S.: It's not that it isn't important. I don't want to lose my teeth, but I also don't want all of that sensitivity. I was thinking that getting my teeth whitened will make me look better and wouldn't hurt as much.

Hygienist: Avoiding pain is important to you. [Responding to sustain talk with reflective listening]

Ms. S.: Yeah, I guess I sound pretty wimpy. My teeth are important but if I have to be in pain for a long time afterward it's not worth it to me.

Hygienist: You want healthy teeth and if you could get your teeth whitened and gum disease treated without a lot of pain afterward, it might be worth doing. [Reflective listening]

Ms. S.: If I knew that I could get my gums healthy and not have to go through what I did before, I might be willing to discuss gum treatments. Is that possible?

Hygienist: There are several things that have worked for others to reduce the temperature sensitivity after deep cleaning. Are you interested in learning a little bit more? [Ask permission before providing information]

Ms. S.: I might be.

Hygienist: All right, let me give you some information and we can talk about strategies for controlling the sensitivity after treatment. We can also talk about a plan for whitening your teeth once we get the gum disease under control. How would that meet your need for appearance and health? [Support autonomy]

Chapter Summary Statement

A key challenge for dental hygiene practitioners is working with patients to foster behavior change. Motivational interviewing provides an empirically supported approach to the challenges of counseling patients for health behavior change. It rests on a foundation of partnership, acceptance, and compassion and uses specific methods such as open-ended questions and reflective listening to evoke patients' own reasons for change. Use of this patient-centered approach to behavior change can enhance the quality of encounters between hygienists and their patients by fostering greater patient motivation for change and strengthening the patient–provider relationship.

Section 4
Focus on Patients

Clinical Patient Care

CASE 1

Refer to the case of Mrs. J. the 50-year-old attorney to answer the following questions:

1. Why does the hygienist begin with the question *"Can you tell me a little about . . . why you are here today?"*
2. Describe Mrs. J's ambivalence regarding behavior change (i.e., what cons AND pros for change does SHE see?).
3. What examples of "change talk" can you identify in the dialogue?

CASE 2

Refer to the case of Mr. A. the 58-year-old banker to answer the following questions:

1. When the conversation first turns to smoking, the hygienist asks Mr. A. *"Are you sufficiently motivated about the implant to consider stopping smoking?"* This is labeled as an example of "developing discrepancy." What discrepancy does this refer to and how is this meant to foster motivation for change?
2. What is Mr. A's ambivalence regarding behavior change (i.e., what cons AND pros for change does HE see?)?
3. Mr. A. provided lots of change talk in the dialogue but what turns out to be the key barrier for change that, if the hygienist can help address, will significantly increase his motivation?

CASE 3

Using the information in the case of Ms. S., the 35-year-old administrative assistant, try the following:

1. With a classmate, take turns assuming the role of Ms. S. and the hygienist. Practice asking an open-ended question to begin the visit followed by a reflection of Ms. S's response.
2. Ms. S. could benefit from information on how to get her gums healthy while reducing sensitivity. With a classmate, practice using the three steps "Elicit, Provide, Elicit" to give her some relevant information.

Ethical Dilemma

Dr. Jasper Greene hired Eden—a recent dental hygiene graduate—to work 4 days a week in his busy dental practice. Dr. Greene employs three other hygienists on a full-time basis, as well as three other dentists.

Dr. Greene was very pleased, as the patients really liked Eden, and he thought she had excellent clinical skills, especially for a new graduate. Eden was quite happy too, and enjoyed the office staff as well as the variety of patients she was treating. She was particularly excited to utilize the method of motivational interviewing, as a means to enhance patient behavior change, specifically as it related to patient self-care. While a student, Eden was praised by her clinical faculty for her exceptional mastery of this technique.

Approximately 3 months later, Dr. Greene had a cancellation, and was walking by Eden's operatory while she was using motivational interviewing, and he stopped to listen to the conversation. Eden was working with a new patient, who was scheduled for periodontal instrumentation of deep periodontal pockets, but had a fear of needles, and refused anesthesia. She spent a significant amount of time counseling in a patient-centered manner. Dr. Greene was not familiar with this approach, and quite frankly, disagreed with the patient "calling the shots."

Later that day, Dr. Greene asked Eden to come to his office. He told her that she was to stop all this "mumbo jumbo," and tell each patient what was best for him/her, as she was the expert. He further told her that none of the other hygienists or dentists in the office utilize this technique, and he requires continuity amongst his office staff.

Eden was very upset, and did not know what to do. On one hand, she loved working for Dr. Greene, but on the other hand, she realized that she was not comfortable compromising her belief of patient-centered counseling and moving her patients naturally toward health.

1. Are there advantages to motivational interviewing?
2. Are there ethical principles in conflict in this dilemma?
3. What is the best way for Eden to handle this ethical dilemma?

References

1. Bandura A. *Self-Efficacy : The Exercise of Control*. New York: W.H. Freeman; 1997:604.
2. Fishbein M. Factors influencing behavior and behavior change. In: Baum A, Revenson T, Singer J, eds. *Handbook of Health Psychology*. Mahwah, N.J.: Lawrence Erlbaum Associates; 2001:961.
3. Ryan RM, Deci EL. Self-determination theory and the facilitation of intrinsic motivation, social development, and well-being. *American Psychol*. 2000;55(1):68–78.
4. Williams GC, McGregor HA, Zeldman A, Freedman ZR, Deci EL. Testing a self-determination theory process model for promoting glycemic control through diabetes self-management. *Health Psychol*. 2004;23(1):58–66.
5. Freeman R. The psychology of dental patient care. 10. Strategies for motivating the non-compliant patient. *Br Dent J*. 1999;187(6):307–312.
6. Miller WR, Rollnick S, MyiLibrary. *Motivational Interviewing Helping People Change*. New York: Guilford Press; 2013. Available from: http://libproxy.temple.edu/login?url=http://lib.myilibrary.com/detail.asp?id=394471Connect to MyiLibrary resource.
7. Resnicow K, DiIorio C, Soet JE, Ernst D, Borrelli B, Hecht J. Motivational interviewing in health promotion: it sounds like something is changing. *Health Psychol*. 2002;21(5):444–451.
8. Shinitzky HE, Kub J. The art of motivating behavior change: the use of motivational interviewing to promote health. *Public Health Nurs*. 2001;18(3):178–185.
9. Misra S, Daly B, Dunne S, Millar B, Packer M, Asimakopoulou K. Dentist-patient communication: what do patients and dentists remember following a consultation? Implications for patient compliance. *Patient Prefer Adherence*. 2013;7:543–549.
10. Prounis C. Doctor-patient communication. Pharmaceutical Executive [Internet]. Available from: http://www.pharmexec.com. Published 2014. Accessed August 29, 2005.
11. Rollnick S, Miller WR, Butler C. *Motivational Interviewing in Health Care: Helping Patients Change Behavior*. New York: Guilford Press; 2008:210.
12. Lundahl B, Moleni T, Burke BL, et al. Motivational interviewing in medical care settings: a systematic review and meta-analysis of randomized controlled trials. *Patient Educ Couns*. 2013;93(2):157–168.

13. Lundahl W, Kunz C, Brownell C, Tollefson D, Burke B. A meta-analysis of motivational interviewing: Twenty-five years of empirical studies. *Res Soc Work Pract*. 2010;20(2):137–160.

14. Gao X, Lo E, Kot S, Chan K. Motivational interviewing in improving oral health: A systematic review of randomized controlled trials. *J Periodontol*. 2014;85:426–437.

15. Weinstein P, Harrison R, Benton T. Motivating parents to prevent caries in their young children: one-year findings. *J Am Dent Assoc*. 2004;135(6):731–738.

16. Weinstein P, Harrison R, Benton T. Motivating mothers to prevent caries: confirming the beneficial effect of counseling. *J Am Dent Assoc*. 2006;137(6):789–793.

17. Ismail A, Ondersma S, Jendele JM, Little R, Lepkowski JM. Evaluation of a brief tailored motivational intervention to prevent early childhood caries. *Community Dent Oral Epidemiol* 2011;39(5):432–448.

18. Almomani F, Williams K, Catley D, Brown C. Effects of an oral health promotion program in people with mental illness. *J Dent Res*. 2009;88(7):648–652.

19. Jonsson B, Ohrn K, Oscarson N, Lindberg P. An individually tailored treatment programme for improved oral hygiene: introduction of a new course of action in health education for patients with periodontitis. *Int J Dent Hyg*. 2009;7(3):166–175.

20. Jonsson B, Ohrn K, Oscarson N, Lindberg P. The effectiveness of an individually tailored oral health educational programme on oral hygiene behaviour in patients with periodontal disease: a blinded randomized-controlled clinical trial (one-year follow-up). *J Clin Periodontol*. 2009;36(12):1025–1034.

21. Brand VS, Bray KK, MacNeill S, Catley D, Williams K. Impact of single-session motivational interviewing on clinical outcomes following periodontal maintenance therapy. *Int J Dent Hyg*. 2013;11(2):134–141.

22. Stenman J, Lundgren J, Wennstrom JL, Ericsson JS, Abrahamsson KH. A single session of motivational interviewing as an additive means to improve adherence in periodontal infection control: a randomized controlled trial. *J Clin Periodontol*. 2012;39(10):947–954.

23. Hedman E, Riis U, Gabre P. The impact of behavioural interventions on young people's attitudes towards tobacco use. *Oral Health Prev Dent*. 2010;8(1):23–32.

24. Lando HA, Hennrikus D, Boyle R, Lazovich D, Stafne E, Rindal B. Promoting tobacco abstinence among older adolescents in dental clinics. *J Smok Cessat*. 2007;2(1):23–30.

25. Bray KK, Catley D, Voelker MA, Liston R, Williams KB. Motivational interviewing in dental hygiene education: curriculum modification and evaluation. *J Dent Educ*. 2013;77(12):1662–1669.

26. Rubak S, Sandbaek A, Lauritzen T, Christensen B. Motivational interviewing: a systematic review and meta-analysis. *Br J Gen Pract*. 2005;55(513):305–312.

27. Amrhein PC, Miller WR, Yahne CE, Palmer M, Fulcher L. Client commitment language during motivational interviewing predicts drug use outcomes. *J Consult Clin Psychol*. 2003;71(5):862–878.

STUDENT ANCILLARY RESOURCES

A wide variety of resources to enhance your learning is available online:

- Audio Glossary
- Book Pages
- Chapter Review Questions and Answers

33 Maintenance for the Periodontal Patient

Clinical Application. Given the chronic nature of periodontitis, an appropriately timed periodontal maintenance program, performed at regular timed intervals, is the most integral part of the entire periodontal treatment approach. A periodontal maintenance program is especially important in preventing future progression or recurrence of the disease after the periodontium has been successfully stabilized following active treatment. At each periodontal maintenance, members of the dental team continuously monitor the patient's oral health, diagnose any incipient signs of recurrent disease, and intercept any unstable/ deteriorating sites with the appropriate supportive therapy. The success of periodontal maintenance care hinges on two major factors: (1) the patient's willingness to maintain plaque biofilm levels that are consistent with health and stability and to adhere to the recommended periodontal maintenance regimen, and (2) the clinician's ability to deliver the appropriate management. As such, the dental hygienist must have a firm understanding of the goals, benefits, and objectives of periodontal maintenance care and the importance of continually reinforcing and motivating the patient to follow the recommended periodontal maintenance regimen at each recall visit. This chapter outlines the fundamental aspects of periodontal maintenance for all members of the dental team to consider during patient care.

Learning Objectives

- List three objectives of periodontal maintenance.
- Describe how periodontal maintenance relates to other phases of periodontal treatment.
- List the typical steps performed during an appointment for periodontal maintenance.
- Explain the term baseline data.
- Describe guidelines for determining whether the general practice office or the periodontal office should provide periodontal maintenance.
- Describe how to establish an appropriate interval between maintenance appointments.
- Define the term recurrence of periodontitis.
- List clinical signs of recurrence of periodontitis.
- List reasons for recurrence of periodontitis.
- Define the term compliance.
- Explain the role compliance plays in maintaining periodontal health and stability.
- List reasons for noncompliance with periodontal maintenance recommendations.
- Explain some strategies that can be used to improve patient compliance.
- Explain the term root caries and list recommendations for use of fluorides in the prevention of root caries.

Key Terms

Periodontal maintenance therapy
Baseline data
Recurrence of periodontitis
Refractory periodontitis

Compliance
Compliant patient
Noncompliant patient
Root caries

Caries management by risk
  assessment (CAMBRA)

Section 1
Introduction to Periodontal Maintenance Therapy

1. **Description of Periodontal Maintenance Therapy.** Long-term successful management of periodontitis requires involvement of patients in post-treatment appointments at regular intervals known as periodontal maintenance therapy. **Periodontal maintenance therapy** is a term that refers to the continuing patient care provided by members of the dental team to help a patient maintain periodontal health following the successful completion of nonsurgical or surgical periodontal therapy.[1-5]

    A. Periodontal maintenance is performed at appropriately timed intervals to assist the patient in maintaining oral health; the precise intervals are selected to meet the needs of the individual patient.

    B. Once begun, periodontal maintenance is routinely continued for the life of the natural dentition (or the life of the dental implant).

    C. Periodontal maintenance can be discontinued temporarily if surgical or nonsurgical therapy must be reinstituted because of the recurrence of periodontitis.

    D. Periodontal maintenance is performed on both natural teeth and dental implants.

    E. Though periodontal maintenance is the preferred term, other terms that have been used for periodontal maintenance are supportive periodontal therapy (SPT) and periodontal recall.

    F. It is important to realize that periodontal maintenance is not synonymous with a dental prophylaxis.

2. **Importance of Periodontal Maintenance**

    A. Periodontal maintenance is one of the most important phases of periodontal treatment. A periodontal maintenance program is key to ensure that the periodontal tissues are maintained in a state of health, with an acceptable degree of disease stability, patient comfort, and function.

    1. With good periodontal maintenance, most periodontitis patients can retain their teeth or implants in function and comfort throughout their lives.[3,5]

    2. In the absence of periodontal maintenance, patients frequently exhibit a recurrence of periodontitis.[6-10]

    3. Periodontal maintenance can be successful regardless of the specific type of periodontal treatment (surgical or nonsurgical) needed by the patient.

    4. The success of periodontal maintenance in reducing tooth loss is well documented in the literature.[9,11-13] Figure 33-1 illustrates some of the outcomes possible with periodontal maintenance.

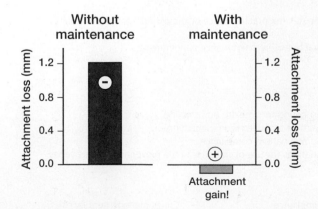

Figure 33-1. Attachment Loss With Maintenance Versus Attachment Loss Without Maintenance. A classic study assessed the efficacy of a periodontal maintenance program to prevent the recurrence of disease in patients treated for advanced periodontitis. Patients who were not in a periodontal maintenance program had progressive attachment loss over a 6-year period. On the other hand, patients who were placed on maintenance every 2 to 3 months over the 6-year period *exhibited attachment gain.*

3. **Goals of Periodontal Maintenance Therapy**
   There are several overlapping goals of periodontal maintenance (Box 33-1).
   A. **To minimize the recurrence and progression of periodontitis**
      1. The primary risk factor for inflammatory periodontal diseases is bacterial plaque biofilm.
         a. In spite of a patient's best self-care efforts, it is common for plaque biofilms to form at some sites and for some calculus to reform at some sites. Periodic professional biofilm and calculus removal is an important part of periodontal maintenance.
         b. It is common for a patient's self-care efforts to become less effective over time. Reinforcement or review of self-care techniques is also an important part of each periodontal maintenance visit.
      2. Secondary risk factors for inflammatory periodontal diseases include plaque-retentive areas (such as restorations with overhangs), smoking, and certain systemic factors.
         a. Whereas these secondary risk factors should always be addressed as part of nonsurgical periodontal therapy, the condition of most patients changes over time.
         b. The dental practitioner should be vigilant for any newly emerging secondary risk factors (such as, recently placed plaque-retentive restorations, or changes in medical history) that might put the patient at a higher risk of disease recurrence.[11,14–16]
   B. **To reduce the incidence of tooth loss.** One of the primary overall goals of all phases of periodontal therapy (including periodontal maintenance) is to reduce the incidence of tooth loss (or reduce the incidence of implant loss).
      1. In a study by Wilson et al., evaluating tooth loss in maintenance patients in a private periodontal practice, tooth loss was shown to be inversely proportional to the frequency of periodontal maintenance.[17]
      2. Other studies have also shown that patients who maintain regular periodontal maintenance lose fewer teeth than patients who receive less frequent periodontal maintenance.[9,12,18]
      3. Even a patient who has lost teeth during the active stage of treatment can prevent additional tooth loss if he/she adheres to the recommended periodontal maintenance regimen.[1,2,11,18]
   C. **To increase the probability of detecting and treating other oral conditions**
      1. As members of the health care community, the dental team must be vigilant for the development of any oral condition that can affect patient welfare. For example, at each periodontal maintenance visit, an oral cancer screening is performed. If oral cancer is identified at its early stage, then interceptive treatment of the pathology can improve the long-term prognosis of the patient and treatment outcomes.
      2. Periodontal maintenance offers an ideal opportunity for ongoing monitoring of the overall oral health of a patient.

Box 33-1. Goals of Periodontal Maintenance

- Minimize the recurrence and progression of periodontitis.
- Reduce the incidence of tooth loss.
- Increase the probability of detecting and treating other oral conditions.

4. **Patient/Clinician Roles in Periodontal Maintenance**
   A. Periodontal maintenance is a team effort that requires commitment from everyone involved. The periodontal maintenance team includes the members of the dental team plus the patient and occasionally other health care providers, such as the patient's physician.
   B. Periodontal maintenance requires considerable effort from the patient in sustaining meticulous self-care and cooperating with regular ongoing professional periodontal maintenance care. Patients must be made aware of the need for this ongoing effort even prior to receiving nonsurgical periodontal therapy.
   C. In addition, periodontal maintenance requires considerable effort on the part of the dental health team for professional care at regular intervals, renewal of patient motivation, instruction in self-care techniques, and elimination or reduction of primary and secondary risk factors.
5. **Relationship of Periodontal Maintenance to Other Phases of Therapy.** It is important for a clinician to understand how periodontal maintenance for a patient that has been treated for periodontal disease relates to other phases of comprehensive periodontal therapy; this relationship is summarized in Figure 33-2.

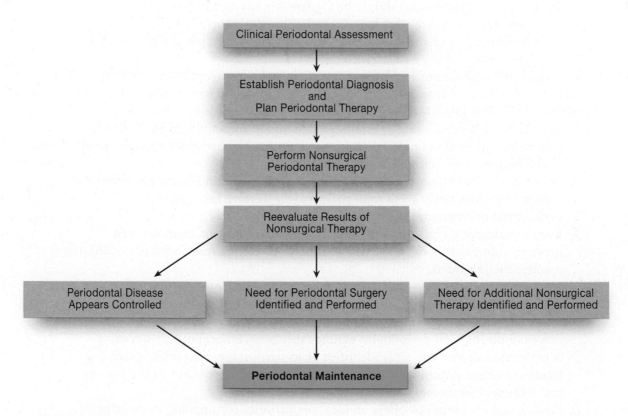

Figure 33-2. Phases of Periodontal Therapy. This flowchart illustrates how periodontal maintenance relates to other phases of periodontal therapy that are frequently provided for patients with periodontal disease.

Section 2
Planning Periodontal Maintenance

1. **When to Implement Periodontal Maintenance.** Following nonsurgical periodontal therapy, a reevaluation of the patient's periodontal status is performed with a particular emphasis on the results obtained from nonsurgical therapy.
   A. Based upon the findings of this reevaluation, additional therapy such as periodontal surgery might be recommended.
   B. At the reevaluation, the dental team also must determine the most appropriate time interval for future periodontal maintenance recall visits.
   C. For most patients, periodontal maintenance will begin following this reevaluation since for many patients no further active therapy is needed at least in selected sites in the dentition that exhibit periodontal stability.
   D. Even though periodontal surgery may be recommended in some sites, the maintenance phase begins following nonsurgical therapy at least for those sites where no further active periodontal therapy is indicated.

2. **Procedures Performed During Periodontal Maintenance.** Successful periodontal maintenance requires the active participation of the patient as well as all members of the dental team. In most dental offices, the dental hygienist plays a major role in each periodontal maintenance visit. A typical patient office visit for periodontal maintenance includes the steps discussed below and outlined in Box 33-2.[19-21]
   A. **Update of Medical Status.** An update of a patient's medical status is always the first step in any clinical appointment.
   B. **Patient Interview**
      1. A patient interview is part of a periodontal maintenance appointment; during the interview, changes in the social or dental status of the patient should be explored and documented.
      2. Examples of social status issues that should be explored would be changes in lifestyle, bereavement, and work status.
      3. The patient interview should also include a review of dental care provided by other clinicians since the previous maintenance visit.
      4. In addition, the patient interview should clarify the patient's perception of his/her oral status including the patient's thoughts about problems encountered during self-care efforts.

Box 33-2. Overview of the Steps Performed During a Periodontal Maintenance Appointment

- Update medical status
- Patient interview
- Clinical assessment
- Evaluation of effectiveness of patient self-care
- Identification of treatment needs
- Periodontal instrumentation
- Patient counseling
- Application of fluorides

C. **Clinical Assessment**
1. Following the patient interview, a thorough clinical assessment should be performed. Results of the clinical assessment should then be compared with previous baseline data. The term baseline data refers to clinical data gathered at the initial visit that is subsequently used for comparison at future maintenance visits.
2. The actual clinical assessment usually includes steps such as those listed below.
   a. Extraoral and Intraoral Examination
   b. Dental Examination
   c. Radiographic Examination, if indicated
   d. Periodontal Examination including the following features:
      1) **Probing Depths**
         a) Probing depths should be recorded with the same attention to detail that was employed during the initial examination.
         b) Disease progression (continuing attachment loss) should be suspected when a 2-mm increase in probing depth is noted at a site.
      2) **Bleeding on Probing**
         a) When present, bleeding on probing is generally visible within a few seconds after gentle periodontal probing.
         b) Research suggests that after a few years of maintenance, a high frequency of bleeding on probing is a predictor of increased risk for progressive attachment loss.[22]
         c) Bleeding sites should be charted because these sites may need more attention during periodontal instrumentation.
      3) **Attachment Level**
         a) Attachment levels should be recorded at all sites in the dentition.
         b) The most reliable way to evaluate periodontal disease control is by sequential comparison of clinical attachment level measurements.
         c) Disease progression is thought to be indicated by a 2-mm increase in clinical attachment loss at a specific site *as measured with a manual periodontal probe*.
      4) **Tooth Mobility**
         a) In the assessment of tooth mobility, mobility can be stable or increasing. Increasing mobility over time is one of the important clinical features to note.
         b) The more severe the mobility measured in a tooth, the greater the risk of eventual tooth loss.
      5) **Furcation Involvement**
         a) Periodontal disease control is more difficult in areas of furcation involvement.
         b) The more advanced the furcation involvement, the greater the risk of tooth loss over time.
      6) **Mucogingival Involvement**
      7) **Levels of Plaque Biofilm and Calculus**

D. **Evaluation of Effectiveness of Self-Care**
1. Patients often spend considerable time on self-care and justifiably expect to be informed about the effectiveness of their efforts.
   a. Plaque scores recorded after using a disclosing solution are good indications of the patient's level of self-care compliance and disclosing solution can be used to allow patients to view the biofilm accumulation.
   b. Plaque scores may reveal that the patient is in need of renewed instruction in self-care methods.
2. Biofilm accumulation can be related to many factors; examples of these factors are listed below.
   a. Patients may lack the manual dexterity needed to carry out the self-care regimen that was recommended previously. When manual dexterity is a problem, alternative self-care techniques should be considered. Older patients can lose skills that they were perfectly capable of performing at a previous maintenance visit.
   b. Unfortunately, it is common for patients to discontinue the use of one or more of the self-care methods recommended previously.
   c. Gingival recession or shrinkage may have occurred following periodontal surgery; introduction of new interdental aids may be indicated for plaque biofilm removal on proximal root surfaces (refer to Chapter 25 to review the many types of interdental aids available to help remove plaque biofilm from interproximal areas).
E. **Identification of Treatment Needs**
1. It is a routine part of periodontal maintenance to perform thorough periodontal instrumentation to remove biofilm and calculus, but other treatment needs can also be identified.
2. Examples of other treatment needs can include local delivery of antimicrobials, restorative therapy, and reinstitution of active periodontal therapy.
3. Selective tooth polishing may be indicated for removal of tooth stains that are visible when the patient smiles.
F. **Biofilm Removal**
1. Biofilms are resistant to topical chemical control; therefore, frequent professional removal of plaque biofilm is an essential component of successful nonsurgical periodontal therapy.
2. Professional biofilm control may be accomplished by hand and/or ultrasonic instrumentation or subgingival glycine powder air polishing.
G. **Periodontal Instrumentation**
1. The goal of periodontal instrumentation is to create an environment that is biologically acceptable to the tissues of the periodontium.
2. Thorough removal of biofilm and calculus deposits should be accomplished using hand and/or ultrasonic instrumentation.
3. The main adverse effect of frequent mechanical instrumentation of the root surface is disturbance of the epithelial attachment and cumulative, irreversible root substance removal,[23–28] and gingival recession.[29,30]
   a. Hard tissue loss is one of the major causes of dentin sensitivity to hot and cold stimuli, as well as sensitivity to toothbrushing.[31–34]

      b. Because periodontal instrumentation is a routine part of nonsurgical periodontal therapy, it is important that removal is accomplished in an efficient manner with minimal hard tissue damage.[35]

          1) Following periodontal therapy, some patients will present for periodontal maintenance with little or no subgingival calculus deposits. In these patients, firm stroke pressure with the instrument against the tooth is not necessary and should be avoided.

          2) Ultrasonic instrumentation with a precision-thin tip has been shown to remove less root substance than hand instrumentation and offers the added benefit of the antimicrobial effect created by the vibrating ultrasonic tip.[36,37]

          3) Plastic curettes (such as those used to debride dental implants) can be effective for deplaquing root surfaces and minimizing trauma to the root during maintenance care when no calculus is present or when implants are involved.

H. Patient Counseling

  1. As already discussed, maintenance patients should always be counseled related to the effectiveness of self-care efforts since biofilm control by the patient is a critical element in preventing recurrence of periodontitis.

      a. Failure to provide this information may give a patient the impression that the dental team is not truly interested in the patient's dental health status.

      b. Most patients will need some reinforcement of motivation for biofilm control in addition to retraining in the complex skills involved. Vatne et al. found that providing the patient with customized information on the pathogenesis, prevention, and treatment as well as maintenance of periodontal diseases resulted in a high degree of patient compliance with maintenance therapy.[38]

  2. It is also prudent to include counseling that explains the need for compliance with the periodontal maintenance regimen, since compliance with the periodontal maintenance regimen will always remain a challenge for some patients.

  3. Other counseling may be indicated for specific patients. Examples of counseling that may be needed are caries prevention counseling, smoking cessation, or dietary changes.

I. Application of Fluorides

  1. Professional application of fluoride treatments during periodontal maintenance care is normally indicated to promote remineralization of tooth surfaces, minimize the risk of root caries on exposed root surfaces, and manage dentinal hypersensitivity. Additionally, patients who are deemed to be highly susceptible to caries (i.e., due to drug-induced xerostomia) may benefit by routine application of fluoride at each periodontal maintenance visit.

  2. Research studies suggest that high concentrations of topical fluorides may also have some antimicrobial properties and may be of some benefit in decreasing plaque biofilm accumulation.

  3. The use of fluorides is discussed in detail in Section 5 of this chapter.

3. Decisions Related to Periodontal Maintenance Therapy

  A. Office Guidelines for Provision of Periodontal Maintenance. For patients treated in a periodontal office, the general dental team should discuss guidelines for how periodontal maintenance should be provided (i.e., either in the general dental practice office or in the periodontal practice). This decision is dependent on the combined clinical judgments of the general practice dental team and the periodontal practice team in determining how to best maintain the health of the patient. Some general guidelines are outlined below:

1. Patients who have been treated previously for Stage I periodontitis and currently display a stable periodontium can usually receive periodontal maintenance in a general dental practice.

2. Patients who have been treated previously for Stage II periodontitis and currently display a stable periodontium can usually be managed by alternating periodontal maintenance visits between the general dental practice and the periodontal practice.

3. Patients with Stage III (severe periodontitis with potential for additional tooth loss) and Stage IV (advanced periodontitis with extensive previous tooth loss and potential for loss of remaining dentition) periodontitis should be monitored and should receive periodontal maintenance in a periodontal practice because of the high risk of tooth loss. In addition, annual or semiannual visits should be scheduled with a general dentist who will provide restorative and other general dental care.

4. Patients who have been treated for Stage IV, Grade C periodontitis should receive all phases of periodontal therapy including periodontal maintenance in a periodontal practice. In addition, annual or semiannual visits should be scheduled with a general dentist who will provide restorative and other general dental care.

B. **Establishing Appropriate Periodontal Maintenance Intervals**
   1. Establishing a periodontal maintenance interval that is appropriate for the patient can be challenging. The frequency of periodontal maintenance visits must be determined on an individual basis.[39,40] A single recall interval (e.g., 6 months) is not suitable for all patients. Some factors to consider in determining the interval between maintenance visits include the following:
      a. **Severity of Periodontitis.** In general, the more severe the periodontitis, the shorter the intervals should be between periodontal maintenance visits.
      b. **Adequacy of Patient Self-Care.** In general, the more effective the patient's self-care, the less frequently the patient needs to be seen. For patients with less than optimal self-care, the intervals between maintenance visits should be shorter.
      c. **Host Response.** Systemic or genetic factors may negatively affect the host response. For example, a patient who continues to smoke or one with poorly controlled diabetes should be seen at shorter intervals.
   2. An important guide for determining the frequency of maintenance care is based on the time interval for the repopulation of periodontal pathogens following thorough periodontal instrumentation.
      a. Studies indicate that following periodontal instrumentation, the subgingival pathogens return to pre-instrumentation levels in approximately 9 to 11 weeks in most patients, though times can vary.[41]
      b. Research evidence shows that periodontal maintenance should be performed at least every 3 months or less for the removal and disruption of subgingival periodontal pathogens. *This 3-month interval is the one most frequently recommended, though this interval may need to be adjusted based on sound clinical judgment.*[40]
      c. Patients who comply with frequent periodontal maintenance experience less attachment loss and tooth loss than patients who have less frequent maintenance care.

Section 3
Periodontal Disease Recurrence

1. **Understanding Periodontal Disease Recurrence**
   A. **Periodontal Disease Recurrence Defined**
      1. The term periodontal disease recurrence refers to the return of the disease in *a patient that has been previously, successfully treated for periodontitis.*
      2. The term disease recurrence implies that the periodontitis was indeed brought under control following active periodontal therapy (nonsurgical periodontal therapy alone or nonsurgical periodontal therapy plus periodontal surgery), but that at some later time the periodontitis once again results in progressive attachment loss.
      3. It should be noted that in spite of having received excellent treatment, patients who have been treated for periodontitis are at risk for future recurrence of periodontitis for as long as teeth (or implants) are present.
      4. Recurrence of periodontitis can occur at specific sites only (not necessarily throughout the dentition). For example, it would be possible for a patient previously treated for periodontitis to exhibit disease recurrence on the mesial surface of a maxillary first premolar tooth (due to the plaque-retentive mesial root concavity) while all other sites on the same aforementioned tooth or all the teeth in the dentition exhibit periodontal stability. It is also possible for disease recurrence to be more generalized and affect the entire dentition.
   B. **Clinical Recognition of Recurrence of Periodontitis.** At present, the most effective way to identify sites of recurrence of periodontitis (i.e., sites of progressive attachment loss) is through thorough periodic clinical assessments. The usual clinical signs of recurrence of periodontitis are listed in Box 33-3.
   C. **Reasons for Disease Recurrence.** Periodontitis recurs in patients for a variety of reasons, and the members of the dental team should be aware that it is not always possible to determine a specific reason for disease recurrence. However, the most common reasons for recurrence of periodontitis are:
      1. Inadequate self-care by the patient and/or poor patient adherence to the recommended periodontal maintenance regimen
      2. Incomplete professional treatment
         a. Incomplete periodontal instrumentation
         b. Failure to control all local risk factors
      3. Failure to control systemic factors
      4. Inadequate control of occlusal contributing factors
      5. Improper periodontal surgical technique
      6. Attempting to treat teeth with a poor prognosis

Box 33-3. Clinical Signs of Recurrence

- Progressive clinical attachment loss
- Pockets that get deeper over time
- Pockets that bleed upon probing
- Pockets that exhibit exudate
- Radiographic evidence of progressing bone loss
- Increasing tooth mobility

D. **Refractory Disease Differentiated From Recurrent Disease.** Refractory periodontal disease should be differentiated from recurrent periodontal disease. Unfortunately, periodontitis in certain patients is difficult or impossible to control even with all the modern therapies currently available and in spite of the best efforts of the most skilled clinicians.

1. As already discussed, the term recurrence of periodontitis refers to *the return of the disease in a patient that has been previously, successfully treated for periodontitis.*

2. The term refractory periodontitis, however, refers to *periodontitis that is resistant to treatment from the outset of therapy even with what appears to be appropriate periodontal therapy.*

3. Referral to a periodontal practice is usually indicated when refractory periodontitis is suspected in a patient.

2. **Options for Management of Patients With Disease Recurrence.** The members of the dental team should be alert for the need for re-treatment that may be identified during any periodontal maintenance visit. When periodontal disease recurrence is identified, several factors should be considered when planning the periodontal re-treatment:

A. If inadequate patient self-care appears to be the fundamental cause of the disease recurrence, then nonsurgical therapy should be reinstituted followed by a reevaluation of the patient's periodontal status after an appropriate healing time.

B. If failure to comply with the schedule of periodontal maintenance appears to be the fundamental cause of the disease recurrence, then nonsurgical therapy should be reinstituted along with further patient education about the need for maintenance followed by a reevaluation of the patient's periodontal status after an appropriate healing time.

C. If there appears to be disease recurrence in limited individual sites in the presence of *adequate* patient self-care, treatment options can include localized periodontal instrumentation, local delivery of antimicrobial agents, or localized surgical therapy.

D. If there appears to be disease recurrence in multiple sites in the presence of adequate patient self-care, periodontal surgical therapy is frequently indicated.

E. If generalized attachment loss has recurred, the systemic condition of the patient should be reassessed with emphasis on the possible need for periodontal surgical intervention, for possible microbial analysis, or for possible local or systemic antimicrobial therapy. Patients of this type should be managed by a periodontist.

Section 4
Patient Compliance With Periodontal Maintenance

1. **Overview of Patient Compliance.** The term compliance is defined as the extent to which a person's behavior coincides with medical or health advice. Compliance also is called adherence or therapeutic alliance, but compliance is the most common term used in the literature.
   A. A patient is described as being compliant if he or she adheres to the recommendations set forth by the health care provider. Examples of compliant patients would be a patient who faithfully takes antihypertensive medications as prescribed by a physician or a patient who cooperates in meeting regularly scheduled periodontal maintenance appointments as recommended by the dental team.
   B. A patient is described as being noncompliant if he or she does *not* follow recommendations set forth by the health care provider. Examples of noncompliant patients would be a patient who does not take prescribed medications daily to control diabetes or a patient who does not perform adequate daily self-care that has been recommended as part of the maintenance regimen.
2. **Patient Compliance During Periodontal Maintenance.** Patient compliance with a program of periodontal maintenance is not easy to achieve. It requires that a patient faithfully adhere to a strict program of recall appointments several times each year and follow very specific recommendations for meticulous daily self-care.
   A. Overall, patient compliance with most medical advice is poor, and it should not be surprising that patient compliance with periodontal maintenance is also poor.
   B. Studies of compliance exhibited by periodontal maintenance patients indicate that only 16% to 30% of the patients are fully compliant with periodontal maintenance.[42–44]
   C. Reasons for noncompliance with periodontal maintenance are complex, and those reasons can be different for each patient and even for the same patient at different times.[18,45–49]
   D. Examples of some reasons that have been suggested for noncompliance with recommended programs of periodontal maintenance include the following:
      1. Patient fear of receiving dental treatment
      2. The expense of the dental treatment involved
      3. The low priority for dental care for some patients in the face of competing demands for time
      4. Denial on the part of some patients related to the periodontal challenges they face
      5. Failure for some patients to understand the implications of noncompliance
      6. Perceived indifference on the part of the dental health care providers
3. **Strategies of Improving Compliance.** The thoughtful dental team will investigate and adopt strategies for improving patient compliance with periodontal maintenance.[45] Some strategies for improving compliance are discussed below and outlined in Figure 33-3.
   A. Give a patient printed self-care instructions, and make sure to supply the instructions written in the patient's native language.
   B. Simplify self-care recommendations as much as possible for each patient.
      1. Patients often perceive self-care instructions as being difficult to follow and as too time-consuming in their busy lives.
      2. Self-care instructions should be as clear and as simple as possible while addressing the specific needs of the patient.

3. Caution should be exercised when recommending multiple types of self-care aids. Patients are less likely to comply with self-care when they are instructed to use multiple aids on a daily basis.

4. When possible, alternatives to traditional dental floss should be considered since compliance with flossing is generally poor.

C. Vary the office approach to patient education and self-care instructions from appointment to appointment. Patients often complain about having to listen to the "same old lecture" from the dental hygienist at each periodontal maintenance appointment.

D. Seek out patient concerns and provide opportunities for communication by asking patients open-ended questions. Examples of open-ended questions appear below.

1. "What are your concerns about this suggestion or treatment?"

2. "How do you think you will fit this self-care recommendation into your daily schedule?"

3. "How would you compare using this powered flossing device to using traditional dental floss?"

E. Accommodate the individual patient's needs whenever possible. A satisfied patient is more likely to comply with self-care and maintenance appointments.

F. Keep patients fully informed about their periodontal condition.

1. At each visit, counsel the patients about their periodontal health status.

2. Explain the benefits of having regularly scheduled periodontal maintenance visits and the risks of infrequent professional care.

G. Monitor compliance with the maintenance appointments and contact patients promptly when compliance seems to become a problem.

H. Provide positive feedback to patients as frequently as possible. Positive reinforcement can help improve compliance.

1. Areas of improvement should be pointed out to the patient (e.g., such as less biofilm accumulation, fewer bleeding sites, or less inflamed tissue).

2. Positive reinforcement should be used to convey a motivational message rather than criticism.

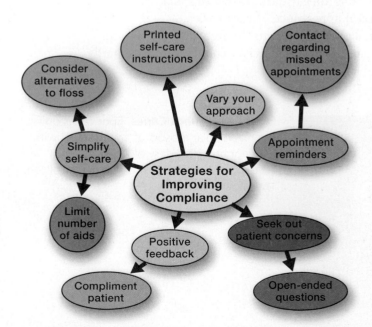

Figure 33-3. Suggestions for Improving Patient Compliance. An idea map of various strategies for improving patient compliance with recommendations for periodontal maintenance.

Section 5
Root Caries as a Complication During Maintenance

1. **Introduction to Root Caries**
   A. **Occurrence of Root Caries in Patients With Periodontitis**
      1. Whereas dental caries frequently occurs on enamel surfaces, the term root caries refers to tooth decay that occurs on the root surfaces of the teeth.
      2. According to the *1999–2004 National Health and Nutrition Examination Survey*:
         a. Root caries is a significant problem for adults: 21.6% of adults aged 50 to 64 years and 31% of adults aged 65 to 74 years had unrestored or restored root caries.
         b. The percentage of adults with root caries increases to 42.3% at age 75.[50]
      3. The Northwest Practice-based Research Collaborative in Evidence-based Dentistry research network recently reported
         a. A total of 19.6% of adults had root caries.
         b. The factors associated with increased prevalence of root caries in middle-aged adults are: being of the male sex, dry mouth, root surfaces exposed to the oral environment, and increased frequency of eating or drinking between meals.[51]
      4. A 2004 systematic review on root caries incidence found that 23.7% of older adults *develop at least one new lesion annually.*[52]
      5. Root caries occurs only if the root surface is exposed to the oral environment due to loss of attachment.[53]
         a. In health, the root surface is protected by the periodontal attachment apparatus and is not exposed to the oral environment.
         b. The root may be exposed to the oral environment due to gingival recession or within a periodontal pocket.
   B. **Clinical Appearance of Root Caries**
      1. Active root caries lesions usually appear yellowish to light brown and may be covered with biofilm. Inactive lesions appear dark brown or black.[53,54] Figure 33-4 shows a typical clinical appearance of root caries.
      2. Root caries usually begins at or slightly coronal to the free gingival margin. The carious lesions can spread laterally and can even extend circumferentially around the root surface.[55]

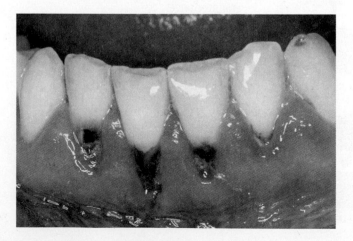

Figure 33-4. Root Caries. Root caries on the mandibular incisors of an individual with periodontitis. (Courtesy of Dr. Richard J. Foster, Guilford Technical Community College, Jamestown, NC.)

C. Etiology of Root Caries

1. No specific microorganisms have been proven to cause root caries. Root caries is most likely the result of a mixed infection or a succession of bacterial populations, such as *Streptococcus mutans* and *Lactobacillus* spp. Recent studies, with few exceptions, fail to find association between *Actinomyces* spp. and root caries.[56]

2. Like enamel caries, root caries requires a susceptible tooth surface, plaque biofilm, and time to initiate and progress. However, root caries differs from enamel caries in some ways:

   a. Root surfaces are more vulnerable to demineralization than enamel surfaces. Root surfaces demineralize at a pH of 6.2 to 6.7.[57]

   b. Mineral loss for the root surface during the process of demineralization is up to 2.5 times greater than enamel.[58]

3. Risk factors for the development of root caries include attachment loss, inadequate patient self-care, a cariogenic diet, infrequent dental visits, past caries experience, inadequate salivary flow, lack of fluoride exposure, and removable partial dentures. A recent review found past root caries, number of surfaces at risk, poor oral hygiene, gender, age, and periodontal disease as the factors most associated with root caries incidence.[59]

4. In addition, individuals who have coronal caries are 2 to 3.5 times more likely to develop root caries.[60]

2. General Recommendations for the Prevention of Root Caries.

Root caries is a common problem in patients with periodontitis. Managing root caries from a restorative standpoint can be quite difficult, and the best strategy for managing root caries is to prevent the root caries from forming.

A. Prevention of Periodontitis.
The prevention of periodontitis and its associated attachment loss is the most effective way to prevent root caries. In patients with existing periodontal disease, prevention of further attachment loss will reduce the surface area susceptible to decay.

B. Fluoride for the Prevention of Root Caries

1. Root lesions can be arrested by remineralization. A 2007 systematic review of fluoride interventions for root caries concluded that fluoride appears to be a preventive and therapeutic treatment for root caries.[61,62]

2. A variety of fluoride products can be helpful in preventing root caries. Figure 33-5 depicts some of these products. A 2011 systematic review recommended 1.1% NaF pastes/gels and fluoride varnishes as the most effective modalities for root caries remineralization.[63]

   a. **Fluoridated Drinking Water.** Several studies have demonstrated that the presence of fluoridated drinking water throughout the lifetime of an individual reduces the development of root surface caries.[64]

   b. **Fluoride Toothpaste**

      1) The use of an 1100 ppm sodium fluoride (NaF) dentifrice results in a significant decrease in root surface caries of 67%.[65]

      2) A recent randomized clinical trial demonstrates that prescription strength fluoride toothpaste, containing 5000 ppm NaF, is significantly more effective in controlling root caries lesion progression and promoting remineralization compared to lower-prescription strength fluoride toothpaste.[66]

      3) Patients using fluoride toothpastes should avoid rinsing with large volumes of water after the use of fluoride toothpaste.[67]

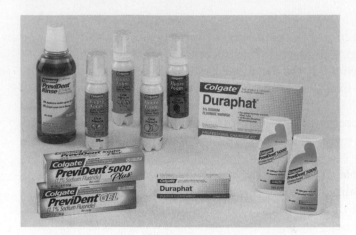

Figure 33-5. Fluoride Products. There are a variety of fluoride products for professional or home use that are helpful in the control of root caries. These include toothpastes, gels, foams, rinses, and varnishes. (Courtesy of Colgate-Palmolive company.)

   c. Fluoride Mouthrinses. Fluoride mouthrinses containing 0.05% NaF have been shown to significantly reduce root caries incidence.[68]

   d. Professional Application of Fluoride

      1) A large long-term clinical study showed that semiannual applications of 1.23% APF gel significantly reduced the formation of new root caries. The number of remineralized lesions was significantly increased by daily rinsing with a 0.05% NaF rinse.[69]

      2) Fluoride varnish applied every 3 months has been shown to reduce new root caries formation by over 50%.[70]

   e. Silver Diamine Fluoride (SDF)

      1) SDF has been widely used outside the United States since 1970. The U.S. Food and Drug Administration (FDA) approved SDF as a desensitizing agent in 2014. Recently, SDF was granted "breakthrough therapy status" by the FDA for caries arrest.

      2) Indications for SDF include extreme caries risk, treatment challenged by behavioral or medical management, and difficult to treat carious lesions.[71,72]

C. Antimicrobial and Supplemental Remineralization Therapies

   1. A recent systematic review found no benefit from the use of chlorhexidine varnish in reducing root caries.[73] There is limited evidence of benefit from the use of a chlorhexidine mouthrinse.[74] High and extreme caries risk adults should rinse with 10 mL of 0.12% chlorhexidine once daily for 1 week per month.

   2. Xylitol containing gums and mints are recommended for high and extreme caries risk patients.

    a. The therapeutic dose of xylitol is 6 to 10 g spread throughout the day.

    b. A recent randomized clinical trial found 40% fewer root caries lesions in the xylitol group compared to placebo. The xylitol group received 5 lozenges containing 1 g of xylitol. The lozenges were consumed across the day.[75]

3. Casein phosphopeptide (CPP)-amorphous calcium phosphate (ACP) pastes are recommended for extreme caries risk patients.
   a. The paste can be applied with a fingertip on a daily basis.
   b. Most research on CPP-ACP is laboratory based rather than in vivo. However, CPP-ACP may promote remineralization in patients with low salivary flow.
   c. A 2008 systematic review concluded that there is insufficient evidence to make conclusions regarding the effectiveness of CPP-ACP in preventing caries.[76]
4. In a clinical practice guideline from the American Dental Association, application of a 1:1 mixture of chlorhexidine and thymol varnish (Cervitec Gel), every 3 months was recommended to reduce the incidence of root caries.[77]

D. **Summary and Best Practices**
   1. Improved oral hygiene, good dietary habits, regular periodontal maintenance visits, and locally applied preventive agents are important to prevent root caries and periodontal disease progression.[78]
   2. Research supports the use of fluoridated water, fluoride toothpastes, fluoride mouth rinses, xylitol, and professional topical fluorides for the prevention of root caries.[79]

3. **Caries Management by Risk Assessment (CAMBRA)**
   A. **Caries Risk Assessment**
      1. Recent research clearly demonstrates that assigning caries risk assessment levels facilitates the effective management of patients for dental caries.[80]
      2. Subsequent to this research, protocols for clinical management of caries risk factor level were developed and employed at a number of dental schools.[81] While complete consensus on these protocols continues to develop, there is strong agreement about treating patients for dental caries based on risk level.[81]
      3. These protocols for clinical management of caries risk are known as "Caries management by risk assessment (CAMBRA)."[80]
      4. The CAMBRA protocols seek to provide practical clinical guidelines for managing dental caries based upon risk group assessment. The protocols are based upon the best evidence at this time and can be used in planning effective caries management for any patient.[80,82]
   B. **CAMBRA Treatment Recommendations**
      1. **A Caries Risk Assessment Form**
         a. In 2002, a group of experts from across the United States produced a caries risk assessment form.[82]
         b. In 2006, outcomes research based upon the use of the form in a large cohort of patients was published, validating the form.[83] The results from this study are the basis for the current version of the caries risk assessment form shown in Figure 33-6.

2. **Caries Risk Determination.** Assigning a "caries risk level" to a patient is the first step in managing the disease process. Table 33-1 presents the four risk levels groups (low, moderate, high, and extreme) and the recommendations for caries management procedures for each level.

   a. Low or moderate caries risk is assigned based on clinical judgment following an evaluation of the risk factors and protective factors of the patient.

   b. High caries risk is signified by the presence of any one of the following: clinical (visible) evidence of cavities or radiographic evidence of caries extending past the dentinoenamel junction and into the dentin, radiographic interproximal enamel lesions, white spots on smooth surfaces, or restorations in the last 3 years.

   c. Extreme caries risk is high caries risk and severe salivary gland hypofunction (salivary flow rate of less than 0.5 mL per minute).

3. **Evidence-Based Treatment Plan.** Following caries risk determination, the next step is to develop an evidence-based treatment plan based upon the patient's risk level.

   a. Low risk patients should use fluoride toothpaste twice daily and professional topical fluoride applications are optional. Bacterial and salivary tests are not necessary. Most periodontal maintenance patients are not considered low risk because exposed roots are a primary risk factor for root caries.

   b. Moderate caries risk patients should use fluoride toothpaste twice daily, rinse with a 0.05% sodium fluoride mouthrinse, and receive fluoride varnish applications at maintenance appointments. Bacterial and salivary tests are optional.

   c. High caries risk patients should use a prescription of 1.1% sodium fluoride toothpaste twice daily and receive 1 to 3 topical fluoride varnish applications during initial therapy. Fluoride varnish should be applied at 3-month intervals. Bacterial and salivary tests are recommended.

   d. Extreme caries risk patients receive the same CAMBRA therapies as high risk. In addition, baking soda rinses, 0.5% sodium fluoride rinses, and calcium/phosphate pastes may be recommended.

Caries Risk Assessment Form - Children Age 6 and Over/Adults

Patient Name: _____ Chart #: _____ Date: _____

Assessment Date: Is this (please circle) base line   or   recall

Disease Indicators (Any one "YES" signifies likely "High Risk" and to do a bacteria test**)	YES = CIRCLE	YES = CIRCLE	YES = CIRCLE
Visible cavities or radiographic penetration of the dentin	YES		
Radiographic approximal enamel lesions (not in dentin)	YES		
White spots on smooth surfaces	YES		
Restorations last 3 years	YES		
Risk Factors (Biological or predisposing factors)			
MS and LB both medium or high (by culture**)		YES	
Visible heavy plaque on teeth		YES	
Frequent snack (>3x daily between meals)		YES	
Deep pits and fissures		YES	
Recreational drug use		YES	
Inadequate saliva flow by observation or measurement (***If measured, note the flow rate below)		YES	
Saliva reducing factors (medications/radiation/systemic)		YES	
Exposed roots		YES	
Orthodontic appliances		YES	
Protective Factors			
Lives/work/school flouridated community			YES
Fluoride toothpaste at least once daily			YES
Fluoride toothpaste at least 2x daily			YES
Fluoride mouthrinse (0.05% NaF) daily			YES
5,000 ppm F fluoride toothpaste daily			YES
Flouride varnish in last 6 months			YES
Office F topical in last 6 months			YES
Chlorhexidine prescribed/used one week each of last 6 months			YES
Xylitol gum/lozenges 4x daily last 6 months			YES
Calcium and phosphate paste during last 6 months			YES
Adequate saliva flow (>1ml/min stimulated)			YES
Bacteria/Saliva Test Results: MS: LB: Flow Rate: ml/min. Date:			

VISUALIZE CARIES BALANCE
(Use circled indicators/factors above)
(EXTREME RISK = HIGH RISK + SEVERE SALIVARY GLAND HYPOFUNCTION)
CARIES RISK ASSESSMENT (CIRCLE): EXTREME   HIGH   MODERATE   LOW

Signature: _____   Date: _____

Figure 33-6. Caries Risk Assessment Form. Used with permission from Featherstone JD, Domejean-Orliaguet S, Jenson L, Wolff M, Young DA. Caries risk assessment in practice for age 6 through adult. *J Calif Dent Assoc.* 2007;35(10):Table 1, 703–707, 710–713.[80]

TABLE 33-1 | CARIES MANAGEMENT BY RISK ASSESSMENT: CLINICAL GUIDELINES

Risk Level[a,b]	Frequency of Radiographs	Frequency of Caries Recall	Saliva Test (Saliva Flow and Bacterial Culture)	Antibacterials Chlorhexidine Xylitol[c]	Fluoride	pH Control	Calcium Phosphate Topical Supplements
Low risk	Bitewing radiographs every 24–36 months	Every 6–12 months to reevaluate caries risk	May be done as a base line reference for new patients	Per saliva test if done	OTC fluoride-containing toothpaste twice daily; Optional NaF varnish if excessive root exposure or sensitivity	Not required	Not required; Optional for excessive root exposure or sensitivity
Moderate risk	Bitewing radiographs every 18–24 months	Every 4–6 months to reevaluate caries risk	May be done as a base line reference for new patients or if there is a suspicion of high bacterial challenge	Per saliva test if done; Xylitol (6–10 g/day) of gum or candies	OTC fluoride-containing toothpaste twice daily plus 0.05% NaF rinse daily. Initially 1–2 app of NaF varnish; 1 app at 4–6-month recall	Not required	Not required; Optional for excessive root exposure or sensitivity
High risk[d]	Bitewing radiographs every 6–18 months or until no cavitated lesions are evident	Every 3–4 months to reevaluate caries risk and apply fluoride varnish	Saliva flow test and bacterial culture initially and at every caries recall appt. to assess efficacy and patient cooperation	Chlorhexidine gluconate 0.12%; 10 mL rinse for 1 minute daily for 1 week each month. Xylitol (6–10 g/day)	1.1% NaF toothpaste twice daily instead of regular fluoride toothpaste; Optional 0.2% NaF rinse daily (1 bottle) then OTC 0.05% NaF rinse 2× daily. Initially 1–3 app of NaF varnish; 1 app at 3–4 month recall	Not required	Optional: Apply calcium/phosphate paste several times daily
Extreme risk[e] (High risk plus dry mouth or special needs	Bitewing radiographs every 6 months or until no cavitated lesions are evident	Every 3 months to reevaluate caries risk and apply fluoride varnish	Saliva flow test and bacterial culture initially and at every caries recall appt. to assess efficacy and patient cooperation	Chlorhexidine gluconate 0.12% (preferably CHX in water base rinse) 10 mL rinse for 1 minute daily for 1 week each month. Xylitol (6–10 g/day)	1.1% NaF toothpaste twice daily instead of regular fluoride toothpaste. OTC 0.05% NaF rinse when mouth feels dry, after snacking, breakfast, and lunch. Initially 1–3 app. NaF varnish; 1 app at 3-month recall	Acid neutralizing rinses as needed if mouth feels dry, after snacking, bedtime, and after breakfast. Baking soda gum as needed	Required. Apply calcium/phosphate paste twice daily

[a]All restorative work to be done with minimally invasive philosophy in mind.
[b]For all risk levels: Patients must maintain good self-care and a diet low in frequency of fermentable carbohydrates.
[c]Xylitol is not good for pets (especially dogs).
[d]Patients with one (or more) cavitated lesion(s) are high-risk patients.
[e]Patients with one (or more) cavitated lesion(s) and severe hyposalivation are extreme-risk patients.
Used with permission from Jenson L, Budenz AW, Featherstone JD, Ramos-Gomez FJ, Spolsky VW, Young DA. Clinical protocols for caries management by risk assessment. *J Calif Dent Assoc.* 2007;35(10):Table 1. 714–723.[73]

Chapter Summary Statement

Periodontal maintenance refers to continuing patient care provided by the dental team to help the periodontitis patient maintain periodontal health following successful completion of nonsurgical or surgical periodontal therapy. In most dental offices, the dental hygienist plays a major role during each periodontal maintenance visit. At each periodontal maintenance visit, the dental hygienist performs a thorough patient interview, clinical assessment, evaluation of effectiveness of self-care, identification of treatment needs, periodontal instrumentation, patient counseling, and application of fluorides. Currently, the most frequently recommended interval for periodontal maintenance is every 3 months. Recurrence of periodontitis in treated patients with the need for additional active periodontal treatment is always a possibility. Patient compliance with periodontal maintenance recommendations is poor, but strategies can be employed to improve compliance. Root caries is a complication in many treated periodontitis patients.

Section 6
Focus on Patients

Clinical Patient Care

CASE 1

Your dental team has just completed a reevaluation of the results of nonsurgical therapy for a patient with generalized Stage I periodontitis. The findings of the reevaluation reveal that the periodontitis appears to be under control and that periodontal maintenance is the next logical step. When should the first maintenance appointment be scheduled and what factors should be considered when assigning this maintenance interval?

CASE 2

One of your dental team's Stage II periodontitis patients has recently undergone periodontal surgery and now has several sites of gingival recession exposing tooth roots. Unfortunately, this patient has had a high incidence of both coronal and root caries over the past few years. What measures might your team take to minimize the risk of further root caries in this patient?

CASE 3

A patient who has been treated for Stage II periodontitis by your team has been followed for periodontal maintenance for more than 3 years. During each maintenance visit, there have been no indications of recurrence of the periodontitis. The patient calls you before her next maintenance visit to inform you that she has just been diagnosed with diabetes mellitus. She looked up diabetes on the Internet and now wants to know if this will affect her periodontal condition. How should your dental team respond to the patient's concern?

References

1. Allen E, Ziada H, Irwin C, Mullally B, Byrne PJ. Periodontics: 10. Maintenance in periodontal therapy. *Dent Update*. 2008;35(3):150–152, 154–156.

2. Ramfjord SP. Maintenance care and supportive periodontal therapy. *Quintessence Int*. 1993;24(7):465–471.

3. Shumaker ND, Metcalf BT, Toscano NT, Holtzclaw DJ. Periodontal and periimplant maintenance: a critical factor in long-term treatment success. *Compend Contin Educ Dent*. 2009;30(7):388–390.

4. Tan AE. Periodontal maintenance. *Aust Dent J*. 2009;54(Suppl 1):S110–S117.

5. Wilson TG, Jr., Valderrama P, Rodrigues DB. The case for routine maintenance of dental implants. *J Periodontol*. 2014;85(5):657–660.

6. Bostanci HS, Arpak MN. Long-term evaluation of surgical periodontal treatment with and without maintenance care. *J Nihon Univ Sch Dent*. 1991;33(3):152–159.

7. Costa FO, Cota LO, Lages EJ, et al. Periodontal risk assessment model in a sample of regular and irregular compliers under maintenance therapy: a 3-year prospective study. *J Periodontol*. 2012;83(3):292–300.

8. Jansson L, Lagervall M. Periodontitis progression in patients subjected to supportive maintenance care. *Swed Dent J*. 2008;32(3):105–114.

9. Lorentz TC, Cota LO, Cortelli JR, Vargas AM, Costa FO. Tooth loss in individuals under periodontal maintenance therapy: prospective study. *Braz Oral Res*. 2010;24(2):231–237.

10. Soolari A. Compliance and its role in successful treatment of an advanced periodontal case: review of the literature and a case report. *Quintessence Int*. 2002;33(5):389–396.

11. Costa FO, Miranda Cota LO, Pereira Lages EJ, et al. Progression of periodontitis and tooth loss associated with glycemic control in individuals undergoing periodontal maintenance therapy: a 5-year follow-up study. *J Periodontol*. 2013;84(5):595–605.

12. Lee CT, Huang HY, Sun TC, Karimbux N. Impact of patient compliance on tooth loss during supportive periodontal therapy: a systematic review and meta-analysis. *J Dent Res*. 2015;94(6):777–786.

13. Nibali L, Farias BC, Vajgel A, Tu YK, Donos N. Tooth loss in aggressive periodontitis: a systematic review. *J Dent Res*. 2013;92(10):868–875.

14. Chambrone L, Chambrone D, Lima LA, Chambrone LA. Predictors of tooth loss during long-term periodontal maintenance: a systematic review of observational studies. *J Clin Periodontol*. 2010;37(7):675–684.

15. Costa FO, Lages EJ, Cota LO, Lorentz TC, Soares RV, Cortelli JR. Tooth loss in individuals under periodontal maintenance therapy: 5-year prospective study. *J Periodontal Res*. 2014;49(1):121–128.

16. Ravald N, Johansson CS. Tooth loss in periodontally treated patients: a long-term study of periodontal disease and root caries. *J Clin Periodontol*. 2012;39(1):73–79.

17. Wilson TG, Jr., Glover ME, Malik AK, Schoen JA, Dorsett D. Tooth loss in maintenance patients in a private periodontal practice. *J Periodontol*. 1987;58(4):231–235.

18. Lorentz TC, Cota LO, Cortelli JR, Vargas AM, Costa FO. Prospective study of complier individuals under periodontal maintenance therapy: analysis of clinical periodontal parameters, risk predictors and the progression of periodontitis. *J Clin Periodontol*. 2009;36(1):58–67.

19. Parameters of Care. American Academy of Periodontology. *J Periodontol*. 2000;71(5 Suppl):i–ii, 847–883.

20. American Academy of Periodontology. Comprehensive periodontal therapy: a statement by the American Academy of Periodontology*. *J Periodontol*. 2011;82(7):943–949.

21. Cohen RE, Research Science and Therapy Committee, American Academy of Periodontology. Position paper: periodontal maintenance. *J Periodontol*. 2003;74(9):1395–1401.

22. Lang NP, Joss A, Tonetti MS. Monitoring disease during supportive periodontal treatment by bleeding on probing. *Periodontol 2000*. 1996;12:44–48.

23. Flemmig TF, Petersilka GJ, Mehl A, Hickel R, Klaiber B. Working parameters of a magnetostrictive ultrasonic scaler influencing root substance removal in vitro. *J Periodontol*. 1998;69(5):547–553.

24. Flemmig TF, Petersilka GJ, Mehl A, Hickel R, Klaiber B. The effect of working parameters on root substance removal using a piezoelectric ultrasonic scaler in vitro. *J Clin Periodontol*. 1998;25(2):158–163.

25. Flemmig TF, Petersilka GJ, Mehl A, Rudiger S, Hickel R, Klaiber B. Working parameters of a sonic scaler influencing root substance removal in vitro. *Clin Oral Investig*. 1997;1(2):55–60.

26. Kocher T, Fanghanel J, Sawaf H, Litz R. Substance loss caused by scaling with different sonic scaler inserts—an in vitro study. *J Clin Periodontol*. 2001;28(1):9–15.

27. Ritz L, Hefti AF, Rateitschak KH. An in vitro investigation on the loss of root substance in scaling with various instruments. *J Clin Periodontol*. 1991;18(9):643–647.

28. Schmidlin PR, Beuchat M, Busslinger A, Lehmann B, Lutz F. Tooth substance loss resulting from mechanical, sonic and ultrasonic root instrumentation assessed by liquid scintillation. *J Clin Periodontol*. 2001;28(11):1058–1066.

29. Badersten A, Nilveus R, Egelberg J. Effect of nonsurgical periodontal therapy. I. Moderately advanced periodontitis. *J Clin Periodontol*. 1981;8(1):57–72.

30. Badersten A, Nilveus R, Egelberg J. Effect of nonsurgical periodontal therapy. II. Severely advanced periodontitis. *J Clin Periodontol*. 1984;11(1):63–76.

31. Chabanski MB, Gillam DG. Aetiology, prevalence and clinical features of cervical dentine sensitivity. *J Oral Rehabil*. 1997;24(1):15–19.

32. Fischer C, Wennberg A, Fischer RG, Attstrom R. Clinical evaluation of pulp and dentine sensitivity after supragingival and subgingival scaling. *Endod Dent Traumatol*. 1991;7(6):259–265.

33. Tammaro S, Wennstrom JL, Bergenholtz G. Root-dentin sensitivity following non-surgical periodontal treatment. *J Clin Periodontol*. 2000;27(9):690–697.

34. von Troil B, Needleman I, Sanz M. A systematic review of the prevalence of root sensitivity following periodontal therapy. *J Clin Periodontol*. 2002;29(Suppl 3):173–177.

35. Moene R, Decaillet F, Andersen E, Mombelli A. Subgingival plaque removal using a new air-polishing device. *J Periodontol*. 2010;81(1):79–88.

36. Jacobson L, Blomlof J, Lindskog S. Root surface texture after different scaling modalities. *Scand J Dent Res*. 1994;102(3):156–160.

37. Mishra MK, Prakash S. A comparative scanning electron microscopy study between hand instrument, ultrasonic scaling and erbium doped:Yttrium aluminum garnet laser on root surface: A morphological and thermal analysis. *Contemp Clin Dent.* 2013;4(2):198–205.

38. Vatne JF, Gjermo P, Sandvik L, Preus HR. Patients' perception of own efforts versus clinically observed outcomes of non-surgical periodontal therapy in a Norwegian population: an observational study. *BMC Oral Health.* 2015;15:61.

39. Armitage GC, Xenoudi P. Post-treatment supportive care for the natural dentition and dental implants. *Periodontol 2000.* 2016;71(1):164–184.

40. Darcey J, Ashley M. See you in three months! The rationale for the three monthly periodontal recall interval: a risk based approach. *Br Dent J.* 2011;211(8):379–385.

41. Shiloah J, Patters MR. Repopulation of periodontal pockets by microbial pathogens in the absence of supportive therapy. *J Periodontol.* 1996;67(2):130–139.

42. Famili P, Short E. Compliance with periodontal maintenance at the University of Pittsburgh: Retrospective analysis of 315 cases. *Gen Dent.* 2010;58(1):e42–e47.

43. Ojima M, Hanioka T, Shizukuishi S. Survival analysis for degree of compliance with supportive periodontal therapy. *J Clin Periodontol.* 2001;28(12):1091–1095.

44. Wilson TG, Jr. Compliance. A review of the literature with possible applications to periodontics. *J Periodontol.* 1987;58(10):706–714.

45. de Carvalho VF, Okuda OS, Bernardo CC, et al. Compliance improvement in periodontal maintenance. *J Appl Oral Sci.* 2010;18(3):215–219.

46. Mendoza AR, Newcomb GM, Nixon KC. Compliance with supportive periodontal therapy. *J Periodontol.* 1991;62(12):731–736.

47. Novaes AB, Jr., Novaes AB. Compliance with supportive periodontal therapy. Part 1. Risk of non-compliance in the first 5-year period. *J Periodontol.* 1999;70(6):679–682.

48. Novaes AB, Jr., Novaes AB. Compliance with supportive periodontal therapy. Part II: Risk of non-compliance in a 10-year period. *Braz Dent J.* 2001;12(1):47–50.

49. Umaki TM, Umaki MR, Cobb CM. The psychology of patient compliance: a focused review of the literature. *J Periodontol.* 2012;83(4):395–400.

50. Dye BA, Tan S, Smith V, et al. Trends in oral health status: United States, 1988–1994 and 1999–2004. *Vital Health Stat 11.* 2007;248:1–92.

51. Chi DL, Berg JH, Kim AS, Scott J; Northwest Practice-based REsearch Collaborative in Evidence-based DENTistry. Correlates of root caries experience in middle-aged and older adults in the Northwest Practice-based REsearch Collaborative in Evidence-based DENTistry research network. *J Am Dent Assoc.* 2013;144(5):507–516.

52. Griffin SO, Griffin PM, Swann JL, Zlobin N. Estimating rates of new root caries in older adults. *J Dent Res.* 2004;83(8):634–638.

53. Pitts N, Ekstrand K; ICDAS Foundation. International Caries Detection and Assessment System (ICDAS) and its International Caries Classification and Management System (ICCMS)—methods for staging of the caries process and enabling dentists to manage caries. *Community Dent Oral Epidemiol.* 2013;41(1):e41–e52.

54. Shivakumar K, Prasad S, Chandu G. International Caries Detection and Assessment System: A new paradigm in detection of dental caries. *J Conserv Dent.* 2009;12(1):10–16.

55. Berry TG, Summitt JB, Sift EJ, Jr. Root caries. *Oper Dent.* 2004;29(6):601–607.

56. Zambon JJ, Kasprzak SA. The microbiology and histopathology of human root caries. *Am J Dent.* 1995;8(6):323–328.

57. Atkinson JC, Wu AJ. Salivary gland dysfunction: causes, symptoms, treatment. *J Am Dent Assoc.* 1994;125(4):409–416.

58. Ogaard B, Arends J, Rolla G. Action of fluoride on initiation of early root surface caries in vivo. *Caries Res.* 1990;24(2):142–144.

59. Lopez R, Smith PC, Gostemeyer G, Schwendicke F. Ageing, dental caries and periodontal diseases. *J Clin Periodontol.* 2017;44(Suppl 18):S145–S152.

60. Papas A, Joshi A, Giunta J. Prevalence and intraoral distribution of coronal and root caries in middle-aged and older adults. *Caries Res.* 1992;26(6):459–465.

61. Griffin SO, Regnier E, Griffin PM, Huntley V. Effectiveness of fluoride in preventing caries in adults. *J Dent Res.* 2007;86(5):410–415.

62. Heijnsbroek M, Paraskevas S, Van der Weijden GA. Fluoride interventions for root caries: a review. *Oral Health Prev Dent.* 2007;5(2):145–152.

63. Gibson G, Jurasic MM, Wehler CJ, Jones JA. Supplemental fluoride use for moderate and high caries risk adults: a systematic review. *J Public Health Dent.* 2011;71(3):171–184.

64. Brustman BA. Impact of exposure to fluoride-adequate water on root surface caries in elderly. *Gerodontics.* 1986;2(6):203–207.

65. Jensen ME, Kohout F. The effect of a fluoridated dentifrice on root and coronal caries in an older adult population. *J Am Dent Assoc.* 1988;117(7):829–832.

66. Ekstrand KR, Poulsen JE, Hede B, Twetman S, Qvist V, Ellwood RP. A randomized clinical trial of the anti-caries efficacy of 5,000 compared to 1,450 ppm fluoridated toothpaste on root caries lesions in elderly disabled nursing home residents. *Caries Res.* 2013;47(5):391–398.

67. Sjogren K, Birkhed D. Factors related to fluoride retention after toothbrushing and possible connection to caries activity. *Caries Res.* 1993;27(6):474–477.

68. Ripa LW, Leske GS, Forte F, Varma A. Effect of a 0.05% neutral NaF mouthrinse on coronal and root caries of adults. *Gerodontology.* 1987;6(4):131–136.

69. Wallace MC, Retief DH, Bradley EL. The 48-month increment of root caries in an urban population of older adults participating in a preventive dental program. *J Public Health Dent.* 1993;53(3):133–137.

70. Hendre AD, Taylor GW, Chavez EM, Hyde S. A systematic review of silver diamine fluoride: Effectiveness and application in older adults. *Gerodontology.* 2017;34(4):411–419.

71. Horst JA, Ellenikiotis H, Milgrom PL. UCSF Protocol for Caries Arrest Using Silver Diamine Fluoride: Rationale, Indications and Consent. *J Calif Dent Assoc.* 2016;44(1):16–28.

72. Schaeken MJ, Keltjens HM, Van Der Hoeven JS. Effects of fluoride and chlorhexidine on the microflora of dental root surfaces and progression of root-surface caries. *J Dent Res.* 1991;70(2):150–153.

73. Slot DE, Vaandrager NC, Van Loveren C, Van Palenstein Helderman WH, Van der Weijden GA. The effect of chlorhexidine varnish on root caries: a systematic review. *Caries Res.* 2011;45(2):162–173.

74. Featherstone JD, White JM, Hoover CI, et al. A randomized clinical trial of anticaries therapies targeted according to risk assessment (caries management by risk assessment). *Caries Res.* 2012;46(2):118–129.

75. Ritter AV, Bader JD, Leo MC, et al. Tooth-surface-specific effects of xylitol: randomized trial results. *J Dent Res.* 2013;92(6):512–517.

76. Azarpazhooh A, Limeback H. Clinical efficacy of casein derivatives: a systematic review of the literature. *J Am Dent Assoc.* 2008;139(7):915–924.

77. Rethman MP, Beltran-Aguilar ED, Billings RJ, et al. Nonfluoride caries-preventive agents: executive summary of evidence-based clinical recommendations. *J Am Dent Assoc.* 2011;142(9):1065–1071.

78. Bignozzi I, Crea A, Capri D, Littarru C, Lajolo C, Tatakis DN. Root caries: a periodontal perspective. *J Periodontal Res.* 2014;49(2):143–163.

79. Wierichs RJ, Meyer-Lueckel H. Systematic review on noninvasive treatment of root caries lesions. *J Dent Res.* 2015;94(2):261–271.

80. Featherstone JD, Domejean-Orliaguet S, Jenson L, Wolff M, Young DA. Caries risk assessment in practice for age 6 through adult. *J Calif Dent Assoc.* 2007;35(10):703–707.

81. Young DA, Featherstone JD, Roth JR. Curing the silent epidemic: caries management in the 21st century and beyond. *J Calif Dent Assoc.* 2007;35(10):681–685.

82. Featherstone JD, Adair SM, Anderson MH, et al. Caries management by risk assessment: consensus statement, April 2002. *J Calif Dent Assoc.* 2003;31(3):257–269.

83. Domejean-Orliaguet S, Gansky SA, Featherstone JD. Caries risk assessment in an educational environment. *J Dent Educ.* 2006;70(12):1346–1354.

 STUDENT ANCILLARY RESOURCES

A wide variety of resources to enhance your learning is available online:

- Audio Glossary
- Book Pages
- Chapter Review Questions and Answers

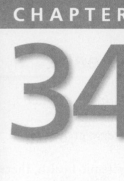

CHAPTER

34 Impact of Periodontitis on Systemic Health

Clinical Application. Over the last several decades, an important bidirectional relationship between periodontal disease and certain systemic diseases has been uncovered, bridging the once-wide gap between medicine and dentistry. On one side of this relationship (as discussed in Chapter 16), it is recognized that certain systemic factors can potentially influence the progression and severity of periodontal disease. On the other side of this relationship (as will be the focus of this chapter), periodontitis has been implicated as a potential contributing factor in the pathogenesis of certain systemic diseases. The possibility of an association between periodontal disease and systemic disease suggests that periodontal therapy may play an important role in decreasing the incidence and severity of certain systemic diseases. Interprofessional relationships between dental team members and other health care providers should be established early to provide the highest standard of care for patients with systemic disease.

Learning Objectives

- Contrast the terms "association" and "causation" between a given factor (A) and a systemic disease (B).
- Educate patients at risk for cardiovascular diseases about the possible impact of periodontal infection on cardiovascular health and encourage oral disease prevention and treatment services.
- Educate pregnant women and those planning pregnancies regarding the possible impact of periodontal infection on pregnancy outcomes and encourage preventive oral care and treatment services.
- Educate patients with diabetes about the probable bidirectional association between periodontal disease and diabetes and encourage oral disease prevention and treatment services.
- Educate family members and caregivers about the association between periodontal disease and pneumonia in health-compromised individuals in hospitals and long-term care facilities.
- Establish collaborative relationships with other health care providers to ensure the highest standard of care for periodontal patients with systemic diseases and conditions.

Key Terms

Association	C-reactive protein	Community-acquired pneumonia
Causation	Preeclampsia	Hospital-acquired pneumonia
Metastatic infection	Glycemic control	Ventilator-associated
Atherosclerosis	HbA1C	pneumonia

Section 1
Linking Periodontitis With Systemic Disease

Recently, it has been recognized that oral infection, especially periodontitis, may alter the course and pathogenesis of a number of systemic diseases/conditions, such as cardiovascular disease, bacterial pneumonia, diabetes mellitus, and adverse pregnancy outcomes.

While there seems to be an association between oral health and systemic health, there is no scientific evidence at this time to suggest a causal relationship between the two. *When reading and interpreting research, great care must be taken to understand exactly what the data and statistics are implying—and more importantly—what they are not implying.* The terms association and causality are two important concepts relevant to medical and dental research. For example, when researchers find an association between a given factor (A) and a health effect (B), this relationship does not necessarily imply that Factor A *causes* the specific disease B. It is important for health care providers to understand the difference between *association* and *causation* and to help patients understand what the research means to their health.

1. **Association Versus Causal Relationships.** Theoretically, the difference between association and a causal relationship is easy to distinguish—variable A can *cause* variable B (e.g., smoking *causes* an increased risk of developing lung cancer), or variable A *is associated* with variable B (e.g., smoking is associated with alcoholism, but smoking does not cause alcoholism).
   A. **Association.** Association indicates that there is a relationship or a connection between two or more variables (the rate of alcoholism is higher in smokers). An association cannot explain why or how the variables are related and *does not necessarily mean that one variable causes the other variable.* More research is necessary before that conclusion can be reached.
   B. **Causation.** Causation means that variable A is certain to cause or lead to variable B (the *Mycobacterium tuberculosis* bacterium causes the disease, tuberculosis). Determining causation of a disease or condition is difficult. Diseases may be caused by a multitude of factors; causation often involves joint actions of several complex mechanisms.
      1. For example, we used to believe that stomach ulcers were *caused* by stress and spicy foods. Yet, current research proves that ulcers are caused by a corkscrew-shaped bacterium, *Helicobacter pylori*. Natural stomach acids and spicy food may have irritated the already damaged stomach lining (association) but never caused the ulcers (causation).
      2. *Based on available research, it is not possible to prove causality between periodontitis and systemic disease.*[1] In 2013, Working Group 4 of *The Joint European Federation of Periodontology (EFP) and American Academy of Periodontology (AAP) Workshop on Periodontitis and Systemic Diseases* was unanimous in their opinion that the reported associations of periodontitis and systemic diseases do not imply causality.[2] The working group further concluded that gaps in knowledge are large. It is possible that the association is the result of common risk factors and not causality.

2. **Possible Mechanisms Linking Periodontitis to Systemic Disease.** *The best evidence suggests that periodontitis is characterized by both infection and pro-inflammatory events and may contribute toward select systemic diseases and disorders.*[2] Three mechanisms have been postulated as to how periodontitis may modify some aspect of certain systemic diseases to make those diseases more severe: (1) metastatic infection, (2) inflammation, and (3) immune response.[3] All three of these mechanisms have the potential to impact the systemic inflammatory/immune response that, in turn, may mediate a range of systemic diseases.

A. **Metastatic Infection.** Metastatic infection is an infectious disease mediated by microorganisms that originate from a distant body site. For example, certain organisms found in the oral microbiome can travel to the lung and possibly cause a lung infection.[4,5]

1. A periodontal infection is not limited to the periodontium or even the oral cavity.[5,6] The everyday acts of chewing and tooth brushing disseminate whole bacteria and their products throughout the body to other nonadjacent organs or body parts.[7]

2. Oral bacteria from periodontal lesions and the DNA of periodontal pathogens can survive in the blood stream and adhere to other sites in the body causing systemic disorders, such as endocarditis, lung infections, abscesses of the brain or liver, and fatty deposits in the carotid arteries.

B. **Inflammation**

1. Infection of the periodontal pocket can stimulate the oral tissues to release pro-inflammatory mediators which can then enter the blood stream and initiate significant systemic inflammation. Leukocytes, hepatocytes, and endothelial cells respond to oral bacteria by releasing pro-inflammatory mediators (cytokines, chemokines, C-reactive protein) that amplify systemic inflammation.[8,9]

2. Pro-inflammatory mediators—such as IL-1β, IL-6, TNF-α, and PGE$_2$—produced locally in the inflamed periodontal tissues disseminate into the blood stream and have a systemic impact.[8,10]

C. **Immune Response**

1. In periodontitis, bacterial antigens are processed and presented to body's immune system and recognized by lymphocytes (T-lymphocytes and B-lymphocytes). In response to a microbial challenge, host immune cells release pro-inflammatory mediators. As discussed in Chapter 15, it is clear that the body's immune response plays a significant role in inflammation and tissue destruction.

2. Systemic inflammation—defined by increased circulating pro-inflammatory mediators such as TNF-α—is associated with obesity, diabetes, and periodontitis and has been proposed as a mechanism for the connection between these conditions.[11,12]

3. A hypercoagulable state is a medical term for an abnormally increased tendency toward coagulation. In atherosclerotic cardiovascular disease, blood coagulation can have an adverse effect when a blood clot forms in a coronary artery, obstructing blood flow to the heart.

4. The coagulation and fibrinolytic systems play important roles in the thickening of the arteries and clot formation.[32,33] *Elevated fibrinogen is a risk factor for atherosclerosis.*

5. The association of periodontitis with blood clotting factors has been reported by a number of investigators.
   a. In an early study, Kweider and colleagues reported that patients with periodontitis have higher plasma fibrinogen levels than age-matched control subjects.[34]
   b. Recent studies note increased fibrinogen levels in patients with periodontitis and an association between the number of periodontal pockets and fibrinogen levels.[35–39]

D. **Periodontitis May Result in Dyslipidemia**
   1. In this fourth proposed pathway, periodontal infections may contribute to atherosclerosis by triggering the host to produce elevated levels of serum cholesterol, as well as low-density lipoproteins (LDLs), triglycerides, and very low-density lipoproteins (vLDL).[17]
   2. Dyslipidemia (dys·lip·id·e·mia) refers to abnormal amounts of lipids ("fats") and lipoproteins in the blood. A lipoprotein is a molecule that is a combination of lipid (fat) and protein. Lipoproteins are the form in which lipids are transported in the blood.
   3. Several studies indicate that blood serum concentrations of inflammatory lipids, including cholesterol, LDLs, triglycerides, and vLDL are elevated in periodontitis patients. These inflammatory lipids may more easily enter the blood vessel wall and therefore are more likely to be incorporated in to the atherosclerotic lesion (thickening of the vessel wall). This would accelerate development of the local lesions.[40–42]

3. **Clinical Relevance: ACVD and Periodontitis**
   A. *The Consensus Report of the EFP/AAP Workshop on Periodontitis and Systemic Diseases* concludes that "there is consistent and strong epidemiologic evidence that periodontitis imparts increased risk for future cardiovascular disease; and while in vitro, animal and clinical studies do support the interaction and biological mechanism, intervention trails to date are not adequate to draw further conclusions."[16]
   B. *It is important to note, however, that insufficient evidence exists to show that the treatment of periodontal disease can reduce the risk for cardiovascular disease.* The impact of treatment for periodontitis on the cardiovascular disease is an area for ongoing research.

4. **Implications for Dental Practice: ACVD and Periodontitis**
   A. Dental health care providers should be aware of the emerging evidence that periodontitis is a risk factor for developing ACVD. All members of the dental team should be prepared to educate patients who are at risk for cardiovascular diseases about the possible impact of periodontal infection on cardiovascular health.[16,43]
   B. There is evidence suggesting that periodontal therapy reduces systemic inflammation, but limited evidence on its effects on cardiovascular health in the long term.[44] Well-designed research studies are needed to clarify associations of poor periodontal health on atherosclerotic cardiovascular disease.[45]

C. Comprehensive periodontal therapy should include patient education and advice on modifiable lifestyle risk factors such as smoking, diet, and exercise. Collaboration with appropriate specialists may facilitate the patient's efforts in making lifestyle modifications.[16,43]

D. Periodontitis patients—with other risk factors for ACVD, such as smoking, hypertension, obesity, etc.—who have not been seen by a physician within the last year should be referred for a physical.[16,43]

E. Table 34-1 summarizes clinical recommendations for the care of individuals with periodontitis and specific risk factors as published in the *American Journal of Cardiology* and the *Journal of Periodontology*.[16,43]

TABLE 34-1	CLINICAL RECOMMENDATIONS: PATIENTS WITH PERIODONTITIS	
Condition	**ACVD Risk Factors**	**Recommendations**
Moderate to severe periodontitis	None	Inform patient that there may be an increased risk for CVD associated with periodontitis
Moderate to severe periodontitis	One known risk factor (smoking, family history of CVD, high cholesterol)	Recommend that patient seek a medical evaluation if he/she has not had one in the last 12 months
Mild, moderate, or severe periodontitis	Two or more known risk factors	Refer patient for a medical evaluation if he/she has not had one in the last 12 months

ADVERSE PREGANCY OUTCOMES

1. Overview of Adverse Pregnancy Outcomes
   A. Adverse pregnancy outcomes that have been associated with periodontitis include preterm birth, low birth weight, and preeclampsia. The strength of this association, however, is modest.[14]
      1. Preterm delivery of low–birth-weight infants is a leading cause of neonatal death and long-term neurodevelopmental disturbances and health problems in children.
      2. Preeclampsia is a serious complication of pregnancy that can have serious (and possibly life-threatening) repercussions on both the mother and the unborn baby. For the unborn baby, preeclampsia can reduce the blood flow to the placenta, thereby decreasing the amount of oxygen and nutrients that flow to the fetus. If preeclampsia occurs prior to 37 weeks, the physician may decide that it is necessary to induce delivery to resolve this serious condition and save both the mother and unborn baby. This would result in the preterm birth of a low-birth-weight infant.
   B. Adverse pregnancy outcomes most likely involve additional shared risk factors with periodontitis, such as tobacco use, alcohol use, obesity, and diabetes.

2. **Two Proposed Biologically Plausible Mechanisms. How is Periodontitis Related to Adverse Pregnancy Outcomes?** Research demonstrates a modest association between periodontal disease and adverse pregnancy outcomes; however, exact mechanisms remain unclear. Two major pathways have been proposed—direct and indirect pathways.[46–48] Figure 34-2A–C shows these proposed biologic pathways.

A. The direct biological pathway proposes that oral microorganisms and/or their components disseminate from the oral cavity and directly travel to the placenta/fetal unit. In turn, the placenta/fetal unit, itself, mounts an inflammatory immune response by releasing increased levels of proinflammatory mediators. While these proinflammatory mediators have a protective role, they also have the potential to trigger a range of adverse pregnancy outcomes, such as hypercontractility of the uterine smooth muscle, cervical dilation, and loss of membrane integrity leading to pre term delivery or, even worse, spontaneous abortion, late miscarriage, or stillbirth (Fig. 34-2A).

B. The indirect pathway may occur via two separate mechanisms:

1. In response to bacterial challenge, the *maternal periodontal tissues* locally produce pro-inflammatory mediators (e.g., PGE_2, TNF-α). These locally produced pro-inflammatory mediators enter the maternal bloodstream to initiate, intensify, and propagate the inflammatory response systemically. Ultimately, the pro-inflammatory mediators travel to the placenta/fetal unit and result in a potentially adverse outcome (Fig. 34-2B).

2. The oral bacteria enter the maternal blood stream and circulate to the liver, enhancing cytokine production (e.g., IL 6) and acute phase protein reactants (e.g., CRP). The cytokines and acute protein reactants then spread systemically to eventually have an adverse impact on the fetal–placental unit (Fig. 34-2C).

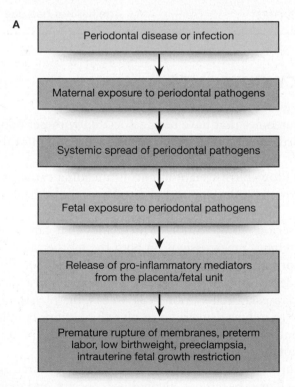

Figure 34-2A. Direct Pathway #1. The oral bacteria travel directly from the maternal periodontal tissues to the placenta/fetal unit.

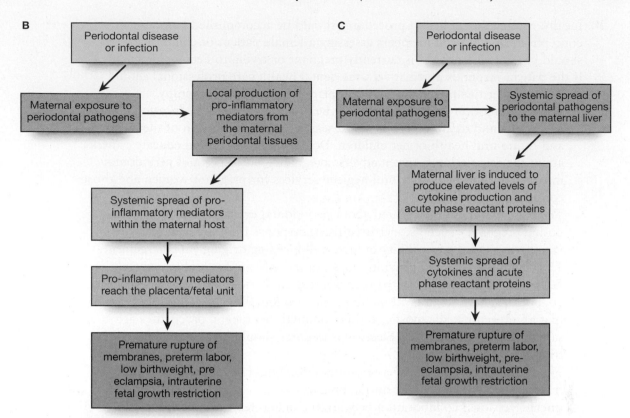

Figure 34-2B. Indirect Pathway #1. Unlike the direct pathway, the oral bacteria do not directly travel to the placenta/fetal unit, but rather induces the *maternal periodontal tissues* to release elevated levels of pro-inflammatory mediators. From there, the pro-inflammatory mediators spread systemically to have an impact on the placenta/fetal unit.

Figure 34-2C. Indirect Pathway #2. The oral bacteria spread systemically within the maternal host and reaches the *maternal liver*. The liver responds by producing elevated levels of pro-inflammatory mediators and acute phase reactant proteins. From there, elevated levels of pro-inflammatory mediators and acute phase reactant proteins spread to the placenta/fetal unit to potentially induce an adverse pregnancy outcome.

3. **Clinical Relevance: Adverse Pregnancy Outcomes and Periodontitis**
   A. Periodontitis may be a significant, modifiable risk factor for adverse pregnancy outcomes. The *Consensus Report of the EFP/AAP Workshop on Periodontitis and Systemic Diseases* concludes that "it is very relevant to understand the extent of these associations, their possible biological mechanisms, and the implications for healthcare."[14]
   B. *It is important to note, however, that nonsurgical treatment of pregnant women does not significantly reduce the risk of preterm birth or low birthweight.*[48]
4. **Implications for Dental Practice: Adverse Pregnancy Outcomes and Periodontitis**
   A. The American Academy of Periodontology issued a statement in 2004 recommending, "Women who are pregnant or planning pregnancy should undergo periodontal examinations. Appropriate preventive or therapeutic services, if indicated, should be provided. Preventive oral care services should be provided as early in pregnancy as possible. However, women should be encouraged to achieve a high level of oral hygiene prior to becoming pregnant and throughout their pregnancies."[49]

B. Ideally, routine dental health procedures should be accomplished before conception. Dental team members assessing a female patient of childbearing age should inquire whether she is currently pregnant or trying to become pregnant. If the patient responds affirmatively, the dental health care professional should always consider this pregnancy status in planning periodontal therapy.

1. Health promotion information should be provided including education about preventing and treating periodontal diseases for the oral health of the patient and future oral health of her children. Dental clinicians should educate patients about the association between adverse pregnancy outcomes and periodontal infection and provide early oral hygiene services for pregnant women and those considering pregnancy.

2. The patient should be educated about periodontal events usually occurring during pregnancy such as: increased tissue response to biofilm, increase in vascularity, and the possibility of increased bleeding or gingival enlargement. The dental team should provide education on self-care for biofilm control.

3. Periodontitis should be treated with nonsurgical periodontal therapy with the goal of reducing subgingival biofilm and periodontal inflammation. Emphasize that all preventive, diagnostic, and periodontal therapeutic procedures are safe throughout pregnancy. Elective procedures should be avoided in the first trimester.

4. The pregnant patient with periodontitis should be scheduled for periodontal maintenance at a later stage during pregnancy.

5. Interprofessional collaboration between the dental team and other health professionals involved with pregnancy care is strongly encouraged. It is important to remember that treatment is being rendered to two patients: mother and fetus. All treatment should be done only after consultation with the patient's obstetrician. It is best to avoid drugs and therapy that would put a fetus at risk.[50]

DIABETES MELLITUS

Over the last several decades, a body of evidence supports significant associations between periodontitis and adverse effects on glycemic control in individuals with diabetes, glycemic status in individuals without diabetes, and complications of diabetes.[13,51-55] The American Diabetes Association's *Standards of Medical Care in Diabetes—2018* emphasizes the importance of taking a history of past and current dental infections as part of the physician's examination.[56]

1. Overview of Glycemic Control in Diabetes
    A. Glycemic control is a medical term referring to the typical blood glucose levels in those with diabetes mellitus.
        1. Optimal management of diabetes involves patients monitoring and recording their own blood glucose levels.
        2. If left unchecked and untreated, prolonged and elevated levels of glucose in the blood will result in serious health complications, or even death.
    B. Blood glucose level is measured by means of a glucose meter, with the result either in mg/dL (milligrams per deciliter in the USA) or mmol/L (millimoles per liter in Canada and Europe) of blood.
        1. A fasting blood glucose level (blood sugar level) *less than* 100 mg/dL (5.6 mmol/L) is normal. A fasting blood glucose level between 100 mg/dL and 125 mg/dL is considered prediabetes.

2. Poor glycemic control refers to persistently elevated fasting blood glucose, greater than or equal to 126 mg/dL (7 mmol/L), or a glycosylated hemoglobin level greater than 7%.

C. **HbA1C** level is the average blood glucose level over the past 2 to 3 months (the lifespan of the red blood cell). The HbA1C test measures the amount of glycosylated hemoglobin in the blood. Glucose in the blood enters the red blood cell and attaches to the hemoglobin. The more glucose in the blood, the more will irreversibly bind to the hemoglobin. A1C is reported as a percentage of total hemoglobin in the blood. For example, an A1C of 8 means that 8% of the hemoglobin has glucose bound to it.

1. A normal HbA1C level for nondiabetics is *below* 5.6%.[57]
2. A reasonable A1C goal for many adults with diabetes is *below* 7%.[58]

2. **Proposed Biologically Plausible Mechanism. How is Periodontitis Related to Diabetes Mellitus?** Diabetes is the pathological consequence of a number of physiological changes and the resulting impairment of metabolic regulation, hyperglycemia, and chronic inflammation that potentially impacts tissue integrity and repair. Figure 34-3 illustrates this potential biologic pathway that provides a helpful perspective but needs further supportive evidence.

A. Periodontal diseases may serve as initiators of insulin resistance, thereby aggravating glycemic control. In this proposed pathway, systemic inflammation induced by periodontitis may increase insulin resistance, adversely affect glycemic control, and contribute to the development of complications in patients with diabetes mellitus.

B. Evidence suggests that periodontitis raises the levels of pro-inflammatory mediators in blood serum.[13,51,59–63]

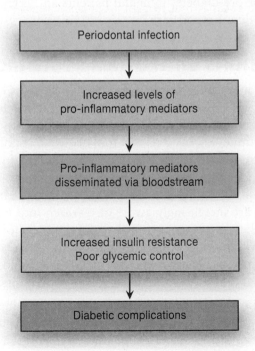

Figure 34-3. Proposed Biological Pathway for the Association Between Periodontal Disease and Diabetes. Periodontal diseases may serve as initiators of insulin resistance, thereby aggravating glycemic control.

3. **Clinical Relevance: Periodontitis and Diabetes Mellitus**
   A. Severe periodontitis adversely effects diabetes control. There is a direct relationship between periodontitis severity and diabetes complications in patients with diabetes and emerging evidence that severe periodontitis may predispose individuals to the development of diabetes.[13]
   B. Several studies indicate that periodontal therapy may result in improved insulin sensitivity, and eventually lead to improved glycemic control and overall outcomes of diabetes mellitus.[64–66]
   C. There is substantial information on potential mechanistic pathways which support a close association between diabetes and periodontitis, but there is a real need for longitudinal clinical studies using larger patient groups.[55]
4. **Implications for Dental Practice: Periodontitis and Diabetes Mellitus**
   A. Members of the dental team should be prepared to educate patients with diabetes about the possible impact of periodontal infection on glycemic control and encourage oral disease prevention and treatment services.
   B. Patients with diabetes should be informed of other associated oral conditions, such as xerostomia, burning mouth syndrome, fungal infections, and slower wound healing.
   C. Collaboration with other health care professionals is encouraged to assist patients in managing diabetes. As our understanding of the relationship between diabetes mellitus and periodontitis deepens, collaboration among medical and dental professionals for the management of affected individuals becomes increasingly important.[51]
   D. Many patients with diabetes remain undiagnosed, and oral findings may offer an opportunity for the identification of affected individuals unaware of their condition. Dental health care professionals have the opportunity to identify unrecognized diabetes or pre-diabetes in dental patients and refer them to a physician for further evaluation and care.[67]

POTENTIAL ASSOCIATIONS WITH OTHER SYSTEMIC CONDITIONS

In recent years, there has been intense interest in potential associations between periodontal disease and various chronic systemic diseases and conditions. Diseases with possible associations to periodontitis include chronic obstructive pulmonary disease (COPD), pneumonia, chronic kidney disease, rheumatoid arthritis, cognitive impairment, obesity, metabolic syndrome, and cancer. Evidence of potential links of periodontitis to these systemic conditions is minimal and *no causal relationships* can be inferred to date, with the exception that organisms found in the oral microbiome cause lung infections.[1,2]

Patients with periodontitis are increasingly aware of research into possible links with systemic diseases. Yet, to be clear, members of the dental team should be aware that while current research demonstrates a weak association, there is no concrete evidence that periodontal disease has a causative role in COPD, chronic kidney disease, rheumatoid arthritis, cognitive impairment, obesity, metabolic syndrome, and cancer.

1. **Pneumonia.** Pneumonia is a serious inflammation of one or both lungs. It is caused by the inhalation of microorganisms and can range in severity from mild to life threatening. There are two types of pneumonia: community-acquired and hospital-acquired.
   A. **Overview of Pneumonia**
      1. Community-acquired pneumonia is pneumonia that is contracted outside of the hospital setting.

    a. Most cases of community-acquired bacterial pneumonia are caused by aspiration of oropharyngeal organisms such as *Streptococcus pneumoniae*, *Haemophilus influenzae*, and *Mycoplasma pneumoniae*.[68]

    b. Community-acquired bacterial pneumonia generally responds well to treatment. There is no evidence that periodontal disease or oral hygiene alters the risk for community-acquired pneumonia.

2. Hospital-acquired pneumonia is an infection of the lungs contracted during a stay in a hospital or long-term care facility.

    a. Hospital-acquired pneumonia usually results from organisms called *potential respiratory pathogens* that are generally found in the gastrointestinal tract but may colonize the mouth and oropharynx. Bacterial plaque biofilms can serve as reservoirs of potential respiratory pathogens, particularly during prolonged hospitalization.[1,2,69-71]

    b. Oral colonization with potential respiratory pathogens increases during hospitalization, and the longer a patient is hospitalized the greater their prevalence.

    c. Ventilator-associated pneumonia is a type of hospital-acquired pneumonia developing after intubation for mechanical ventilation.

        1. In ventilator-associated pneumonia, placement of the endotracheal tube can transport oropharyngeal organisms into the lower airway.

        2. The oral cavity may serve as an important reservoir of infection for ventilator-associated pneumonia.[1,2,70,72,73]

B. Proposed Biologically Plausible Mechanisms. How is Periodontitis Related to Pneumonia? There are four biologically plausible mechanisms to explain the possible role of oral pathogens in the onset and pathogenesis of respiratory infection.[74] These potential mechanisms are depicted in Figure 34-4.

1. *Direct Aspiration of Oral Pathogens into the Lung.* Oral bacteria are constantly shedding from the plaque biofilm into the saliva and subsequently aspirated into the lungs. In individuals with a competent immune system, this event ordinarily has no deleterious effect since the immune system is capable of neutralizing the oral bacteria invading the lungs. However, immunocompromised patients lack a capable immune system to ward off the bacterial invasion. As a result, these types of individuals may be more susceptible to developing a lung infection.

2. *Modification of Oral Mucosal Surfaces by Periodontal Disease-Associated Bacteria.* Patients with poor self-care and/or a deficient immune system have elevated levels of oral pathogens which have the ability to release proteolytic enzymes. The actions of the proteolytic enzymes alter the environment of the surface epithelium so as to favor the adhesion and colonization of potential respiratory pathogens to the mucosal surface. Subsequently, the potential respiratory pathogens can be aspirated into the lungs.

3. *Reduction of Protective Salivary Pellicle by Oral Bacteria.* Not only can bacterial-derived proteolytic enzymes alter the oral mucosal surface, but it can also have damaging effects on the salivary pellicle. Ordinarily, the salivary pellicle plays a role in defending the host by "sticking" to pathogens before they have a chance to adhere to oral mucosal tissue. In patients with poor oral hygiene, the increased bacterial levels result in elevated production of proteolytic enzymes which enter the saliva from the gingival sulcus. Exposure of the salivary pellicle to these proteolytic enzymes will cause pellicle destruction. As a result, the host has lost a means of limiting the adhesion of potential respiratory pathogens to the oral mucosa tissue. Periodontal pathogens, such as *Porphyromonas gingivalis* have the capability to produce these damaging enzymes.

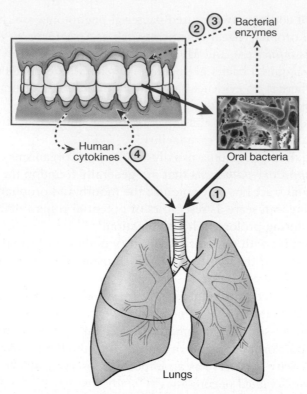

Figure 34-4. Biologically Plausible Mechanisms by Which Oral Bacteria Play a Role in Respiratory Infection. (*1*) Oral pathogens may be directly inhaled into the lungs. (*2*) Oral microorganisms may release enzymes that may damage oral mucosal surfaces causing increased colonization by pathogenic bacteria. (*3*) Oral bacterial enzymes may reduce the protection of the protective salivary pellicle resulting in increased colonization by pathogenic bacteria. (*4*) Salivary cytokines may alter the respiratory epithelium, promoting respiratory infection.

4. *Alteration of Respiratory Epithelium by Salivary Cytokines.* Patients with poor oral hygiene have increased levels of plaque biofilm which, in turn, stimulates cells of the periodontium and oral tissues to deploy a wide array of pro-inflammatory mediators. It is possible that the pro-inflammatory mediators originating from the host oral tissues may exit from the gingival sulcus and be mixed with the whole saliva. The contaminated saliva may travel to the respiratory epithelium and stimulate the respiratory cells to release more cytokines that have the potential to damage respiratory epithelium and make it more susceptible to colonization by both oral pathogens and respiratory pathogens.

C. **Implications for Dental Practice: Pneumonia and Periodontitis**
1. There is ample evidence that improved patient self-care and frequent professional care reduce respiratory diseases among high-risk elderly patients living in nursing homes and those in intensive care units.[69,75]
2. Poor oral hygiene is common in patients residing in hospitals or long-term care facilities, especially in patients who are chronically ill. Dental health care providers should advocate for programs that enhance the access of dental care services to long-term care residents and collaborate with medical health care providers on the importance of improving daily oral hygiene care to this population.
3. Application of 0.2% chlorhexidine gel to the teeth, gingiva, and other oral mucosal surfaces has been shown to significantly decrease the risk for pneumonia, especially in patients who are on ventilators.[76] Clinicians should take these findings into account when providing oral care to intubated patients.

2. **Chronic Obstructive Pulmonary Disease.** COPD is a group of lung diseases, mainly emphysema and chronic bronchitis, characterized by an obstruction of airflow during exhalation. Several investigators have hypothesized that periodontal infections may increase the risk of COPD. Reviews of the current evidence, however, indicate that *at present there is not sufficient evidence for an association between periodontal disease and COPD.*[1,69,71]

3. **Chronic Kidney Disease.** Chronic kidney disease is a progressive loss of kidney function, sometimes over years, leading to permanent kidney failure. Several studies report an association between chronic kidney disease and periodontitis.[77–81] The complex pathogenesis of chronic kidney disease makes studies of the role of periodontitis challenging.

4. **Rheumatoid Arthritis.** Rheumatoid arthritis is an autoimmune disease that causes redness, warmth, swelling, and pain of the joints. There is currently little evidence of an association between periodontitis and rheumatoid arthritis.[82,83]

5. **Cognitive Impairment.** Mild cognitive impairment is a slight but noticeable and measurable decline in cognitive abilities, including memory and thinking skills. The evidence from currently published studies for an association between periodontitis and cognitive impairment is weak.[1]

6. **Obesity.** Obesity is defined by the National Institutes of Health as a Body Mass Index (BMI) of 30 and above. A BMI of 30 is about 30 pounds overweight. Two systematic reviews suggest a weak association between periodontitis and obesity.[84,85] In clinical practice, a higher prevalence of periodontal disease should be expected among obese adults. Overweight/obese individuals are more likely to suffer from periodontitis compared to normal weight individuals.[86]

7. **Metabolic Syndrome.** Metabolic syndrome is a cluster of conditions—increased blood pressure, high blood sugar, excess body fat around the waist, and abnormal cholesterol or triglyceride levels—that occur together, increasing the risk of heart disease, stroke, and diabetes. Currently, there is little evidence to support an association between metabolic syndrome and periodontitis.[1] The strong increased risk of diabetes for individuals with metabolic syndrome further confuses any association with periodontitis.

8. **Cancer.** Cancer is a group of diseases involving abnormal cell growth with the potential to invade or spread to other parts of the body. Periodontitis has been identified as a possible risk factor for oral and oropharyngeal cancer.[1]

CHAPTER SUMMARY STATEMENT

Periodontitis is a chronic oral infection that may be a risk factor for a myriad of systemic diseases/disorders. Research shows an association between periodontitis and various systemic diseases and conditions, albeit supported by modest evidence. Well-designed research studies are still needed to better clarify associations; clinicians should keep abreast of the emerging evidence. Better patient education that emphasizes periodontal health and reinforces the importance of patient self-care and periodontal therapy may play roles in improving overall systemic health.

Section 3
Focus on Patients

Clinical Patient Care

A new patient in your dental office is 3-months pregnant with her first child. She is 38 years old and has periodontitis. What counsel would you provide this patient about the association between adverse pregnancy outcomes and periodontitis?

Evidence in Action

You are a dental hygienist in a periodontal practice. Mr. O—a 45-year-old insurance executive—has been referred to the periodontal practice from his general dentist for treatment of periodontitis. Today is his initial appointment with you.

Mr. O tells you that there is a history of heart attacks in his family and that he has been reading all about "how gum disease causes heart attacks." In addition, Mr. O states that he wants the periodontist to prescribe antibiotics for his gum disease, as he is quite convinced that the antibiotics will eliminate the gum disease and prevent him from having a heart attack when he gets older.

What education would you provide on the association between periodontitis and cardiovascular diseases? What information would you provide to Mr. O. on use of antibiotic therapy for the treatment of chronic periodontitis?

References

1. Linden GJ, Lyons A, Scannapieco FA. Periodontal systemic associations: review of the evidence. *J Clin Periodontol*. 2013;40 Suppl 14:S8–S19.
2. Linden GJ, Herzberg MC; Working group 4 of joint EFP/AAP workshop. Periodontitis and systemic diseases: a record of discussions of working group 4 of the Joint EFP/AAP Workshop on Periodontitis and Systemic Diseases. *J Clin Periodontol*. 2013;40 Suppl 14:S20–S23.
3. Van Dyke TE, van Winkelhoff AJ. Infection and inflammatory mechanisms. *J Clin Periodontol*. 2013;40 Suppl 14:S1–S7.
4. Raghavendran K, Mylotte JM, Scannapieco FA. Nursing home-associated pneumonia, hospital-acquired pneumonia and ventilator-associated pneumonia: the contribution of dental biofilms and periodontal inflammation. *Periodontol 2000*. 2007;44:164–177.
5. van Winkelhoff AJ, Slots J. Actinobacillus actinomycetemcomitans and Porphyromonas gingivalis in nonoral infections. *Periodontol 2000*. 1999;20:122–135.
6. Chiang AC, Massague J. Molecular basis of metastasis. *N Engl J Med*. 2008;359(26):2814–2823.
7. Kinane DF, Riggio MP, Walker KF, MacKenzie D, Shearer B. Bacteraemia following periodontal procedures. *J Clin Periodontol*. 2005;32(7):708–713.
8. Amar S, Gokce N, Morgan S, Loukideli M, Van Dyke TE, Vita JA. Periodontal disease is associated with brachial artery endothelial dysfunction and systemic inflammation. *Arterioscler Thromb Vasc Biol*. 2003;23(7):1245–1249.
9. Li X, Kolltveit KM, Tronstad L, Olsen I. Systemic diseases caused by oral infection. *Clin Microbiol Rev*. 2000;13(4):547–558.
10. Elter JR, Hinderliter AL, Offenbacher S, et al. The effects of periodontal therapy on vascular endothelial function: a pilot trial. *Am Heart J*. 2006;151(1):47.
11. Al-Zahrani MS, Bissada NF, Borawskit EA. Obesity and periodontal disease in young, middle-aged, and older adults. *J Periodontol*. 2003;74(5):610–615.
12. Genco RJ, Grossi SG, Ho A, Nishimura F, Murayama Y. A proposed model linking inflammation to obesity, diabetes, and periodontal infections. *J Periodontol*. 2005;76(11 Suppl):2075–2084.
13. Chapple IL, Genco R; Working group 2 of joint EFP/AAP workshop. Diabetes and periodontal diseases: consensus report of the Joint EFP/AAP Workshop on Periodontitis and Systemic Diseases. *J Clin Periodontol*. 2013;40 Suppl 14:S106–S112.
14. Sanz M, Kornman K; Working group 3 of joint EFP/AAP workshop. Periodontitis and adverse pregnancy outcomes: consensus report of the Joint EFP/AAP Workshop on Periodontitis and Systemic Diseases. *J Clin Periodontol*. 2013;40 Suppl 14:S164–S169.
15. Teng YT, Taylor GW, Scannapieco F, et al. Periodontal health and systemic disorders. *J Can Dent Assoc*. 2002;68(3):188–192.
16. Tonetti MS, Van Dyke TE; Working group 1 of the joint EFP/AAP workshop. Periodontitis and atherosclerotic cardiovascular disease: consensus report of the Joint EFP/AAP Workshop on Periodontitis and Systemic Diseases. *J Periodontol*. 2013;84(4 Suppl):S24–S29.

17. Schenkein HA, Loos BG. Inflammatory mechanisms linking periodontal diseases to cardiovascular diseases. *J Periodontol.* 2013;84(4 Suppl):S51–S69.

18. Preshaw PM, Taylor JJ. How has research into cytokine interactions and their role in driving immune responses impacted our understanding of periodontitis? *J Clin Periodontol.* 2011;38 Suppl 11:60–84.

19. Reyes L, Herrera D, Kozarov E, Rolda S, Progulske-Fox A. Periodontal bacterial invasion and infection: contribution to atherosclerotic pathology. *J Periodontol.* 2013;84(4 Suppl):S30–S50.

20. Gibson FC, 3rd, Genco CA. Porphyromonas gingivalis mediated periodontal disease and atherosclerosis: disparate diseases with commonalities in pathogenesis through TLRs. *Curr Pharm Des.* 2007;13(36):3665–3675.

21. Gibson FC, 3rd, Yumoto H, Takahashi Y, Chou HH, Genco CA. Innate immune signaling and Porphyromonas gingivalis-accelerated atherosclerosis. *J Dent Res.* 2006;85(2):106–121.

22. Hayashi C, Gudino CV, Gibson FC, 3rd, Genco CA. Review: Pathogen-induced inflammation at sites distant from oral infection: bacterial persistence and induction of cell-specific innate immune inflammatory pathways. *Mol Oral Microbiol.* 2010;25(5):305–316.

23. Teles R, Wang CY. Mechanisms involved in the association between periodontal diseases and cardiovascular disease. *Oral Dis.* 2011;17(5):450–461.

24. Van Dyke TE, Kornman KS. Inflammation and factors that may regulate inflammatory response. *J Periodontol.* 2008;79 (8 Suppl):1503–1507.

25. Haverkate F, Thompson SG, Pyke SD, Gallimore JR, Pepys MB. Production of C-reactive protein and risk of coronary events in stable and unstable angina. European Concerted Action on Thrombosis and Disabilities Angina Pectoris Study Group. *Lancet.* 1997;349(9050):462–466.

26. Liuzzo G, Biasucci LM, Gallimore JR, et al. The prognostic value of C-reactive protein and serum amyloid a protein in severe unstable angina. *N Engl J Med.* 1994;331(7):417–424.

27. Ridker PM, Rifai N, Rose L, Buring JE, Cook NR. Comparison of C-reactive protein and low-density lipoprotein cholesterol levels in the prediction of first cardiovascular events. *N Engl J Med.* 2002;347(20):1557–1565.

28. Ridker PM, Silvertown JD. Inflammation, C-reactive protein, and atherothrombosis. *J Periodontol.* 2008;79(8 Suppl): 1544–1551.

29. Slade GD, Offenbacher S, Beck JD, Heiss G, Pankow JS. Acute-phase inflammatory response to periodontal disease in the US population. *J Dent Res.* 2000;79(1):49–57.

30. Wu T, Trevisan M, Genco RJ, Dorn JP, Falkner KL, Sempos CT. Periodontal disease and risk of cerebrovascular disease: the first national health and nutrition examination survey and its follow-up study. *Arch Intern Med.* 2000;160(18):2749–2755.

31. Wu T, Trevisan M, Genco RJ, Falkner KL, Dorn JP, Sempos CT. Examination of the relation between periodontal health status and cardiovascular risk factors: serum total and high density lipoprotein cholesterol, C-reactive protein, and plasma fibrinogen. *Am J Epidemiol.* 2000;151(3):273–282.

32. Davalos D, Akassoglou K. Fibrinogen as a key regulator of inflammation in disease. *Semin Immunopathol.* 2012;34(1):43–62.

33. Popovic M, Smiljanic K, Dobutovic B, Syrovets T, Simmet T, Isenovic ER. Thrombin and vascular inflammation. *Mol Cell Biochem.* 2012;359(1-2):301–313.

34. Kweider M, Lowe GD, Murray GD, Kinane DF, McGowan DA. Dental disease, fibrinogen and white cell count; links with myocardial infarction? *Scott Med J.* 1993;38(3):73–74.

35. Amabile N, Susini G, Pettenati-Soubayroux I, et al. Severity of periodontal disease correlates to inflammatory systemic status and independently predicts the presence and angiographic extent of stable coronary artery disease. *J Intern Med.* 2008;263(6):644–652.

36. Buhlin K, Hultin M, Norderyd O, et al. Risk factors for atherosclerosis in cases with severe periodontitis. *J Clin Periodontol.* 2009;36(7):541–549.

37. Sahingur SE, Sharma A, Genco RJ, De Nardin E. Association of increased levels of fibrinogen and the -455G/A fibrinogen gene polymorphism with chronic periodontitis. *J Periodontol.* 2003;74(3):329–337.

38. Schwahn C, Volzke H, Robinson DM, et al. Periodontal disease, but not edentulism, is independently associated with increased plasma fibrinogen levels. Results from a population-based study. *Thromb Haemost.* 2004;92(2):244–252.

39. Vidal F, Figueredo CM, Cordovil I, Fischer RG. Periodontal therapy reduces plasma levels of interleukin-6, C-reactive protein, and fibrinogen in patients with severe periodontitis and refractory arterial hypertension. *J Periodontol.* 2009;80(5):786–791.

40. Katz J, Chaushu G, Sharabi Y. On the association between hypercholesterolemia, cardiovascular disease and severe periodontal disease. *J Clin Periodontol.* 2001;28(9):865–868.

41. Monteiro AM, Jardini MA, Alves S, et al. Cardiovascular disease parameters in periodontitis. *J Periodontol.* 2009;80(3): 378–388.

42. Pussinen PJ, Vilkuna-Rautiainen T, Alfthan G, et al. Severe periodontitis enhances macrophage activation via increased serum lipopolysaccharide. *Arterioscler Thromb Vasc Biol.* 2004;24(11):2174–2180.

43. Friedewald VE, Kornman KS, Beck JD, et al. The American Journal of Cardiology and Journal of Periodontology editors' consensus: periodontitis and atherosclerotic cardiovascular disease. *J Periodontol.* 2009;80(7):1021–1032.

44. D'Aiuto F, Orlandi M, Gunsolley JC. Evidence that periodontal treatment improves biomarkers and CVD outcomes. *J Periodontol.* 2013;84(4 Suppl):S85–S105.

45. Dietrich T, Sharma P, Walter C, Weston P, Beck J. The epidemiological evidence behind the association between periodontitis and incident atherosclerotic cardiovascular disease. *J Periodontol.* 2013;84(4 Suppl):S70–S84.

46. Ide M, Papapanou PN. Epidemiology of association between maternal periodontal disease and adverse pregnancy outcomes—systematic review. *J Periodontol.* 2013;84(4 Suppl):S181–S194.

47. Madianos PN, Bobetsis YA, Offenbacher S. Adverse pregnancy outcomes (APOs) and periodontal disease: pathogenic mechanisms. *J Periodontol.* 2013;84(4 Suppl):S170–S180.

48. Michalowicz BS, Gustafsson A, Thumbigere-Math V, Buhlin K. The effects of periodontal treatment on pregnancy outcomes. *J Periodontol.* 2013;84(4 Suppl):S195–S208.

49. Task Force on Periodontal Treatment of Pregnant Women, American Academy of Periodontology. American Academy of Periodontology statement regarding periodontal management of the pregnant patient. *J Periodontol.* 2004;75(3):495.

50. Kurien S, Kattimani VS, Sriram RR, et al. Management of pregnant patient in dentistry. *J Int Oral Health.* 2013;5(1):88–97.

51. Lalla E, Papapanou PN. Diabetes mellitus and periodontitis: a tale of two common interrelated diseases. *Nat Rev Endocrinol.* 2011;7(12):738–748.

52. Mealey BL, Ocampo GL. Diabetes mellitus and periodontal disease. *Periodontol 2000*. 2007;44:127–153.

53. Preshaw PM, Alba AL, Herrera D, et al. Periodontitis and diabetes: a two-way relationship. *Diabetologia*. 2012;55(1):21–31.

54. Taylor GW, Burt BA, Becker MP, et al. Severe periodontitis and risk for poor glycemic control in patients with non-insulin-dependent diabetes mellitus. *J Periodontol*. 1996;67(10 Suppl):1085–1093.

55. Taylor JJ, Preshaw PM, Lalla E. A review of the evidence for pathogenic mechanisms that may link periodontitis and diabetes. *J Periodontol*. 2013;84(4 Suppl):S113–S134.

56. American Diabetes Association. Standards of Medical Care in Diabetes—2018 Abridged for Primary Care Providers. *Clin Diabetes*. 2018;36(1):14–37.

57. American Diabetes Association. Classification and Diagnosis of Diabetes: Standards of Medical Care in Diabetes—2018. *Diabetes Care*. 2018;41(Suppl 1):S13–S27.

58. American Diabetes Association. Glycemic Targets: Standards of Medical Care in Diabetes—2018. *Diabetes Care*. 2018;41(Suppl 1):S55–S64.

59. Engebretson S, Chertog R, Nichols A, Hey-Hadavi J, Celenti R, Grbic J. Plasma levels of tumour necrosis factor-alpha in patients with chronic periodontitis and type 2 diabetes. *J Clin Periodontol*. 2007;34(1):18–24.

60. Gupta A, Ten S, Anhalt H. Serum levels of soluble tumor necrosis factor-alpha receptor 2 are linked to insulin resistance and glucose intolerance in children. *J Pediatr Endocrinol Metab*. 2005;18(1):75–82.

61. King GL. The role of inflammatory cytokines in diabetes and its complications. *J Periodontol*. 2008;79(8 Suppl):1527–1534.

62. Pickup JC. Inflammation and activated innate immunity in the pathogenesis of type 2 diabetes. *Diabetes Care*. 2004;27(3):813–823.

63. Shoelson SE, Lee J, Goldfine AB. Inflammation and insulin resistance. *J Clin Invest*. 2006;116(7):1793–1801.

64. Engebretson S, Kocher T. Evidence that periodontal treatment improves diabetes outcomes: a systematic review and meta-analysis. *J Periodontol*. 2013;84(4 Suppl):S153–S169.

65. Simpson TC, Needleman I, Wild SH, Moles DR, Mills EJ. Treatment of periodontal disease for glycaemic control in people with diabetes. *Cochrane Database Syst Rev*. 2010;(5):CD004714.

66. Teeuw WJ, Gerdes VE, Loos BG. Effect of periodontal treatment on glycemic control of diabetic patients: a systematic review and meta-analysis. *Diabetes Care*. 2010;33(2):421–427.

67. Lalla E, Kunzel C, Burkett S, Cheng B, Lamster IB. Identification of unrecognized diabetes and pre-diabetes in a dental setting. *J Dent Res*. 2011;90(7):855–860.

68. Ostergaard L, Andersen PL. Etiology of community-acquired pneumonia. Evaluation by transtracheal aspiration, blood culture, or serology. *Chest*. 1993;104(5):1400–1407.

69. Azarpazhooh A, Leake JL. Systematic review of the association between respiratory diseases and oral health. *J Periodontol*. 2006;77(9):1465–1482.

70. Paju S, Scannapieco FA. Oral biofilms, periodontitis, and pulmonary infections. *Oral Dis*. 2007;13(6):508–512.

71. Scannapieco FA, Bush RB, Paju S. Associations between periodontal disease and risk for nosocomial bacterial pneumonia and chronic obstructive pulmonary disease. A systematic review. *Ann Periodontol*. 2003;8(1):54–69.

72. Craven DE. Preventing ventilator-associated pneumonia in adults: sowing seeds of change. *Chest*. 2006;130(1):251–260.

73. Scannapieco FA, Stewart EM, Mylotte JM. Colonization of dental plaque by respiratory pathogens in medical intensive care patients. *Crit Care Med*. 1992;20(6):740–745.

74. Scannapieco FA. Role of oral bacteria in respiratory infection. *J Periodontol*. 1999;70(7):793–802.

75. Sjogren P, Nilsson E, Forsell M, Johansson O, Hoogstraate J. A systematic review of the preventive effect of oral hygiene on pneumonia and respiratory tract infection in elderly people in hospitals and nursing homes: effect estimates and methodological quality of randomized controlled trials. *J Am Geriatr Soc*. 2008;56(11):2124–2130.

76. Labeau SO, Van de Vyver K, Brusselaers N, Vogelaers D, Blot SI. Prevention of ventilator-associated pneumonia with oral antiseptics: a systematic review and meta-analysis. *Lancet Infect Dis*. 2011;11(11):845–854.

77. Fisher MA, Taylor GW, West BT, McCarthy ET. Bidirectional relationship between chronic kidney and periodontal disease: a study using structural equation modeling. *Kidney Int*. 2011;79(3):347–355.

78. Grubbs V, Garcia F, Jue BL, et al. The Kidney and Periodontal Disease (KAPD) study: A pilot randomized controlled trial testing the effect of non-surgical periodontal therapy on chronic kidney disease. *Contemp Clin Trials*. 2017;53:143–150.

79. Grubbs V, Plantinga LC, Crews DC, et al. Vulnerable populations and the association between periodontal and chronic kidney disease. *Clin J Am Soc Nephrol*. 2011;6(4):711–717.

80. Ioannidou E, Hall Y, Swede H, Himmelfarb J. Periodontitis associated with chronic kidney disease among Mexican Americans. *J Public Health Dent*. 2013;73(2):112–119.

81. Ioannidou E, Swede H. Disparities in periodontitis prevalence among chronic kidney disease patients. *J Dent Res*. 2011;90(6):730–734.

82. Arkema EV, Karlson EW, Costenbader KH. A prospective study of periodontal disease and risk of rheumatoid arthritis. *J Rheumatol*. 2010;37(9):1800–1804.

83. Demmer RT, Molitor JA, Jacobs DR, Jr., Michalowicz BS. Periodontal disease, tooth loss and incident rheumatoid arthritis: results from the First National Health and Nutrition Examination Survey and its epidemiological follow-up study. *J Clin Periodontol*. 2011;38(11):998–1006.

84. Chaffee BW, Weston SJ. Association between chronic periodontal disease and obesity: a systematic review and meta-analysis. *J Periodontol*. 2010;81(12):1708–1724.

85. Suvan J, D'Aiuto F, Moles DR, Petrie A, Donos N. Association between overweight/obesity and periodontitis in adults. A systematic review. *Obes Rev*. 2011;12(5):e381–e404.

86. Suvan JE, Petrie A, Nibali L, et al. Association between overweight/obesity and increased risk of periodontitis. *J Clin Periodontol*. 2015;42(8):733–739.

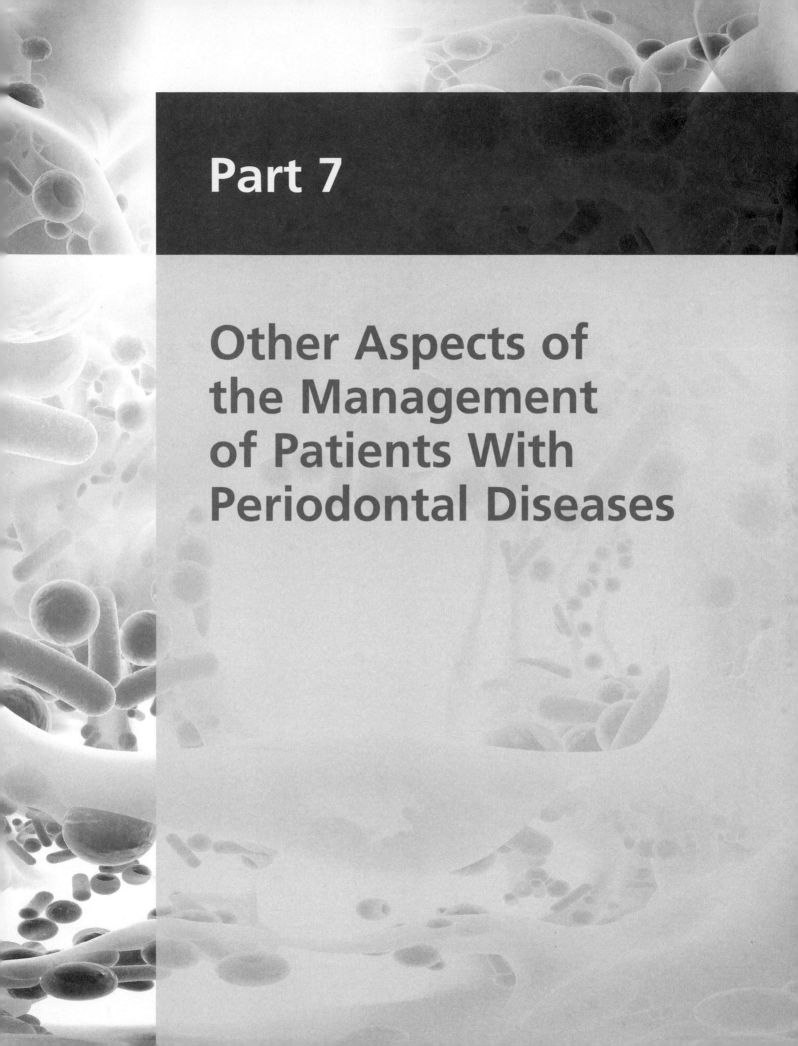

Part 7

Other Aspects of the Management of Patients With Periodontal Diseases

35 Documentation and Insurance Reporting of Periodontal Care

Clinical Application. The maxim "*Sloppy documentation is equated with sloppy care*" rings true when it comes to the ethical and professional responsibility of all dental clinicians to properly record a thorough and accurate written or typed report in each patient's record as a routine part of periodontal care. A complete and accurate entry in the patient's records is essential for fostering continuity of care and ensuring the continual delivery of quality dental care. It also provides a standard means of communication between two different providers and/or between a provider and patient about the health status, recommended treatment options, and anticipated outcomes of treatment. Moreover, legal ramifications related to the quality of the documentation in patients' records require dental clinicians to have a thorough understanding of how to document patient interactions accurately. Additionally, this chapter provides guidance in the use of ADA approved terminology for insurance reporting related to delivery of care for periodontal patients.

Learning Objectives

- Explain the foundations of tort law and how it applies to the profession of dentistry.

- Define the term liability as it applies to the provision of periodontal care.

- Describe situations in the dental office that trigger liability for dental hygienists.

- Define the terms intentional torts and negligence and give examples of each.

- In the clinical setting, thoroughly document all periodontal treatment including treatment options, cancellations, patient noncompliance, refusal of treatment, and follow-up telephone calls.

- Explain the use of insurance codes and forms in periodontal care.

Key Terms

Standard of care	Tort	Upcoding
Liability	Intentional torts	Insurance codes
Malpractice	Negligence	Insurance forms

Section 1
Legal Issues in the Provision and Documentation of Care

It is important for every dental clinician to practice to the highest established standards of care, not only to ensure the safety of the patient receiving treatment but also to avoid costly malpractice litigation.[1] Potential liability is a reality for every health care provider. While patients can sue a dentist or dental hygienist for many reasons, the success of such a suit often depends on the quality of the chart notes. The dental practitioner has a moral and ethical obligation not only to deliver high quality care, but also to maintain thorough and accurate chart notes for each patient visit to protect the practice against liability.

CONCEPTS OF MALPRACTICE AND TORT LAW

1. **Standard of Care.** The legal definition of standard of care varies in North America. In general terms, dental health care providers are required to exercise the same degree of skill and care as could reasonably be expected of a prudent dental health care provider of the same experience and standing.[1,2]
2. **Liability.** In the context of health care, liability is a health care provider's obligation or responsibility to provide services to another person (the patient). The health care provider's liability entails the possibility of being sued if the person receiving the services feels as if he or she has been treated improperly or negligently.
3. **Malpractice.** Malpractice is the improper or negligent treatment by a health care provider that results in injury or damage to the patient.[3,4]
4. **Tort.** The legal basis for most lawsuits in dental and dental hygiene practice is founded on tort law. A tort is a civil wrong where a person has breached a duty to another. A tort is the law that permits an injured person to recover compensation from the person who caused the injury.
5. **Intentional Torts.** Intentional torts are actions designed to injure another person or that person's property. There are many specific types of intentional torts, including the following:
   A. Battery is the unlawful and unwanted touching or striking of one person by another, with the intention of bringing about a harmful or offensive contact. Forceful discipline of unruly children in the dental chair could be construed as battery.
   B. Assault is an unlawful threat or attempt to do bodily injury to another. A doctor who treats a minor patient without proper parental or guardian informed consent could be charged with assault or battery.
   C. Infliction of emotional distress. An example is talking in a loud or harsh voice to an unruly child.
   D. Fraud is deception carried out for the purpose of achieving personal gain while causing injury to another party.
   E. Misrepresentation occurs when a health care provider deliberately deceives a patient about possible outcomes.
   F. Defamation is communication to third parties of false statements about a person that injure the reputation of or deter others from associating with that person. For example, a dental hygienist learns that another hygienist has been making disparaging comments about the quality of care that he or she provides. The hygienist being disparaged could sue for defamation.

G. Trespass is to infringe on the privacy, time, or attention of another. An example is discussing a patient's personal information with someone without the patient's permission.

H. Defamation by computer. Email correspondence and other written documents are discoverable in court, so avoid disparaging remarks in email communications.

6. **Negligence.** Negligence is a failure to exercise reasonable care to avoid injuring others. It is the failure to do something that a reasonable person would do under the same circumstances, or the doing of something a reasonable person would not do. Negligence is characterized by carelessness, inattentiveness, and neglectfulness rather than by a positive intent to cause injury.[2]

A. Negligence is different from an intentional tort in that negligence does not require *the intent* to commit a wrongful action; instead, the wrongful action itself is sufficient to constitute negligence.

B. Examples of negligence include accidentally spilling a chemical on a patient, not updating the patient's health history resulting in the patient's health being jeopardized, and incorrect treatment of periodontal disease. Professional liability insurance typically covers only unintentional torts or negligence.

7. **Upcoding.** Upcoding refers to reporting a higher level of service than was actually performed. A good example of upcoding would be performing an adult prophylaxis (code D1110) procedure but recording the scaling and root planning code (D4341). The purpose of upcoding is to charge a higher fee. The fee for a quadrant of scaling and root planning is about three times the fee for a prophylaxis. Upcoding is unethical and dishonest. Dental boards have been known to levy serious disciplinary measures, including revocation of license, for clinicians that have been found guilty of upcoding.

AREAS OF POTENTIAL LIABILITY

In judging whether a professional has been negligent, the courts use a standard called the "*reasonable prudent person or professional.*" This means the court compares what a reasonably prudent person or professional would have done in a similar situation. For example, the standard of care for periodontal charting is that every adult patient will have a six-point periodontal charting with all numbers recorded at least once per year. Failure to include a service because the dental hygienist is unaware of the current standard of care will not hold up in court. The top ten areas of potential liability for dental hygienists are summarized below in Box 35-1.

Box 35-1. Top Ten Areas of Potential Liability for Dental Hygienists

1. Failure to ask and document whether the patient has taken his or her premedication.
2. Failure to detect and document oral cancer.
3. Failure to update the patient's medical history.
4. Failure to detect and thoroughly document the presence of periodontal disease.
5. Injuring a patient.
6. Failure to document treatment thoroughly in the patient chart or computerized record.
7. Failure to protect patient privacy or divulging confidential patient information.
8. Failure to inform the patient about treatment options and the consequences of nontreatment.
9. Practicing outside the legal scope of practice. All dental hygienists should be well informed about the state practice act and follow the rules and regulations explicitly.
10. Failure to provide care that meets the established standards of care.

Section 2
Documentation of Periodontal Care

The dental chart is a **legal document**. It is the first line of defense in a malpractice suit. *When a patient decides to file a lawsuit, the dental chart becomes the single most important piece of information relative to the suit. Faulty records can be the most important reason for the loss of a lawsuit.*[5] All periodontal assessment, educational, and treatment services should be documented in the patient chart or computerized record. Recommendations for thorough documentation are summarized in (Table 35-1 and Box 35-2).

PRINCIPLES FOR THOROUGH DOCUMENTATION

TABLE 35-1	DOCUMENTATION GUIDELINES
Action	**Why It Is Recommended**
Format: • Write on the proper form or computer document. • Write or print legibly in blue or black ink. • Use correct grammar, spelling, and standard dental terminology. • Date each entry correctly.	• It is important to write or print legibly to avoid miscommunication. (Some lawyers infer sloppy care from sloppy entries or charting.) • The date that actions occur, or observations are made is a legal account of care provided.

Content:
• Only record care that you have given or observations that you have made. Do not make entries for another care provider.
• Enter information in a complete, accurate, concise, and factual manner.
• Entries may include the:
  • Reason for today's appointment
  • Through documentation of medical and dental history
  • Patient's chief complaint
  • Symptoms reported by the patient
  • Findings from the clinical periodontal assessment
  • Treatment options and recommendations
  • Patient treatment options
  • All assessment, educational, and treatment services
  • Items given to patient, such as home care aids
  • Date or interval of next appointment
• Remember that in a liability situation, care or recommendations not recorded was not provided.
	• By making an entry in a dental record, you accept legal responsibility for that entry.
	• Use only commonly accepted dental terminology and standard abbreviations and symbols. Do not create your own abbreviations. Using correct terminology and abbreviations will prevent others from having to second-guess your meaning.
	• Proper and conscientious recording protects the patient, your employer, and you.

TABLE 35-1	DOCUMENTATION GUIDELINES (*Continued*)

Action	Why It Is Recommended
Accountability: • Check the patient's name on the dental record and on the form where you are recording. • Always sign your first initial, last name and title to each entry. • All entries should be written on the lines. No entries should be made in the margins or below the last line on the page. No lines should be skipped. • Do not use dittos, erasures, or correcting fluids. A single line should be drawn through an incorrect entry and words "mistaken entry" or "error in charting" should be printed above or beside the entry and signed. The entry should then be rewritten correctly. • Identify each page of the record with the patient's name and chart identification number. • Recognize that a patient record (chart) is permanent.	• By verifying the patient's identification information, you ensure that you are recording the person's information on the correct record. • By signing your entry, you indicate that you are the person who needs to be consulted if further clarification of the information is needed. Additionally, signing your entry indicates that you accept legal responsibility for what you have written. • All lines should be used so that there is no opportunity for anyone to add information after a lawsuit is initiated. Making entries in the margins or below the last line on a page can cause juries to wonder if the entry was made at a later date. • Striking through an error is the only legal way to indicate a change in the dental record. Erasing or using correction fluid could be seen as an attempt to hide or change existing information.
Timing: • Record information in a timely manner. • Document care as closely as possible to the time of rendering treatment. • Do not record care as given before you have provided the care.	• If you wait until the end of the day to record, you may forget important information. • Something may occur that prevents you from providing the anticipated care (the patient may become ill halfway through the appointment; the patient may refuse a fluoride treatment). If you record care as "provided" in the dental record, but then do not actually complete this care, you will have committed fraud.
Confidentiality: • Clinicians using patient records are bound professionally and ethically to keep in strict confidence all information they learn by reading patient records.	• Individuals have a moral and legal right to expect that the information contained in their patient dental record will be kept private.

Box 35-2. Determining How Much to Write—The Amnesia Test

Imagine that you have amnesia and cannot remember any of the treatment that you have performed for any of your patients since you started to work in a periodontal practice 5 years ago! Would you be able to read any one of your patient charts and be able to:

- *Know every assessment, educational, and treatment procedure that the patient has undergone and why this treatment was necessary.*
- *Know what additional treatment has been recommended and accepted by the patient and know why this treatment is recommended.*

Two Criteria should dictate how much to write:

1. Write sufficient information that would allow you or any other clinician to determine *exactly* which assessment, educational, and treatment procedures were performed at each appointment; why that treatment was necessary; and what treatment is next—based solely on your documentation.
2. Write sufficient information that meets all the record keeping requirements of your state board.

1. **Recommendations for Thorough Documentation.** Tonner[6] recommends several principles that every dental professional should follow when documenting periodontal treatment in the patient chart or computerized record.
   A. **General Guidelines for Chart Entries**
      1. All entries should be complete and accurate using accepted dental terminology and abbreviations. **Chart Entry-1** is an example of a complete chart entry.
      2. It is helpful to organize the services documented in sequential order so that no information is omitted.
      3. If handwritten, entries should be legible and in *permanent* ink.
      4. The health care provider making the entry should sign the entry with his or her first initial, last name, and title. Since many different people write in the patient chart, it is important that each entry be signed. If there are multiple dentists in the practice, the dentist that examines the hygienist's patient should be identified also.
      5. Thorough chart entries provide valuable information for the next clinician that treats this patient.
      6. The patient should be thoroughly interviewed regarding his or her medical status at each visit. Patients do not usually volunteer information when they are taking a new medicine or if there has been a change in their medical history. The medical status should be thoroughly documented at each visit.
   B. **Treatment Options.** The health care provider should document all treatment options presented to the patient.
   C. **Appointment Schedule and Chart Entries**
      1. Chart entries should be consistent with the appointment schedule.
         a. With most dental software and computer scheduling, the patient's name must be on the schedule in order to make a chart entry.
         b. With manual appointment books, however, entries can be erased and changed.

2. In the event of a lawsuit, doubt may be cast on the reliability of the office's records if the treatment dates in the chart do not match the appointment book entries.

3. If the patient is being seen on an emergency basis, this circumstance should be recorded in the chart.

D. **Cancellations and Missed Appointments.** All cancellations and missed appointments should be recorded in the patient chart. Infrequent periodontal maintenance appointments can lead to a recurrence and progression of periodontal disease. **Chart Entry-2** and **Chart Entry-3** provide examples of how to document missed and cancelled appointments.

E. **Patient Noncompliance and Refusal of Treatment**

1. Patient noncompliance with recommendations, such as (1) inadequate self-care, (2) continued smoking, (3) failure to regulate diabetes, or (4) failure to follow specific instructions, can lead to disease progression. Noncompliance should be noted in the chart (**Chart Entry-4**).

2. Instances when a patient opts not to have recommended treatment or declines a referral to a specialist should be documented. In such situations, it is recommended that patients sign a "Refusal of Treatment Recommendation" document. An example of a refusal of treatment form is shown in Figure 35-1. Further, when a patient is referred to a specialist, it is recommended that a copy of the referral letter be kept in the patient chart. **Chart Entry-5** provides an example of documentation of inadequate self-care.

F. **Follow-up Telephone Calls.** Patients appreciate a follow-up telephone call from the dentist or hygienist following a long or difficult treatment procedure. For hygienists, a good rule of thumb is to call any patient that required anesthesia for periodontal instrumentation. Follow-up telephone calls should be documented (**Chart Entry-6**).

Date	Treatment Rendered
1/10/18	Reason for visit: 3-month periodontal maintenance. Medical history update: pat. now taking 1 aspirin a day per his physician's recommendation. Chief complaint: none. Oral cancer exam: normal. Periodontal probing: changes noted in charting. Plaque: light, calculus: light, bleeding areas noted on periodontal chart. Perio maintenance: perio instrumentation of all 4 quads; ultrasonic and hand instrumentation. Plaque removal by patient using toothbrush and interdental brush. Patient tolerated all procedures well. Patient education: reviewed use of tufted dental floss around distal surfaces of maxillary and mandibular molars. Tray fluoride application 1.23% APF gel for sensitivity. 4 bitewing radiographs. Next maintenance visit in 3 months. *R. Zimmer, RDH*

Chart Entry-1. Complete Chart Entry. This chart entry is an example of a thorough chart entry that documents all the events of the patient's appointment.

Date	Treatment Rendered
1/10/18	Patient missed maintenance appointment because of illness. *R. Zimmer, RDH*

Chart Entry-2. Missed Appointment. This chart entry is an example of documentation of a missed appointment due to illness.

Date	Treatment Rendered
1/10/18	Telephoned patient to confirm her 3-month maintenance appt. Patient cancelled and said that she would call to reschedule later. I reminded her of the importance of regular maintenance. *R. Zimmer, RDH*

Chart Entry-3. Cancelled Maintenance Appointment. This chart entry provides an example of the documentation for a cancelled periodontal maintenance appointment.

Date	Treatment Rendered
1/10/18	Discussed options for smoking cessation. Patient stated that "he is not interested in quitting smoking." *R. Zimmer, RDH*

Chart Entry-4. Patient Noncompliance. This chart entry provides an example of the documentation for patient noncompliance with recommendations.

Date	Treatment Rendered
1/10/18	Patient reports brushing twice daily but "does not have time to use an interdental brush." Showed patient signs of periodontal inflammation in the interdental areas. Explained benefits of interdental plaque removal and several alternatives for interdental self-care. Patient decided that he was not interested and stated that "he only wants to brush." *R. Zimmer, RDH*

Chart Entry-5. Inadequate Self-Care. This chart entry is an example of documentation of inadequate self-care by a patient.

Date	Treatment Rendered
1/10/18	Telephoned patient at home this evening to check on her. Patient reports that she "has no bleeding and rates her pain as a 2, on a scale of 1 to 10." Reminded her to use warm saltwater rinse before bedtime. *R. Zimmer, RDH*

Chart Entry-6. Follow-up Telephone Call. This chart entry is an example of documentation of a follow-up telephone call after a long or difficult treatment procedure.

Date	Treatment Rendered
1/10/18	Px, Ex

Chart Entry-7. Incomplete Chart Entry. Although this hygienist may have been quite thorough in delivering care, the chart does not reflect that.

Date	Treatment Rendered
1/10/18	Patient reports that his "gums no longer bleed during brushing." Tissue color, tone, and texture are much improved from 3 weeks ago. *R. Zimmer, RDH*

Chart Entry-8. Patient Comments. This chart entry is an example of how to include a patient's comments at a periodontal maintenance visit.

Refusal of Treatment Recommendation

Patient Name _____ Date of Birth _____

                              Last   First   M.I.

I am being provided with this information and refusal form so I may better understand the treatment recommended for me and the consequences of my refusal of the recommended treatment. I understand that I may ask any questions I wish regarding the recommended treatment.

It has been recommended that I have the following treatment: _____
_____

This recommendation is based on visual examination, on any X-rays, models, photos and other diagnostic tests taken, and on my doctor's knowledge of my medical and dental history. The treatment is necessary because of:

☐ Decay   ☐ Broken tooth/teeth   ☐ Infection   ☐ Periodontal disease   ☐ Pain   ☐ Other

Note: _____
_____

_____ I have had an opportunity to ask questions about the recommended treatment.
Patient's Initials

I understand that complications to my teeth, mouth, and/or general health may occur if I do not proceed with the recommended treatment. These complications include: _____
_____

Acknowledgement

Note: _____ , have received information about the proposed treatment. I have discussed my treatment with Dr. _____ and have been given an opportunity to ask questions and have them fully answered. I understand the nature of the recommended treatment and the risks of my refusal of the recommended treatment.

I personally assume the risks and consequences of my refusal. I have read this document in its entirety.

I do NOT wish to proceed with the recommended treatment.

Signed: _____ Date: _____
                          Patient or Guardian

Signed: _____ Date: _____
                          Treating Dentist

Signed: _____ Date: _____
                          Witness

Figure 35-1. Refusal of Treatment Form. Shown above is one example of a Refusal of Recommended Treatment Form.

PITFALLS IN DOCUMENTATION

1. **Common Problems in Documentation.** Tonner[6] outlines four common pitfalls in documentation.
   A. **Making Entries in Haste. Chart Entry-7** is an example of an *inadequate* chart entry. For example, in her haste to stay on schedule, the dental hygienist simply forgets to record that she did a periodontal charting and evaluation. Later, if the patient develops periodontal disease, he may accuse the dental practitioner of failure to diagnose. The dentist or hygienist may state to a jury that a periodontal evaluation is done on every patient. *In the eyes of a jury, however, if a procedure is not recorded in the patient chart, it was not performed.*
   B. **Skipping Lines Between Entries or Writing in Margins**
      1. Keeping in the lines or skipping lines.
         a. Chart entries should be written with small enough strokes to be contained within the space provided.
         b. No lines should be skipped on a treatment record form. All lines should be used so that there is no opportunity for anyone to add information *after* a lawsuit is initiated.
      2. Writing in margins or below the last line. All entries should be written on the lines, and no entries should be written in the margins or below the last line on the page. Doing so can cause juries to wonder if the entry was made at a later date.
   C. **Altering Chart Entries.** *The single most common cause of punitive damages in a dental malpractice suit is altering the chart.*
      1. Correction fluid should never be used to correct an entry. If an error is made, a single line should be drawn through the incorrect entry so that it can still be read, the words *charting error or mistaken entry* written above it, and the correct entry made on the next available line. The revised entry should be signed.
      2. Additional information should never be added to an entry from a previous appointment. Juries perceive such added entries to be fraudulent and deceptive.
      3. Forensic ink dating analysis allows an expert to determine the date that ink was used on a particular document. Therefore, it is foolhardy to add things at a later date to a patient chart in an attempt to avoid or win a lawsuit.
   D. **Not Clearly Indicating Patient Comments.** Quotation marks should be used to indicate patient comments. This is especially important when making follow-up telephone calls after a difficult or invasive procedure. A sample chart entry is shown in **Chart Entry-8.**

Section 3
Computer-Based Patient Records

The development, implementation, and evaluation of computer-based dental records present both challenges and opportunities for the periodontal dental office.[7,8]

ADVANTAGES OF COMPUTERIZED PATIENT RECORDS

1. **Organization and Data Gathering**
   - *Standardization of clinical data* where all staff members use the same templates for gathering data and the same abbreviations.
   - *Greater legibility.* Handwriting can often be illegible, which increases liability risk for the clinician.
   - *Easier and faster access to information.* Information is only a few keystrokes away.
   - *Enhanced use of clinical images and radiographs.*
   - *Provision of new ways to analyze clinical information.* For example, digital radiography allows the clinician to view radiographs with digital tools designed to enhance the image and visualize bone levels around teeth.
   - *Potential for greater security of patient data.* Paper records are vulnerable to fire, earthquake, and water damage from flooding. Computer-based patient records can be backed up offsite to preserve data. Note that computerized data is more secure only if it is continuously backed up to an offsite location separate from the dental office.
2. **Processing of Information**
   - *Patient information is accessible across the network simultaneously.* For example, business assistants can read input from clinicians and be ready for patient check-out before the patient reaches the business office.
   - *Facilitates submission of insurance claims.* Computerized information facilitates submission of dental insurance claim forms to insurance companies.
3. **Communication**
   - *Faster and better multidisciplinary interaction with specialists.* Successful treatment of periodontitis requires a team approach involving the primary care (general) dental team, the periodontal dental team, and often, other dental specialists or physicians.
   - Continuous communication among health care providers is critical to the success of diagnosis, treatment, and maintenance. Ongoing communication is needed because it is common for the patient to be treated in phases, going back and forth between the primary care dental practice and the periodontal practice. A computer-based patient record can greatly increase the effectiveness of communication among dental health care providers.

CAUTIONS REGARDING COMPUTERIZED RECORDS

Even with advancing technologies, practitioners and staff must realize that the transition to computer-based patient records is not seamless, totally safe, or problem-free.

1. **Data Backup.** Anyone who has ever used a computer recognizes that computers crash, freeze-up, and frequently loose data. Computer-based patient records can be backed up offsite to preserve data. Data should be continuously backed up to a secure offsite location.
2. **State Regulations.** In some states, computerized records may not eliminate the need to keep paper records due to legal requirements in those states. In such cases, the dental office may need to maintain patient data on paper and in computerized versions.

Section 4
Insurance Codes for Periodontal Treatment

This section highlights the importance of understanding various numeric and alphanumeric codes for accurately billing dental-related services to private pay or third-party insurance carriers. Claim submissions for dental care are submitted either electronically or by means of paper forms. An example of a completed dental insurance claim form is shown in Figure 35-2.

DENTAL CLAIM FORM

Check One:
☐ Dentist's pre-treatment estimate
☐ Dentist's statement of actual services

If the cost of treatment is expected to exceed $300, a pre-treatment estimate should be completed.
The physician or dentist must indicate: A list of every recommented dental procedure; and the charge for each procedure and provide supporting pre-treatment radiographs.

1. Patient name & address: **Mr. Boyd Bogus** **22 S. Green St. Ardendale, NC 28759**	2. Relationship to employee ☒ Self ☐ Spouse ☐ Child	3. Sex (M) / F	4. Patient birthdate **05 / 14 / 50**	5. Is dependent a full time Student? ___ Yes ___ No
6. Employee's name (Last, First, Middle Initial) **UUP Benefit Trust Fund**	7. Employee's SSN **001-00-1-1000**	7. Group number/Name **3214192**		

9. Employee'smailing address **22 S. Green Street** — 10. City, State, Zip **Ardendale, NC 28759**

11. Other family members employed? If yes, member's name **Brenda Bogus** — SSN# **002-02-0000** — Spouse Birthdate: **09 / 05 / 53** — 12. Name and address of employer **22 S. Green Street Ardendale, NC 28759**

11. Is patient covered by another dental plan? ___ Yes _X_ No — Dental plan name — Group number — 14. Name and address of employer

I have reviewed the following treatment plan, I authorize release of any information relating to this claim.
Signed (patient or parent if minor) ______ Date ______

I authorize direct **payment** of benefits to the dentist or supplier.
Signed (employee) ______ Date ______

14. Dentist's name **Harry M. Montigue**

22. Is treatment result of Occupational illness or injury? ___ Yes _X_ No
If **yes**, give brief description and dates

15. Dentist's address **1212 Upward Avenue** **Ardendale, NC 28759**

23. Is treatment result of Auto Accident? ___ Yes _X_ No
Other accident? ___ Yes ___ No
24. If **yes**, give brief description and dates

16. Dentist's SSN or TIN — 17. License# — 18. Phone#

25. If Prosthesis, is this initial placement? ___ Yes _X_ No
If **no**, reason for placement
28. Date of placement

19. First visit date Current series — 20. Place of treatment ☐Office ☐Hospital ☐ECF ☐Other ______ — 21. Radiographs or models enclosed? ___ Yes ___ No How many? ______

27. Is treatment for Orthodontics? ___ Yes _X_ No
28. If services already commenced:
Date appliances applied: ______ Months of treatment remaining: ______

19. Identify missing teeth with **"X"**

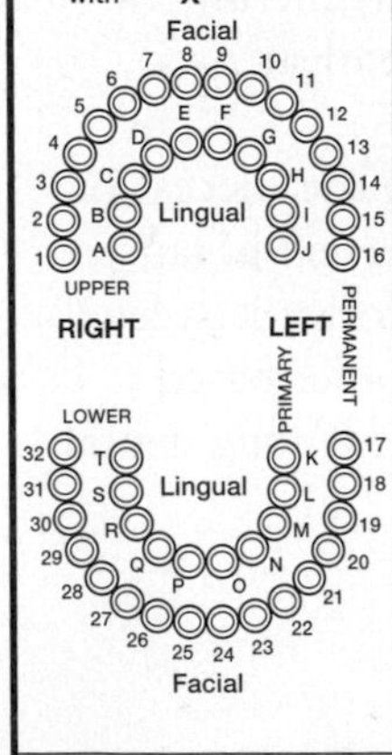

30. EXAMINATION & TREATMENT PLAN. LIST IN ORDER FROM TOOTH NO. 1 THROUGH TOOTH NO. 32
USE CHARTING SYSTEM SHOWN

TOOTH No. or Letter	SURFACE	DESCRIPTION OF SERVICE (Including X-rays, prophylaxis, materials used, etc.)	Date service performed Mo. Day Year	Procedure Code	FEE
		Complete intraoral radiographic series	3 / 28 / 19	D0210	
		Periodontal maintenance	3 / 28 / 19	D4910	
31	D	**Localized delivery antimicrobial agent**	3 / 28 / 19	D4381	
		Fluoride varnish	3 / 28 / 19	D1208	
		Oral hygiene instructions	3 / 28 / 19	D1330	
			/ /		
			/ /		
			/ /		
			/ /		

I hereby certify that the procedures as indicated by Date ☐Will be ☐Have been completed
Signed ______ Date ______

REMARKS:

TOTAL FEE CHARGED	
MAXIMUM ALLOWABLE	
DEDUCTIBLE	
PLAN %	
PLAN PAYS	
PATIENT PAYS	

Figure 35-2. Insurance Claim Form. An example of a completed dental insurance claim form.

INSURANCE CODING OVERVIEW

In the United States, dental health care providers most commonly use **Common Dental Terminology (CDT) codes** to submit insurance claims.[9] **Insurance codes** are numeric codes used by insurance companies and the government to classify different dental procedures.[10] For example, periodontal maintenance procedures are designated by the insurance code D4910. The most important use of codes is for insurance billing purposes. Insurance codes are entered on **insurance forms**. Dental treatment is listed under the appropriate procedure number. These codes are very specific and should be reviewed carefully before specific dental treatment is coded.[10] Claim submissions for care provided can be completed electronically or by means of paper forms. An example of a completed dental insurance claim form is shown in Figure 35-2.

INSURANCE CODES FOR NONSURGICAL PERIODONTAL SERVICES

1. **Evolution of Dental Terminology**
   A. Members of the dental team should be aware that there is a continuous evolution of terminology used in dentistry and medicine.
      1. Changes in terminology occur as a natural result of scientific advances and improved understanding of disease pathogenesis.
      2. Terminology related to nonsurgical periodontal therapy is currently undergoing one such a change.
   B. Traditionally in the dental literature, two terms have been used to describe the therapies employed to remove deposits from tooth surfaces. These terms are (1) *dental prophylaxis* and (2) *scaling and root planing*.
   C. Recently in the dental hygiene literature, increasing numbers of authors are using new terminology to describe periodontal instrumentation.
      1. The term "*periodontal instrumentation*" or "*periodontal debridement*" is suggested to replace the older terms dental prophylaxis and scaling and root planing.
      2. *In dental hygiene literature, periodontal instrumentation is defined as the removal or disruption of plaque biofilm, its by-products, and biofilm-retentive calculus deposits from coronal surfaces, root surfaces, and within the pocket space, as indicated, for periodontal healing and repair.*
2. **Codes for Insurance Reporting.** The ADA Current Dental Terminology continues to use the terms "prophylaxis" and "scaling and root planing" to describe periodontal instrumentation. *Dental team members will have to use the currently accepted insurance codes when filling out insurance forms and in communications with insurance companies or other third-party payers.*
   A. **Examination Codes**
      1. D0120—Periodic Oral Evaluation. An evaluation performed on a patient of record to determine any changes in the patient's dental and medical health status since a previous comprehensive or periodic evaluation. This includes periodontal screening and may require interpretation of information acquired through additional diagnostic procedures.
      2. D0180—Comprehensive Periodontal Evaluation—New or Established Patient. This code is used for patients showing signs or symptoms of periodontal disease and for patients with risk factors such as smoking or diabetes. This examination code may be used when the hygienist performs a comprehensive periodontal evaluation including full-mouth, six-point probing and recording, charting of recession, furcations, tooth mobility, or tissue abnormalities once per year.

B. **Currently Accepted Insurance Codes Pertaining to Periodontal Instrumentation**
1. D1110—Adult Prophylaxis (four quadrants). Removal of plaque, calculus, and stains from the tooth structures in the permanent and transitional dentition. It is intended to control local irritating factors. *This code usually is used for healthy patients and patients with gingivitis.* Supragingival and subgingival scaling on this type of patient usually can be completed in a single appointment. This code may also be used to describe and report the cleaning of complete dentures in edentulous patients.
2. D4341—Periodontal Scaling and Root Planing—Four or More Teeth Per Quadrant. This procedure involves instrumentation of the crown and root surfaces to remove plaque and calculus from these surfaces. *It is indicated for patients with periodonitits and is a therapeutic code, not preventive in nature.* This procedure may be used as a definitive treatment in some stages of periodontitis and/or as a part of pre-surgical procedures in others.
3. D4342—Periodontal Scaling and Root Planing—One to Three Teeth Per Quadrant. This code is essentially the same as the D4341 code, the difference being the number of teeth that are treated in a quadrant.
4. D4910—Periodontal Maintenance. *This procedure is instituted following periodontal therapy and continues at varying intervals for the life of the dentition or implant replacements.* It includes the removal of the bacterial plaque and calculus from supragingival and subgingival regions, site specific scaling and root planing where indicated, and polishing of the teeth.
5. D4381—Localized Delivery of Antimicrobial Agents via a Controlled Release Vehicle. Synthetic fibers or other approved delivery devices containing controlled-release chemotherapeutic agents are inserted into a periodontal pocket.
6. D4355—Full Mouth Debridement to Enable Comprehensive Evaluation and Diagnosis. **This code should not be confused with the term "periodontal debridement" as used in dental hygiene literature.** Full mouth debridement is the gross removal of plaque and calculus that interfere with the ability of the dentist to perform a comprehensive oral evaluation. Full mouth debridement refers to an *incomplete* removal of heavy supragingival calculus deposits only. This is a preliminary procedure that will necessitate the need for additional periodontal instrumentation.
7. D4921—Gingival Irrigation: Per Quadrant. Irrigation of gingival pockets with medicinal agent. Not to be used to report use of mouth rinses or noninvasive chemical debridement.
8. D5994—Periodontal Medicament Carrier with Peripheral Seal: Laboratory Processed. A custom fabricated laboratory-processed carrier that covers the teeth and alveolar mucosa. Used as a vehicle to deliver prescribed medicaments for sustained contact with the gingiva, alveolar mucosa, and into the periodontal sulcus or pocket.
9. **D4346—Scaling in presence of generalized moderate or severe gingival inflammation--full mouth, after oral evaluation.**
   The removal of plaque, calculus, and stains from supra- and subgingival tooth surfaces when there is *generalized moderate or severe gingival inflammation* in the *absence* of periodontitis. It is indicated for patients who have swollen, inflamed gingiva, generalized suprabony pockets, and moderate to severe bleeding on probing. Should not be reported in conjunction with prophylaxis, scaling and root planing, or debridement procedures. The definition of **"...generalized moderate to severe gingival inflammation..."** when 30% or more of the patient's teeth at one or more sites are involved. If gingivitis is localized, the correct code is D1110. Note that unlike a dental prophylaxis, this type of care is therapeutic not preventive.

10. **D0414**—Laboratory processing of microbial specimen to include culture and sensitivity studies, preparation and transmission of written report.
11. **D0600**—Nonionizing diagnostic procedure capable of quantifying, monitoring, and recording changes in structure of enamel, dentin, and cementum. An example would be the use of a tool such as DIAGNOdent to aid in detection of caries.
12. **D6081**—Scaling and debridement in the presence of inflammation or mucositis of a single implant, including cleaning of the implant surface, without flap entry and closure.

C. **Codes for Radiographs.** The most common dental radiographs are:
1. **D0210**—a complete intraoral radiographic series including bitewings
2. **D0220**—an intraoral periapical (first film)
3. **D0230**—an intraoral periapical film (each additional film)
4. **D0240**—an intraoral occlusal film
5. **D0250**—an extraoral first film, such as a cephalometric film
6. **D0260**—an extraoral film (each additional film)
7. **D0270**—a single bitewing film
8. **D0272**—two bitewing films
9. **D0274**—four bitewing films
10. **D0330**—a panoramic film
11. **D0277**—vertical bitewings—7 to 8 films
12. **D0350**—oral/facial images. The oral/facial image code includes traditional photographs or digital images obtained by intraoral cameras.

D. **Codes for Topical Fluoride**
1. **D1206**—topical application of fluoride varnish
2. **D1208**—topical application of fluoride. This code used to report prescription strength fluoride swishes, trays, isolates, or paint on fluorides, but not varnishes

E. **Codes for Patient Counseling**
1. **D1310**—nutritional counseling for control of dental disease. Counseling on food selection and dietary habits as a part of treatment and control of periodontal disease and caries.
2. **D1320**—tobacco cessation counseling for control and prevention of oral disease.
3. **D1330**—oral hygiene (self-care) instructions. Examples include tooth brushing technique, flossing, and the use of special oral hygiene aids.

Chapter Summary Statement

In judging whether a professional has been negligent, the courts use a standard called the *reasonable prudent person or professional*. Thus, providing and documenting periodontal care that meets or exceeds the standard of care is extremely important for dental health professionals.

The dental chart is a legal document. All periodontal assessment, educational, and treatment services should be documented in the patient chart or computerized record. When a patient decides to file a lawsuit, the dental chart becomes the single most important piece of information relative to the suit.

Insurance coding was developed to speed and simplify the reporting of dental treatments to third parties such as insurance companies and the government. These codes are very specific and should be reviewed carefully before specific dental treatment is coded.

Section 5
Focus on Patients

Clinical Patient Care

CASE 1

During a social gathering one evening, a dental hygienist tells her friend about an HIV-positive patient she had treated that day. As the news traveled down the grapevine and the patient learned that the hygienist had revealed his HIV status, he sued her. What specific charge could he bring against the hygienist? Would she be covered under the dentist/employer's malpractice coverage or her own personal malpractice coverage?

CASE 2

The dental hygienist performed an oral cancer screening on every patient, but she never wrote it in her progress notes. When a patient found out he had oral cancer, he sued his dentist and the dental hygienist. The patient had been seen for a prophylaxis and restorative care 6 months before his diagnosis of oral cancer, and the basis for his suit was that he felt the hygienist and dentist had been negligent in failing to detect the lesion. Why is it likely that the patient will win his suit against the dental practice?

CASE 3

During the informed consent process, the patient is informed of (1) his diagnosis; (2) purpose, description, benefits, and risks of the proposed treatment; (3) alternative treatment options; (4) prognosis of no treatment; and (5) costs. The patient asks questions and demonstrates that he understands all information presented during the discussion. Then the patient refuses any treatment. What, if anything, should the dental hygienist do?

Ethical Dilemma

Winnie RDH has been working as a dental hygienist for Dr. Mooney for the last year. It is her first job after graduation. She is very happy with her working arrangements, enjoys her co-workers and patients, and has been given increased office responsibilities, as well as a pay increase.

Winnie RDH has been instructed to review all the patients' chart entries—for all the clinicians in the office—at the end of each business day for accuracy and make corrections as needed. Dr. Mooney has authorized Winnie RDH, to write and sign all of his patient notes, to maximize his time with patient treatments.

Dr. Mooney has also instructed each of the four other hygienists in his employ, as well as Winnie RDH, to bill each cleaning as "quadrant periodontal instrumentation" as opposed to a prophylaxis, so every patient will receive the ultimate dental hygiene experience. He also requires that all patients receive localized delivery of antimicrobial agents, and that the respective hygienists enter the proper insurance code for that service.

Dr. Mooney sent Winnie RDH, to a practice management seminar, to help improve the management of the office. At the course, Winnie RDH learned that many of the above office practices were unethical. Winnie RDH wants to continue working for Dr. Mooney but is concerned about her liability.

1. Discuss Winnie's potential liability with Dr. Mooney's current office practices and documentation of the care provided by the hygienists in the office.
2. Are there ethical principles in conflict in this dilemma?

References

1. Graskemper JP. *Professional Responsibility in Dentistry: A Practical Guide to Law and Ethics*. Chichester, West Sussex, UK; Ames, Iowa: Wiley-Blackwell; 2011:205.
2. Lai B, Lebuis A, Emami E, Feine JS. New technologies in health care. Part 2: a legal and professional dilemma. *J Can Dent Assoc.* 2008;74(7):637–640.
3. Morse D. Dealing with dental malpractice, Part 2. Malpractice prevention. *Dent Today.* 2004;23(3):116–121.
4. Morse DR. Dealing with dental malpractice, Part 1. *Dent Today.* 2004;23(2):140–143.
5. Hapcook CP, Sr. Dental malpractice claims: percentages and procedures. *J Am Dent Assoc.* 2006;137(10):1444–1445.
6. Tonner JJ. *Malpractice: What They Don't Teach You in Dental School*. Tulsa, OK: PennWell; 1996:218.
7. Schleyer T, Spallek H. Dental informatics. A cornerstone of dental practice. *J Am Dent Assoc.* 2001;132(5):605–613.
8. Schleyer TK, Thyvalikakath TP, Spallek H, Dziabiak MP, Johnson LA. From information technology to informatics: the information revolution in dental education. *J Dent Educ.* 2012;76(1):142–153.
9. American Dental Association. *CDT 2014: Dental Procedure Codes*. 1st ed. Chicago, IL: American Dental Association; 2013:180.
10. Napier RH, Bruelheide LS, Demann ET, Haug RH. Insurance billing and coding. *Dent Clin North Am.* 2008;52(3):507–527.

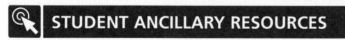 **STUDENT ANCILLARY RESOURCES**

A wide variety of resources to enhance your learning is available online:

- Audio Glossary
- Book Pages
- Chapter Review Questions and Answers

36 Future Directions for Management of Periodontal Patients

Clinical Application. All dental health care providers should be excited about what the future holds for the management of patients with periodontal diseases. There are not many absolutes in periodontics, but there is undoubtedly one—the simple fact that strategies for management of patients with periodontal diseases will continue to evolve and change over time. Dental hygienists must be prepared for changes in recommendations for management of patients with periodontal diseases as research into these diseases continues. This chapter explores a few relevant topics that point to the direction of ongoing and future dental research.

Learning Objective

• Describe some strategies in the management of patients with periodontal diseases that are likely to evolve in the future.

Key Terms

Computed tomography
Medical lasers
Genetic testing

Stem cells
Undifferentiated (cells)
Dental stem cells

Section 1
Contemporary and Evolving Diagnostic Technology

1. **Computer-Linked Periodontal Probes**
   A. **Traditional Manual Probes.** The diagnosis and monitoring of patients with periodontal diseases has been based on traditional clinical assessment methods for many years. Many of these traditional clinical assessment methods involve the use of manual periodontal probes to measure both probing depths and attachment levels.
      1. An experienced clinician can record probing depths fairly rapidly, and in many patients probing depths provide a reasonable assessment of periodontal health.
      2. On the other hand, attachment levels provide a more accurate assessment of the precise condition of the periodontium, but attachment levels are difficult to measure and record using manual periodontal probes.
   B. **Computer-Linked Probes.** Computer-linked, controlled-force, electronic periodontal probes are already available to clinicians.[1-3]
      1. These computer-linked probes can make it possible to measure both probing depths and attachment levels quickly, as well as provide automatic data entry features.
      2. This technology of computer-linked periodontal probes will continue to improve. As this technology improves, the use of these computer-linked probes in dental offices will undoubtedly become universal, making it much easier for clinicians to measure and record attachment levels while caring for patients with periodontal diseases.

2. **Digital Radiographs**
   A. **Film Radiography.** While conventional (film) radiography is still widely used today, advances in diagnostic imaging technology are transforming the way that we take and interpret radiographic images. Digital radiography is a new type of diagnostic imaging technology that provides an enhanced image quality with better spatial resolution compared to conventional radiographs. Furthermore, unlike conventional radiographic techniques, digital radiography images are instantly available for distribution to the clinical services without the time and physical effort needed to either archive or retrieve film packets.[1,4-6]
   B. **Digital Radiography.** Digital (filmless) radiographic techniques have developed to the stage where they are now being used by most clinicians.
      1. Digital radiographic techniques allow members of the dental team to collect radiographic information using special sensors instead of printing the radiographic image on a film.
      2. These digital images are then stored on a computer and can be viewed on a computer screen or even printed when needed.
      3. Modern technology for viewing these images on computer screens has substantial advantages over the traditional use of radiographic film.
      4. Software for viewing these digitized images can eliminate distortion that is seen with traditional film, can allow for easy magnification of details, and can provide precise, anatomically correct measurements.
      5. The same software can also allow for enhancing aspects of a digitized image, providing members of the dental team with more details of the actual status of a tooth or of the periodontium.
      6. In addition, these digital images can be shared with other health care providers quite readily—as might be indicated during a patient referral or during consultation with a specialist.

3. **Computed Tomographic Radiography.** Another evolutionary diagnostic imaging modality is computed tomographic techniques.
   A. Computed tomography is a radiologic procedure using a machine called a scanner to examine a body site by taking a series of cross-sectional images one slice at a time in a full circle rotation (Fig. 36-1).
      1. Computed tomographic techniques provide clinicians with the ability to study minute details and precise dimensions of the jaws in a three-dimensional (3-D) perspective on a computer screen.
      2. These details can be so precise that they can include a three-dimensional radiographic image of a thin slice made through the jaws at any specific location. For this reason, computed tomographic techniques are currently in use by many clinicians when planning for the placement of dental implants.
   B. Presently, the routine use of 3-D imaging to diagnose and treat periodontal disease is not warranted from a radiation exposure and cost perspective. However, in the future, if technological advancements in 3-D imaging are able to minimize radiation exposure and cost, 3-D imaging may become more widely accepted for routine use.[7]
4. **Other Technologies of Interest in the Future.** There are a variety of other technologies that are related to the diagnosis and treatment of patients with periodontal disease that may indeed become more important as the results of further research become available. Examples of these other technologies include the following:
   • Improved means of identification of the microbes populating periodontal pockets
   • Enhanced testing for genetic predispositions for developing periodontal diseases
   • Improved mechanisms for identifying the content of the gingival crevicular fluid as a means of understanding underlying periodontal disease processes, such as infrared spectral analysis
   • Development of techniques for using infrared spectroscopy to obtain diagnostic profiles of periodontal diseases
   • Increased utilization of noninvasive ultrasound imaging in the assessment of the status of the periodontium and other oral tissues[8]

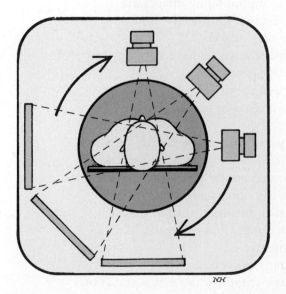

Figure 36-1. Computed Tomography. Computed tomography is a radiologic procedure using a machine called a scanner to examine a body site by taking a series of cross-sectional images one slice at a time in a full circle rotation. A computer then calculates and converts rates of absorption and density of the x-rays into a 3-dimensional image which can be viewed by the dental clinician.

Section 2
Periodontal Disease/Systemic Disease Connections

Dental and medical researchers have been studying the connection between periodontitis and certain systemic diseases for some time. Research into this critical topic is ongoing and continues to offer insights into these connections.[9-17] Review of the dental literature will reveal many studies about how systemic conditions may be linked to periodontal diseases, but all of these areas will require further scientific study. *For review, the complex bidirectional relationship between periodontal inflammation and systemic health is discussed in Chapters 16 and 34.*

1. **Systemic Diseases With a Link to Periodontal Disease**
   A. Some examples of systemic diseases or conditions that may have a connection to periodontitis are atherosclerotic cardiovascular disease, adverse pregnancy outcomes, and diabetes mellitus.
   B. Discussion of these systemic conditions is included in Chapters 16 and 34 of this book, but it is of interest to review some of the relationships between one specific condition—diabetes mellitus—and periodontal disease.

2. **Diabetes Mellitus in Periodontal Patients**
   A. **Need for Additional Research.** It is clear that our current understanding into the connection between diabetes and periodontal disease is still limited. Nevertheless, ongoing research contributions in this field will indeed impact the practice of dentistry.
      1. As discussed in other chapters of this book, research has demonstrated that patients with poorly controlled diabetes have an increased risk for periodontitis.[18-23]
      2. Since periodontitis is a type of infection, and since diabetes can lower the body's resistance to infections in general, it is not surprising that there is a connection between poorly controlled diabetes and periodontitis in some susceptible patients.
      3. In addition, research suggests that periodontal infection and the elimination of the periodontal infection through proper periodontal therapy have the potential to alter the body's control of blood sugar levels.
      4. It has even been suggested that thorough treatment of periodontitis in a diabetic patient may potentially lower the HbA1c levels and make it easier for a patient to manage his diabetic condition.[24]
   B. **Research Questions.** There are many research questions that need to be answered related to the periodontitis/diabetes connection, but a few of those questions that can have a direct impact on the practice of dentistry are outlined below.
      1. Are the measures used to prevent or control periodontitis in the patient without diabetes mellitus adequate for the patient with diabetes mellitus?
      2. Since wound healing appears altered in patients with diabetes, are there adjustments clinicians need to make when delivering dental hygiene therapy to maximize the potential for healing in these patients?
      3. What precise periodontal maintenance protocols are the most effective for patients with diabetes?
      4. When a dental clinician treats a patient with diabetes, what communication protocols can be most effective in ensuring that the patient's physician is aware of the patient's periodontal status so that adjustments in the therapy for diabetes can be made where needed?

C. **Use of Intensive Therapies for Diabetes Mellitus.** In examining the periodontitis/diabetes connection there is another line of inquiry that will also affect dental practice—the type of medical therapy used in diabetic patients.[24]

1. In medicine, there have been dramatic improvements in the treatment regimens for patients with diabetes, and these regimens now frequently include intensive treatment with oral agents and with insulin.

2. Unfortunately, some of these medical treatments have increased the risk for medical emergencies (such as hypoglycemia) during dental office treatment of a patient with diabetes.

3. This medical trend in intensive therapies for patients with diabetes will continue.

4. As physicians use more intensive therapies to manage patients with diabetes, all members of the dental team will need to have more knowledge about these therapies, about how to manage these patients in a dental setting, and about how to respond when a medical emergency arises.

Section 3
Research in Dental Implantology

1. **State of Dental Implantology.** In modern dentistry, dental implants are a viable option as one alternative for replacing most missing teeth. It should be noted that dental implants available today have a high success rate. Even though dental implantology has been intensively studied for several decades, there are still many unanswered questions related to this field, and research will continue. Since implants are susceptible to breakdown in the presence of inflammation, patient selection and the proper maintenance of the peri-implant tissues in a state of health are of paramount importance. The reader is referred to Chapter 9 to review the many widely accepted and evidence-based treatment protocols available to maintain dental implants.

2. **Research Questions Related to Maintenance of Dental Implants.** Much additional investigation is needed in the area of dental implantology, and some examples of questions related to dental hygiene that are in need of further study are listed below. Answering these types of questions with appropriate scientific investigation is quite likely to have a substantial impact on clinical care delivered by the dental hygienist.

   A. What self-care measures can best prevent peri-implant infections?

   B. What are the most effective protocols for effective maintenance of implants?

   C. Should clinicians recommend the same techniques for minimizing the bacterial challenge to an implant that apply to a natural tooth?

   D. When treating dental implants patients, what types of instruments provide the greatest chance of maintaining periodontal health?

Section 4
Treatment Modalities in Periodontal Care

Treatment modalities for patients with periodontal diseases are constantly evolving. This section outlines some treatment modalities that can be expected to enhance more effective periodontal therapy as they evolve further.

1. **Lasers in Periodontal Care**
    A. Lasers have been widely used in many fields of medicine since the early 1960s. Medical lasers are medical devices that use precisely focused light sources to treat or remove tissues. Lasers produce a narrow beam of light with a single wavelength that can produce intense energy at precise locations.
        1. In dentistry, these intense light beams are passed down a narrow optical tubing and can be focused on a small area of tissue within the mouth and within the periodontium.
        2. Some laser beams are so intense that they can actually be used to remove oral soft tissue or to cut tissues in the mouth.
        3. There are different types of lasers that have been studied for use in dentistry, and each type has a somewhat different effect on soft tissue, enamel, dentin, pulp, and bone.
    B. Lasers have been suggested for use in dentistry for a variety of dental applications. Some of these devices even have Food and Drug Administration (FDA) safety clearance for some intraoral soft tissue procedures (Fig. 36-2).
        1. More study is needed, however, to clarify how these devices can be used appropriately in subgingival applications in patients with periodontal diseases, and some of these studies are in progress.[25,26]
        2. Some investigations have suggested a possible combined use of lasers as with conventional manual instruments to debride periodontally diseased root surfaces.
        3. Additional research will clarify appropriate uses for these devices in patients with periodontal diseases and may impact some of the therapy provided by dental hygienists for patients with periodontitis and for those with peri-implantitis.
        4. If further study of these devices confirms that patients with periodontal diseases do benefit from their use, lasers may one day be a routine part of the care of patients with periodontitis, peri-implantitis,[27] and perhaps even a part of the practice of dental hygiene.
    C. *Currently, however, an American Academy of Periodontology statement on the efficiency of lasers in the nonsurgical treatment of inflammatory periodontal disease states that there is minimal evidence to support use of a laser for the purpose of subgingival periodontal instrumentation, either as a monotherapy or adjunctive to SRP.[28] Additionally, for the treatment and management of peri-implantitis, a recent systemic review and meta-analysis concluded that laser therapy only produced identical reductions in probing depths, amount of radiographic bone fill, and clinical attachment level gains compared to other commonly used surface detoxification methods.[29]*

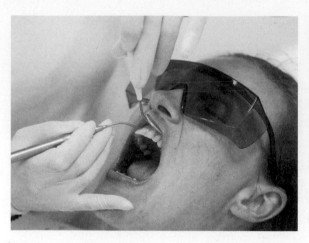
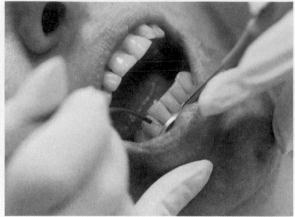

Figure 36-2. Lasers Being Used in Periodontal Therapy. These two photographs show a laser being used in periodontal therapy. The application of lasers in dentistry has grown in the last few decades. Lasers may prove to be an effective instrument to have in the periodontal armamentarium since it has the potential to improve on efficiency, specificity, ease, and cost and comfort for the patient. However, at this time, investigations are still ongoing to compare the effectiveness of lasers vs. conventional periodontal instrumentation.

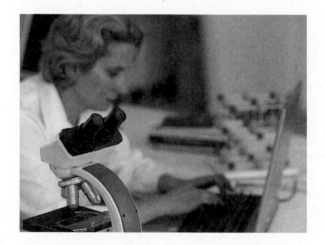

Figure 36-3. Genetic Testing. Scientific studies also indicate that certain genetic factors determine how an individual patient's host defenses actually react to an increased bacterial challenge. Much more study into the genetic factors that increase the risk for periodontitis is needed, but it is already possible to use some types of genetic information to guide clinical decision-making in a small group of selected patients.

2. **Genetic Technology in Periodontal Care.** Genetic testing is a type of medical test that identifies changes in chromosomes, genes, or proteins. The results of a genetic test can confirm or rule out a suspected genetic condition or help determine a person's chance of developing or passing on a genetic disorder.
   A. Clinicians have known for a long time that there are many factors that can increase the risk of developing periodontitis.
      1. One factor that is known to increase the risk of developing periodontitis is failure to control bacterial plaque growth on the teeth, thereby increasing the bacterial challenge to the periodontium.
      2. Scientific studies also indicate that certain genetic factors determine how an individual patient's host defenses actually react to an increased bacterial challenge.
      3. Based upon the current research literature available, it now appears that a key factor in determining whether a patient develops periodontitis in response to the bacterial challenge is how the body reacts to that bacterial challenge.
      4. One major determinant of how the body reacts to the bacterial challenge is genetics (or inherited characteristics).

B. Much more study into the genetic factors that increase the risk for periodontitis is needed, but it is already possible to use some types of genetic information to guide clinical decision-making in a small group of selected patients.

1. Genetic testing can identify patients carrying gene mutations for several rare syndromes that are often accompanied by a form of periodontal disease (Fig. 36-3).

2. In addition to identifying patients with rare syndromes, there is already a commercially available genetic susceptibility test for severe chronic periodontitis.

3. In this test, specific gene polymorphisms (forms) that have been associated with the development of periodontitis can be detected.

4. Ongoing scientific investigations will undoubtedly clarify how such genetic testing can be used in periodontitis patient management.

C. As more and more scientific information about identifying genetic control of host defenses becomes available, it is quite likely that this information will impact how we manage patients with periodontal diseases and will impact the practice of dental hygiene.

3. **Local Delivery Mechanisms in Periodontal Care**

A. As already discussed in Chapter 27, research has demonstrated that using local delivery mechanisms for antimicrobial chemicals in patients with periodontitis has a small but measurable impact upon clinical parameters, such as attachment levels.[30] Reported analyses of the long-term effects of chemotherapeutic agents usually do not extend beyond a few months to a year. Nonsurgical periodontal instrumentation remains the gold standard for the treatment of inflammatory periodontitis.[26]

B. There are several areas of research investigation that are needed related to these local delivery mechanisms, and some examples of research questions about this topic that need to be answered are listed below.

1. Can future local delivery mechanisms be designed that have a greater clinical impact than those currently available for clinical use?

2. What specific local delivery treatment protocols should be followed to produce the most benefit for individual patients?

3. Are there additional antimicrobial agents that can be delivered safely using the local delivery concept?

4. Can other therapy provided by the dental hygienist be enhanced by using some of these local delivery mechanisms?

C. Research into the modification of polymers, manufacturing technologies, and carrier systems will undoubtedly lead to vastly improved drug delivery systems that may have an impact on periodontal therapy strategies.

D. Research into the use of local delivery mechanisms for antimicrobial agents continues. It is probable that as this modality improves in clinical effectiveness, using local delivery mechanisms may become more and more useful in the care of the periodontal patient by the dental hygienist.

4. **Host Modulation Therapies in Periodontal Care**

A. As already discussed in Chapter 28, research has demonstrated that host defenses can play a significant role in the actual development of attachment loss and alveolar bone loss in patients with periodontitis.

1. A variety of host modulation therapies have been investigated that could be used as adjunctive (supplemental) treatment in patients with periodontitis.[31-33]

2. Host modulation therapies usually involve using medications that can alter biochemical pathways in a manner that will (1) slow attachment loss, (2) slow alveolar bone loss, or (3) decrease inflammation.

B. Investigations into possible host modulation therapies have already resulted in one commercially available medication (low-dose doxycycline hyclate) that can be used as adjunctive treatment in patients with chronic periodontitis.
   1. This medication can be used to lower levels of collagenase, an enzyme involved in the destruction of collagen.
   2. Collagen is one of the components of many of the structures that make up the periodontium. Thus, lowering the levels of collagenase can slow the progress of periodontitis.
   3. Investigations are ongoing into a number of other possible host modulation therapies that include studies into (1) modulation of cytokines (chemicals involved in periodontitis that can result in increased periodontal disease progression), (2) reduction of prostaglandins (chemicals that enhance inflammation in the gingiva and in the periodontium), and (3) slowing alveolar bone loss with chemical agents.
C. In addition, an interesting future direction for research will include local delivery systems that can deliver varied concentrations of host modulating agents over a sustained period of time. Variable concentrations could be used to achieve the maximum therapeutic effects when planning individualized nonsurgical treatment for patients with periodontal disease.
D. As further scientific investigations improve our understanding of host modulation therapies, there are likely to be a variety of new therapeutic options for members of the dental team to use in patient management.

Box 36-1. Examples of Factors That May Help Predict Periodontal Disease Activity

- Smoking
- Poorly controlled diabetes
- Poor patient self-care
- Severity of alveolar bone loss
- Positive family history
- Presence of pocket depths >6 mm
- Age
- Gender
- Gingival bleeding/Bleeding on probing
- Number of missing teeth
- Specific periodontal pathogens

---

5. Disease Risk Assessment in Periodontal Care
   A. Recently, there has been increased interest in identifying clinical tools that can be used to quantify a patient's risk for developing periodontitis.[34–36]
      1. Traditionally, clinicians have assessed the risk of developing periodontitis subjectively, but studies have shown that subjective risk assessment is surprisingly variable even among clinicians who are experts.[36]
      2. Objective periodontal disease risk assessment tools would be quite useful to members of the dental team if they provided a method of risk assessment that could accurately predict which patients are most likely to develop periodontitis.
      3. Examples of risk factors that have been suggested to be predictive of periodontal disease activity are listed in Box 36-1.

4. Using risk assessment tools to identify the patients with the highest risk for developing periodontitis would allow members of the dental team to provide more aggressive treatment for those patients.

5. In addition, these tools might identify which periodontal patients should be referred to a specialist early in their treatment and which patients can best be managed in a general dental setting.

B. Studies show that some of these risk assessment tools are reasonable predictors of alveolar bone loss and loss of periodontally affected teeth.

1. It is likely that some of these tools for quantifying a patient's risk will soon be in widespread use in dental offices.

2. Guidelines from the American Academy of Periodontology indicate that periodontal disease risk assessment should be part of every comprehensive dental and periodontal evaluation.

3. The American Academy of Periodontology has even developed a simplified form of risk assessment for use by patients. This web-based patient self-assessment can be viewed at www.perio.org.

4. These risk assessment tools would be useful to the dental hygienist and the dentist in planning therapy and in identifying patients in need of immediate referral.

6. **Advances Based on Stem Cell Biology**

A. **Introduction to Stem Cell Biology.** Stem cell biology is an emerging field of medical research that can have a profound effect on medical therapy available for certain systemic diseases and that may have utility in regeneration of periodontal tissues in the future.[37–42]

1. Stem cells are the "master cells" of the human body that have the ability to develop into any one of the body's more than 200 cell types.

2. Stem cells are unspecialized (undifferentiated) cells. When a stem cell divides, each new cell has the potential either to remain a stem cell or become another type of cell with a more specialized function, such as a muscle cell, a red blood cell, or a brain cell. Figure 36-4 depicts the process of cellular differentiation.

3. Stem cells retain the ability to divide throughout life and give rise to cells that can become highly specialized and take the place of cells that die or are lost. Stem cells contribute to the body's ability to renew and repair its tissues.

B. **Dental Stem Cell Research**

1. Human stem cells have already been isolated from the periodontal ligament, dental pulp tissue, exfoliated deciduous teeth, dental papillae, and dental follicles.

2. Dental stem cells apparently can differentiate into specific components of the periodontium (such as periodontal ligament and cementum).

3. Given their unique regenerative abilities, stem cells offer new potentials for treating diseases such as diabetes, and to influence periodontal treatment strategies. However, much work remains to be done in the laboratory and the clinic to understand how to use these cells for cell-based therapies to treat disease, which is also referred to as regenerative or reparative medicine.

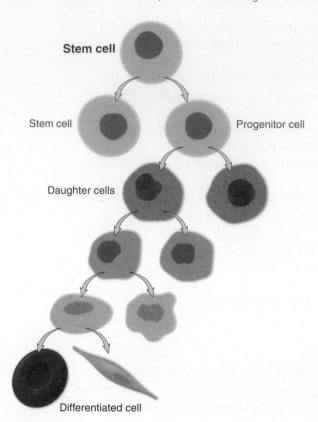

Stem cell

Stem cell
Progenitor cell

Daughter cells

Differentiated cell

Figure 36-4. Cellular Differentiation. Cellular differentiation is the process by which cells become more specialized. Undifferentiated stem cells divide into like stem cells and parent (progenitor) cells, which continue to divide and further differentiate into highly specialized and functional cells.

Chapter Summary Statement

All members of the dental team should expect many changes to take place in recommendations for management of patients with periodontal diseases as research continues. This chapter presented a brief overview of a few of the possibilities for future directions in the management of patients with periodontal diseases by dental hygienists.

References

1. Armitage GC; Research, Science and Therapy Committee of the American Academy of Periodontology. Diagnosis of periodontal diseases. *J Periodontol.* 2003;74(8):1237–1247.
2. Renatus A, Trentzsch L, Schonfelder A, Schwarzenberger F, Jentsch H. Evaluation of an electronic periodontal probe versus a manual probe. *J Clin Diagn Res.* 2016;10(11):ZH03–ZH07.
3. Wang SF, Leknes KN, Zimmerman GJ, Sigurdsson TJ, Wikesjo UM, Selvig KA. Reproducibility of periodontal probing using a conventional manual and an automated force-controlled electronic probe. *J Periodontol.* 1995;66(1):38–46.
4. Eickholz P, Kim TS, Benn DK, Staehle HJ. Validity of radiographic measurement of interproximal bone loss. *Oral Surg Oral Med Oral Pathol Oral Radiol Endod.* 1998;85(1):99–106.
5. Jeffcoat MK, Reddy MS. Digital subtraction radiography for longitudinal assessment of peri-implant bone change: method and validation. *Adv Dent Res.* 1993;7(2):196–201.
6. Jeffcoat MK, Wang IC, Reddy MS. Radiographic diagnosis in periodontics. *Periodontol 2000.* 1995;7:54–68.
7. Kim DM, Bassir SH. When is cone-beam computed tomography imaging appropriate for diagnostic inquiry in the management of inflammatory periodontitis? An American Academy of Periodontology best evidence review. *J Periodontol.* 2017;88(10):978–998.
8. Xiang X, Sowa MG, Iacopino AM, et al. An update on novel non-invasive approaches for periodontal diagnosis. *J Periodontol.* 2010;81(2):186–198.
9. Parameter on systemic conditions affected by periodontal diseases. American Academy of Periodontology. *J Periodontol.* 2000;71(5 Suppl):880–883.
10. El-Shinnawi U, Soory M. Associations between periodontitis and systemic inflammatory diseases: response to treatment. *Recent Pat Endocr Metab Immune Drug Discov.* 2013;7(3):169–188.
11. Gulati M, Anand V, Jain N, et al. Essentials of periodontal medicine in preventive medicine. *Int J Prev Med.* 2013;4(9): 988–994.
12. Gurav AN. The association of periodontitis and metabolic syndrome. *Dent Res J (Isfahan).* 2014;11(1):1–10.

13. Huck O, Tenenbaum H, Davideau JL. Relationship between periodontal diseases and preterm birth: recent epidemiological and biological data. *J Pregnancy*. 2011;2011:164654.

14. Jeffcoat MK. Osteoporosis: a possible modifying factor in oral bone loss. *Ann Periodontol*. 1998;3(1):312–321.

15. Otomo-Corgel J, Pucher JJ, Rethman MP, Reynolds MA. State of the science: chronic periodontitis and systemic health. *J Evid Based Dent Pract*. 2012;12(3 Suppl):20–28.

16. Shangase SL, Mohangi GU, Hassam-Essa S, Wood NH. The association between periodontitis and systemic health: an overview. *SADJ*. 2013;68(1):8, 10–12.

17. Zhu M, Nikolajczyk BS. Immune cells link obesity-associated type 2 diabetes and periodontitis. *J Dent Res*. 2014;93(4):346–352.

18. Gurav AN. Advanced glycation end products: a link between periodontitis and diabetes mellitus? *Curr Diabetes Rev*. 2013;9(5):355–361.

19. Leite RS, Marlow NM, Fernandes JK, Hermayer K. Oral health and type 2 diabetes. *Am J Med Sci*. 2013;345(4):271–273.

20. Loe H. Periodontal disease. The sixth complication of diabetes mellitus. *Diabetes Care*. 1993;16(1):329–334.

21. Mealey BL, Oates TW; American Academy of Periodontology. Diabetes mellitus and periodontal diseases. *J Periodontol*. 2006;77(8):1289–1303.

22. Pradhan S, Goel K. Interrelationship between diabetes and periodontitis: a review. *JNMA J Nepal Med Assoc*. 2011;51(183):144–153.

23. Taylor GW. Bidirectional interrelationships between diabetes and periodontal diseases: an epidemiologic perspective. *Ann Periodontol*. 2001;6(1):99–112.

24. Mealey BL. Periodontal implications: medically compromised patients. *Ann Periodontol*. 1996;1(1):256–321.

25. Cobb CM. Lasers in periodontics: a review of the literature. *J Periodontol*. 2006;77(4):545–564.

26. Drisko CL. Periodontal debridement: still the treatment of choice. *J Evid Based Dent Pract*. 2014;14 Suppl:33–41.e1.

27. Romanos GE, Javed F, Delgado-Ruiz RA, Calvo-Guirado JL. Peri-implant diseases: a review of treatment interventions. *Dent Clin North Am*. 2015;59(1):157–178.

28. American Academy of Periodontology statement on the efficacy of lasers in the non-surgical treatment of inflammatory periodontal disease. *J Periodontol*. 2011;82(4):513–514.

29. Mailoa J, Lin GH, Chan HL, MacEachern M, Wang HL. Clinical outcomes of using lasers for peri-implantitis surface detoxification: a systematic review and meta-analysis. *J Periodontol*. 2014;85(9):1194–1202.

30. Finkelman RD, Polson AM. Evidence-based considerations for the clinical use of locally delivered, controlled-release antimicrobials in periodontal therapy. *J Dent Hyg*. 2013;87(5):249–264.

31. Bhatavadekar NB, Williams RC. New directions in host modulation for the management of periodontal disease. *J Clin Periodontol*. 2009;36(2):124–126.

32. Gokhale SR, Padhye AM. Future prospects of systemic host modulatory agents in periodontal therapy. *Br Dent J*. 2013;214(9):467–471.

33. Oringer RJ; Research, Science, and Therapy Committee of the American Academy of Periodontology. Modulation of the host response in periodontal therapy. *J Periodontol*. 2002;73(4):460–470.

34. American Academy of Periodontology. American Academy of Periodontology statement on risk assessment. *J Periodontol*. 2008;79(2):202.

35. Page RC, Martin J, Krall EA, Mancl L, Garcia R. Longitudinal validation of a risk calculator for periodontal disease. *J Clin Periodontol*. 2003;30(9):819–827.

36. Persson GR, Mancl LA, Martin J, Page RC. Assessing periodontal disease risk: a comparison of clinicians' assessment versus a computerized tool. *J Am Dent Assoc*. 2003;134(5):575–582.

37. Fawzy El-Sayed KM, Dorfer C, Fandrich F, Gieseler F, Moustafa MH, Ungefroren H. Adult mesenchymal stem cells explored in the dental field. *Adv Biochem Eng Biotechnol*. 2013;130:89–103.

38. Feng R, Lengner C. Application of stem cell technology in dental regenerative medicine. *Adv Wound Care*. 2013;2(6):296–305.

39. Han J, Menicanin D, Gronthos S, Bartold PM. Stem cells, tissue engineering and periodontal regeneration. *Aust Dent J*. 2014;59 Suppl 1:117–130.

40. Hynes K, Menicanin D, Gronthos S, Bartold PM. Clinical utility of stem cells for periodontal regeneration. *Periodontol 2000*. 2012;59(1):203–227.

41. Research, Science and Therapy Committee of American Academy of Periodontology. Informational paper: implications of genetic technology for the management of periodontal diseases. *J Periodontol*. 2005;76(5):850–857.

42. Ulmer FL, Winkel A, Kohorst P, Stiesch M. Stem cells—prospects in dentistry. *Schweiz Monatsschr Zahnmed*. 2010;120(10):860–883.

 STUDENT ANCILLARY RESOURCES

A wide variety of resources to enhance your learning is available online:

- Audio Glossary
- Book Pages
- Chapter Review Questions and Answers

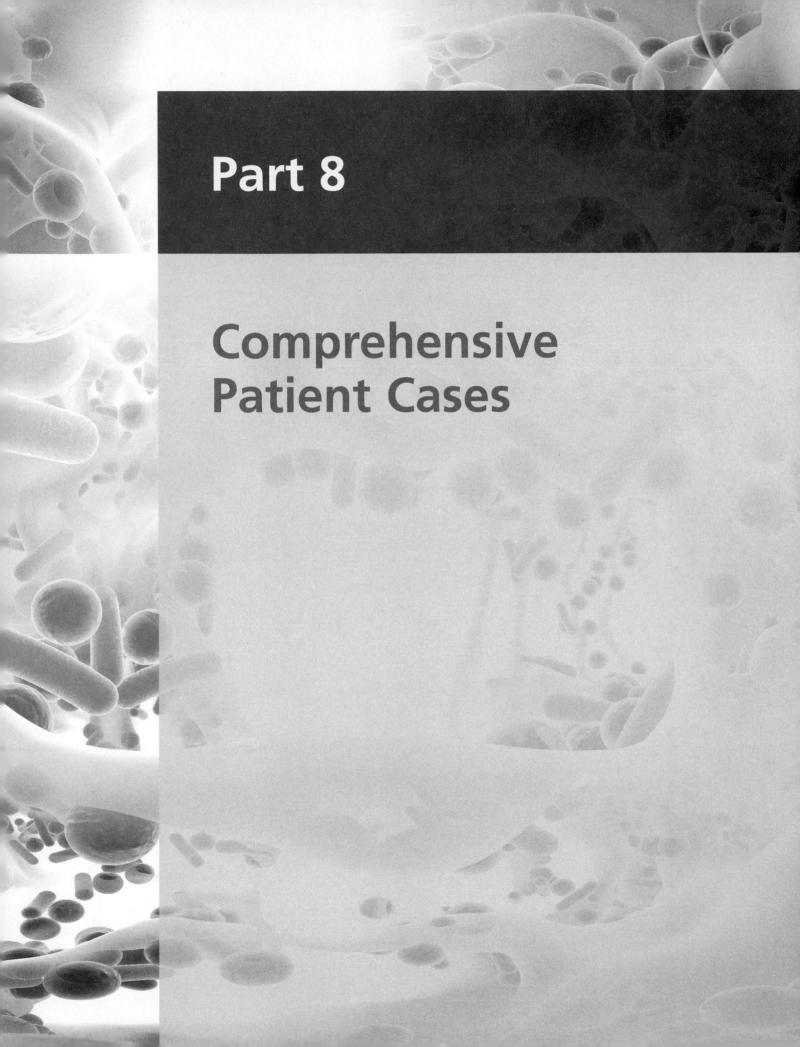

Part 8

Comprehensive Patient Cases

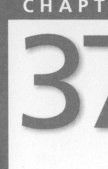

37 Comprehensive Patient Cases

Learning Objective

- Apply the content from the chapters in this book to answer the decision-making questions for the hypothetical case scenarios presented in this chapter.

Fictitious Patient Case 1—Mr. Karn

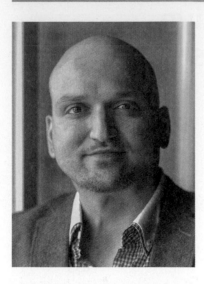

PATIENT PROFILE

Mr. Karn is a 47-year-old high school administrator who has recently moved to your city. He came to the dental office because he would like to know if it is possible to replace his missing upper right first molar tooth with a dental implant.

During Mr. Karn's first office visit, he informs you that he has been too busy lately to get a dental check-up and that he has not seen a dentist for quite a few years. Mr. Karn states that he brushes his teeth twice daily when he has time and that he does not floss regularly even though he knows that he should. He also uses an over-the-counter mouth rinse occasionally.

PATIENT HEALTH HISTORY

- On the day of his first visit to your dental office Mr. Karn's blood pressure is 130/80 mm Hg and his pulse is 62 beats/min.
- A review of Mr. Karn's health history reveals that he takes two medications: Zocor and Nifedipine.
- Mr. Karn also states that he smokes between one half and one pack of cigarettes each day.

Clinical Photographs for Mr. Karn

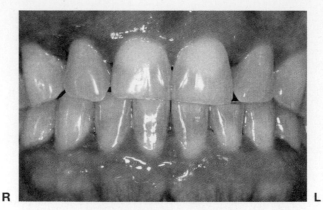

Figure 37-1. Anterior Teeth, Facial View.

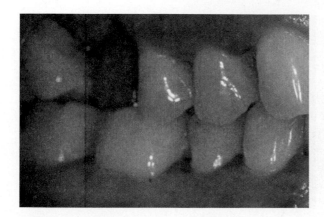

Figure 37-2. Right Side, Facial View.

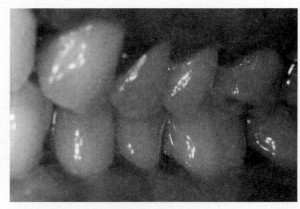

Figure 37-3. Left Side, Facial View.

Clinical Photographs for Mr. Karn

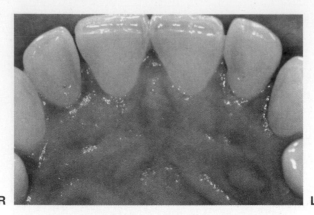

Figure 37-4. Maxillary Anterior, Lingual View.

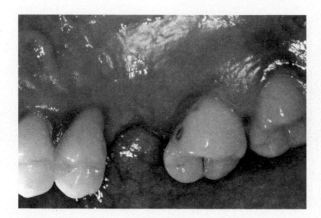

Figure 37-5. Maxillary Right, Lingual View.

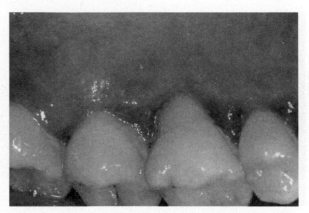

Figure 37-6. Maxillary Left, Lingual View.

Clinical Photographs for Mr. Karn

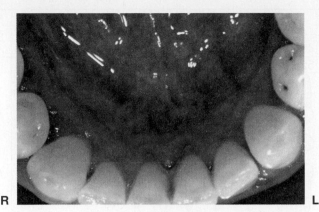

Figure 37-7. Mandibular Anterior, Lingual View.

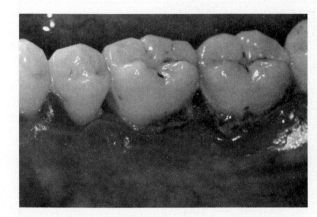

Figure 37-8. Mandibular Right, Lingual View.

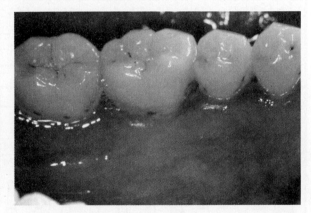

Figure 37-9. Mandibular Left, Lingual View.

CASE #1

1	2	3	4	5	6	7	8	9	10	11	12	13	14	15	16	Maxilla
					I	I						I			I	Mobility (I, II, III)
+	+		+	+	+	+			+	+	+	+	+	+	+	Bleeding/Purulence (+)
646	647		535	536	415	322	322	334	425	435	536	626	638	846	746	Attachment Level (CEJ to BP)
646	635		325	536	525	435	433	334	425	435	536	626	638	846	746	Probing Depth (FGM to BP)

Facial / *Palatal*

1	2	3	4	5	6	7	8	9	10	11	12	13	14	15	16	
+	+		+	+	+	+	+	+	+	+	+	+	+	+	+	Bleeding/Purulence (+)
646	646		546	526	536	425	443	324	424	525	535	626	859	937	736	Attachment Level (CEJ to BP)
636	525		335	526	536	425	443	324	424	525	535	626	627	827	736	Probing Depth (FGM to BP)
																F/P Plaque
	✓		✓	✓					✓	✓			✓	✓	✓	Supragingival Calculus
✓	✓		✓	✓	✓	✓	✓	✓	✓	✓	✓	✓	✓	✓	✓	Subgingival Calculus
		4					3					4				PSR Code

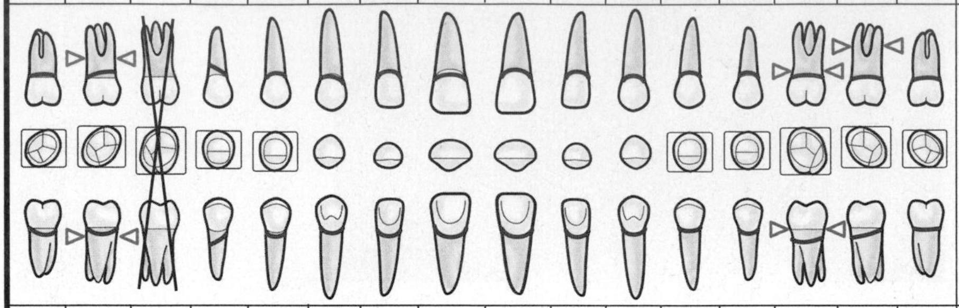

Right / *Left*

32	31	30	29	28	27	26	25	24	23	22	21	20	19	18	17	Mandible
			I			I	I									Mobility (I, II, III)
+		+	+	+	+			+		+	+	+		+	+	Bleeding/Purulence (+)
546	746	736	635	435	534	324	534	434	324	324	434	435	536	746	635	Attachment Level (CEJ to BP)
546	736	626	635	535	534	324	423	323	324	324	434	435	536	746	635	Probing Depth (FGM to BP)

Lingual / *Facial*

32	31	30	29	28	27	26	25	24	23	22	21	20	19	18	17	
+	+	+	+	+		+	+	+		+	+	+		+	+	Bleeding/Purulence (+)
546	736	625	535	635	534	324	423	323	324	324	434	435	526	736	625	Attachment Level (CEJ to BP)
546	736	625	535	635	534	324	423	323	324	324	434	435	526	736	625	Probing Depth (FGM to BP)
																L/F Plaque
					✓	✓	✓	✓	✓				✓	✓		Supragingival Calculus
✓	✓	✓	✓	✓	✓	✓	✓	✓	✓	✓	✓	✓	✓	✓	✓	Subgingival Calculus
		4					3					4				PSR Code

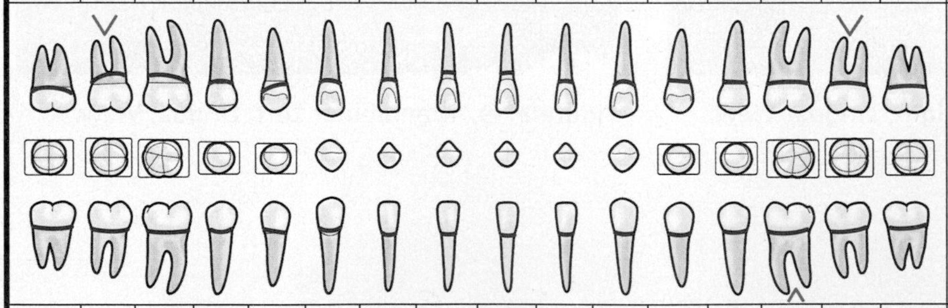

Figure 37-10. Mr. Karn's Periodontal Chart.

Radiographic Series for Mr. Karn

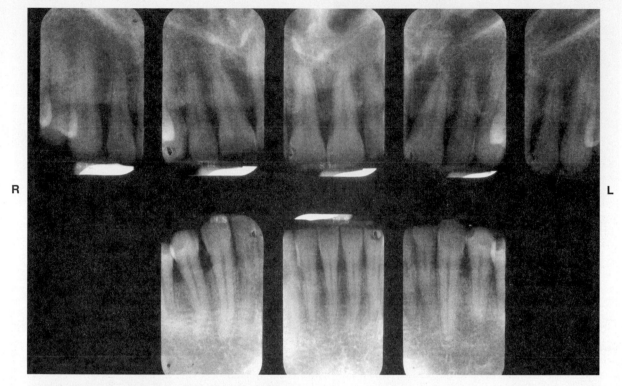

R   L

Figure 37-11A. Radiographs: Anterior Teeth.

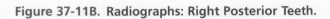

Figure 37-11B. Radiographs: Right Posterior Teeth.

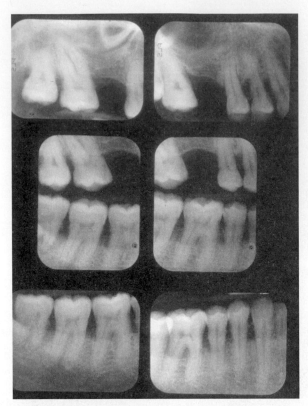

Figure 37-11C. Radiographs: Left Posterior Teeth.

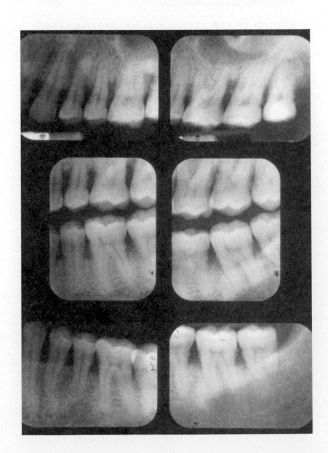

DECISION-MAKING QUESTIONS FOR CASE 1: MR. KARN

1. What should Mr. Karn be told about the possibility of replacing his maxillary right first molar tooth with a dental implant? Note that this question was what prompted Mr. Karn to make an appointment in your dental office.
2. What factors in Mr. Karn's profile indicate that achieving an acceptable level of patient self-care may be a problem for the dental team?
3. What factors revealed in Mr. Karn's health history will be critical for the dental team to consider during treatment?
4. What signs of gingival inflammation are evident in Mr. Karn's clinical photographs?
5. What etiologic risk factors for gingival and periodontal diseases are evident in Mr. Karn's clinical photographs?
6. How might the presence of the furcation involvements found during Mr. Karn's periodontal evaluation affect his periodontal treatment?
7. Does Mr. Karn's periodontal evaluation indicate that he has attachment loss present on some teeth?
8. What etiologic factors for gingival and periodontal diseases are evident in Mr. Karn's dental radiographs?
9. On Mr. Karn's radiographs what specific findings indicate that he has alveolar bone loss present?
10. How would you characterize Mr. Karn's periodontal condition? Do you think that he has gingivitis, periodontitis, neither, or both? What clinical or radiographic findings did you use to reach your conclusion?
11. Develop a suggested step-by-step plan for nonsurgical periodontal therapy for Mr. Karn.
12. What information should your team give Mr. Karn about his periodontal condition?
13. What should Mr. Karn be told about the possible need for periodontal surgery later in the treatment?
14. What should Mr. Karn be told about the need for continuing treatment such as periodontal maintenance?

Fictitious Patient Case 2—Mr. Wilton

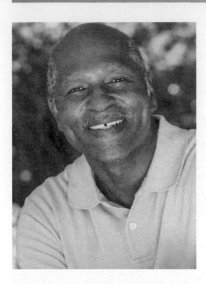

PATIENT PROFILE

Mr. Wilton is a 52-year-old manager of a local gardening store who has come to your dental office for an initial visit. During his patient interview, Mr. Wilton informs you that he made this appointment at his wife's insistence. He states that his wife wants to know if there is anything that can be done about his bad breath. Mr. Wilton informs you that he cannot seem to get his bad breath under control using mouth rinses.

PATIENT HEALTH HISTORY

- At the time of his initial visit, Mr. Wilton's blood pressure is 164/100 mm Hg and his pulse rate is 74 per minute.
- Mr. Wilton informs you that he is taking Amoxicillin prescribed by his physician for an ear infection.
- Mr. Wilton tells you that he had high blood pressure once and that he did take a prescribed medication a few years ago for that condition. He tells you that he was feeling just fine so he stopped taking the prescribed blood pressure medication.

Clinical Photographs for Mr. Wilton

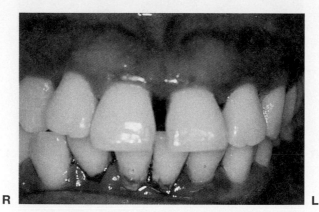

Figure 37-12. Anterior Teeth, Facial View.

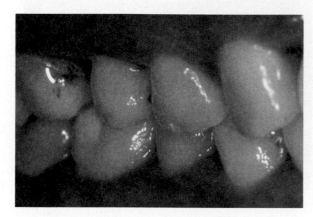

Figure 37-13. Right Side, Facial View.

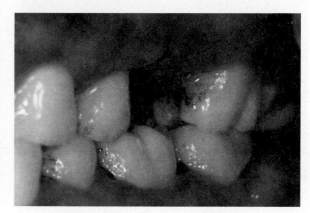

Figure 37-14. Left Side, Facial View.

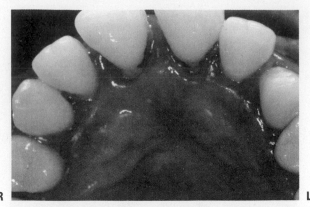

R   L

Figure 37-15. Maxillary Anteriors, Lingual View.

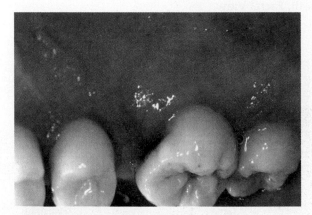

Figure 37-16. Maxillary Right, Lingual View.

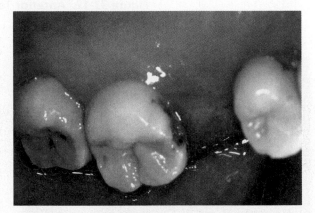

Figure 37-17. Maxillary Left, Lingual View.

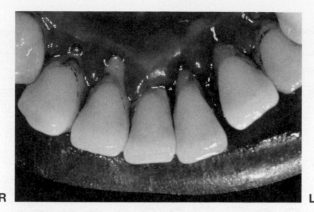

Figure 37-18. Mandibular Anteriors, Lingual View.

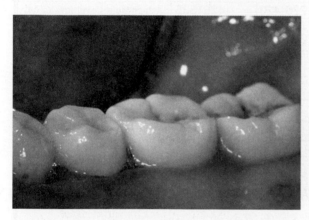

Figure 37-19. Mandibular Right, Lingual View.

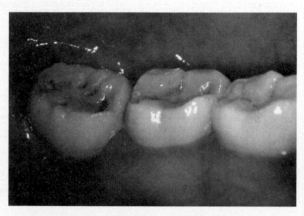

Figure 37-20. Mandibular Left, Lingual View.

CASE #2

Maxilla

	1	2	3	4	5	6	7	8	9	10	11	12	13	14	15	16
Mobility (I, II, III)				I			I	I	II	I		I				
Bleeding/Purulence (+)	+	+			+		+	+	+		+	+	+		+	+
Attachment Level (CEJ to BP)	635	634		338	535	537	626	736	537	625	536	725	524		435	535
Probing Depth (FGM to BP)	635	634		338	535	537	626	625	537	625	536	725	524		435	535

(Facial tooth diagrams; teeth 3 and 14 crossed/marked)

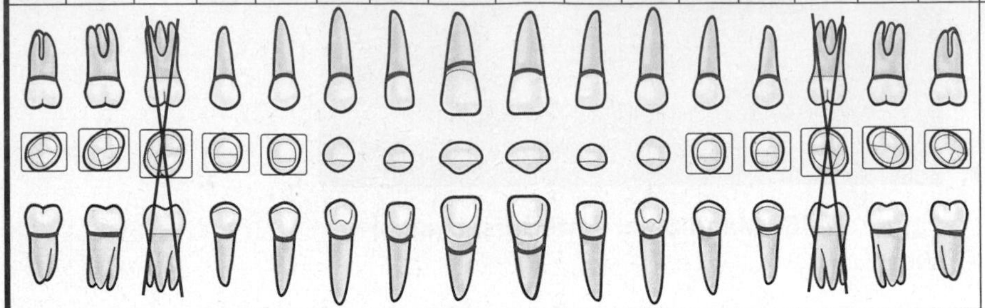

(Palatal tooth diagrams)

	1	2	3	4	5	6	7	8	9	10	11	12	13	14	15	16
Bleeding/Purulence (+)	+	+		+	+	+		+	+		+	+	+		+	
Attachment Level (CEJ to BP)	535	634		438	534	636	536	646	746	535	536	726	423		426	535
Probing Depth (FGM to BP)	535	634		438	534	636	536	535	635	535	536	726	534		426	535
Plaque (F/P)	••	••	✕	••	••	••	••	••	••	••	••	••	••	✕	••	••
Supragingival Calculus		✓				✓	✓	✓	✓	✓	✓		✓		✓	✓
Subgingival Calculus	✓	✓		✓	✓	✓	✓	✓	✓	✓	✓	✓	✓	✓	✓	✓
PSR Code		4					4						4			

Right — Left

Mandible

	32	31	30	29	28	27	26	25	24	23	22	21	20	19	18	17
Mobility (I, II, III)			I				II	II	II	II						
Bleeding/Purulence (+)		+	+	+		+	+	+	+	+	+	+	+		+	+
Attachment Level (CEJ to BP)		435	536	545	524	535	746	656	647	748	635	524	535	535	636	645
Probing Depth (FGM to BP)		535	536	545	524	535	635	545	536	637	635	524	535	635	636	635

(Lingual tooth diagrams; tooth 32 crossed/marked)

(Facial tooth diagrams)

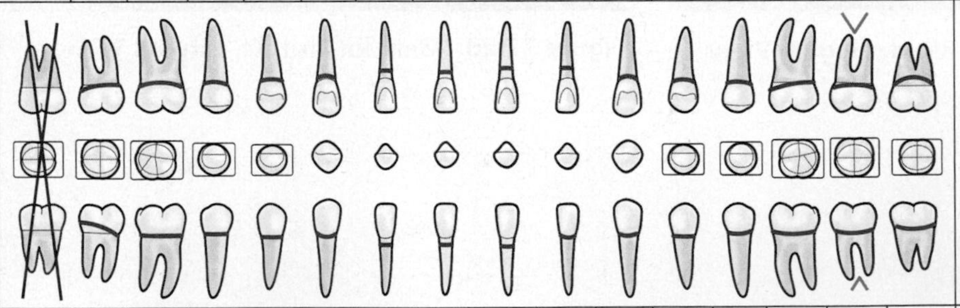

	32	31	30	29	28	27	26	25	24	23	22	21	20	19	18	17
Bleeding/Purulence (+)		+	+		+	+	+	+	+	+	+		+	+	+	+
Attachment Level (CEJ to BP)		435	526	535	424	535	735	646	636	536	524	525	425	525	526	625
Probing Depth (FGM to BP)		535	526	535	424	535	624	535	525	536	524	525	425	525	526	625
Plaque (L/F)	✕	••	••	••	••	••	••	••	••	••	••	✕	••	✕	••	••
Supragingival Calculus						✓	✓	✓	✓	✓	✓					✓
Subgingival Calculus		✓	✓	✓	✓	✓	✓	✓	✓	✓	✓	✓	✓	✓	✓	✓
PSR Code			4				4						4			

Figure 37-21. Mr. Wilton's Periodontal Chart.

Radiographic Series for Mr. Wilton

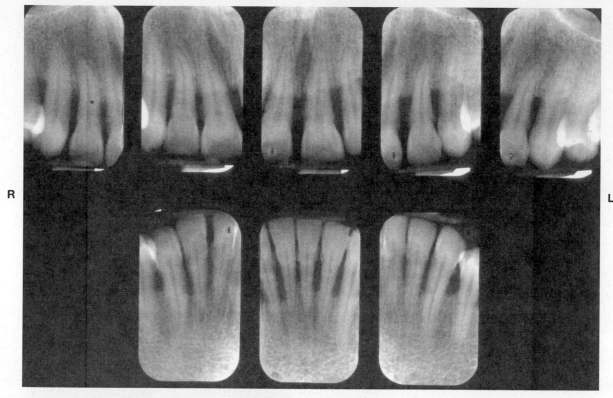

Figure 37-22A. Radiographs: Anterior Teeth.

R

L

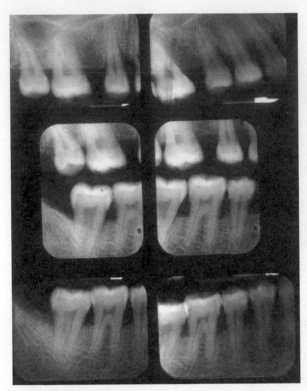

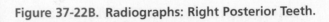

Figure 37-22B. Radiographs: Right Posterior Teeth.

Figure 37-22C. Radiographs: Left Posterior Teeth.

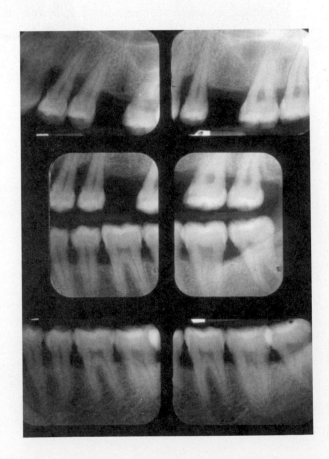

DECISION-MAKING QUESTIONS FOR CASE 2: MR. WILTON

1. What information should your team give Mr. Wilton regarding his wife's concern about his bad breath? Note that this was the complaint that prompted Mr. Wilton to make an appointment in your office.

2. What factors in Mr. Wilton's profile indicate that achieving an acceptable level of patient self-care may be a problem for the dental team?

3. What factors revealed in Mr. Wilton's health history will be critical for the dental team to consider during periodontal evaluation or treatment?

4. What signs of gingival inflammation are evident in Mr. Wilton's clinical photographs?

5. What etiologic risk factors for gingival and periodontal diseases are evident in Mr. Wilton's clinical photographs?

6. Does Mr. Wilton's periodontal evaluation indicate that he has attachment loss present on some teeth?

7. In response to your questions, Mr. Wilton informs you that the spaces between his front teeth were not there a few years ago. What do you think may be causing these spaces between his teeth to appear?

8. What etiologic factors for gingival and periodontal diseases are evident in Mr. Wilton's dental radiographs?

9. On Mr. Wilton's radiographs, what specific findings indicate that he has alveolar bone loss present?

10. How would you characterize Mr. Wilton's periodontal condition? Do you think that he has gingivitis, periodontitis, neither, or both? What clinical or radiographic findings did you use to reach your conclusion?

11. Write a suggested step-by-step plan for nonsurgical periodontal therapy for Mr. Wilton.

12. What information should your team give Mr. Wilton about his periodontal condition?

13. What should Mr. Wilton be told about the possible need for periodontal surgery later in the treatment?

14. What should Mr. Wilton be told about the need for continuing treatment such as periodontal maintenance?

15. What should your team tell Mr. Wilton if he refuses your team's recommendations for periodontal therapy?

Fictitious Patient Case 3—Ms. Sandsky

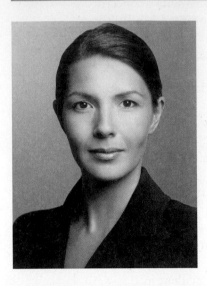

PATIENT PROFILE

Ms. Sandsky is a 42-year-old department store manager who has come to your dental office to get her dental condition in order. She states that she has neglected her dental care because she has been taking care of the dental needs of her children for many years, but now she is ready to take care of herself.

She informs your dental team that some years ago she was told that she had a gum disease, but elected not to receive any care for that condition at the time. She states that she brushes and flosses daily now in hopes that these actions can help her keep her teeth.

PATIENT HEALTH HISTORY

- At the time of Ms. Sandsky's initial dental visit, her blood pressure measures 130/83 mm Hg and her pulse is 75 beats/min.
- She explains that she has problems with gastroesophageal reflux disease and elevated cholesterol level.
- She reports that currently she is taking Omeprazole and Simvastatin prescribed by her physician and that she is also taking multivitamin tablets because she thinks she needs them.
- Ms. Sandsky informs you that she smoked 1 pack of cigarettes daily for about 8 years when she was younger, but that she quit smoking 10 years ago and has not smoked since that time.

Clinical Photographs for Ms. Sandsky

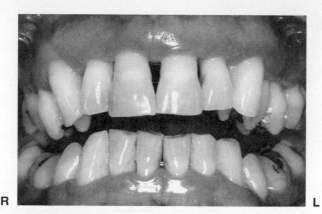

R   L

Figure 37-23. Anterior Teeth, Facial View..

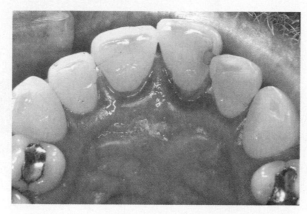

Figure 37-24. Maxillary Anterior Teeth, Lingual View.

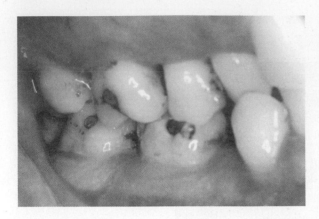

Figure 37-25. Right Side, Facial View.

Figure 37-26. Left Side, Facial View.

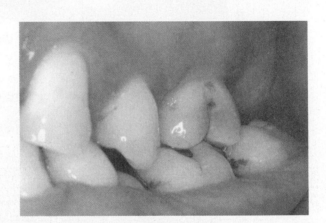

CASE #3

	1	2	3	4	5	6	7	8	9	10	11	12	13	14	15	16	Maxilla
Mobility (I, II, III)								I	I			I					
Bleeding/Purulence (+)		+	+	+	+		+	+	+		+	+		+			
Attachment Level (CEJ to BP)		646	544	535	545	646	656	656	656	756	655	646		545			
Probing Depth (FGM to BP)		646	545	535	545	535	545	545	545	645	545	635		545			

Facial / Palatal (tooth diagrams)

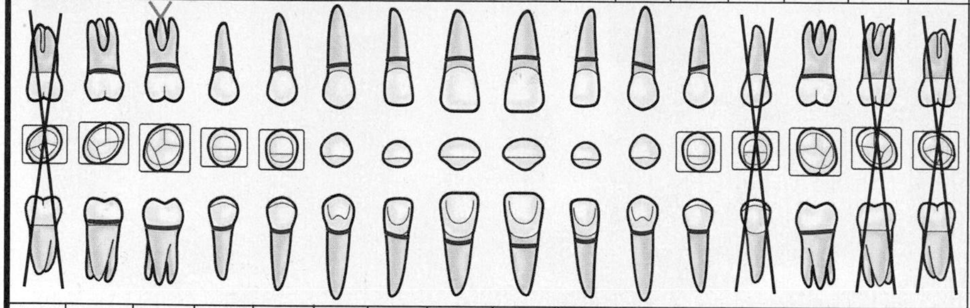

	1	2	3	4	5	6	7	8	9	10	11	12	13	14	15	16	
Bleeding/Purulence (+)		+	+	+	+	+	+	+	+	+	+	+		+			
Attachment Level (CEJ to BP)		645	545	543	545	545	645	656	656	666	545	535		545			
Probing Depth (FGM to BP)		645	545	545	545	545	645	545	545	555	545	535		545			
^F_P Plaque																	
Supragingival Calculus		✓	✓	✓	✓		✓			✓	✓			✓			
Subgingival Calculus		✓	✓	✓	✓	✓	✓	✓	✓		✓	✓		✓			
PSR Code																	

Right .... *Left*

	32	31	30	29	28	27	26	25	24	23	22	21	20	19	18	17	Mandible
Mobility (I, II, III)																	
Bleeding/Purulence (+)		+	+	+	+	+	+	+	+	+	+	+	+	+	+		
Attachment Level (CEJ to BP)		455	545		545	545	544	444	544	545	543	543	434	545	545		
Probing Depth (FGM to BP)		455	545		545	545	544	444	544	545	545	434	434	545	545		

Lingual / Facial (tooth diagrams)

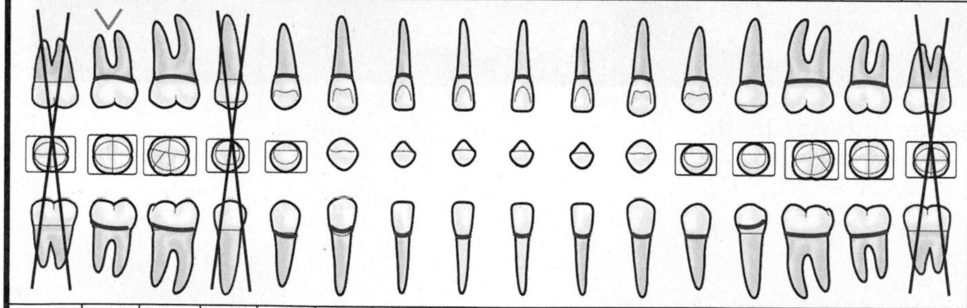

	32	31	30	29	28	27	26	25	24	23	22	21	20	19	18	17	
Bleeding/Purulence (+)												I					
Attachment Level (CEJ to BP)		355	545		545	544	444	444	445	545	545	535	525	545	545		
Probing Depth (FGM to BP)		455	545		544	544	444	444	445	545	545	535	646	545	545		
^L_F Plaque																	
Supragingival Calculus		✓	✓		✓	✓	✓	✓	✓	✓	✓	✓	✓	✓	✓		
Subgingival Calculus		✓	✓		✓	✓	✓	✓	✓	✓	✓	✓	✓	✓	✓		
PSR Code																	

Figure 37-27. Ms. Sandsky's Periodontal Chart.

Radiographic Series for Ms. Sandsky

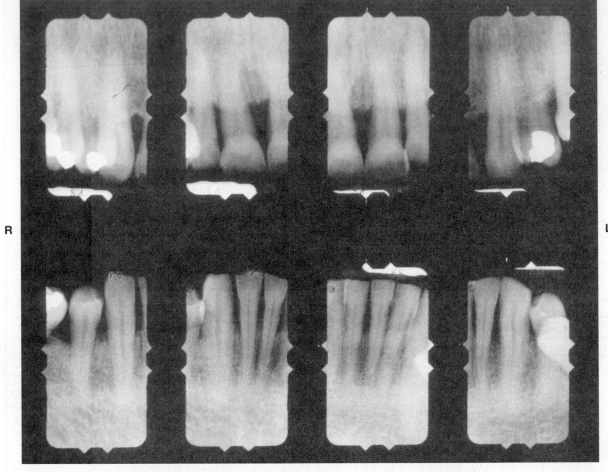

R

L

Figure 37-28A. Radiographs: Anterior Teeth.

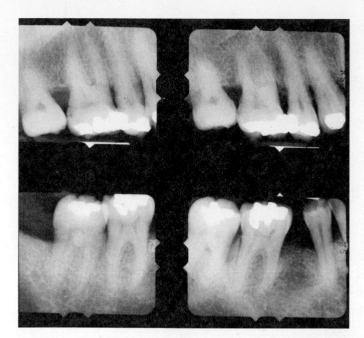

Figure 37-28B. Radiographs: Right Posterior Teeth.

Figure 37-28C. Radiographs: Left Posterior Teeth.

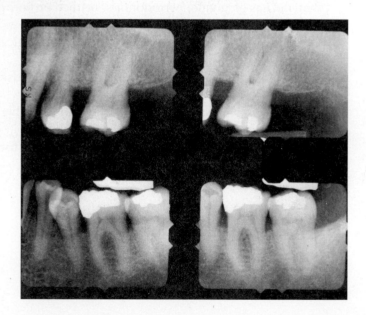

DECISION-MAKING QUESTIONS FOR CASE 3: MS. SANDSKY

1. What factors in Ms. Sandsky's profile indicate that achieving an acceptable level of patient self-care may *not* be as difficult for her as it is for many patients?
2. Will the medications being taken by Ms. Sandsky require any special precautions during treatment by the members of the dental team?
3. How might the history of smoking relate to Ms. Sandsky's past and current risk for periodontal disease?
4. What signs of gingival inflammation are evident in Ms. Sandsky's clinical photographs?
5. What etiologic risk factors for gingival and periodontal diseases are evident in Ms. Sandsky's clinical photographs?
6. Does Ms. Sandsky's periodontal evaluation indicate that she has attachment loss present on some teeth?
7. In response to your questions, Ms. Sandsky informs you that the open triangular space between her upper front teeth was not there a few years ago. What do you think may be causing this space between her teeth to appear?
8. What etiologic factors for gingival and periodontal diseases are evident in Ms. Sandsky's dental radiographs?
9. How would you characterize Ms. Sandsky's periodontal condition? Do you think that she has gingivitis, periodontitis, neither, or both? What clinical or radiographic findings did you use to reach your conclusion?
10. Develop a suggested step-by-step plan for nonsurgical periodontal therapy for Ms. Sandsky.
11. What information should your team give Ms. Sandsky about her periodontal condition?
12. What should Ms. Sandsky be told about the possible need for periodontal surgery later in the treatment?
13. What should Ms. Sandsky be told about the need for continuing treatment such as periodontal maintenance?

Fictitious Patient Case 4—Mr. Verosky

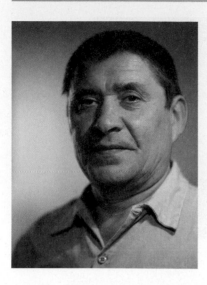

PATIENT PROFILE

Mr. Verosky is a 62-year-old recently elected to a local city council. He has become very interested in getting his oral health up to par following his election.

During his initial visit, Mr. Verosky explains that he has always had spaces between his front teeth and is not really worried about that. He tells you that his major concern is that he has been told he has periodontal disease, and he does not want to lose his teeth.

PATIENT HEALTH HISTORY

- On the day of his first visit to your dental office Mr. Verosky's blood pressure is 142/90 mm Hg and his pulse is 66 beats/min.
- Review of Mr. Verosky's health history reveals that he is supposed to be taking two medications: losartan/hydrochlorothiazide tablets and low-dose aspirin, but he readily admits that he frequently "forgets" to take his medications.
- Mr. Verosky also states that he smoked cigarettes prior to the age 40, but that he quit smoking during his early 40s.

Clinical Photographs for Mr. Verosky

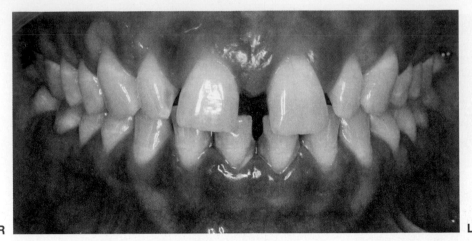

Figure 37-29. Anterior Teeth, Facial View.

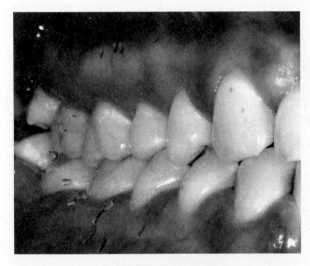

Figure 37-30. Right Side, Facial View.

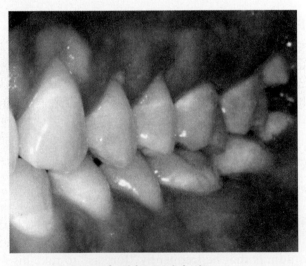

Figure 37-31. Left Side, Facial View.

Clinical Photographs for Mr. Verosky

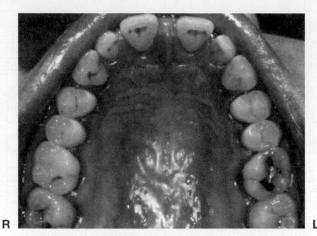

R   L

Figure 37-32. Maxillary Arch, Lingual View.

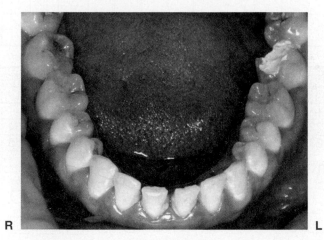

R   L

Figure 37-33. Mandibular Arch.

CASE #4

1	2	3	4	5	6	7	8	9	10	11	12	13	14	15	16	**Maxilla**
	I												I			Mobility (I, II, III)
+	+	+	+	+	+	+	+	+	+	+	+	+	+	+	+	Bleeding/Purulence (+)
336	867	646	241	342	151	242	111	111	233	232	234	313	425	447	544	Attachment Level (CEJ to BP)
558	756	535	322	423	222	323	313	313	324	323	325	424	425	446	655	Probing Depth (FGM to BP)

Facial

Palatal

+	+	+	+	+	+	+	+	+	+	+	+	+	+	+	+	Bleeding/Purulence (+)
233	665	676	212	222	444	222	223	323	222	222	223	312	555	558	410	Attachment Level (CEJ to BP)
555	654	545	323	333	555	333	334	434	333	333	334	423	424	437	633	Probing Depth (FGM to BP)
																ᶠ/ₚPlaque
✓	✓	✓											✓	✓	✓	Supragingival Calculus
✓	✓	✓	✓	✓					✓		✓	✓	✓	✓	✓	Subgingival Calculus
			4					3					4			PSR Code

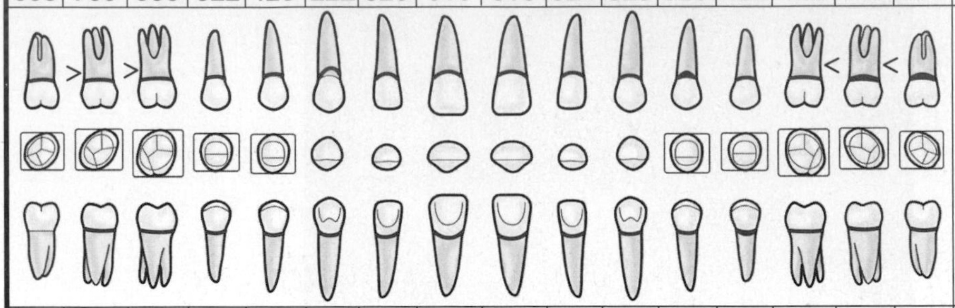

Right   *Left*

32	31	30	29	28	27	26	25	24	23	22	21	20	19	18	17	**Mandible**
I															I	Mobility (I, II, III)
+	+	+	+	+	+	+	+	+	+	+	+	+	+	+	+	Bleeding/Purulence (+)
336	444	433	333	222	222	222	221	122	331	121	232	244	443	534	434	Attachment Level (CEJ to BP)
547	555	544	434	323	323	323	322	223	422	222	333	345	544	545	655	Probing Depth (FGM to BP)

Lingual

Facial

+	+	+	+	+	+	+	+	+	+	+	+	+	+	+	+	Bleeding/Purulence (+)
344	444	432	222	222	222	232	222	232	222	222	232	232	233	435	423	Attachment Level (CEJ to BP)
555	525	523	323	323	323	333	323	333	323	323	323	323	324	526	533	Probing Depth (FGM to BP)
																ᴸ/ꜰPlaque
					✓	✓	✓	✓	✓	✓						Supragingival Calculus
✓	✓	✓	✓		✓	✓	✓	✓	✓	✓	✓		✓	✓	✓	Subgingival Calculus
			3					3					4			PSR Code

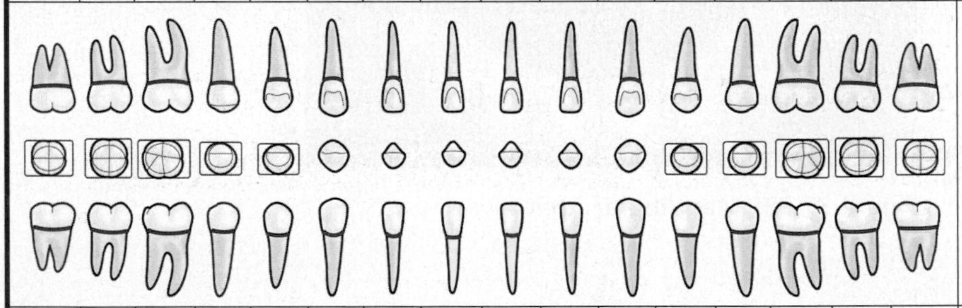

Figure 37-34. Mr. Verosky's Periodontal Chart.

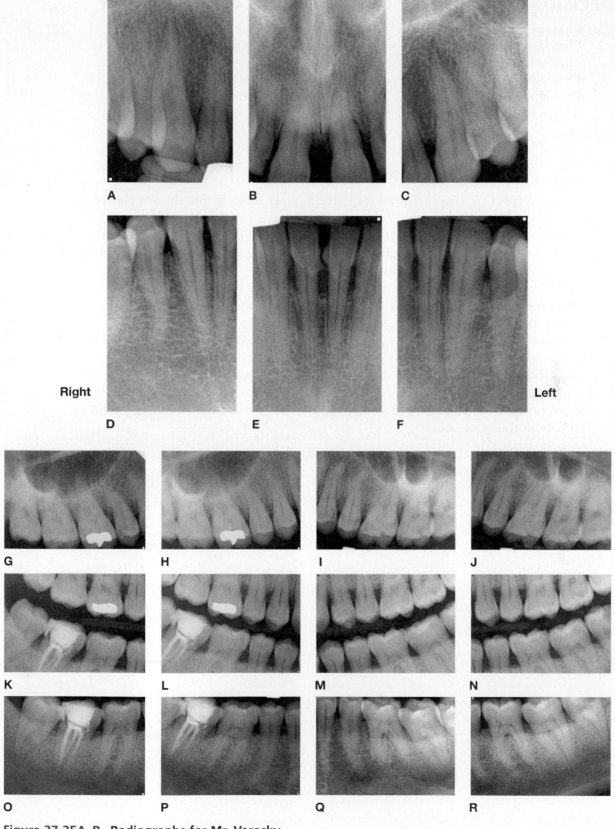

Right   Left

Figure 37-35A–R. Radiographs for Mr. Verosky.

DECISION-MAKING QUESTIONS FOR CASE 4: MR. VEROSKY

1. What should Mr. Verosky be told about the spaces between his anterior teeth?
2. What factors in Mr. Verosky's health history will be critical for the dental team to consider during treatment?
3. What signs of inflammation are evident on Mr. Verosky's clinical photographs?
4. What etiologic risk factors for gingival and periodontal diseases are evident on Mr. Verosky's clinical evaluation?
5. Does Mr. Verosky's periodontal evaluation indicate that he has attachment loss on some of his teeth? How did you arrive at your conclusion?
6. What etiologic risk factors for gingival and periodontal diseases are evident from Mr. Verosky's radiographs?
7. On Mr. Verosky's radiographs, what specific findings indicate that the alveolar bone level is normal or abnormal?
8. How should you characterize Mr. Verosky's periodontal condition? Do you think that he has gingivitis, periodontitis, neither, or both? What clinical or radiographic findings did you use to reach your conclusion?
9. Develop a step-by-step plan for nonsurgical periodontal therapy for Mr. Verosky.
10. What information should your team give Mr. Verosky about his periodontal condition?
11. What should Mr. Verosky be told about the possible need for periodontal surgery later in his treatment?
12. What should Mr. Verosky be told about the need for continuing treatment such as periodontal maintenance?
13. Mr. Verosky has a temporary restoration in a lower molar tooth. What should he be told about this restoration?

Fictitious Patient Case 5—Mr. Tomlinson

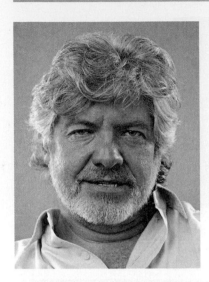

PATIENT PROFILE

Mr. Tomlinson is a 48-year-old patient who is new to your dental office. He works as a computer technician in a large local firm. This is his first job following an extended tour of military duty.

During his initial visit, Mr. Tomlinson explains that he has no dental problems, but he decided to make an appointment for a "cleaning" since he has a new dental insurance plan. He tells you that everyone in his family has always had pretty good teeth, so he is certain that you will not find anything wrong with his teeth or with his old fillings.

PATIENT HEALTH HISTORY

- On the day of his first visit to your dental office, Mr. Tomlinson's blood pressure is 132/82 mm Hg and his pulse is 64 beats/min.
- Review of Mr. Tomlinson's health history reveals that he is taking two medications: atorvastatin tablets and fluticasone propionate nasal spray.
- He states that he is currently under treatment for post-traumatic stress disorder (PTSD) that has resulted from his multiple military deployments.

Clinical Photographs for Mr. Tomlinson

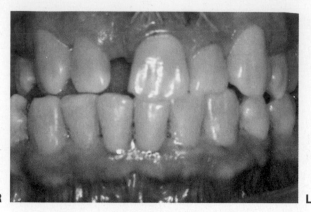

Figure 37-36. Anterior Teeth, Facial View.

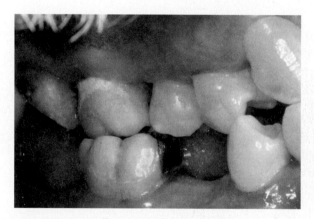

Figure 37-37. Right Side, Facial View.

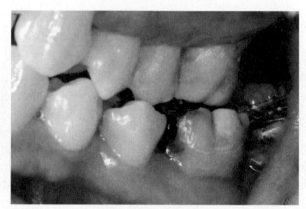

Figure 37-38. Left Side, Facial View.

Clinical Photographs for Mr. Tomlinson

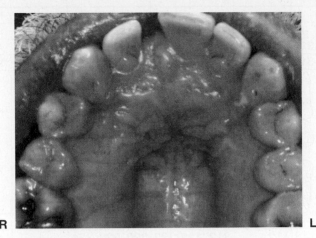

Figure 37-39. Maxillary Arch, Lingual View.

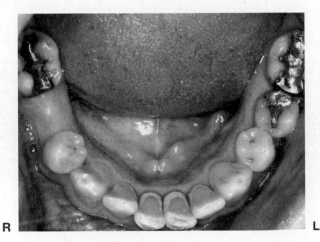

Figure 37-40. Mandibular Arch.

CASE #5

Maxilla

Measurement	1	2	3	4	5	6	7	8	9	10	11	12	13	14	15	16
Mobility (I, II, III)														I		
Bleeding/Purulence (+)		+	+	+	+	+	+				+	+	+	+		
Attachment Level (CEJ to BP)		546	745	323	312	312	311		112	213	213	424	447	747		
Probing Depth (FGM to BP)		324	523	323	312	312	311		112	213	213	424	447	747		

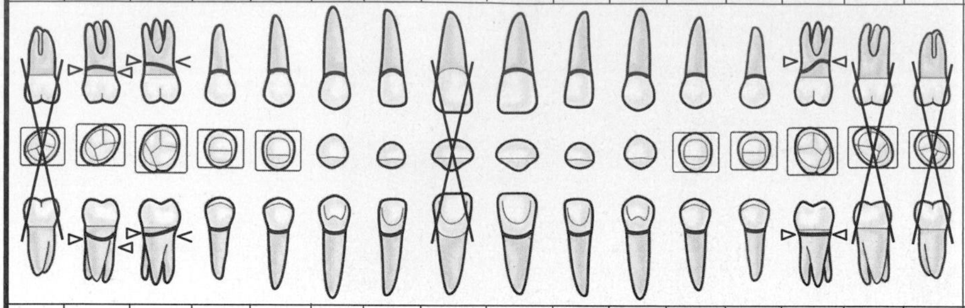

Facial / *Palatal*

Measurement	1	2	3	4	5	6	7	8	9	10	11	12	13	14	15	16
Bleeding/Purulence (+)		+		+	+	+	+			+	+	+	+	+		
Attachment Level (CEJ to BP)		766	654	223	321	113	112		312	122	322	222	222	334		
Probing Depth (FGM to BP)		513	423	223	321	113	112		312	122	322	222	222	223		
^F_P Plaque	✕	✕	✕	✕	✕	✕	✕	✕	✕	✕	✕	✕	✕	✕	✕	✕
Supragingival Calculus		✓	✓	✓	✓	✓	✓							✓		
Subgingival Calculus		✓	✓	✓	✓	✓	✓				✓	✓	✓	✓		
PSR Code		4						2				4				

Right | *Left*

Mandible

Measurement	32	31	30	29	28	27	26	25	24	23	22	21	20	19	18	17
Mobility (I, II, III)																
Bleeding/Purulence (+)			+		+	+	+	+	+	+	+	+	+	+		+
Attachment Level (CEJ to BP)			645		323	323	323	222	223	323	444	323	323	536		556
Probing Depth (FGM to BP)			423		323	323	323	222	223	323	333	323	323	424		334

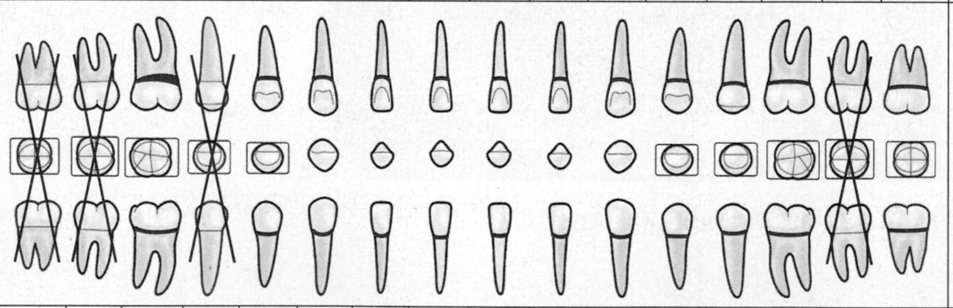

Lingual / *Facial*

Measurement	32	31	30	29	28	27	26	25	24	23	22	21	20	19	18	17
Bleeding/Purulence (+)			+			+	+	+		+	+	+	+	+		+
Attachment Level (CEJ to BP)			545		434	423	334	424	224	223	223	212	124	755		334
Probing Depth (FGM to BP)			323		324	423	334	424	224	223	223	212	113	533		223
^L_F Plaque	✕	✕	✕	✕	✕	✕	✕	✕	✕	✕	✕	✕	✕	✕	✕	✕
Supragingival Calculus					✓	✓	✓	✓	✓					✓		✓
Subgingival Calculus			✓		✓	✓	✓	✓	✓	✓	✓	✓	✓	✓		✓
PSR Code			4				3					4				

Figure 37-41. Mr. Tomlinson's Periodontal Chart.

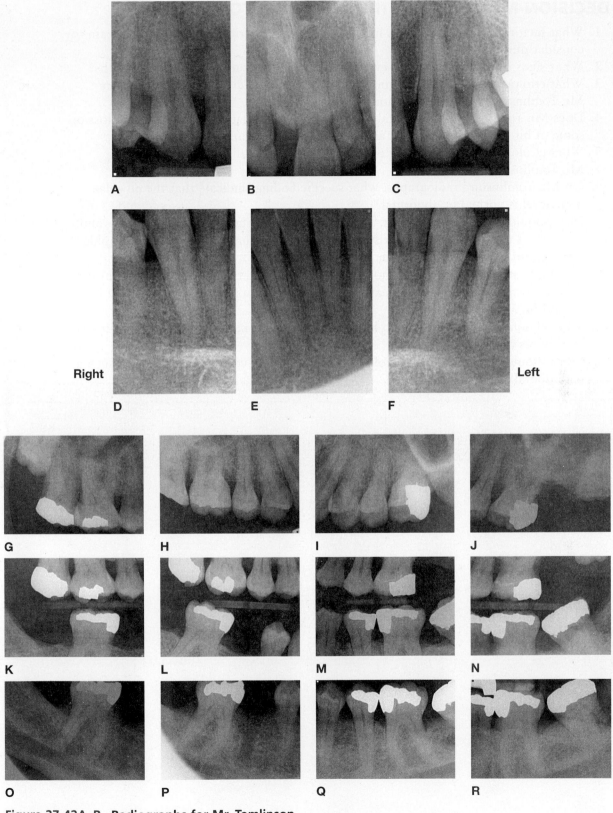

Figure 37-42A–R. Radiographs for Mr. Tomlinson.

DECISION-MAKING QUESTIONS FOR MR. TOMLINSON

1. What factors in Mr. Tomlinson's health history will be critical for the dental team to consider during treatment?

2. What signs of inflammation are evident on Mr. Tomlinson's clinical photographs?

3. What etiologic risk factors for gingival and periodontal diseases are evident from Mr. Tomlinson's clinical evaluation?

4. Does Mr. Tomlinson's periodontal evaluation indicate that he has attachment loss on some of his teeth? How did you arrive at your conclusion?

5. What etiologic risk factors for gingival and periodontal diseases are evident Mr. Tomlinson's radiographs?

6. On Mr. Tomlinson's radiographs, what specific findings indicate that the alveolar bone level is normal or abnormal?

7. How should you characterize Mr. Tomlinson's periodontal condition? Do you think that he has gingivitis, periodontitis, neither, or both? What clinical or radiographic findings did you use to reach your conclusion?

8. Develop a step-by-step plan for nonsurgical periodontal therapy for Mr. Tomlinson.

9. What information should your team give Mr. Tomlinson about his periodontal condition?

10. What should Mr. Tomlinson be told about the possible need for periodontal surgery later in his treatment?

11. What should Mr. Tomlinson be told about the need for continuing treatment such as periodontal maintenance?

Glossary

Aggregatibacter actinomycetemcomitans: an important periodontal pathogen.

Abscess of the periodontium: an acute infection involving a circumscribed collection of pus in the periodontium. Also see gingival abscess, periodontal abscess, pericoronal abscess.

Absorbable suture: a suture made from a material designed to dissolve harmlessly in body fluids over time; though absorbable sutures do not normally require removal by the dental team, some absorbable sutures do not dissolve well and thus may require removal by a dental provider 1 to 2 weeks following the surgery. Also see nonabsorbable suture.

Abutment: a component of a dental implant; the titanium post that attaches to the implant body and protrudes partially or completely through the gingival tissue into the mouth.

Abutment: see implant abutment.

Acquired immunodeficiency syndrome (AIDS): a communicable disease caused by human immunodeficiency virus (HIV). People with acquired immunodeficiency syndrome are at an increased risk for developing certain cancers and for infections that usually occur only in individuals with a weak immune system.

Acquired pellicle: a film composed of a variety of salivary glycoproteins and antibodies that forms within minutes after cleaning a tooth surface; its purpose is to protect the enamel from acidic activity.

Active disease site: an area of tissue destruction that shows continued apical migration of the junctional epithelium over time.

Acute gingivitis: gingivitis of a short duration, after which professional care and patient self-care returns the gingiva to a healthy state. Also see gingivitis and chronic gingivitis.

Acute inflammation: is a short-term, normal inflammatory response that protects and heals the body following physical injury or infection. Also see inflammation and chronic inflammation.

Acute periodontal conditions: periodontal conditions that are commonly characterized by a rapid onset and rapid course, that are frequently accompanied by pain and discomfort, and that may be unrelated to the presence of pre-existing gingivitis or periodontitis. One example is an abscess of the periodontium.

Aerobic bacteria: bacteria that require oxygen to live. Also see facultative bacteria and anaerobic bacteria.

AIDS: see acquired immunodeficiency syndrome.

Allografts: bone replacement grafts taken from individuals that are genetically dissimilar to the donor (i.e., another human donor); these grafting materials must be modified to eliminate the potential for rejection. Also see autographs, xenografts, and alloplasts.

Alloplasts: bone replacement grafts that are synthetic materials or inert foreign materials. Also see autografts, allografts, and xenografts.

Alveolar bone: the bone that surrounds the roots of the teeth. It forms the bony sockets that support and protect the roots of the teeth.

Alveolar bone loss: is the resorption of alveolar bone as a result of periodontitis. Also see horizontal bone loss and vertical bone loss.

Alveolar bone proper: the thin layer of bone that lines the socket to surround the root of the tooth (also called the cribriform plate); the ends of the periodontal ligament fibers are embedded in the alveolar bone proper.

Alveolar crest: the most coronal portion of the alveolar process. In health, the alveolar crest is located 1 to 2 mm apical to (below) the cementoenamel junctions (CEJs) of the teeth.

Alveolar mucosa: the apical boundary, or lower edge, of the gingiva; it can be distinguished easily from the gingiva by its dark red color and smooth, shiny surface.

Alveolar process: the bone of the upper or lower jaw that surrounds and supports the roots of the teeth.

Alveolus: the bony socket; a cavity in the alveolar bone that houses the root of a tooth.

Ambivalence: having mixed feelings and attitudes about something, such as a behavior change.

American Academy of Periodontology (AAP): an association of dental professionals specializing in the prevention, diagnosis, and treatment of diseases affecting the periodontium.

Anaerobic bacteria: bacteria that cannot live in the presence of oxygen. Also see aerobic bacteria and facultative bacteria.

Anastomose: to join together; in the periodontium a complex system of blood vessels supply blood to the periodontal tissues.

Antibiotics: medications used to help fight infections either because they kill bacteria or because they can inhibit the growth of bacteria. Also see antibiotic resistance.

Antibiotic resistance: the ability of a bacterium to withstand the effects of an antibiotic by developing mechanisms to protect the bacterium from the killing or inhibiting effects of the antibiotic.

Antibodies: Y-shaped proteins; one end of the Y binds to the outside of the B cell and the other end binds to a microorganism and helps to kill it. Antibodies are known collectively as immunoglobulins.

Anti-inflammatory biochemical mediators: biologically active compounds secreted by immune cells that are protective and keep the bacterial infection from doing serious harm to the periodontium, such as the cytokines IL-4 (interleukin-4) and IL-10 (interleukin-10).

Antioxidants: substances that occur naturally in the body and in certain foods; antioxidants can inhibit oxidation and thereby block damage to cells by free radicals.

Apical migration: the movement of the cells of the junctional epithelium from their normal position to a position apical to the CEJ.

Apical migration of the junctional epithelium: the movement of the junctional epithelium apical to its normal location.

Apically positioned flap with osseous resective surgery: a periodontal surgical procedure involving a combination of a displaced flap (displaced in an apical direction) plus resective osseous surgery; this procedure is ideal for minimizing periodontal pocket depths in patients with osseous craters caused by moderate periodontitis. Also see displaced flap.

Ascorbic acid-deficiency gingivitis: an inflammatory response of the gingiva caused by dental plaque that is aggravated by chronically low vitamin C (ascorbic acid) levels; manifests clinically as bright red, swollen, ulcerated gingival tissue that bleeds with the slightest provocation.

"Ask. Advise. Refer.": the American Dental Hygiene Association's national Smoking Cessation Initiative designed to promote smoking cessation intervention by dental hygienists.

Association: a relationship between two or more variables. Association does not imply a causal relationship between two different variables and is therefore not synonymous with causation. See causation.

Atherosclerosis: a process characterized by a thickening of artery walls.

Attached gingiva: the part of the gingiva that is firm, dense, and tightly connected to the cementum on the cervical-third of the root or to the periosteum (connective tissue cover) of the alveolar bone.

Attachment loss: the destruction of the tooth supporting structures have been destroyed around a tooth; characterized by: relocation of the junctional epithelium to the tooth root, destruction of the fibers of the gingiva, destruction of the periodontal ligament fibers, and loss of alveolar bone support from around the tooth. Also see clinical attachment loss.

Autografts: bone replacement materials taken from the patient that is receiving the graft; periodontal autografts can be taken from sites in the patient's own jaws or occasionally from other areas of the patient's body. Also see allografts, xenografts, and alloplasts.

Autonomy: freedom to determine one's own actions, behaviors, etc.; placing responsibility for behavior change or treatment decisions with the patient.

Bacteria: the simplest organisms and can be seen only through a microscope. Also see innocuous and pathogenic.

Bacterial blooms: periods when specific species or groups of species grow at rapidly accelerated rates with a dental plaque biofilm.

Bacterial enzymes: agents that are harmful or destructive to host cells; a variety of enzymes produced by periodontal pathogens are important in tissue destruction.

Basal lamina: a thin, tough sheet that separates the epithelial cells from the underlying connective tissue. Also see external basal lamina and internal basal lamina.

Baseline data: clinical data gathered at the beginning of the periodontal treatment that is subsequently used for comparison to clinical information gathered at subsequent appointments.

B-cells: see B-lymphocytes.

Best evidence: the highest level of evidence available for a specific clinical question. Also see best practices and levels of evidence.

Best practices: are clinical practices, treatments, and interventions that result in the best possible outcome for the patient. Also see best evidence and levels of evidence.

Biochemical mediators: biologically active compounds secreted by immune cells that activate the body's inflammatory response; inflammatory mediators of importance in periodontitis are the cytokines, prostaglandins, and matrix metalloproteinases. Also see anti-inflammatory biochemical mediators and pro-inflammatory biochemical mediators.

Biocompatible: a non-biologic material that is not rejected by the body. Titanium is a biocompatible metal that allows tissue healing around an implant abutment.

Biofilm: a well-organized community of bacteria that adheres to a surface and is embedded in an extracellular slime layer; forms rapidly on almost any surface that is wet. See extracellular slime layer and fluid channels.

Biologic equilibrium: a state of balance in the internal environment of the body.

Biologic seal: the union of the epithelial cells to the surface of a dental implant.

Biologic width (also known as supracrestal tissue attachment): the space on the tooth surface occupied by the junctional epithelium and the connective tissue attachment fibers immediately apical to (below) the junctional epithelium.

Biomechanical forces: the biologic and mechanical forces placed on an osseointegrated dental implant; controlling these forces is vital to achieve long-term success with implants.

Bisphosphonates: drugs that can inhibit the resorption of bone by altering osteoclastic activity. One of the possible side effects of these drugs is osteonecrosis of the jaws following their extended use. Also see osteonecrosis of the jaw, bleeding on gentle probing, tooth mobility, or loss of alveolar bone support.

Blunt dissection: elevation of a flap during periodontal surgery using tools that are not sharpened on the edge (i.e., blunted or slightly rounded); blunt dissection minimizes the chance of accidental damage to the flap. In this type of flap elevation the flap is lifted or pried up using surgical tools called periosteal elevators, and it is elevated in a manner quite similar to lifting the peeling off an orange. Also see sharp dissection.

Blunted papilla: a papilla is flat and does not fill the interproximal space.

B-lymphocytes: small leukocytes that help in the defense against bacteria, viruses, and fungi; principal function is to make antibodies. B-lymphocytes can further differentiate into one of the two types of cells: plasma B-cells and memory B-cells.

Bone morphogenetic proteins (BMP): a group of regulatory glycoproteins that have been studied for possible use in the field of periodontal regeneration.

Bone remodeling: throughout its lifetime, bone will undergo continuous turnover of the bone matrix that first involves bone resorption followed by bone formation.

Bone replacement graft: a periodontal surgical procedure used to encourage the body to rebuild alveolar bone that has been lost usually as a result of periodontal disease.

Bruxism: the forceful grinding of the teeth.

Bulbous papilla: an enlarged papilla that appears to bulge out of the interproximal space.

Calcium channel blocker: a class of drugs that block the influx of calcium ions through cardiac and vascular smooth muscle cell membranes resulting in the dilation of the main coronary and systemic arteries. Also see cyclosporine.

CAMBRA (Caries Management by Risk Assessment): protocols that seek to provide practical clinical guidelines for managing dental caries based upon risk group assessment. The protocols are based upon the best evidence at this time and can be used in planning effective caries management for any patient.

Cancellous bone: the lattice-like bone that fills the interior portion of the alveolar process between the cortical bone and the alveolar bone proper; cancellous bone is oriented around the tooth to form support for the alveolar bone proper.

Caries Management by Risk Assessment: see CAMBRA.

Catabasis: a highly regulated process that occurs following removal of microbial challenge and leads to resolution of inflammation and a return to homeostasis.

Causation: one variable directly causes changes in another variable.

Cell junctions: cellular structures that mechanically attach a cell and its cytoskeleton to its neighboring cells or to the basal lamina. Also see desmosome and hemidesmosome.

Cells: the smallest structural unit of living matter capable of functioning independently: cells group together to form a tissue.

Cementum: a mineralized layer of connective tissue that covers the root of the tooth; anatomically, cementum is part of the tooth, however it also part of the periodontium.

Cervical enamel projection (CEP): an apical extension of the coronal enamel beyond the CEJ that is projected toward the furcation entrance. A localized furcation invasion may be attributed to the presence of a CEP.

Change talk: encouraging the expression of statements in the direction of change; evoking, facilitating, and strengthening a patient's desire for change. Change talk can be elicited with simple open-ended questions such as "What advantages do you see of cutting back on sugary foods?"

Chemokines: a major subgroup of cytokines that cause additional immune cells to be attracted to the site of infection or injury. Also see cytokines.

Chemotaxis: the process whereby leukocytes are attracted to an infection site in response to biochemical compounds released by invading microorganisms.

Chronic gingivitis: long-lasting gingivitis; gingivitis may exist for years without ever progressing to periodontitis. Also see gingivitis and acute gingivitis.

Chronic inflammation: is a long-lived, out-of-control inflammatory response that continues for more than a few weeks; it is a pathologic condition characterized by active inflammation, tissue destruction, and attempts at repair. Also see inflammation and acute inflammation.

Circumscribed: localized or confined to a specific site.

Clenching: the continuous or intermittent forceful closure of the maxillary teeth against the mandibular teeth.

Clinical attachment level (CAL): an estimate of the true periodontal support around the tooth as measured with a periodontal probe. This measurement is only an estimation of the actual histologic level of attachment still present. It is a means of estimating the level of the junctional epithelium.

Clinical attachment loss: an estimate of the extent that the tooth supporting structures have been destroyed around a tooth. Also see attachment loss.

Clinical periodontal assessment: a fact-gathering process designed to provide a comprehensive picture of the patient's periodontal health status. Also see comprehensive periodontal assessment and periodontal screening examination.

Coaggregation: the cell-to-cell adherence of one oral bacterium to another; the ability to adhere and coaggregate is an important determinant in the development of oral bacterial biofilms.

Cochrane Database of Systematic Reviews: a database of systematic reviews of health care interventions.

Collaborate: to work together, such as a patient and health care provider working together to obtain the best possible health for the patient.

Collagen fibers: protein fibers that form a dense network of strong, rope-like cables that secure and hold the gingival connective tissues together.

Co-management: the shared responsibility of the care of patient between two different providers. A common example of co-management is a patient who alternates his/her periodontal maintenance visits between a periodontist and a general practitioner.

Commensal microorganisms: the indigenous, resident bacteria of the healthy mouth. They are considered to be part of the normal, healthy oral microflora and do not cause disease.

Communicable: a disease that may be passed from one person to another by direct or indirect contact via substances such as inanimate objects; there is little or no evidence that periodontal infections are communicable.

Complement System: a complex series of proteins circulating in the blood that works to facilitate phagocytosis or kill bacteria directly by puncturing bacterial cell membranes.

Complexity of Management: accounts for factors that help to define the level of clinical competence and experience a periodontitis case is likely to require for optimal outcomes.

Compliance: the extent to which a person's behavior coincides with health advice. Examples of compliant patients would be a patient who faithfully takes antihypertensive medications as prescribed by a physician or a patient who cooperates in meeting regularly scheduled periodontal maintenance appointments as recommended by the dental team. Also see noncompliant patients.

Comprehensive periodontal assessment: an intensive evaluation used to gather information about the periodontium; normally includes clinical features such as probing depth measurements, bleeding on probing, presence of exudate, level of the free gingival margin and the mucogingival junction, tooth mobility, furcation involvement, presence of calculus and bacterial plaque, gingival inflammation, radiographic evidence of alveolar bone loss, and presence of local contributing factors.

Concavity: a trench-like depression in the root surface; commonly occur on the proximal surfaces of anterior and posterior teeth and the facial and lingual surfaces of molar teeth.

Computed tomography (CT): an emerging imaging technique that emits cone-shaped x-ray beams which are then recaptured by the scanning machine to reconstruct a 3-dimensional image of the patient's anatomy.

Confirmation bias: a human tendency to look for or interpret information that confirms our beliefs.

Connective tissue: tissue that fills the spaces between the tissues and organs in the body; it consists of cells and collagen fibers separated by abundant extracellular substance.

Connective tissue papillae: finger-like extensions of connective tissue that extend up into the epithelium.

Controlled-release delivery device: in dentistry, usually consists of an antibacterial chemical that is imbedded in a carrier material; it is designed to be placed directly into the periodontal pocket where the carried material attaches to the tooth surface and dissolves slowly, producing a sustained release of the antimicrobial agent over a period of several days within the periodontal pocket.

Conventional mechanical periodontal therapy: a term that refers to self-care, periodontal instrumentation, and control of local contributing factors.

Coronally positioned flap: a periodontal plastic surgical procedure that can be used to repair gingival recession if the recession is not advanced; the coronally positioned flap is a displaced flap (displaced in a coronal direction in this case). Also see laterally positioned flap and semilunar flap.

Cortical bone: a layer of compact bone that forms the hard, outside wall of the mandible and maxilla on the facial and lingual aspects; cortical bone surrounds the alveolar bone proper and gives support to the socket.

Co-therapist: the concept of referring to a patient as co-therapist strengthens the notion that the patient plays an active role in the treatment and management of their periodontal condition.

Cratered papillae: a papilla appears to have been "scooped out" leaving a concave depression in the mid-proximal area. Cratered papillae are associated with necrotizing periodontal disease.

C-reactive protein: a special type of plasma protein that is present during episodes of acute inflammation or infection: CRP is an important cardiovascular risk predictor.

Crestal irregularities: the appearance on a dental radiographic of breaks or fuzziness instead of a clear, distinct radiopaque line at the crest of the interdental alveolar bone.

Crevicular fluid: see gingival crevicular fluid.

Crevicular incision: one type of horizontal incision employed during periodontal flap surgery in which the surgical scalpel is simply placed into the gingival crevice or sulcus and the tissues are incised apically to bone. Also see horizontal incision and internal bevel incision.

Crown lengthening surgery: a periodontal plastic surgical procedure designed to create a longer clinical crown for a tooth by removing some of the gingiva and usually by removing some alveolar bone from the necks of the teeth. Also see functional crown lengthening and esthetic crown lengthening.

Cyclosporine: an immunosuppressive agent used for prevention of transplant rejection as well as for management of a number of autoimmune conditions such as rheumatoid arthritis; associated with drug-influenced gingival enlargement.

Cytokines: a general name for powerful regulatory proteins released by immune cells that influence the behavior of other nearby cells: cytokines signal the immune system to send additional phagocytic cells to the site of an infection.

Databases: online indexes that list all articles published in a given period of time by journals in a particular profession or group of professions, such as PubMed, MEDLINE, or CINAHL (Cumulative Index of Nursing and Allied Health Literature).

Dehiscence: loss of alveolar bone on one aspect of the tooth, typically the facial aspect, that leaves the area of the root covered by soft tissue only.

Dental biofilm-induced gingivitis: periodontal disease involving inflammation of the gingiva in response to bacteria located at the gingival margin; the most common form of gingival disease.

Dental calculus: mineralized bacterial plaque, covered on its external surface by nonmineralized, living bacterial plaque.

Dental implant: a non-biologic (artificial) device surgically inserted into the jawbone to replace a missing tooth or provide support for a prosthetic denture.

Dental prosthesis: see prosthesis.

Dental water jet: a generic term for a device that delivers a pulsed irrigation of water or other solution around and between teeth and into the gingival sulcus or periodontal pocket.

Dentinal hypersensitivity: a short, sharp painful reaction that occurs when some areas of exposed dentin are subjected to mechanical, thermal, or chemical stimuli. See also hydrodynamic theory.

Dentinal tubule: a microscopic tube within dentin that spreads outward from the pulp throughout the dentin.

Dentogingival unit: is comprised of the junctional epithelium and the gingival fibers; the dentogingival unit acts to provide structural support to the gingival tissue.

Deplaquing: the disruption or removal of subgingival microbial plaque and its byproducts from cemental surfaces and the pocket space.

Desmosome: a specialized cell junction that connects two neighboring epithelial cells and their cytoskeletons together.

Diabetes mellitus: a disease in which the body does not produce or properly use insulin. Insulin is a hormone that is needed to convert sugar, starches and other food into energy that the body uses to sustain life. Also see type I diabetes mellitus and type II diabetes mellitus.

Dilantin: see phenytoin.

Disease progression: the change or advancement of periodontal destruction. Also see intermittent disease progression.

Disease site: an area of tissue destruction. A disease site may involve only a single surface of a tooth, for example, the distal surface of a tooth. The disease site may involve several surfaces of the tooth or all four surfaces (mesial, distal, facial, and lingual). Also see inactive disease site and active disease site.

Disengagement behavior: behavior characterized by a patient's disinterest, defensiveness, lack of warmth, or negative demeanor. A patient exhibiting disengagement behavior may be a sign of anxiousness or disinterest. See engagement behavior.

Displaced flap: a periodontal flap that is sutured with the margin of the flap placed at a position other than its original position in relationship to the CEJ of the tooth; a displaced flap can be positioned apically, coronally, or laterally in relationship to its original position. Also see nondisplaced flap.

Dissection: the process of cutting apart or separating tissue. Also see blunt dissection and sharp dissection.

Distraction: a common iatrosedation technique used to calm an anxious child. Distraction relies on diverting the patient's attention away from a procedure that the child may perceive as unpleasant.

Doxycycline: an antibiotic drug that is used to treat a variety of infections. Doxycycline at low doses is used as a host-modulating agent to inhibit part of the destruction occurs in periodontitis. See sub-antibacterial dose.

Drug-influenced gingival enlargement: an esthetically disfiguring overgrowth of the gingiva that is a side effect associated with certain medications such as anticonvulsants, calcium channel blockers, and immunosuppressants.

Dysbiosis: a microbial imbalance that results in a disruption of the microbial homeostasis inside the biofilm. Dysbiosis is the direct opposite of symbiosis.

Elevation: separating the surface tissues from the underlying tooth root and alveolar bone during periodontal surgery; the term elevation is used to convey the concept of lifting the surface tissues away from the tooth roots and away from the alveolar bone.

Elicit: encouraging the patient to talk about his or her opinions, behaviors, attitudes.

Embrasure space: see gingival embrasure space.

Empathy: the ability to identify with and understand another person's feelings or difficulties.

Enamel matrix derivative (EMD): a preparation of proteins extracted from porcine tooth buds; enamel matrix derivative has been used to enhance periodontal regeneration.

Enamel pearl: a ectopic, spherical formation of enamel that is located on the root surface. The presence of an enamel pearl can be a local contributing factor to periodontal inflammation.

Endothelium: the thin layer of epithelial cells that line the interior surface of the blood vessels.

Engagement behavior: behavior characterized by a patient's attentiveness, receptivity, warmth, and positive demeanor. See disengagement behavior.

Environmental tobacco smoke: refers to being exposed to tobacco smoke from someone else's cigarette, cigar, or pipe. Also known as secondhand smoke.

Epidemiology: the study of the health and disease within the total population (rather than an individual) and the risk factors that influence health and disease.

Epithelial-connective tissue interface: the boundary where the epithelial and connective tissues meet.

Epithelial tissue: the tissue that makes up the outer surface of the body (skin) and lines the body cavities such as the mouth, stomach, and intestines.

Eruption gingivitis: a transient form of gingivitis that is seen in young children as the teeth erupt out of the gingiva.

Essential oil: an active ingredient in some mouth rinses such as thymol, menthol, eucalyptol, and methyl salicylate. Listerine is an example of an essential oil.

Esthetic crown lengthening: a crown lengthening performed on teeth to improve the appearance of the teeth where there is excessive gingiva or a "gummy smile" as it is sometimes called. Also see functional crown lengthening.

European Academy of Periodontology (EFP): an association of dental professionals specializing in the prevention, diagnosis, and treatment of diseases affecting the periodontium.

Evidence-based health care: the conscientious, explicit, and judicious use of current best evidence in making decisions about the care of individual patients; requires the integration of individual clinical expertise and patient preferences with the best available external clinical evidence from systematic research.

Evidence levels: see levels of evidence.

Exotoxins: harmful proteins released from the bacterial cell that act on the body's host cells at a distance.

Extent: the degree or amount of periodontal destruction and can be characterized based on the number of sites that have experienced tissue destruction. Also see severity.

External basal lamina: a thin mat of extracellular matrix between the epithelial cells of the junctional epithelium and the gingival connective tissue. Also see internal basal lamina.

Extracellular matrix: a mesh-like material that surrounds the cells; this material helps to hold cells together and provides a framework within which cells can migrate and interact with one another.

Extracellular slime layer: a protective barrier that surrounds the mushroom-shaped bacterial microcolonies of a biofilm; protects the bacterial microcolonies from antibiotics, antimicrobials, and the body's immune system. Also see biofilm and fluid channels.

Exudate: pus that can be expressed from a periodontal pocket; sometimes called suppuration.

Facultative anaerobic bacteria: bacteria that can exist either with or without oxygen. Also see aerobic bacteria and anaerobic bacteria.

Familial aggregation: clustering of certain traits, behaviors, or disorders within a given family.

Fenestration: a "window" of bone loss bordered by alveolar bone on its coronal aspect.

Fictitious injury: self-inflicting injury. An example of a fictitious injury is improper use of a toothpick which traumatizes the gingiva.

Fimbriae: hair-like structures possessed by some bacteria that enable them to attach rapidly upon contact with the tooth surface.

Flap: see periodontal flap.

Flap curettage: see open flap debridement.

Flap for access: a periodontal surgical technique used to provide access to the tooth roots for improved root preparation. In this surgical procedure the gingival tissue is incised and temporarily elevated (lifted away) from the tooth roots. Also see open flap debridement.

Fluid channels: a series of channels that penetrate the extracellular slime layer of a biofilm that provide nutrients and oxygen for the bacterial microcolonies and facilitate movement of bacterial metabolites, waste products, and enzymes within the biofilm structure. Also see biofilm and extracellular slime layer.

Food impaction: forcing food (such as pieces of tough meat) between teeth during chewing, trapping the food in the interdental area.

Free gingiva: the unattached portion of the gingiva that surrounds the tooth in the region of the cementoenamel junction; also known as the unattached gingiva or the marginal gingiva.

Free soft tissue autograft (previously known as free gingival graft): a type of periodontal plastic surgery that was one of the first procedures used to augment the width of attached gingiva. The free gingival graft requires harvesting a donor section of tissue, usually from the palate, so there are two intraoral wounds that are created during this surgery: the donor site and the recipient site.

Free gingival groove: a shallow linear depression that separates the free and attached gingiva; this line may be visible clinically but is not obvious in many instances.

Fremitus: a palpable or visible movement of a tooth when in function.

Frenectomy: a periodontal plastic surgical procedure that results in removal of a frenum, including the attachment of the frenum to bone.

Full-thickness flap: a periodontal surgical procedure that includes elevation of entire thickness of the soft tissue (including epithelium, connective tissue, and periosteum); the full-thickness flap provides the complete access to underlying bone that might be needed when bone replacement grafting or periodontal regeneration procedures are anticipated.

Functional crown lengthening: a periodontal plastic surgical procedure performed on a tooth where the remaining tooth structure is inadequate to support a needed restoration; can be used to make a restorative dental procedure (such as a crown) possible when the only sensible alternative might be to remove the tooth. Also see esthetic crown lengthening.

Functional occlusal forces: normal occlusal forces produced during the act of chewing food. Also see parafunctional occlusal forces.

Furcation involvement: an osseous defect that results in a loss of alveolar bone between the roots of a multi-rooted tooth.

Genetic test: see PST genetic susceptibility test.

Gestational diabetes: a form of diabetes that occurs during pregnancy in women who have never had diabetes before pregnancy. Also see diabetes mellitus.

Gingival abscess: an abscess of the periodontium that is primarily limited to the gingival margin or interdental papilla without involvement of the deeper structures of the periodontium. Also see periodontal abscess, pericoronal abscess.

Gingival crevicular fluid: a fluid that flows into the sulcus from the adjacent gingival connective tissue; the flow is slight in health and increases in disease.

Gingival curettage: an older type of periodontal surgical procedure that involves an attempt to scrape away the lining of the periodontal pocket usually using a periodontal curet, often a Gracey curet. Research has demonstrated that normally the same benefits from gingival curettage can be derived from thorough periodontal instrumentation by the clinician plus meticulous self-care by the patient. Thus, curettage is rarely needed as a separate periodontal surgical procedure in modern dentistry.

Gingival diseases: a category of periodontal diseases that usually involve inflammation of the gingival tissues, most often in response to bacterial plaque. Also see gingivitis, dental biofilm-induced gingivitis, non–plaque-induced gingivitis, acute gingivitis, and chronic gingivitis.

Gingival embrasure space: the small triangular open space (apical to the contact area) between the curved proximal surfaces of two teeth. In health, the interdental papilla fills the gingival embrasure space. Also see type I, type II, and type III gingival embrasure.

Gingival epithelium: a specialized stratified squamous epithelium that functions well in the wet environment of the oral cavity; the microscopic anatomy of the gingival epithelium is similar to the epithelium of the skin. Also see oral epithelium, sulcular epithelium, and junctional epithelium.

Gingival fibers: see supragingival fiber bundles.

Gingival margin: the thin, rounded edge of free gingiva that forms the coronal boundary, or upper edge, of the gingiva. In health, the gingival margin contacts the tooth slightly coronal to the cementoenamel junction.

Gingival pocket: a deepening of the gingival sulcus as a result of swelling or enlargement of the gingival tissue. Also see periodontal pocket.

Gingival sulcular fluid: see gingival crevicular fluid.

Gingival sulcus: the *space* between the free gingiva and the tooth surface.

Gingiva: the part of the mucosa that surrounds the cervical portions of the teeth and covers the alveolar processes of the jaws.

Gingival health: a periodontium is deemed to be healthy if the pockets are 3 mm or less and there is a bleeding score less than 10%.

Gingivectomy: a resective periodontal surgical procedure designed to excise (cut away) and to remove some of the gingival tissue. Historically the gingivectomy was used for many years in periodontics as a primary treatment modality, but it plays a greatly reduced role in modern dentistry. Also see gingivoplasty.

Gingivitis: an inflammation of the periodontium that is confined to the gingiva resulting in damage to the gingival tissue that is reversible. Also see gingival diseases, acute gingivitis, chronic gingivitis and periodontitis.

Gingivoplasty: a periodontal surgical procedure used to reshape the surface of the gingiva to create a natural form and contour to the gingiva. Unlike the gingivectomy, gingivoplasty implies reshaping the surface of the gingiva without removing any of the gingiva actually attached to the tooth surface. Also see gingivectomy.

Glycemic control: a medical term referring to the typical levels of blood sugar (glucose) in a person with diabetes mellitus; optimal management of diabetes involves patients measuring and recording their own blood glucose levels.

Grading: periodontitis grading is one of two diagnostic parameters (along with periodontitis staging), that is used to define an individual's periodontitis condition. Grading provides an estimate of the potential future risk of disease progression and potential risk of systemic impact of an individual patient's periodontitis.

Gram staining: a laboratory method that reveals differences in the chemical and physical properties of bacterial cell walls that divides bacteria into gram-positive (purple color) and gram-negative (red color) bacterial cell wall types. See gram-positive bacteria and gram-negative bacteria.

Gram-negative bacteria: bacteria with a thin cell wall which is surrounded by an outer membrane and an inner membrane that shows a red stain under the microscope; believed to play an important role in inflammatory periodontitis. See Gram staining and gram-positive bacteria.

Gram-positive bacteria: bacteria with a single, thick cell wall that show a purple stain under the microscope; most of the bacteria associated with a healthy periodontium are gram-positive. See Gram staining and gram-negative bacteria.

Growth factors: naturally occurring proteins that regulate both cell growth and development. Several growth factors are being studied for their effect in enhancing the predictability of periodontal regeneration.

Guided tissue regeneration (GTR): a periodontal surgical procedure employed to encourage regeneration of lost periodontal structures (i.e., to regrow lost cementum, lost periodontal ligament, and lost alveolar bone).

Heat shock proteins: a group of proteins that are induced when a cell undergoes various types of environmental stresses like heat, cold, and oxygen deprivation.

Hemidesmosome: a specialized cell junction that connects the epithelial cells to the basal lamina. Hemidesmosomes also attach the junctional epithelium to the enamel in teeth without gingival recession.

Histology: a branch of anatomy concerned with the study of the microscopic structures of tissues.

HIV: human immunodeficiency virus. Also see acquired immunodeficiency syndrome.

HIV-associated gingivitis: see linear gingival erythema.

Homeostasis: an internal equilibrium/ balance; such as an internal equilibrium within the biofilm that ensures the safety and survival of all microorganisms living in the biofilm community without harming the host.

Horizontal bone loss: a common pattern of bone loss resulting in a fairly even, overall reduction in the height of the alveolar bone with the margin of the alveolar crest more or less perpendicular to the long axis of the tooth. Also see alveolar bone loss and vertical bone loss.

Horizontal incision: an incision that runs parallel to the gingival margins in a mesio-distal direction. Also see incision and vertical incision.

Hospital-acquired pneumonia: an infection of the lungs contracted during a stay in a hospital or long-term care facility. Hospital-acquired pneumonia is not caused by the same organisms that cause community-acquired pneumonia.

Host: a human in or on which another organism lives; in the case of periodontal disease, bacterial pathogens infect the host (individual with periodontal disease).

Host modulation: in dentistry, altering the host's (patient's) defense responses to help the body limit damage to the periodontium from infections such as periodontitis.

Host response: the way that an individual's body responds to an infection. Also see immune system and inflammation.

Hydrodynamic theory: the prevailing theory that explains dentinal hypersensitivity. Under this theory, a thermal or mechanical stimuli causes movement of the dentinal fluid in the dentinal tubules. In turn, this movement is transmitted to the pain fibers in the dental pulp to induce the short, sharp pain associated with dentinal hypersensitivity.

Hydrokinetic activity: the energy created by fluids in motion; in dentistry the pulsating fluid delivered by dental water jet creates two zones of fluid movement.

Iatrosedation: the act of making a patient calm based on the doctor's behavior. Also see pharmacosedation.

Immune system: a collection of responses that protects the body against infections by bacteria, viruses, fungi, toxins, and parasites; the immune system defends the body against invading microorganisms, as well as toxins in the environment.

Immunoglobulins: Y-shaped proteins; the five major classes of immunoglobulin are immunoglobulin M (IgM), immunoglobulin D (IgD), immunoglobulin G (IgG), immunoglobulin A (IgA), and immunoglobulin E (IgE).

Implant: see dental implant and implant body.

Implant abutment: a titanium post that attaches to the implant body and protrudes partially or completely through the gingival tissue into the mouth.

Implant body: the portion of the implant system that is surgically placed into the living alveolar bone; sometimes referred to as the implant fixture or implant.

Implant fixture: see implant body.

Inactive disease site: an area of tissue destruction that is stable, with the attachment level of the junctional epithelium remaining the same over time.

Incidence: the number of new disease cases in a population that occur over a given period of time. Also see prevalence.

Incision: a cut into a body tissue or organ, especially one made during surgery. Also see horizontal incision, crevicular incision, internal l bevel incision, and vertical incision.

Inflammation: the body's reaction to injury or invasion by disease-producing organisms that focuses host defense components at the site of the infection to eliminate microorganisms and heal damaged tissue. Inflammation is part of the immune response. Also see acute inflammation and chronic inflammation.

Inflammatory biochemical mediators: biologically active compounds secreted by cells that activate the body's inflammatory response; inflammatory mediators of importance in periodontitis are the cytokines, prostaglandins, and matrix metalloproteinases.

Informed consent: a patient's voluntary agreement to proposed treatment after achieving an understanding of the relevant facts, benefits, and risks involved. Also see informed refusal.

Informed refusal: a person's right to refuse all or a portion of the proposed treatment after the recommended treatment, alternate treatment options, and the likely consequences of declining treatment have been explained in language understood by the patient. Also see informed consent.

Infrabony defect: an osseous defect in the alveolar bone resulting in bone resorption that occurs in an uneven, oblique direction.

Infrabony pocket: a periodontal pocket in which there is vertical bone loss and the junctional epithelium, forming the base of the pocket, is located *apical* to the crest of the alveolar bone. The base of the pocket is located within the cratered-out area of the bone alongside of the root surface. Also see periodontal pocket and suprabony pocket.

Innervation: nerve supply; innervation to the periodontium occurs via the branches of the trigeminal nerve.

Innocuous: species of bacteria that are not harmful. Also see pathogenic bacteria.

Insurance codes: numeric codes used by insurance companies and the government to classify different dental procedures. For example, periodontal maintenance procedures are designated by the insurance code D4910.

Intact periodontium: a periodontium with an absence of detectable attachment and/or bone loss.

Intentional torts: actions designed to injure another person or that person's property.

Interdental gingiva: the portion of the gingiva that fills the interdental embrasure between two adjacent teeth apical to the contact area. The interdental gingiva consists of two interdental papillae.

Interdisciplinary care: the close collaboration of two or more health care providers from different disciplines to address the needs of the patient and establish an optimal care plan that results in enhanced health outcomes.

Intermittent disease progression theory: states that periodontal disease is characterized by periods of disease activity and inactivity (remission).

Internal basal lamina: a thin mat of extracellular matrix between the epithelial cells of the junctional epithelium and the tooth surface. Also see external basal lamina.

Internal bevel incision: one type of horizontal incision employed during periodontal flap surgery in which the surgical scalpel enters the marginal gingiva, but is not placed directly into the crevice or sulcus; the scalpel blade enters the gingival margin approximately 0.5 to 1.0 mm away from the margin and follows the general contour of the scalloped marginal gingiva. Also see horizontal incision and crevicular incision.

Irrigation: see oral irrigation.

Junctional epithelium (JE): the specialized epithelium that forms the base of the sulcus and joins the gingiva to the tooth surface. Also see gingival epithelium.

Keratinization: the process by which epithelial cells on the surface of the skin become stronger and waterproof. Also see keratinized epithelial cells and nonkeratinized epithelial cells.

Keratinized epithelial cells: cells that have no nuclei and form a tough, resistant layer on the surface of the skin.

Knee to knee position: a common approach to performing a dental examination on a young infant patient. The provider sits knee-to-knee with the caregiver and the infant patient lays on his/her back on the provider's lap.

Kwashiorkor: a severe protein deficiency that can result in a shift in subgingival oral bacteria to include more periodontal pathogens.

Laterally positioned flap: a periodontal plastic surgery technique that can be used to cover root surfaces with gingiva in isolated sites of gingival recession. Also see coronally positioned flap and semilunar flap.

Leukemia: a type of cancer that begins in blood cells in which the bone marrow produces a large number of abnormal white blood cells, that do not function properly.

Leukocytes: white blood cells that act much like independent single-cell organisms able to move and capture microorganisms on their own.

Levels of evidence: a ranking system used in evidence-based health care to describe the strength of the results measured in a clinical trial or research study.

Liability: a health care provider's obligation or responsibility to provide services to another person (the patient). The health care provider's liability entails the possibility of being sued if the person receiving the services feels as if he has been treated improperly or negligently.

Linear gingival erythema (LGE): a gingival manifestation of immunosuppression characterized by a distinct linear erythematous (red) band that is limited to the free gingiva; formerly known as HIV-associated gingivitis.

Lipopolysaccharide (LPS): a major component of the cell membranes of gram-negative bacteria (also known as endotoxin). LPS was previously thought to play a role in the inflammation seen in periodontal disease, however recent research has shown that this theory is not correct. Also see peptides.

Long junctional epithelium: a form of periodontal repair that is characterized by the apical downgrowth of the junctional epithelium. This type of healing primarily occurs following periodontal instrumentation of a diseased root surface. Healing by long junctional epithelium is not the same as periodontal regeneration.

Lymph nodes: small bean-shaped structures located on either side of the head, neck, armpits, and groin; these nodes filter out and trap bacteria, fungi, viruses, and other unwanted substances to safely eliminate them from the body.

Lymphatic system: a network of lymph nodes connected by lymphatic vessels that plays an important role in the body's defense against infection.

Lymphocytes: small leukocytes that play an important role in recognizing and controlling foreign invaders; two main types of lymphocytes are important in defense against periodontal pathogens are B-lymphocytes and T-lymphocytes. Also see B-lymphocytes and T-lymphocytes.

Lysosomes: granules found in the cytoplasm of PMNs that are filled with strong bactericidal and digestive enzymes; these granules can kill and digest bacterial cells after phagocytosis. Also see phagocytosis.

Macronutrients: a type of food required in large amounts in the diet. Fats, proteins, and carbohydrates are macronutrients.

Macrophages: large phagocytic leukocytes (located in the tissue) that have one kidney-shaped nucleus and some granules. Also see monocytes.

Malpractice: the improper or negligent treatment by a health care provider that results in injury or damage to the patient.

Matrix metalloproteinases (MMP): a family of at least 12 different enzymes produced by various cells of the body that can act together to break down the connective tissue matrix; the presence of increased MMP levels causes extensive collagen destruction in the periodontal tissues.

Medical lasers: a device that produces an intense, narrow beam of light with a single wavelength which can be focused at a precise location. Investigations are still ongoing to determine the effectiveness of using lasers to treat and manage periodontal disease.

MEDLINE (PubMed): a free online index that enables quick access to locate relevant clinical evidence in the published medical, dental, and allied health literature; hosted by the National Library of Medicine.

Membrane attack complex: a protein unit created by the complement system that is capable of puncturing the cell membranes of certain bacteria. Also see complement system.

Memory B-cells: see B-lymphocytes.

Menopausal gingivostomatitis: decreased levels of circulating hormones in women who are menopausal or postmenopausal that may result in oral changes, such as thinning of the oral mucosa, dry mouth, burning sensations, altered taste, gingival recession, and alveolar bone loss.

Metabolic syndrome: a group of risk factors that place an individual at increased risk of developing several major chronic disorders, such as heart disease, diabetes, and stroke.

Metastatic infection: the spread of a pathogen from its initial site to a different secondary site inside the host's body. Periodontal pathogens have the potential to travel to distant sites in the body and cause infections, such as a lung infection or endocarditis.

Microbial reservoir: a niche or secure place in the oral cavity that can allow periodontal pathogens to live undisturbed during routine therapy and subsequently repopulate periodontal pockets quickly.

Micronutrients: nutrients that are needed in trace quantities for normal growth and development of living organisms. Vitamins and calcium are examples of micronutrients.

Mobility: the loosening of a tooth in its socket that may result from loss of bone support to the tooth.

Modeling: an iatrosedation technique used to calm an anxious child. This approach relies on the caregiver or another patient to function as a model for the child by exhibiting the specific behavior that needs to be imitated.

Modified Widman flap surgery: see flap for access.

Monocytes: phagocytic leukocytes located in the bloodstream. Also see macrophages.

Morphology: the study of the anatomic surface features of the teeth.

Motivational interviewing (MI): defined as a patient-centered method for enhancing a patient's motivation for behavior change by exploring the patient's mixed feelings about change.

Mucogingival junction: the clinically visible boundary where the pink-attached gingiva meets the red, shiny alveolar mucosa.

Mucogingival surgery: terminology used in the past to describe periodontal surgical procedures that alter the relationship between gingiva and mucosa. Some of the periodontal plastic surgical procedures utilized in modern dentistry were previously described as mucogingival surgical procedures and this older terminology can still be encountered. Also see periodontal plastic surgery.

Mucoperiosteal flap: see full-thickness flap.

Multifactorial etiology: when one or more factors cause a disease. The etiology of

periodontitis, for instance is considered to be multifactorial since its etiology involves multiple factors, such as bacteria, host susceptibility, and genetic/environmental factors.

Necrosis: cell death. For example, in the case of necrotizing ulcerative gingivitis, necrosis refers to the death of the cells comprising the gingival epithelium.

Necrotizing periodontal diseases: a unique type of periodontal disease that involves tissue necrosis (localized tissue death); characterized by painful infection with ulceration, swelling, and sloughing off of dead epithelial tissue from the gingiva. Also see necrotizing gingivitis and necrotizing periodontitis.

Necrotizing gingivitis (NG): tissue necrosis that is limited to the gingival tissues.

Necrotizing periodontitis (NP): tissue necrosis of the gingival tissues combined with loss of attachment and alveolar bone loss.

Negligence: a failure to exercise reasonable care to avoid injuring others. It is the failure to do something that a reasonable person would do under the same circumstances, or the doing of something a reasonable person would not do. Negligence is characterized by carelessness, inattentiveness, and neglectfulness rather than by a deliberate intent to cause injury.

Neutropenia: a polymorphonuclear leukocyte (PMN) count of less than 1,000 cells/mL of blood; indicates an increased risk of infection.

Neutrophils: are phagocytic cells that actively engulf and destroy microorganisms; PMNs play a vital role in combating the pathogenic bacteria responsible for periodontal disease; also known as polymorphonuclear leukocytes.

New attachment: a term used to describe the union of a *pathologically exposed root* with connective tissue or epithelium. Also see reattachment.

NHANES: abbreviation for the National Health and Nutrition Examination Survey.

Nifedipine: a calcium channel blocker used as a coronary vasodilator in the treatment of hypertension, angina, and cardiac arrhythmias; associated with drug-influenced gingival enlargement. Also see calcium channel blocker.

Nonabsorbable suture: a suture made from a material that does not dissolve in body fluids; a clinician must remove the nonabsorbable sutures after some healing of the wound has occurred. Also see absorbable suture.

Noncompliant patients: patients who do not follow recommendations for health care advice. Examples of noncompliant patients would be a patient that does not take medications daily to control diabetes as prescribed by a physician or a patient that does not follow instructions for performing daily self-care. Also see compliance.

Nondisplaced flap: a periodontal flap that is sutured with the margin of the flap at its original position in relationship to the CEJ on the tooth. Also see displaced flap.

Nonpharmacological therapy: any type of therapy that calms the patient without the use of medication. Iatrosedation is an example of nonpharmacological therapy.

Nonkeratinized epithelial cells: cells that have nuclei and act as a cushion against mechanical stress and wear. Nonkeratinized epithelial cells are softer and more flexible.

Non–plaque-induced gingival diseases: are periodontal diseases that are not caused by bacterial plaque and do not disappear after plaque removal; however, the presence of dental plaque could increase the severity of the gingival inflammation in non–plaque-induced lesions. See plaque-induced gingival diseases.

Nonresponsive disease sites: areas in the periodontium that show deeper probing depths, continuing loss of attachment, or continuing clinical signs of inflammation in spite of thorough therapy.

Nonsteroidal anti-inflammatory drugs (NSAIDs): medications used for many years in medical care to treat pain, acute inflammation, and chronic inflammatory conditions. NSAIDs have been evaluated for their effect on periodontitis (a disease intimately associated with inflammation). NSAIDs can reduce tissue inflammation by inhibiting prostaglandins including PGE_2 and when administered daily over 3 years, have been shown to slow the rate of alveolar bone loss associated with periodontitis.

Nonsurgical periodontal therapy: a phase of periodontal therapy that includes self-care measures, periodontal instrumentation, and use of chemical agents to prevent or control plaque-induced gingivitis or periodontitis.

Occlusal adjustment: a clinical therapy involving minor adjustments in an individual's bite that can be used to help control the damage from trauma from occlusion.

Odontoblastic process: a thin tail of cytoplasm from a cell in the tooth pulp called an odontoblast.

Omega-3 fatty acids: a type of polyunsaturated fat found in leafy green vegetables, vegetable oils, and cold-water fish; omega-3 fatty acids are capable of reducing serum cholesterol levels and having anticoagulant properties.

Open flap debridement: a periodontal surgical procedure that is quite similar in concept and execution to flap for access surgery; usually includes more extensive flap elevation than flap for access—providing access not only to the tooth roots but also to all of the alveolar bone defects. Also see flap for access.

Open-ended questions: questions that cannot be answered with a simple yes or no response.

Open margin: a space or gap between the edge of a restoration and the tooth structure. An open margin is considered to be a local contributing factor since it is an area that can harbor biofilm.

Operculum: a flap of gingival tissue covering part of the occlusal surface of a partially erupted tooth. This tissue flap can become infected and this type of infection under the flap of tissue is referred to as a pericoronal abscess.

Opsonization: coating of the surface of a microorganism by complement components to facilitate the engulfment and destruction by phagocytes.

Oral epithelium (OE): portion of the gingival epithelium that covers the outer surface of the free gingiva and attached gingiva; it extends from the crest of the gingival margin to the mucogingival junction. The oral epithelium is the only part of the periodontium that is visible to the unaided eye. Also see gingival epithelium.

Oral irrigation: the in-home use of a pulsating water stream created by a mechanized device. Also see dental water jet.

Osseointegration: the direct contact of living alveolar bone with the surface of the dental implant body (with no intervening periodontal ligament). Osseointegration is a major requirement for implant success.

Osseous crater: a bowl-shaped osseous defect in the interdental alveolar bone with bone loss nearly equal on the roots of two adjacent teeth. Also see infrabony defect.

Osseous defect: a deformity in the tooth supporting alveolar bone usually resulting from periodontitis. Also see infrabony defect, osseous crater, and furcation involvement.

Osseous resective surgery: a periodontal surgical procedure employed to correct many of the irregular deformities of the alveolar bone that often result from advancing periodontitis. Osseous resective surgery entails removal of bone to correct the bony deformities. It does not result in periodontal regeneration. Also see ostectomy and osteoplasty.

Osseous surgery: see osseous resective surgery.

Ostectomy: removal of alveolar bone that is attached to the tooth via the PDL fibers (i.e., that is still providing some support for the tooth). The removal of small amounts of supporting bone is justified by the attainment of alveolar bone contours that are compatible with the natural contours of the gingiva. Also see osteoplasty.

Osteoblasts: bone-forming cells.

Osteoclasts: bone resorbing cells.

Osteoconductive grafting materials: grafting materials that form a framework for bone cells. Also see osteoinductive grafting materials.

Osteoectomy: see ostectomy.

Osteogenesis: the production of new bone; in periodontal surgery, osteogenesis is the potential for new bone cells and new bone to form following bone grafting.

Osteoinductive grafting materials: grafting materials that release chemical mediators (such as BMP) to draw in host osteoprogenitor cells to the site. Also see osteoconductive grafting materials.

Osteonecrosis of the jaw: a rare condition in which there are painful areas of exposed bone in the mouth that fail to heal after an extraction or oral surgery procedure.

Osteopenia: a condition in which there is a decrease in bone density but not necessarily an increase in the risk or incidence of bone fracture; most commonly seen in people over the age of 50 that have lower than average bone density but do not have osteoporosis. Also see osteoporosis.

Osteoplasty: reshaping the surface of alveolar bone without actually removing any of the supporting bone. Also see ostectomy.

Osteoporosis: a reduction in bone mass that causes an increased susceptibility to fractures; occurs most frequently in postmenopausal women, in sedentary or bedridden individuals, and in patients receiving long-term steroid therapy. Also see osteopenia.

Overhanging restoration: a dental restoration that is not smoothly contoured with the tooth surfaces (also called an overhang).

Porphyromonas gingivalis: an important periodontal pathogen.

Palatogingival groove: a developmental defect that forms on the palatal surface of a tooth and is most frequently seen on maxillary lateral incisors. Plaque retention is a common problem associated with a palatogingival groove since the groove is often difficult or impossible to clean effectively.

Papilla: see interdental gingiva.

Parafunctional occlusal forces: occlusal forces that result from tooth-to-tooth contact made when not in the act of eating. Also see functional occlusal forces.

Partial-thickness flap: or split-thickness flap as it is also called, includes elevation of only the epithelium and a thin layer of the underlying connective tissue rather than the entire thickness of the underlying soft tissues.

Pathogenesis: the sequence of events that occur during the development of a disease or abnormal condition.

Pathogenic: a species of bacteria that are capable of causing disease; also called virulent bacteria.

Pathogenicity: the ability of the dental plaque biofilm to cause periodontal disease.

Patient-centered: a philosophy of health care that recognizes the patient's dignity, and right of choice in all matters, without exception, related to health care; for example, consideration of behavior changes and treatment planning is viewed from the patient's perspective rather than the clinician's perspective.

Pediatric dentistry triad: a collaborative teamwork effort that involves close interaction between the dental clinician, child patient, and parent (or caregiver). Establishing this relationship builds trust between all participants of the triad and serves to facilitate a positive outcome for the child.

Peer-reviewed journal: a journal that uses a panel of experts to review research articles for study design, statistics, and conclusions.

Pellicle: a thin, bacteria-free membrane that forms on the surface of the tooth during the late stages of eruption.

Peptide: short chains of amino acids found in living bacterial cell membranes control the transport of molecules in and out of the bacterial cell. T-cells recognize these peptides and alert the immune system to the presence of bacteria.

Pericoronal abscess: an abscess of the periodontium that involves tissues around the crown of a partially erupted tooth. The pericoronal abscess is also referred to as pericoronitis.

Pericoronitis: see pericoronal abscess.

Peri-implant health: the healthy soft tissue surrounding an implant with no visual signs of inflammation, absence of profuse bleeding on probing, and stable pocket depths that do not increase over time.

Peri-implant gingivitis: see peri-implant mucositis.

Peri-implant mucositis (also called peri-implant gingivitis): plaque-induced gingivitis that is localized in the gingival tissues surrounding a dental implant. Also see peri-implantitis.

Peri-implant tissues: the periodontal tissues that surround the dental implant.

Peri-implantitis: periodontitis in the tissues surrounding an osseointegrated dental implant, resulting in loss of alveolar bone. Also see peri-implant mucositis.

Periodontal abscess: a localized collection of pus that forms in a circumscribed area of the periodontal tissues.

Periodontal abscess: a localized collection of pus that forms in a circumscribed area of the periodontal tissues that affects the deeper structures of the periodontium as well as the gingival tissues. Also see gingival abscess, pericoronal abscess.

Periodontal assessment: see clinical periodontal assessment.

Periodontal disease: refers to inflammation of the periodontium.

Periodontal dressing: a protective material applied over a periodontal surgical wound and used somewhat like using a bandage to cover a finger wound. Periodontal flaps that are well adapted to the alveolar bone and tooth roots may not always require a periodontal dressing. Periodontal dressings can be placed to facilitate flap adaptation and are frequently indicated when the surgical procedures have created varying tissue levels or when displaced flaps are used.

Periodontal flap: a surgical procedure in which incisions are made in the gingiva or mucosa to allow for separation of the surface tissues (epithelium and connective tissue) from the underlying tooth roots and underlying alveolar bone. Also see full-thickness flap, partial-thickness flap, nondisplaced flap, and displaced flap.

Periodontal ligament: the fibers that surround the root of the tooth. These fibers attach to the bone of the socket on one side and to the cementum of the root on the other side.

Periodontal maintenance: continuing patient care provided by the dental team to help the periodontitis patient maintain periodontal health following complete nonsurgical or surgical periodontal therapy. The term periodontal maintenance applies specifically to treated periodontitis patients. It is normally not appropriate to use the term periodontal maintenance for patients treated for other conditions such as those treated for the various types of gingivitis.

Periodontal microsurgery: a periodontal surgical procedure performed with the aid of a surgical microscope.

Periodontal osseous surgery: see osseous resective surgery.

Periodontal pack: see periodontal dressing.

Periodontal plastic surgery: periodontal surgery that is directed toward correcting problems with attached gingiva, aberrant frenum, or vestibular depth; includes an array of periodontal surgical procedures that can be used to improve esthetics of the dentition and to enhance prosthetic dentistry as well as to deal with damage resulting from periodontitis. Also see free gingival graft, subepithelial connective tissue graft, coronally positioned flap, frenectomy, and crown lengthening surgery.

Periodontal pocket: a pathologic deepening of the gingival sulcus as the result of the apical migration of the junctional epithelium, destruction of the periodontal ligament fibers, and destruction of alveolar bone. Also see apical migration.

Periodontal Screening and Recording (PSR): an efficient, easy-to-use screening system for the detection of periodontal disease.

Periodontal screening examination: a periodontal assessment used to determine the periodontal health status of the patient and identify patients needing a more comprehensive periodontal assessment.

Periodontitis associated with endodontic lesions: a category of periodontal disease that involves infection or death of the tissues of the dental pulp.

Periodontitis: a bacterial infection of the periodontium resulting in destruction of all parts of the periodontium including the gingiva, periodontal ligament, bone, and cementum; results in irreversible destruction to the tissues of the periodontium.

Periodontium: the functional system of tissues that surrounds the teeth and attaches them to the jawbone. The periodontium is also called the "supporting tissues of the teeth" and "the attachment apparatus."

Periosteum: a dense membrane composed of fibrous connective tissue that closely wraps the outer surface of the alveolar bone; it consists of an outer layer of collagenous tissue and an inner layer of fine elastic fibers.

Phagocytosis: the process by which leukocytes engulf and digest microorganisms.

Pharmacosedation: the act of making a patient calm with the use of medications, such as a anxiolytic agent.

Phenytoin: one of the most commonly used anticonvulsant medications used to control convulsions or seizures in the treatment of epilepsy; associated with drug-influenced gingival enlargement.

PICO Process: a structure for formulating questions that the PICO entails four critical components: Patient, Intervention, Comparison, and Outcome.

Plaque-induced gingival diseases: Older terminology for dental biofilm induced gingivitis.

Plasma B-cells: see B-lymphocytes.

Plastic surgery: see periodontal plastic surgery.

Polymicrobial: a microbial community that is composed of many different species of microorganisms; plaque biofilm is a polymicrobial community.

Polymorphonuclear leukocytes (PMNs): are phagocytic cells that actively engulf and destroy microorganisms; PMNs play a vital role in combating the pathogenic bacteria responsible for periodontal disease; also known as neutrophils.

Positive reinforcement: a method of behavioral modification that reinforces positive behavior and encourages the reoccurrence of such desire behaviors.

Postmenopausal osteoporosis: a disorder caused by the cessation of estrogen production and is characterized by bone fractures.

Preeclampsia: a condition that occurs only during pregnancy. If not treated properly, preeclampsia can affect fetal growth and development.

Pregnancy gingivitis: gingival inflammation initiated by plaque, and exacerbated by hormonal changes in the second and third trimesters of pregnancy.

Pregnancy tumor: see pregnancy-associated pyogenic granuloma.

Pregnancy-associated pyogenic granuloma: a localized, mushroom-shaped gingival mass projecting from the gingival margin or more commonly from a gingival papilla during pregnancy.

Prevalence: the number of all cases (both old and new) of a disease that can be identified within a specified population at a given point in time. Also see incidence.

Primary herpetic gingivostomatitis: is a painful oral condition that results from the initial infection with the herpes simplex virus (HSV).

Primary intention: healing that occurs when wound margins or edges are closely adapted to each other; an example of primary intention healing would be seen in a small wound in a finger that required stitches. Also see secondary and tertiary intention.

Primary trauma from occlusion: excessive occlusal forces on a sound (healthy) periodontium.

Professional subgingival irrigation: the in-office flushing of pockets performed by the dental hygienist or dentist using one of three systems: a blunt-tipped irrigating cannula, an ultrasonic unit equipped with a fluid reservoir, or a specialized air-driven handpiece.

Pro-inflammatory mediators: biologically active compounds secreted by immune cells that can damage the periodontium; such as prostaglandin E_2, IL-1α (interleukin-1 alpha), IL-1β (interleukin-1 beta), IL–6 (interleukin-6), and tumor necrosis factor alpha. Also see biochemical mediators.

Pro-resolving mediators: specialized chemical mediators that are released by the body during the resolution phase of acute inflammation.

Prostaglandins: a series of powerful biochemical mediators, of which prostaglandins D, E, F, G, H, and I are the most important biologically; prostaglandins of the E series (PGE) play an important role in the bone destruction seen in periodontitis.

Prosthesis: an appliance used to replace missing teeth. Also see removable prosthesis.

Pseudomembrane: a yellowish white or grayish tissue slough that covers the necrotic areas of the gingiva in necrotizing periodontal diseases. Also see necrotizing periodontal diseases.

PST genetic susceptibility test: a test for genetic susceptibility to periodontal disease.

Pulpal abscess: an abscess that results from an infection of the tooth pulp. A pulpal abscess can be caused by death of the tooth pulp from trauma to the tooth or from deep dental decay.

Puberty gingivitis: common form of gingivitis seen in children between 9 to 14 years of age. Most likely associated with hormone changes that intensify the inflammatory response to plaque biofilm.

Pus: collections of dead white blood cells that can result when body defense mechanisms are involved in attempting to control an infection.

Pyogenic granuloma: see pregnancy-associated pyogenic granuloma.

Quorum sensing: the ability of one microbe to communicate with other microorganisms living within the plaque biofilm by sending signaling molecules.

Radiolucent: materials and structures that are easily penetrated by x-rays and appear as dark gray to black on the radiograph; examples of radiolucent structures are the tooth pulp, periodontal ligament space, a periapical abscess, marrow spaces in the bone, and bone loss defects.

Radiopaque: materials and structures absorb or resist the passage of x-rays and appear light gray to white on the radiograph; examples of radiopaque structures and materials are metallic silver (amalgam restorations) and newer composite restorations, enamel, dentin, pulp stones, and compact or cortical bone.

Reasonable person standard: a standard that is based on the premise that the health care practitioner must disclose all information that may help a reasonable patient decide to proceed or decline treatment.

Reattachment: healing of a periodontal wound by the reunion of the connective tissue and roots where these two tissues have been separated by incision or injury but *not by disease*. Also see new attachment.

Reactive oxygen species (ROS): highly unstable molecules that are contributors to oxidative stress which can lead to various disorders, such as cardiovascular disorders, cancer, and various neurodegenerative diseases.

Recurrence of periodontitis: the return of periodontitis in a patient that has been previously, successfully treated for periodontitis. The term recurrence implies that the periodontitis was brought under control during nonsurgical periodontal therapy (or nonsurgical periodontal therapy plus periodontal surgery) and that the periodontitis is once again resulting in progressive attachment loss.

Recurrent disease: new signs and symptoms of destructive periodontitis that reappear after periodontal therapy because the disease was not adequately treated and/or the patient did not practice adequate self-care.

Re-evaluation: a formal step at the completion of nonsurgical therapy. During the re-evaluation appointment, the members of the dental team perform another periodontal assessment to gather information about the patient's periodontal status.

Reduced periodontium: a periodontium with a presence of detectable attachment and/or bone loss. Note that a reduced periodontium can be stable (periodontitis in remission) or it can exhibit signs of active disease.

Refereed journal: see peer-reviewed journal.

Reflective listening: the process in which the health care provider listens to the patient's remarks and then paraphrases what the clinician heard the patient say. This allows the clinician to check with the patient that he or she is "getting the patient's message right," ensuring that the clinician is developing a good picture of the patient's perspective.

Refractory form of periodontitis: destructive periodontitis in a patient who, when monitored over time, exhibits additional attachment loss at one or more sites, despite appropriate, repeated professional periodontal therapy and a patient who practices satisfactory self-care and follows the recommended program of periodontal maintenance visits.

Regeneration: the biologic process by which the architecture and function of lost tissue is *completely* restored. Also see repair.

Relative contraindications: conditions that may make periodontal surgery inadvisable for some patients when the conditions or situations are severe or extreme; these same conditions may not be contraindications when the conditions are mild.

Removable prosthesis: an appliance used to replace missing teeth that the patient can remove for cleaning and before going to bed; commonly called a partial denture.

Repair: the healing of a wound by formation of tissues that do not precisely restore the original architecture or original function of the body part. Also see regeneration.

Resective periodontal surgery: periodontal surgical procedures that simply cut away and remove damaged periodontal tissues.

Risk assessment: the process of identifying risk factors that increase an individual's probability of disease.

Risk factors: factors that modify or amplify the likelihood of developing periodontal disease; major established risk factors for periodontitis are specific bacterial pathogens, cigarette smoking, and diabetes mellitus.

Root caries: tooth decay that occurs on the tooth root surfaces.

Root concavity: a trench-like depression in the root surface.

Scurvy: a systemic disorder caused by severe and prolonged deprivation of vitamin C; scurvy can be accompanied by changes in the periodontium.

Secondary intention: healing that takes place when the margins or edges of the wound are not closely adapted (i.e., the two wound edges are not in close contact with each other). When healing by secondary intention takes place, granulation tissue must form to close the space between the wound margins prior to growth of epithelial cells over the surface of the wound. Also see primary intention and tertiary intention.

Secondary trauma from occlusion: defined as normal occlusal forces on an unhealthy periodontium previously weakened by periodontitis.

Self-efficacy: a person's belief in his or her ability to perform specific tasks (e.g., public speaking, studying, etc.) to attain a goal.

Semilunar flap: a periodontal plastic surgical procedure that can be used to cover gingival recession where the recession is not far advanced and where the keratinized tissues have an adequate thickness. The semilunar flap is a variation of a coronally positioned flap.

Sequestrum: a fragment of necrotic (dead) alveolar bone. Necrotizing periodontitis can be accompanied by the formation of bone sequestra.

Severity: the seriousness, of periodontal tissue destruction as determined by the rate of disease progression over time and the response of the tissues to treatment; severity is one factor involved in classifying a patient's periodontitis stage. Also see extent.

Shared decision-making: a collaborative process that recognizes a patient's right to make decisions about his/her care once fully informed about the treatment options.

Sharp dissection; sharp dissection: elevation of a flap by incising the underlying connective tissue in such a manner as to separate the epithelial surface plus a small portion of the connective tissue from the periosteum; use of this technique would leave the periosteal tissues covering the bone.

Sharpey fibers: the ends of the periodontal ligament fibers that are embedded in the cementum and alveolar bone.

Signs: the features of a disease that can be observed or are measurable by a clinician such as bleeding, gingival erythema (redness), and gingival edema (swelling).

Smear layer: crystalline debris from the tooth surface that covers or plugs the dentinal tubules and inhibits fluid flow, thus preventing the sensitivity.

Split-thickness flap: see partial-thickness flap.

Standard of care: the degree of prudence, caution, and attention that a reasonable health care practitioner is expected to exercise when caring for a patient.

Stage: one of two diagnostic parameters (along with periodontitis grading) that is used to define an individual patient's periodontitis. It provides a way of classifying the extent, severity, and complexity of managing the periodontitis case.

Stippling: the dimpled appearance, similar to an orange peel, that may be visible on the surface of the attached gingiva.

Stratified squamous epithelium: a type of epithelium that is comprised of flat cells arranged in several layers that makes up the skin and the mucosa of the oral cavity.

Stem cells: a class of undifferentiated (precursor) cells that have the capability to differentiate into specialized cell types.

Sub-antibacterial doses: doses of an antibiotic that are below the normal bacterial killing or inhibiting doses. Doxycycline at low doses is used as a host-modulating agent to inhibit part of the destruction that occurs in periodontitis.

Subepithelial connective tissue graft: a periodontal plastic surgical procedure that can also be used to augment the width of attached gingiva and to cover areas of gingival recession. In addition to gingival augmentation, the subepithelial connective tissue graft is used to alter the contour of alveolar ridges to improve the esthetics of some types of dental prostheses.

Substantivity: the property of a chemical to adhere to a target and be released slowly over time.

Sulcular epithelium (SE): the epithelial lining of the gingival sulcus; it extends from the crest of the gingival margin to the coronal edge of the junctional epithelium. Also see gingival epithelium.

Sulcular fluid: see gingival crevicular fluid.

Sulcular incision: see crevicular incision.

Surgical periodontal therapy: a part of periodontal therapy that entails elevating a flap to obtain improved visibility and better access to the underlying root surfaces so as to remove subgingival plaque and calculus. It is also indicated in cases that require correction of osseous contours or mucogingival deformities.

Suppuration: see exudate.

Suprabony pocket: a periodontal pocket in which there is horizontal bone loss and the junctional epithelium, forming the base of the pocket, is located *coronal* to the crest of the alveolar bone. Also see periodontal pocket and infrabony pocket.

Supragingival fiber bundles (gingival fibers): a network of rope-like collagen fiber bundles in the gingival connective tissue located coronal to (above) the crest of the alveolar bone.

Suture: a stitch; a device placed by a surgeon to hold tissues together during healing. Also see nonabsorbable suture and absorbable suture.

Symbiosis: a beneficial interaction between microorganisms living in close association, typically to the advantage of each other. The direct opposite is dysbiosis.

Symptoms: the features of a disease that can be noticed by the patient such as itching gums, blood on the bed pillow, or a bad taste in the mouth.

Systematic desensitization: a common iatrosedation technique used to calm an anxious child. This approach relies on initially presenting a situation that evokes a little fear, and then progressively presenting stimuli that are more fear-provoking.

Systematic review: a concise summary of individual research studies on a treatment or device to determine the overall validity and clinical applicability of that treatment or device.

Systemic delivery: in dentistry, usually refers to administering chemical agents in the form of a tablet or capsule. When a tablet is taken by the patient, the chemical agent contained is released as the tablet dissolves, and the agent subsequently enters the blood stream – thus the chemical agent is circulated "systemically" throughout the body.

Systemic risk factors: conditions or diseases that increase an individual's susceptibility to periodontal infection by modifying or amplifying the host response to the bacterial infection; proven systemic risk factors include diabetes mellitus, osteoporosis, hormone alteration, medications, tobacco use, and genetic influences.

Tannerella forsythia: an important periodontal pathogen.

T-cells: see T-lymphocytes.

Tell-show-do: an iatrosedation technique that works to alleviate the anxiety of apprehensive children receiving dental care. Tell-show-do involves: 'Tell': the health care provider explains what they are planning to do to the child patient; 'Show': the health care provider shows the instruments to the child patient and demonstrates it on a finger; and 'Do': the health care provider performs the procedure.

Tertiary intention: healing of a wound that is temporarily left open with the specific intent of surgically closing that wound at a later date; healing by tertiary intention is not normally a type of healing that applies to healing of periodontal surgical procedures. Also see primary intention and secondary intention.

Therapeutic mouth rinse: a mouth rinse that has some actual benefit (provides some therapeutic action) to the patient in addition to the simple goal of making the breath smell a bit better.

Tissue: a group of interconnected cells that perform a similar function within an organism. For example, muscle cells group together to form muscle tissue that functions to move parts of the body. Also see connective tissue and epithelial tissue.

Tissue-associated plaque: bacteria that adhere loosely to the epithelium of the pocket wall that can invade the gingival connective tissue and be found within the periodontal connective tissues and on the surface of the alveolar bone.

Tissue inhibitor of metalloproteinases (TIMP): an inhibitory enzyme that is released by the host to regulate the activity of MMPs. TIMPs and MMPs work in concert to maintain tissue function and form, extracellular matrix integrity, and wound healing.

Titanium: a biocompatible, light-weight metal which makes it a material-of-choice for conventional dental implants.

T-lymphocytes: small leukocytes whose main function is to intensify the response of other immune cells—such as B-lymphocytes and macrophages—to the bacterial invasion.

Tongue coating: an accumulation of bacteria, food debris and desquamated epithelial cells on the dorsal surface of the tongue and is a source of oral malodor.

Tongue thrusting: the application of forceful pressure against the anterior teeth with the tongue an example of a parafunctional habit.

Tooth-associated plaque: bacteria that attach to an area of the tooth surface that extends from the gingival margin almost to the junctional epithelium at the base of the pocket.

Topical delivery: in dentistry, usually refers to placing a chemical agent into the mouth or even into a periodontal pocket where the chemical agent then comes into contact with plaque forming either on the teeth or in the periodontal pocket.

Tort: an act that injures someone in some way, and for which the injured individual may sue the wrongdoer for damages.

Trans-endothelial migration: the process of immune cells exiting the vessels and entering the tissues.

Transmission: the transfer of periodontal pathogens from the oral cavity of one person to another.

Trauma from occlusion: excessive occlusal forces that cause damage to the periodontium. Also see primary trauma from occlusion and secondary trauma from occlusion.

Treatment plan: a sequential outline of the measures to be carried out by the dentist, the dental hygienist, or the patient to eliminate disease and restore a healthy periodontal environment.

Triangulation: the appearance on a dental radiographic of widening of the periodontal ligament space; triangulation is caused by the resorption of bone along either the mesial or distal aspect of the interdental (interseptal) crestal bone.

Type I diabetes mellitus: a type of diabetes mellitus caused by destruction of the insulin-producing cells of the pancreas. Also see diabetes mellitus and type II diabetes mellitus.

Type II diabetes mellitus: a type of diabetes mellitus that occurs when the body does not make enough insulin hormone and/or the body cells ignore the insulin and fail to use it to help bring glucose into the cells; the most common form of diabetes. Also see diabetes mellitus and type I diabetes mellitus.

Type I gingival embrasure: space filled by the interdental papilla.

Type II gingival embrasure: height of interdental papilla is reduced so that there is some open space visible between two teeth.

Type III gingival embrasure: interdental papilla is missing so that there is an open triangular space visible between two teeth.

Upcoding: an illegal practice where the health care practitioner reports a higher-level of service or procedure than was actually performed.

Ulceration: the loss of the epithelium normally covering underlying connective tissue.

Unattached plaque: bacteria that are free floating within the pocket environment.

Unconventional dentistry: alternative, holistic practices that are scientifically unproven and do not conform to generally accepted dental practices of evaluation, diagnosis, or treatment of diseases.

Vertical bone loss (also known as vertical defect or angular defect): a less common pattern of bone loss resulting in an uneven reduction in the height of the alveolar bone. In vertical bone loss, the resorption progresses *more rapidly* in the bone next to the root surface leaving a trench-like area of missing bone alongside the root. Also see alveolar bone loss and horizontal bone loss.

Vertical incision: an incision that runs perpendicular to the gingival margin in an apico-occlusal direction: primarily used to allow elevation of the flap during the surgical procedure without stretching or damaging the soft tissues during flap elevation.

Virulence factors: the mechanisms that enable biofilm bacteria to colonize, invade, and damage the tissues of the periodontium.

Virulent: species of bacteria that are capable of causing disease; another term for pathogenic.

Volatile sulfur compounds: a family of gases that is responsible for oral malodor.

Xenografts: bone replacement grafts taken from another species, such as bovine bone replacement graft material; these materials must be modified to eliminate the potential for rejection. Also see autografts, allografts, and alloplasts.

Index

Note: Page numbers followed by "f" denote figures, "t" denote tables, and "b" box, respectively.